NURSING CARE PLANS
NURSING DIAGNOSIS & INTERVENTION

NURSING CARE PLANS
NURSING DIAGNOSIS & INTERVENTION

MICHAEL REESE HOSPITAL AND MEDICAL CENTER
Department of Nursing
Chicago, Illinois

Edited by

MEG GULANICK, RN, PHD
Clinical Nurse Specialist

AUDREY KLOPP, RN, PHD, ET
Clinical Nurse Specialist

SUSAN GALANES, RN, MS, CCRN
Clinical Nurse Specialist

DEIDRA GRADISHAR, RNC, BS
Nurse Clinician

MICHELE KNOLL PUZAS, RN,C, MHPE
Nurse Clinician

Second Edition

THE C. V. MOSBY COMPANY
St. Louis • Baltimore • Philadelphia • Toronto   1990

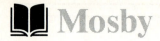

Editor: William Grayson Brottmiller
Senior Developmental Editor: Sally Adkisson
Project Manager: Carol Sullivan Wiseman
Senior Production Editor: Barbara Bowes Merritt
Designer: Liz Fett

Second edition

Previous edition copyrighted 1986

Printed in the United States of America

The C.V. Mosby Company
11830 Westline Industrial Drive, St. Louis, Missouri 63146

Library of Congress Cataloging-in-Publication Data

Nursing care plans: nursing diagnosis & intervention / Michael Reese
  Hospital and Medical Center, Department of Nursing, Chicago,
  Illinois; edited by Meg Gulanick . . . [et al.].—2nd ed.

    p.   cm.

  ISBN 0-8016-6238-9
  1. Nursing care plans. 2. Nursing—Planning. 3. Nursing
assessment. I. Gulanick, Meg. II. Michael Reese Hospital and
Medical Center. Dept. of Nursing.
  [DNLM: 1. Nursing Assessment—handbooks. 2. Patient Care
Planning—handbooks.   WY 39 N9746]
RT49.N87 1990
610.73—dc20
DNLM/DLC
for Library of Congress   89-13726
                                         CIP

C/C/VHP 9 8 7 6 5 4 3

Clinical Consultants

NURSING DIAGNOSES

Meg Gulanick, RN, PhD
Clinical Nurse Specialist, Cardiology/Rehabilitation
Audrey Klopp, RN, PhD, ET
Clinical Nurse Specialist and Enterostomal Therapist
Susan Galanes, RN, MS, CCRN
Clinical Nurse Specialist, Critical Care
Michele Knoll Puzas, RN,C, MHPE
Nurse Clinician, Pediatrics
Deidra Gradishar, RNC, BS
Nurse Clinician, Labor and Delivery
Linda Arsenault, RN, MSN, CNRN
Clinical Nurse Specialist, Neurosurgery
Linda Muzio, RN, MSN
Clinical Nurse Specialist, Rheumatology

CARDIOVASCULAR

Meg Gulanick, RN, PhD
Clinical Nurse Specialist, Cardiology/Rehabilitation
Carol Ruback, RN, MSN, CCRN
Clinical Nurse Specialist, Cardiology

PULMONARY

Susan Galanes, RN, MS, CCRN
Clinical Nurse Specialist, Critical Care
Michele Knoll Puzas, RN,C, MHPE
Nurse Clinician, Pediatrics

NEUROLOGIC/NEUROSURGERY

Linda Arsenault, RN, MSN, CNRN
Clinical Nurse Specialist, Neurosurgery

GASTROINTESTINAL

Audrey Klopp, RN, PhD, ET
Clinical Nurse Specialist and Enterostomal Therapist
Michele Knoll Puzas, RN,C, MHPE
Nurse Clinician, Pediatrics

RENAL

Susan Galanes, RN, MS, CCRN
Clinical Nurse Specialist, Critical Care
Michele Knoll Puzas, RN,C, MHPE
Nurse Clinician, Pediatrics

GENITOURINARY

Audrey Klopp, RN, PhD, ET
Clinical Nurse Specialist and Enterostomal Therapist
Nancy Ruppman, RN, BSN, CURN
Nurse Clinician, Urology

ENDOCRINE

Audrey Klopp, RN, PhD, ET
Clinical Nurse Specialist and Enterostomal Therapist
Michele Knoll Puzas, RN,C, MHPE
Nurse Clinician, Pediatrics
Linda Arsenault, RN, MSN, CNRN
Clinical Nurse Specialist, Neurosurgery

ORTHOPEDIC

Marilyn Magafas, RN,C, BSN, MBA
Nurse Manager, Orthopedics
Linda Muzio, RN, MSN
Clinical Nurse Specialist, Rheumatology
Michele Knoll Puzas, RN,C, MHPE
Nurse Clinician, Pediatrics

HEMATOLOGY/NEOPLASTIC

Christa M. Schroeder, RN, MSN
Clinical Nurse Specialist, Hematology/Oncology
Michele Knoll Puzas, RN,C, MHPE
Nurse Clinician, Pediatrics

SEXUALLY TRANSMITTED DISEASES

Jeffrey Zurlinden, RN, MS
Nursing Education, Evaluation, and Research
Deidra Gradishar, RNC, BS
Nurse Clinician, Labor and Delivery

GYNECOLOGIC

Deidra Gradishar, RNC, BS
Nurse Clinician, Labor and Delivery
Charlotte Razvi, RN, MSN
Clinical Nurse Specialist, Obstetrics/Gynecology
A.S.P.O. Certified Childbirth Educator
Certified Lactation Consultant

PSYCHOSOCIAL

Ann Filipski, RN, MSN, CS, Psy.D. Candidate
Clinical Nurse Specialist, Liaison Psychiatry
Deidra Gradishar, RNC, BS
Nurse Clinician, Labor and Delivery

EMERGENCY/TRAUMA

Helen Snow-Jackson, RN, BSN, TNS, CEN
Nurse Clinician, Ambulatory and Acute Care
Michele Knoll Puzas, RN,C, MHPE
Nurse Clinician, Pediatrics

Contributors

Verda Abernathy, RN, MA

Sherry Adams, RN, ADN

Kristine Alessandrini, RN, BSN

Kathy Alexander, RN

Josephine C. Anderson, RN

Pat Anderson, RN

Cynthia Antonio, RN, BSN

Linda Arsenault, RN, MSN, CNRN

Lou Ann Ary, RN, BSN

Laura Baratta, RN, MSN

Marina Bautista, RN, BSN

Margaret Bell, RN

Lisa Berti, RN

Bella Biag, RN, BSN

Caramen Billheimer, RN, BSN

Denise Birkner, RN, BSN

Carolyn Bolton, RN, BS

Neil Rey B. Bonje, RN, BSN

Janice Borman, RN, MSN, PhD
Candidate

Carol Boyd, RN

Paulette E. Brevard, RN, BSN

Monalisa S. Bron, RN, BSN

Kathryn S. Bronstein, RN, PhD, CS

Debbie Brooks, RN, MS

Catherine Brown, RN, BSN

Ursula Brozek, RN, MSN

Maretha Bryant, RN,C

Reneau Buckner, RN,C, BSN

Jean L. Burke, RN,C, BSN

Carol Burkhart, RN, BSN, CCRN

Virginia Cabongon, RN, BSN

Loretta Cabell, RN

Marian D. Cachero-Salavrakos, RN,
BSN

Mary Leslie Caldwell, RN

Urakay Campbell, RN

Sharon Canariato, RN, BSN

Elicita Chavez, RN

Vicki Chester, RN, BSN, MBA

Carol Clark, RN

Sarah Cohen, RN

Joanne Coleman, RN, BSN

Dawnetta Collins, RN,C

Sue A. Conneighton, RN, MSN,
Psy.D. Candidate

Adrian Cooney, RN, BSN

Nancy J. Cooney, RN, BSN, MBA

Donna Creachbaum, RN, BS, CCRN

Cathy Croke, RN, MSN

Margaret A. Cunningham, RN, MS

Maria Dacanay, RN

Susanne DeFabiis, RN, MSN

Marlene T. de la Cruz, RN, BSN

Leona Dempsey, RN, MSN, CS

Martha Dickerson, RN, MS, CCRN

Dadi Ding, RN

Gail L. Dykstra, RN

Linda Escobar, RN, BSN

Sandra Eungard, RN, MS

Martina Evans, RN, BS

Yvonne Evans-Wordell, RN, MSN

Imelda Fahy, RN

Patricia Farrell, RN,C

Ann Filipski, RN, MSN, CS, Psy.D.
Candidate

Sharon Flucus, RN, BSN

Victoria Frazier-Jones, RN, BSN

Raquel Gabriel-Bennewitz, RN, BSN,
CCRN

Susan Galanes, RN, MS, CCRN

Barbara Gallagher, RN, BSN

Diane Gallagher, RN, BSN

Remedios S. Garces, RN, BSN

Diane Garcia, RN, BSN

Carol Gawron, RN, MSN, ET

Susan Geoghegan, RN, BSN

Margaret Gleason, RN, BSN

Lorraine Goodwin, RN, MSN, CS

Cynthia Gordon, RN, BSN

Deidra Gradishar, RNC, BS

Terry Griffin, RN, BSN

Meg Gulanick, RN, PhD

Patricia A. Hannon, RN, BS

Frankie Harper, RN

Antoinette Harris-Hardy, RN, BSN

Pam Harston, RN

Patricia Hasbrouck-Aschliman, RN,
CCRN

Lorraine M. Heaney, RN

Ruth Hemmeter, RN, BSN

Margaret Hixson, RN, BSN

Hope Hlinka, RN

Barbara J. Hobbs, RN, MSN

Corea Hodge, RN

Anita C. Houtsma, RN

Jean M. Hughes, RN

Christine Hunt, RN

Kathleen Hurst-Delia, RN, BSN

Min Inawat, RN

Florencia Isidro-Sanchez, RN, BSN

Kathleen Jaffry, RN

Annie F. Jenkins, RN

Deborah Jezuit, RN, MS

Nola D. Johnson, RN

Linda M. Jones, RN, BSN

Vivian Jones, RN

Agnes Jones-Perry, RN

Christine Jutzi-Kosmos, RN, MS

Linda Kamenjarin, RN, BSN, CCRN

Maureen Kangleon, RN

Susan Kansas, RN,C

Karen Kavanaugh, RN, MSN, PhD Candidate

Carol Keeler, RN, MSN

Paulette N. Kelleher, RN,C BSN

Bernadette Keller, RNC, BSN

Judith Kenney, RN, MSN

Cheryl A. King, RN, BSN

Audrey Klopp, RN, PhD, ET

Vanida Komutanon, RN

Mary P. Knoezer, RN, BSN

Eileen Kringle, RPT

Sylvia Kupferer, RN, MS

Karen Kushibab, RN, BSN

Susan R. Laub, RN, MEd, CS

Phyllis Lawlor-Klean, RN, BSN

Mary Lawson-Carney, RN

Olga Lazala, RN

Deborah Lazzara, RN, MS, CCRN

Dorothy Lewis, RN,C BSN

Digna Limjoco, RN

Janet I. Linder, RPT

Marie Lindsey, RN,C MS, FNP

Maureen T. Linehan, RN

Chris Loftus, RN, BS

Lori Luke, RN

Evelyn Lyons, RN, BSN

Kim Mackey, RN, BS

Marilyn Magafas, RN,C, BSN, MBA

Ofelia Mallari, RN

Revelyn Manabat, RN, BSN

Beth Manglal-Lan, RN, BSN

Remedios R. Manuel, RN

Mary Martinat, RN, BSN

Marie G. Mazurek, RN, BSN

Janet McCants, RN, BSN

Mary Christine McCarthy, RN, BSN

Patsy McDonald, RN

Michelle McGhee, RN, BSN

Doris M. McNear, RN, BSN

Ellen T. McSwiney, RN, BSN

Encarnacion Mendoza, RN, BSN

Fe Corazon R. Mendoza, RN, BSN

Andrea Merkler, RN, BSN

Janice L. Miller, RN,C, MSN

Melissa Moline, RN, BA

Jacqueline Monaco, RN

Anita D. Morris, RN

Karen Moyer, RN, MS, CCRN, CNA

Marleen Mrozek, RN, BSN

Mary Mullee, RN, BSN

Mary Muse, RN,C, BSN

Linda Muzio, RN, MSN

Denise Myles, RN,C

Mary Ann Naccarato, RN, BSN

Lillian Navarrete, RN

Carol Nawrocki, RN, BSN

Charlotte Niznik, RN, BSN, CDE

Ruth E. Novitt-Schumacher, RN,C, MSN

Joanne O'Connor, RN, BSN

Mary O'Leary, RN, BSN

Manie Omsin, RN, BSN

Sonia Ortaliza, RN

Anne Paglinawan, RN, BSN

Denise Pang, RN, BSN

Pamela Paramore, RN, BSN

Jane Parker, RNC, BAN

Lumie L. Perez, RN, BSN, CCRN

Karen Peterson, RN, BSN

Gina Marie Petruzzelli, RN, BSN

Evangeline Pintag, RN, BSN

Susan Pische, RN, BSN, MBA

Judith Popovich, RN, MS, CCRN

Connie Powell, RN, MSN

Linda Powless, RN, CCRN, CNA

Catherine Provenzano, RN, BSN

Michele Knoll Puzas, RN,C MHPE

Eileen Raebig, RN,C

Vanessa Randle, RN

Donna Raymer, RN, BSN, CCRN

Charlotte Razvi, RN, MSN, PhD

Dorothy Rhodes, RN

Debby Rickard, RN, BSN

Lacy Roach, RN

Yvette Roberts, RN,C, BSN, MHA

Carol Ann Rooks, RN, BSN

Linda Rosen-Walsh, RN, BSN

Mayda T. Roseta, RN

Ruby Rotor-Cajiados, RN, BSN

Marilyn Rousseau, RN

Geraldine Rowden, RN

Robert Rowlands, RN

Rosaline L. Roxas, RN

Fannie Royster, RN,C

Carol Ruback, RN, MSN, CCRN

Nancy Ruppman, RN, BSN, CURN

Terri L. Russell, RN

Laura L. Rybicki, RN, BSN

Louise Rzeszewski, RN, BSN

Teodorina M. Saez, RN, BSN

Mary Sandelski, RN, MSN

Rosetonia Sapaula, RN, BSN

Caroline Sarmiento, RN, BSN

Paula Schipiour, RN, MS

Christa M. Schroeder, RN, MSN

Michael K. Schroyer, RN, BSN, CCRN

Lydia Serra, RN, BSN

Joanne Shearer, RN, MSN

Therese Sineni, RN,C, BSN

Nedra Skale, RN, MS, CNA

Susan Smalheiser, RN, MSN

Helen Snow-Jackson, RN, BSN, TNS, CEN

Andrea So, RN, BSN

Concordia Solita, RN, BSN

Rosita Sortijas, RN, BSN

Nancy Staples, RN, BSN

Lela Starnes, RN

Kathy V. Stewart, RN

Linda Marie St. Julien, RN, MS

Virginia M. Storey, RN, ET

Salvacion P. Sulit, RN, BSN, CCRN

Jackie Suprenant, RN, BSN

Terry Takemoto, RN, MSN, CCRN

Denise Talley-Lacy, RN

Debra Terry, RN

Kevin Tetsworth, MD

Apolonia Tinio, RN

Christine Todd, RN, GBS

Maripat Tomaszkiewicz, RN, BSN

Marisa C. Trybula, RN, BSN

Laurie VadeBoncouer, RN, BSN

Christine L. Valenta, RN, BS

Theresa Vanderhei, RN

Laura Vieceli-Brooks, RN, BSN

Maiu N. Viloria, RN, BSN

Marion C. Wallis, RN, CCRN

Kevin Walsh, MD

Laura Watanabe, RN

Sherry Webber, RN

Maureen Weber, RN, BSN

Sandra P. Wilks, RN, BS

Janet Williams, RN

Margaret Williams, RN

Cynthia R. Wilson, RN, BSN

Sheila Winfield, RN, BSN

Valerie A. Wolf, RN, BSN, FNP

Katie Wyatt, RN

Gloria Young, RN, BS

Ofelia Zafra, RN, BSN

Jeffrey Zurlinden, RN, MS

Preface

Going into the 1990s, the nursing profession is facing a tremendous challenge to provide quality patient care amidst intensive cost containment efforts and a diminishing supply of nurses. This challenge demands that nurses be creative and efficient in planning for their patients' needs. The use of comprehensive care plan guides that serve as reference standards from which nurses can individualize patient care is now recognized as a valuable solution to this problem.

Michael Reese Hospital and Medical Center's Department of Nursing has been a leader in the development of such care plan guides since publication of its *Comprehensive Nursing Care Plan Guidebook* in 1984. That initial book contained 75 guides, and attracted the attention of The C.V. Mosby Co. which subsequently published the first edition of *Nursing Care Plans: Nursing Diagnosis and Intervention.* This nationally acclaimed book is a compilation of over 180 care plans for clinical problems and treatments most widely encountered at major teaching hospitals. Now Michael Reese is proudly presenting an even more comprehensive edition—which includes over 100 additional "state-of-the-art" care plan guides. Over 300 staff nurses participated in the development of these care plans, with input and guidance from Michael Reese's own nationally recognized clinical nursing experts.

An important feature of this book is the unique blend of both nursing diagnoses and medical problems. Chapter One, the core of the book, specifically addresses 44 NANDA-approved nursing diagnosis. This chapter allows a "pure" approach to nursing diagnosis—and ensures that any patient care issue can be addressed. The subsequent chapters are organized by body system or clinical specialty, and include the latest trends in nursing and medical practice. To assist the reader in planning truly comprehensive care, one care plan may include references to several other related care plan guides. In addition, a very clear table of contents makes it easy to locate the needed care plans.

This comprehensive text has something to offer nurses working in all health care settings—hospital, critical care, home care, and clinic. Some examples of newly developed topics include Alzheimers' disease; cardiac, renal, and bone marrow transplant; ventricular assist device; valvuloplasty; scleroderma; tumor lysis syndrome; anorexia/bulimia; penile prosthesis, rape-trauma syndrome. A new chapter on "Sexually Transmitted Diseases" has also been added, reflecting the timely health care issues addressed in this second edition.

This book sports a new design, which makes the content clear, concise, and extremely readable. Definitions for both nursing and medical diagnoses are now included. Both related factors and defining characteristics are listed under each nursing diagnosis. The intervention section includes "ongoing" as well as initial nursing assessments. Moreover, an exciting addition to this book is the inclusion of rationales for particular nursing interventions. These explanations serve as helpful teaching aids, and may eliminate the need for an additional reference book. Finally, an introductory section has been added to provide clarification of the various components of care plans and suggestions on how to use these guides.

This book's format aids both the student and the practitioner in deriving the appropriate nursing diagnoses and formulating the plan of care. A concerted effort was made to maintain a strict separation of the components of nursing process. Ongoing assessments and defining characteristics are clearly separated from therapeutic interventions and expected outcomes. Likewise, defining characteristics are separated from related factors.

Nursing Care Plans reflects the evolution of nursing practice and nursing diagnosis. The care plan guides simultaneously incorporate both independent and collaborative nursing interventions according to priority need, depicting nursing practice in the "real world." Nurses of all levels of expertise will find this book helpful. Its content serves as a self-contained teaching guide and source of support for the novice nurse, while serving as a review or organizational tool for the experienced nurse.

Reflecting the clinical expertise of hundreds of nurses, this clinical reference is truly one of a kind—a book developed *by* nurses, *for* nurses.

MEG GULANICK

Contents

How to Individualize Nursing Care Plans

Nursing is defined as the diagnosis and treatment of human responses to actual or potential health problems. Gordon defines a nursing diagnosis as "an actual or potential health problem which a nurse, by education and experience, is capable and licensed to treat." Inherent in these definitions is the nurse's ability to identify actual or potential problems, and to identify methods of assisting the patient to a resolution of those problems.

Nurses care for large numbers of patients, many or all of whom have complex care needs. Some nursing activities are independent interventions, such as teaching and comfort measures. The nursing process (assessment, diagnosis, planning, implementation, and evaluation) is the organizing framework for these activities. Other activities represent interdependent activities, in which nurses carry out the physician's plan of care and address the patient's response to those interventions. Medication administration is an example of an interdependent activity. Both independent and interdependent activities take place in a complex health care environment, where nurses function as coordinators, arranging the various aspects of health care delivery in a way which best meets patients' needs. Tremendous amounts of information for large numbers of patients must be available to the nurse in a concise, well-organized format.

While nursing diagnosis is clearly an exciting development for nursing, nurses at the bedside are often acutely reminded that the state-of-the-nursing-diagnosis-art is still very much a state of becoming. Most research related to nursing diagnosis has addressed only the label, etiologic factors, and defining characteristics; the interventional strategies have not yet been widely addressed. This situation leaves the bedside nurse with a label (or diagnosis), possible related factors, and defining characteristics, but without the plan of care related to the diagnoses which pertain to the patient's needs. The nursing care plan guides in this book have recognized both the independent and interdependent role of the nurse, have clustered groups of nursing diagnoses in such a manner as to facilitate the nurse's coordinative role in today's complex health care environment, and provide structure and substance for the complex set of behaviors known as the nursing process. Most importantly, these nursing care plan guides assist the nurse in planning comprehensive, individualized care.

COMPONENTS OF THE CARE PLAN

Each care plan guide throughout this book includes the following information: actual or potential nursing diagnoses, related factors, defining characteristics, expected outcomes, and nursing interventions.

Nursing Diagnosis

The nursing diagnosis is the summary judgment which the professional nurse makes about the data gathered during the nursing assessment. Almost all nursing diagnoses used throughout this book have been approved by NANDA (North American Nursing Diagnosis Association, an organization charged with the responsibility of classifying and developing nursing diagnoses) and are expressed in NANDA's nomenclature. This standardization assists nurses in developing a common language to improve professional communication. However, some original diagnostic labels have been incorporated into the care plan guides formulated for medical diagnoses at the discretion of the clinical nurse. Definitions of the NANDA diagnoses are included with each care plan guide in Chapter One. Some definitions were developed by NANDA; others were created by the clinical nurse authors based on review of the literature and their clinical expertise.

Related Factors

Prior to developing a treatment plan for a nursing diagnosis, an evaluation must be made of those factors thought to be related to or the probable cause of the problem. Such factors may be physical, psychological, environmental, social, or spiritual. Each diagnosis in this book lists several contributing factors which may be related to the diagnosis. These related factors serve to direct the selection of subsequent nursing interventions.

Defining Characteristics

Each nursing diagnosis in this book lists observable signs and symptoms that are usually present when the health problem exists; these descriptive signs are known as the defining characteristics for that diagnosis. Some characteristics are quite specific, must be present before a diagnosis can be made, and are considered critical data. Other characteristics are less precise, appear in several diagnoses, and are considered supportive data. The defining characteristics are gathered during the nursing assessment. A valid diagnosis must be based on actual assessment, not assumptions, regarding defining characteristics. Accuracy of a diagnosis can be verified by comparing the assessed defining characteristics with those listed for the standard care plan.

The defining characteristics in this book are a representative, though not an exhaustive listing of the common characteristics associated with a nursing problem. Many of the identified characteristics were modified from NANDA's listing for each diagnosis.

Expected Outcomes

Expected outcomes are concise statements that should identify a specific, observable, realistic, and measurable goal. An example is: "In 24 hours, the patient will have relief or minimization of pain, as evidenced by comfortable appearance and verbalization of comfort." Though it would be possible to write such a specific outcome for each nursing diagnosis identified throughout this book, the editors felt that the repetition of the observable, measurable criteria for each goal, namely a listing of the defining characteristics, was too repetitious. Therefore, the expected outcome section simply includes one broad outcome statement per nursing diagnosis, such as: "Pain will be reduced or relieved", or "Optimal physical mobility will be achieved". Since these care plans serve as guides for actual nursing practice, nurses can individualize outcomes for patients using absence of each defining characteristic as a criterion for achievement.

Expected outcomes must be evaluated within a specific time frame to assist in determining whether the plan of care needs revision or resolution. Because of the individuality and complexities of patient care, no standard time frames were identified in these guides. The readers will have to make this adaptation based on professional judgment.

Nursing Interventions

Nursing interventions are those actions or prescriptions which assist in meeting the defined goal or outcome. They include two components of the nursing process: assessments and planned interventions. The *ongoing assessments* listed for each diagnosis are related to the defining characteristics. Since the presence of a specific cluster of characteristics represents an actual problem, ongoing assessments are needed both to validate actual presence of the problem and to measure or document progress in treating or alleviating the problem. *Therapeutic interventions* are those measures required to accomplish the desired outcome. Since these are orders, they begin with a verb and clearly direct the nurses' actions. They include actual nursing therapies, documentation of actions and results, and consultation and communication with other health professionals. Most interventions reflect treatments which nurses can perform independently. However, the editors did include collaborative (interdependent) practice measures commonly observed in practice (e.g., "Insert foley catheter as needed"; "Give atropine per protocol"). Many of these therapeutic interventions reflect changing national trends in nurses' professional responsibilities, and, in some practice areas, nurses already perform them independently. This is nursing practice in the "real world".

Not every suggested intervention is appropriate for all patients throughout their hospitalization or illness. A broad range of nursing actions are presented here to provide the practitioner with options when adapting the care plan to specific patient needs. As a patient's condition changes, some of the interventions for a specific nursing diagnosis will assume higher priority than others. For example, during the acute phase of "Ineffective Breathing Pattern", immediate physical therapies supercede follow-up care concerns.

The nursing intervention section also includes patient education. These actions are presented in several different formats throughout the book. In the generic nursing diagnosis section in Chapter One, patient education interventions are listed in a separate column. In the chapters which contain medical diagnoses and procedures, some teaching interventions are included in many of the subcategories of nursing diagnoses found in that standard care plan.

Rationales

Rationales are incorporated into the nursing interventions to explain the purpose for or necessity of particular nursing actions; these rationales serve as learning tools for both the novice and experienced practitioner. Inclusion of such rationale eliminates the need for an additional reference book.

General vs. Specific Care Plan Guides

Chapter One includes general, comprehensive care plan guides for the NANDA-approved nursing diagnoses most commonly used in clinical practice. These guides provide a framework for designing an individual patient's care plan. Patients may present with one or several nursing diagnoses; careful initial nursing assessment is required for selection of the most appropriate diagnoses. The nursing interventions for these general care plan guides are comprehensive, reflecting several approaches to treating the health problem. Not all interventions may be appropriate for a specific patient. An extensive listing of possible related or risk factors is provided to direct selection of appropriate nursing activities.

While these general guides allow almost any patient care issue to be addressed, MRH nurses identified the need to develop additional guides for those medical problems and treatments most commonly encountered in their daily practices. While recognizing that all patients are individuals with unique health needs, most patients do share common concerns and problems. These specific care plans focus on similarity among patients, and their use can therefore optimize efficient delivery of nursing care. Working with a clinical resource person (clinical nurse specialist or nurse clinician with expertise in the content area), staff nurses developed the specific care plan guides found in Chapters 2-17. These guides include clustering of the common nursing diagnoses most frequently assessed with each medical problem.

In these guides, nursing diagnoses are presented according to priority needs. For example, airway problems or pre-op teaching needs tend to be first. Actual problems are presented before potential problems; discharge teaching and planning concerns are usually addressed last. Since the nursing diagnosis is now related to a more specific etiology, the nursing interventions are more specific and concise. For example, interventions for decreased cardiac output related to pacemaker failure include many interventions not found in the general decreased cardiac output care plan guide in Chapter One. Many care plans also contain procedural interventions (e.g., complex cardiac care plans) to assist the novice nurse in providing optimal care. When appropriate, references to other pertinent care plans are made within a specific care plan to assist the nurse in providing truly comprehensive care.

Use of the Care Plan Guides

These care plans were written to be used both as guides for nursing practice and as tools to assist nurses and institutions in meeting J.C.A.H.O. state and local requirements. While expectations that individualized plans of care be developed and used for each patient exist, other responsibilities and time constraints often limit care planning efforts.

There are a variety of ways in which *Nursing Care Plans* can be utilized both individually by nurses and collectively by institutions; uses include clinical practice, teaching/education, quality assurance, and research. On the clinical units, standardized care plans can be used to write a plan of care for a particular patient, or they can serve as a guide to the care of a patient population in general. Nurses can use the care plan guides as quick references, especially when caring for new or infrequently encountered types of patients. Using these care plans increases efficiency by allowing nurses to spend their scarce time individualizing and adapting care plans rather than creating new ones. Highlighting applicable information, lining out inappropriate information, or writing in parameters and dates particular to one patient are quick methods of individualization.

The care plan guides in this book are educational tools; each guide encapsulates the plan of care in a logical, rational manner. Establishing the information contained in the care plan guides as standards on a particular unit or for a specific population of patients allows for assessment of staff learning needs, and may be used with students, new staff members, and other health care team members as instructional guides to patient care. The guides can also be used to evaluate individual nursing practice or to address deficiencies noted in nursing care following quality assurance activities.

These care plan guides are also unique quality assurance tools. Quality assurance activities are based on locally, regionally, and nationally accepted standards of care and practice; this collection of care plan guides reflects the expertise of hundreds of practicing staff nurses as well as nationally recognized advanced practice nurses who served as resources in the development of these guides. Individual guides can be used to identify and define standards, so that nurses involved in quality assurance activities, as well as nurse managers, can identify problem areas in specific aspects of care. Documentation issues, often the focus of quality assurance activities, may be addressed using the care plan guides as the basis for evaluating care given. The importance of such monitoring activities is increasing as third party payers and certifying/surveying agencies require increasing amounts of evidence of the plan of care, as well as care provided.

The care plan guides also provide a framework for research. The development, refinement, and validation of nursing diagnoses, efficacy of therapeutic interventions, validity of expected outcomes, acuity systems' reliability, and issues of nurse-generated revenue and direct reimbursement for nursing care rendered are applicable topics for research activities.

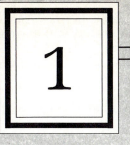

Nursing Diagnosis Care Plans

Activity intolerance
Airway clearance, ineffective
Anxiety
Body image disturbance
Body temperature, altered, potential
Breathing pattern, ineffective
Cardiac output, decreased
Communication, impaired verbal
Constipation/impaction
Coping, ineffective family
Coping, ineffective family
Coping, ineffective individual
Diarrhea
Diversional activity deficit
Family processes, altered
Fear

Fluid volume deficit
Gas exchange, impaired
Grieving, anticipatory
Grieving, dysfunctional
Growth and development, altered
Health maintenance, altered
Home maintenance/management, impaired
Hopelessness
Hyperthermia
Hypothermia
Injury, potential for
Knowledge deficit
Mobility, impaired physical
Noncompliance
Nutrition, altered: less than body
   requirements

Nutrition, altered: more than body
   requirements
Pain
Parenting, altered (actual/potential)
Powerlessness
Self-care deficit
Self concept disturbance (personal identity
   disturbance, self-esteem disturbance)
Sexuality patterns, altered
Skin integrity, impaired
Sleep pattern disturbance
Spiritual distress
Thought processes, altered
Tissue perfusion, altered (peripheral)
Urinary elimination, altered patterns of
Urinary retention

Activity intolerance

A state in which a person has insufficient physical or psychological energy to endure or perform desired physical activities

RELATED FACTORS / DEFINING CHARACTERISTICS	NURSING INTERVENTIONS / *RATIONALES*	EXPECTED OUTCOMES

RELATED FACTORS

Generalized weakness
Deconditioned state
Sedentary life-style
Insufficient sleep or rest periods
Lack of motivation/ depression
Prolonged bedrest
Imposed activity restriction
Imbalance between O_2 supply and demand
Pain

DEFINING CHARACTERISTICS

Verbal report of fatigue or weakness
Inability to begin/ perform activity
Abnormal heart rate or BP response to activity
Exertional discomfort or dyspnea
Electrocardiographic changes reflecting arrhythmias or ischemia

ONGOING ASSESSMENT

- Assess patient's respiratory status before activity:
  Respiratory quality and quantity
  Need for O_2 with increased activity
- Assess patient's cardiac function before activity:
  Pulse: rate, rhythm, volume
  BP: baseline, orthostatic changes
  Skin: color, temperature, moisture, perfusion
  How Valsalva maneuver affects heart rate when patient moves in bed.
    Valsalva maneuver, which requires breath holding and bearing down, can cause bradycardia and related reduced cardiac output.
- Assess patient's level of mobility (see Mobility, impaired physical, p. 35).
- Observe and document response to activity. *Close monitoring serves as a guide for optimal progression of activity.*
  Report to physician:
  Rapid pulse (>20 beats over resting rate or 120 BPM)
  Palpitations
  Significant increase in systolic BP (>20 mm Hg)
  Significant decrease in systolic BP (drop of ≥20 mm Hg)
  Dyspnea, labored breathing, wheezing
  Weakness, fatigue
  Chest pain, lightheadedness, dizziness, pallor, cold sweats
- Assess nutritional status (see Nutrition, altered: less than body requirements, p. 37).
- Assess potential for physical injury with activity.
- Assess need for ambulation aids.
- Assess understanding by patient/significant others of change in activity tolerance.

THERAPEUTIC INTERVENTIONS

- Assist with ADL as indicated *to reduce energy expenditure.*
- Provide bedside commode as indicated *to reduce energy expenditure. Note: bedpans require more energy than commode.*
- Encourage adequate rest periods, especially before ambulation, diagnostic procedure, meals, *to reduce cardiac workload.*
- Refrain from performing nonessential procedures *to promote rest.*
- Anticipate patient's need (e.g., keep telephone, tissues within reach).
- Provide small, frequent meals.
- Program activity gradually *to prevent overexerting the heart and to promote attainment of short-range goals:*
  Dangling 10-15 min t.i.d.
  Deep breathing exercises t.i.d.
  Sitting up in chair 30 min t.i.d.
  Walking in room 1-2 min t.i.d.
  Walking in hall 25 ft, then slowly progressing, saving energy for return trip.
- Encourage active ROM exercises t.i.d. *to maintain muscle strength;* if further reconditioning needed, confer with rehabilitation medicine personnel.
- Provide emotional support while increasing activity. Promote a positive attitude regarding abilities.

PATIENT EDUCATION

- Teach patient/significant others signs of physical overactivity.
- Involve patient/significant others in activity, goal setting, and care planning. *Setting small attainable goals can increase self-confidence and self-esteem.*
- Encourage significant others to bring ambulation aide: walker or cane.

Activity level will be maintained within limits of patient's capabilities.

Activity intolerance—cont'd

RELATED FACTORS / DEFINING CHARACTERISTICS	NURSING INTERVENTIONS / *RATIONALES*	EXPECTED OUTCOMES
	• Teach appropriate use of environmental aides (e.g., bed rails, elevation of head of bed when patient gets out of bed, chair in bathroom, hall rails) *to conserve energy and prevent injury from fall*. • Teach ROM exercises. • Encourage patient to verbalize concerns about discharge and home environment. • Involve patient/significant others in discharge planning.	

Originated by: Michael K. Schroyer, RN, BSN, CCRN

Airway clearance, ineffective

A state in which an individual is unable to clear secretions or obstructions from the respiratory tract to maintain airway patency.

RELATED FACTORS / DEFINING CHARACTERISTICS	NURSING INTERVENTIONS / *RATIONALES*	EXPECTED OUTCOMES

RELATED FACTORS
Decreased energy and fatigue
Tracheobronchial: infection, obstruction, secretion
Perceptual/cognitive impairment
Trauma
 	
DEFINING CHARACTERISTICS
Abnormal breath sounds (rales, rhonchi, wheezes)
Changes in respiratory rate or depth
Cough
Cyanosis
Dyspnea
Fever
	ONGOING ASSESSMENT
	• Auscultate lungs for presence of breath sounds every shift (or as needed). *Routine assessment of breath sounds allows for early detection and correction of abnormalities.*
	• Assess respirations; note quality, rate, pattern, depth, flaring of nostrils, dyspnea on exertion, evidence of splinting, use of accessory muscles, position for breathing.
	• Assess changes in orientation and behavior pattern.
	• Assess changes in vital signs and temperature.
	• Assess patient's present knowledge base of disease process.
	• Assess cough:
	    Effectiveness
	    Productivity
	• Note presence of sputum; assess quality, color, consistency (patient may use a sputum container).
	• Monitor arterial blood gases (ABGs); note changes.
	
	THERAPEUTIC INTERVENTIONS
	• Position patient with proper body alignment for optimal breathing pattern (if tolerated, head of bed at >45 degrees). *This promotes better lung expansion and improved air exchange.*
	• If abnormal breath sounds are present:
	  Assist patient with coughing:
	    Administer pain relief medications before the attempt.
	    Splint any incisional/injured area.
	    Coach the patient through the process.
	  If cough is ineffective, then use oropharyngeal or tracheal suction as needed:
	    Explain procedure to patient.
	    Utilize soft rubber catheters *to prevent trauma to mucous membranes.*
	    Use curved tip catheters and head positioning (if not contraindicated) *to facilitate secretion removal from a specific side.*
	• Provide humidity (when appropriate) via bedside humidifier (positioned near patient) and humidified O_2 therapy *to prevent drying of secretions.*
	• Encourage oral intake/fluids within the limits of cardiac reserve *to maintain hydration.*
	• Instruct and/or change patient's position (e.g., ambulate, turn every 2 hr). *This will help to facilitate secretion movement and drainage.*
		Secretions will be mobilized and airway will be maintained free of secretions.

Continued.

Airway clearance, ineffective—cont'd

RELATED FACTORS / DEFINING CHARACTERISTICS	NURSING INTERVENTIONS / *RATIONALES*	EXPECTED OUTCOMES
	• Administer medications (antibiotics, bronchodilators, diuretics) as ordered, noting effectiveness and side effects. • Assist with oral hygiene every 4 hr or as needed *to decrease oral flora*. • Maintain adequate airway. Anticipate the need for an artificial airway (intubation) if secretions cannot be cleared. • Coordinate with respiratory therapy department optimal time for postural drainage and percussion, i.e., at least 1 hr after eating *to prevent aspiration*. • Pace activities *to prevent fatigue*. • Maintain planned rest periods. • Instruct patient to avoid restrictive clothing *that could prevent adequate respiratory excursion*. **PATIENT EDUCATION** • Demonstrate and teach coughing, deep breathing, and splinting techniques *so patient will understand the rationale and appropriate techniques to keep the airway clear of secretions*. • Instruct patient on indications for, frequency of, and side effects of medications. • Teach patient about environmental factors that can precipitate respiratory problems. • Explain effects of smoking. • Instruct patient on warning signs of pending/recurring pulmonary problems. • Consult with pulmonary clinical nurse specialist as appropriate.	

Originated by: Lorraine Goodwin, RN, MSN, CS
Helen Snow-Jackson, RN, BSN, TNS, CEN
Remedios S. Garces RN, BSN
Janice L. Miller, RN,C, MSN

Anxiety

An apprehensive, uneasy feeling which usually stems from an impending or anticipated circumstance or event. It can be focused on an activity, object, or situation or unfocused and more generalized. It is believed to be primarily internally motivated, and its source may be nonspecific or unknown to the person experiencing it. The feeling may be experienced as diffuse and is generally categorized into four levels: mild, moderate, severe, and panic.

RELATED FACTORS / DEFINING CHARACTERISTICS	NURSING INTERVENTIONS / *RATIONALES*	EXPECTED OUTCOMES
RELATED FACTORS Threat or perceived threat to physical and emotional integrity Change in health status and associated changes in role function Intrusive diagnostic and surgical tests and procedures Changes in environment and routines	**ONGOING ASSESSMENT** • Assess the patient's level of anxiety. *Mild anxiety enhances a patient's awareness and ability to identify and solve problems. Moderate anxiety limits awareness of environmental stimuli. Problem solving can occur but may be more difficult, and the patient may need help. Severe anxiety decreases the patient's ability to integrate information and solve problems. Panic is severe anxiety. The patient is unable to follow directions. Hyperactivity, agitation, and immobilization may be observed.* • Assess the patient's coping mechanisms in handling anxiety. *This can be done by interviewing the patient and significant others. This assessment helps determine the effectiveness of coping strategies currently used by the patient.*	Anxiety will be managed or relieved.

RELATED FACTORS / DEFINING CHARACTERISTICS	NURSING INTERVENTIONS / *RATIONALES*	EXPECTED OUTCOMES

Trauma sustained from assault

Threat or perceived threat to self-esteem

Threat to (or change in) socioeconomic status

Situational and maturational crises

Intrapersonal conflicts caused by unmet needs and/or emotional fixation at an earlier level of development

Interpersonal conflicts

DEFINING CHARACTERISTICS

Autonomic symptoms:
Increase in blood pressure, pulse, respirations
Paresthesia in extremities
Dizziness, lightheadedness
Diaphoresis
Frequent urination
Flushing or pallor
Dyspnea
Palpitations and/or chest pain
Hot or cold flashes
Dry mouth
Blurred vision
Headaches
Nausea and/or diarrhea

Motor tension:
Restlessness
Insomnia, nightmares
Trembling, shaking
Muscle tension
Choking or smothering sensations
Fatigability
Jitteriness, sighing respirations

Impairment in cognitive and emotional status:
Hyperattentiveness
Excessive worry; impatience
Feelings of helplessness and discomfort

THERAPEUTIC INTERVENTIONS

- Document behavioral and verbal expressions of anxiety. *Symptoms often provide information regarding the degree of anxiety. Physiological symptoms and/or complaints intensify as the level of anxiety increases.*
- Acknowledge awareness of the patient's anxiety. *Acknowledgment of the patient's feelings validates the feelings and communicates acceptance of those feelings.*
- Reassure the patient that he/she is safe. Stay with the patient if this appears necessary. *The presence of a trusted person assures the patient of his security and safety during a period of anxiety.*
- Maintain a calm and tolerant manner while interacting with the patient. *Staff's anxiety may be easily perceived by the patient. The patient's feeling of stability increases in a calm and nonthreatening atmosphere.*
- Establish a working relationship with the patient through continuity of care. *An ongoing relationship establishes a basis for communicating anxious feelings.*
- Orient to the environment as needed. *The patient's orientation and awareness of his surroundings promotes comfort and a decrease in anxiety.*
- When possible, adjust the patient's treatment and care to his routines. Reduce requests made of the patient. *Adjustments in care based on the patient's needs reflect awareness of him as an individual with special needs.*
- Use simple language and brief statements when instructing the patient about diagnostic and surgical tests. *When experiencing moderate to severe anxiety, patients are unable to comprehend anything more than simple, clear, and brief instructions.*
- Reduce sensory stimuli by maintaining a quiet environment. *Anxiety may escalate with excessive conversation, noise, and equipment around the patient.*
- Encourage the patient to notify staff when anxious feelings occur. *Staff availability reinforces a feeling of security for the patient.*
- Encourage patient to talk about anxious feelings and examine the anxiety-provoking situation. Assist the patient in assessing the situation realistically and recognizing factors leading to the anxious feelings.
- Avoid false reassurances. As the patient's anxiety subsides, encourage the patient to explore specific events preceding the onset of the anxious feelings. *Recognition and exploration of factors leading to anxious feelings are important steps in developing alternative responses. The patient may be unaware of the relationship between emotional concerns and anxiety.*
- Assist the patient in developing his problem-solving abilities. *Learning to identify a problem and evaluate alternatives to resolve it help the patient to cope.* Emphasize the logical strategies the patient can use when experiencing anxious feelings.
- Administer antianxiety medications as ordered.

PATIENT EDUCATION

- Assist the patient in recognizing symptoms of increasing anxiety; explore alternatives the patient may use to prevent the anxiety from immobilizing him. *The patient will be able to use his problem-solving abilities more effectively when his level of anxiety is low.*
- Remind the patient that anxiety at a mild level can encourage growth and development and is important in mobilizing changes.
- Instruct the patient in the proper use of medications and educate the patient to recognize adverse reactions. *Medication may be used if the patient's anxiety continues to escalate and the anxiety becomes disabling.*

Continued.

■ Anxiety—cont'd

RELATED FACTORS / DEFINING CHARACTERISTICS	NURSING INTERVENTIONS / *RATIONALES*	EXPECTED OUTCOMES
Poor impulse control Exaggerated startle response Rumination and apprehension Decreased ability to express feelings caused by impaired verbal communication		

Originated by: Ursula Brozek, RN, MSN
              Meg Gulanick, RN, PhD
              Janice Borman, RN, MSN, PhD Candidate
              Leona Dempsey, RN, MSN, CS

Body image disturbance

A disturbance or alteration in the attitude a person has about the actual or perceived structure or function of all or part of the body; this attitude is dynamic and altered through interaction with other persons and situations.

RELATED FACTORS / DEFINING CHARACTERISTICS	NURSING INTERVENTIONS / *RATIONALES*	EXPECTED OUTCOMES
RELATED FACTORS Situational changes (e.g., pregnancy, temporary presence of a visible drain/tube, dressing, attached equipment) Permanent alterations in structure and/or function (e.g., mutilating surgery, removal of body part [internal or external]) Malodorous lesions, change in voice quality **DEFINING CHARACTERISTICS** Verbal identification of feeling about altered structure/ function of a body part Verbal preoccupation with changed body part or function	**ONGOING ASSESSMENT** • Assess perception of change in structure/function of body part (also proposed change). *Extent of response is more related to the value or importance the patient places on the part or function than the actual value or importance.* • Assess perceived impact of change on ADL, social behavior, personal relationships, occupational activities. • Note patient's behavior regarding actual or perceived changed body part/function. **THERAPEUTIC INTERVENTIONS** • Acknowledge normalcy of emotional response to actual or perceived change in body structure/function. • Help patient identify actual changes. • Help patient identify concerns regarding actual or perceived changes. • Encourage verbalization of positive or negative feelings about actual or perceived change. • Assist patient in incorporating actual changes into ADL, social life, interpersonal relationships, occupational activities. • Encourage use of support groups. **PATIENT EDUCATION** • Teach patient adaptive behavior to compensate for actual changed body structure/function. • Help patient identify ways of coping that have been useful in the past.	Body image and self-concept will be enhanced through appropriate intervention.

Body image disturbance—cont'd

RELATED FACTORS / DEFINING CHARACTERISTICS	NURSING INTERVENTIONS / *RATIONALES*	EXPECTED OUTCOMES
Naming changed body part or function Refusal to discuss/acknowledge change Focusing behavior on changed body part and/or function Actual change in structure/function Refusal to look at, touch, or care for altered body part Change in social behavior (withdrawal, isolation, flamboyancy) Compensatory use of concealing clothing, other devices		

Originated by: Audrey Klopp, RN, PhD, ET

Body temperature, altered, potential

A state in which an individual is at risk for failure to maintain a normal body temperature caused by one or more factors that cause a physiologic response and a change in body temperature.

RISK FACTORS / DEFINING CHARACTERISTICS	NURSING INTERVENTIONS / *RATIONALES*	EXPECTED OUTCOMES

RISK FACTORS
Extremes of weight or age
Dehydration
Illness
Trauma
Drugs
Environmental temperature
Inappropriate clothing
 	
DEFINING CHARACTERISTICS
Premature birth
Advanced age
Head trauma
Infectious process
Medications:
  Vasodilators
  Vasoconstrictors
  Sedatives
Chemical substance abuse
Recent surgery
	ONGOING ASSESSMENT
	· Assess for presence of risk factors.
	· Assess for precipitating event.
	· Measure temperature at frequent intervals. Use the same instrument and method at each interval. If method is changed (e.g., axillary versus rectal), document route. *A change of this type usually causes a variance in the temperature obtained.*
	· Monitor other physical indicators:
	  Heart and respiratory rate
	  Blood pressure
	  Skin condition
	  Fluid balance
	  Electrolytes
	  Mental status
	
	THERAPEUTIC INTERVENTIONS
	· Provide preventive measures as necessary:
	  Control environment.
	  Provide appropriate clothing/covering.
	  Provide adequate fluid and dietary intake.
	  Administer medications as ordered.
	· Notify physician of changes in physical status, especially temperature.
	· If altered body temperature becomes a problem, refer to appropriate care plan:
	  Hypothermia, p.31
	  Hyperthermia, p. 31
		Body temperature will be maintained within a normal range.

Continued.

7

RELATED FACTORS / DEFINING CHARACTERISTICS	NURSING INTERVENTIONS / *RATIONALES*	EXPECTED OUTCOMES
Vomiting/diarrhea Environmental temperature versus attire	**PATIENT EDUCATION** • Explain risk factors and rationale for temperature measurement. • Explain prevention of risk factors and consequences of development of temperature alterations. • Provide community resources, consultants as needed.	

Originated by: Michele Knoll Puzas, RN,C, MHPE

Breathing pattern, ineffective

A state in which an individual's respiratory pattern (cycles of inhalation and/or exhalation) does not allow adequate ventilation.

RELATED FACTORS / DEFINING CHARACTERISTICS	NURSING INTERVENTIONS / *RATIONALES*	EXPECTED OUTCOMES

RELATED FACTORS
Neuromuscular impairment
Pain
Musculoskeletal impairment
Perception or cognitive impairment
Anxiety
Decreased energy and fatigue
Inflammatory process
Decreased lung expansion
Tracheobronchial obstruction
 	
DEFINING CHARACTERISTICS
Dyspnea
Shortness of breath
Tachypnea
Fremitus
Cyanosis
Cough
Nasal flaring
Respiratory depth changes
Altered chest excursion
Use of accessory muscles
Pursed-lip breathing/prolonged expiratory phase
Increased anteroposterior chest diameter
	ONGOING ASSESSMENT
	• Assess respiratory rate and depth by listening to breath sounds at least every shift. *Respiratory rate and rhythm changes are early warning signs to impending respiratory difficulties.*
	• Assess presence of breath sounds every shift.
	• Assess for dyspnea and quantify (i.e., note how many words per breath patient can say); relate dyspnea to precipitating factors.
	• Note breathing pattern (e.g., Cheyne-Stokes; Kussmaul).
	• Note use of muscles used for breathing (i.e., sternocleidomastoid, abdominal, diaphragmatic).
	• Note retractions, flaring of nostrils.
	• Assess position patient assumes for normal/easy breathing.
	• Monitor ABGs; note differences.
	• Assess for changes in orientation, restlessness.
	• Assess skin color, temperature, capillary refill; note central versus peripheral cyanosis.
	• Check position of portable chest radiograph plate (when needed) *so that entire lung field can be examined; check that patient's position allows for optimal lung expansion.*
	• Assess presence of sputum for quantity, color, consistency.
	• Note changes in activity tolerance.
	• Assess anxiety level.
	• Assure that O_2 delivery system is applied to the patient *so that the appropriate amount of oxygen is continuously delivered and the patient does not desaturate.*
	
	THERAPEUTIC INTERVENTIONS
	• Position patient with proper body alignment for optimal breathing pattern. *If not contraindicated, a sitting position allows for good lung excursion and chest expansion.*
	• Encourage sustained deep breaths by:
	   Demonstration (emphasizing slow inhalation, holding end inspiration for a few seconds, and passive exhalation)
	   Use of incentive spirometer (place close for convenient patient use)
	   Asking patient to yawn, *to promote deep inspiration*
	• Suction as needed *to clear secretions.*
	• Pace and schedule activities *to prevent dyspnea resulting from fatigue.*
	• Provide reassurance and allay anxiety by staying with patient during acute episodes of respiratory distress. *Air hunger can produce an extremely anxious state.*
		Optimal respiratory status within the limits of the disease will be achieved.

RELATED FACTORS / DEFINING CHARACTERISTICS	NURSING INTERVENTIONS / *RATIONALES*	EXPECTED OUTCOMES
	· Encourage diaphragmatic breathing for patient with chronic disease. · Anticipate the need for intubation and mechanical ventilation if the patient is unable to maintain adequate gas exchange with the present breathing pattern. **PATIENT EDUCATION** · Explain effects of wearing restrictive clothing *so that respiratory excursion is not compromised.* · Explain use of O_2 therapy. · Instruct patient/significant others in the O_2 therapy to be used at home. · Explain environmental factors that may worsen patient's pulmonary condition (e.g., pollen, smoking). · Explain symptoms of a "cold" and impending problems. *A respiratory infection would increase the work of breathing.* · Teach patient/significant others appropriate breathing, coughing, and splinting techniques *to facilitate adequate clearance of secretions.* · Teach patient how to count own respirations and relate respiratory rate to activity tolerance. *Patient will then know when to limit activities in terms of his/her own limitations.* · Teach patient when to inhale and exhale while doing strenuous activities. *Appropriate breathing techniques during exercise are important in maintaining adequate gas exchange.*	

Originated by: Lorraine Goodwin, RN, MSN, CS
              Helen Snow-Jackson, RN, BSN, TNS, CEN
              Lumie L. Perez, RN, BSN, CCRN

Cardiac output, decreased

A state in which the left and/or right ventricle is unable to maintain a cardiac output sufficient to meet the needs of the body. Common causes of reduced cardiac output include myocardial infarction, hypertension, valvular heart disease, congenital heart disease, cardiomyopathy, arrhythmias, drug effects, fluid overload, decreased fluid volume, and electrolyte imbalance.

RELATED FACTORS / DEFINING CHARACTERISTICS	NURSING INTERVENTIONS / *RATIONALES*	EXPECTED OUTCOMES

RELATED FACTORS
Increased/decreased ventricular filling (preload)
Impaired contractility
Alteration in heart rate/rhythm/ conduction
Decreased oxygenation
Cardiac muscle disease
	ONGOING ASSESSMENT
	· Assess physical status closely, document changes, report significant changes in parameters.
	    Arterial BP, orthostatic changes, pulses paradoxus
	    Apical/radial pulses; peripheral pulses (strength, equality)
	    Heart rate
	    Respirations, breath sounds
	    Heart sounds, murmurs, rubs
	    Jugular venous distention, pulmonary artery pressure
	    Skin color, temperature, moisture
	    Fluid balance, presence of peripheral edema
	    I & O, weight
	    Change in mental status
	    Pain
	    Diagnostic studies (e.g., ECG changes, ABGs, CBC, chest radiographic examination)
		Optimal hemodynamic function will be maintained.

Continued.

RELATED FACTORS / DEFINING CHARACTERISTICS	NURSING INTERVENTIONS / *RATIONALES*	EXPECTED OUTCOMES

DEFINING CHARACTERISTICS

Variations in hemodynamic parameters (BP, heart rate, CVP, pulmonary artery pressures, cardiac output, neck veins)

Arrhythmias, ECG changes

Rales, tachypnea, dyspnea, orthopnea, cough, abnormal ABGs, frothy sputum

Weight gain, edema, decreased urine output

Anxiety, restlessness

Syncope, dizziness

Weakness, fatigue

Abnormal heart sounds

Decreased peripheral pulses, cold clammy skin

Confusion, change in mental status

- Monitor ECG for rate, rhythm, ectopy, and change in PR, QRS, and QT intervals. *Tachycardia, bradycardia, and ectopic beats can compromise cardiac output.*
- Assess patient's response to increased activity. *Physical activity increases the demands placed on the heart. Close monitoring of patient's response serves as a guide for optimal progression of activity.*
- Assess contributing factors *so appropriate plan of care can be initiated.* (Also see Fluid volume deficit, p. 20, Myocardial infarction, p. 105; Cardiogenic shock, p. 81; Cardiac dysrhythmias, p. 74, Chest trauma, p. 636, etc.).

THERAPEUTIC INTERVENTIONS

- Administer medication as ordered, noting response and watching for side effects and toxicity. Clarify with physician parameters for withholding medications. (Common medications include digitalis therapy, diuretics, vasodilator therapy, and inotropic agents).
- Maintain optimal fluid balance:
    Administer fluid challenge as ordered, closely monitoring effects.
    Maintain hemodynamic parameters at prescribed levels.
    Restrict fluid and Na as ordered.
- Maintain adequate ventilation/perfusion:
    Place patient in semi-Fowler's position *to reduce preload and ventricular filling; supine position to increase venous return, promote diuresis.*
    Administer O_2 as ordered.
- Maintain physical and emotional rest:
    Restrict activity *to reduce O_2 demands.*
    Provide quiet, relaxed environment. *Emotional stress increases cardiac demands.*
    Provide explanations to patient's questions *to allay anxiety.*
    Organize nursing and medical care *to allow rest periods.*
    Monitor progressive activity within limits of cardiac function.
    Administer stool softeners p.r.n..
    Monitor sleep patterns; administer sedative p.r.n.
- If arrhythmia occurs, determine patient response, document, and report if significant or symptomatic. *Both tachy- and bradyarrhythmias can reduce cardiac output and myocardial tissue perfusion.*
- Have antiarrhythmic drugs readily available.
- Treat arrhythmias according to medical orders or protocol and evaluate response. See Treatment under Myocardial infarction: acute phase, p. 105.
- If invasive adjunct therapies are indicated (e.g., intra-aortic balloon pump, pacemaker), maintain within prescribed protocol.

PATIENT EDUCATION

- Explain symptoms and interventions for decreased cardiac output related to etiology.
- Explain drug regimen, purpose, dose, and side effects.
- Explain progressive activity schedule and signs of overexertion.
- Explain diet program.

Originated by: Meg Gulanick, RN, PhD
Karen Moyer, RN, MS, CCRN, CNA

Communication, impaired verbal

(APHASIA, DYSARTHRIA, SLURRED SPEECH)

A state in which the person experiences a decreased ability to speak appropriately or to understand the meaning of words. Aphasia is an impairment of the understanding or use of language. Several types may occur alone or in combination. Motor aphasia is characterized by slow speech, difficulty in articulating words, and deletion of small words. Usually understanding of the spoken or written word is intact, as is ability to write. Auditory receptive aphasia is characterized by inability to understand spoken words and to repeat test phrases. Speech is usually intact. Nominal aphasia is characterized by inability to name common objects, although recognition is intact. Dysarthria is a disorder of speech caused by loss of coordination or power of the muscle needed to speak words. Slurred speech is characterized by difficulty pronouncing words distinctly.

RELATED FACTORS / DEFINING CHARACTERISTICS	NURSING INTERVENTIONS / *RATIONALES*	EXPECTED OUTCOMES

RELATED FACTORS
 	
Impaired cerebral tissue perfusion secondary to stroke, head injury, or brain tumor
 	
DEFINING CHARACTERISTICS
 	
Inability to recognize or understand spoken/written words
Difficulty in articulating words
Inability to recall familiar words, phrases, or names of known persons, objects, and places
	ONGOING ASSESSMENT
	
	• Determine the type and degree of aphasia the patient has by assessing the following:
	  Ability to speak spontaneously
	  Ability to understand spoken word
	  Ability to understand written words, pictures, gestures
	  Ability to express ideas
	  Ability to name objects
	• Assess need for speech specialist and neurologist.
	
	THERAPEUTIC INTERVENTIONS
	
	• Treat patient as an intelligent adult. *Impaired speech does not indicate lack of intelligence.* Explain all diagnostic, therapeutic, and comfort measures before initiating them.
	• Maintain eye contact with patient when speaking. Stand close, within patient's line of vision, generally midline. *Patient may have defect in field of vision. Nurse's eye contact and position provide support and encouragement; facilitate use of body language.*
	• Keep distractions such as television, radio at a minimum when talking to patient to *keep patient focused and assist nurse's ability to listen.*
	• Anticipate needs to *decrease feelings of helplessness.*
	• Place call light within reach.
	• When patient cannot understand spoken word, repeat simple directions until understood. Supplement with gestures, if necessary. *Provide as many sensory channels as possible.*
	• When patient cannot identify objects by name, give practice in receiving word images (e.g., point to an object and clearly enunciate its name: "cup," "pen").
	• Speak slowly and distinctly, repeating key words. *Prevents confusion.*
	• Give concrete directions that the patient is physically capable of doing (e.g., "Point to _____"; "Open your mouth"; "Turn your head").
	• Use short sentences. Ask only one question at a time. *Allows patient to stay focused on one thought.*
	• Do not speak loudly unless patient is hearing-impaired.
	• When patient has difficulty with verbal expressions, give practice in repeating words after you. Begin with simple words, then progress (e.g., "Yes"; "No"; "This is a cup").
	• Encourage patient to speak.
	• Give ample time to respond. *It is difficult for patient to respond under pressure; allow time to organize responses.*
	• Avoid finishing sentences for patient. Say word slowly and distinctly if help is requested. *Be calm and accepting during attempts; do not say you understand if you do not, for this may increase frustration and decrease trust.*
		Optimal communication skills will be achieved within limits of disease.

Continued.

Communication, impaired verbal—cont'd

RELATED FACTORS / DEFINING CHARACTERISTICS	NURSING INTERVENTIONS / *RATIONALES*	EXPECTED OUTCOMES
	- Listen attentively when patient attempts to communicate. - Provide with word-and-phrase cards, writing pad, and pencil. - Provide list of words patient can say; add new words to it. - If vocabulary is limited to yes and no answers, try to phrase questions so that patient can use these responses. - Orient patient to time by placing a clock and calendar at bedside. - Never talk in front of patient as though he/she comprehends nothing. *This will increase frustration and sense of helplessness.* - Praise patient's accomplishments. Acknowledge his/her frustrations. - Consult speech therapist for additional help. - See that patient is well rested before each session with speech therapist. *Fatigue may have an adverse effect on learning ability.* **PATIENT EDUCATION** - Offer significant others the opportunity to ask questions about patient's communication problem. - Inform patient/significant others of the type of aphasia patient has and how it affects speech, language skills, and understanding. - Explain that because of associated brain injury, patient's attention span may be limited. - Encourage patient to socialize with family and friends. Explain that communication should be encouraged despite impairment. - Provide patient with an appointment with a speech therapist. - Inform patient/significant others to seek information about aphasia from the American Speech-Language-Hearing Association, 10810 Rockwell Pike, Rockville, Maryland 20852.	

Originated by: Maria Dacanay, RN
Connie Powell, RN, MSN

Constipation/impaction

A change in normal bowel habits characterized by a decrease in the frequency and/or passage of hard, dry stool, or oozing of liquid stool past a collection of hard, dry stool.

RELATED FACTORS / DEFINING CHARACTERISTICS	NURSING INTERVENTIONS / *RATIONALES*	EXPECTED OUTCOMES
RELATED FACTORS Inadequate fluid intake Low-fiber diet Immobility Fear of pain Medication use Lack of privacy Pain Laxative abuse Pregnancy Tumor or other obstructing mass **DEFINING CHARACTERISTICS** Straining at stools Passage of liquid fecal seepage	**ONGOING ASSESSMENT** - Assess home pattern of elimination; compare to present pattern. Include size, frequency, color, and quality. - Evaluate laxative use, type, and frequency. - Evaluate reliance on enemas for elimination. *Abuse/overuse of cathartics and enemas can result in dependence on them for evacuation.* - Evaluate usual dietary habits, eating habits, eating schedule, and liquid intake; compare with hospital regimen. - Assess food preferences. - Assess activity level. *Prolonged bed rest and lack of exercise contribute to constipation.* - Auscultate for bowel sounds every shift. - Evaluate current medication usage, *which may contribute to constipation.* - Assess privacy for elimination (i.e., enforced use of bedpan). - Evaluate fear of pain. - Assess degree to which patient's procrastination contributes to constipation. - Assess for hemorrhoids. - Check for history of bowel obstruction. - Check for history of paralytic ileus.	Constipation/impaction will be relieved and recurrence prevented.

RELATED FACTORS / DEFINING CHARACTERISTICS	NURSING INTERVENTIONS / *RATIONALES*	EXPECTED OUTCOMES

Frequent but nonproductive desire to defecate
Anorexia
Abdominal distention
Nausea and vomiting
Dull headache, restlessness, and depression
Verbalized pain/fear of pain
	THERAPEUTIC INTERVENTIONS
	• Encourage and provide daily fluid intake of 2000-3000 ml/day, if not contraindicated medically.
	• Encourage increased bulk in diet (e.g., raw fruits, fresh vegetables [if appropriate]).
	• Consult dietitian if appropriate.
	• Encourage patient to eat prunes, prune juices, cold cereal, bean products, etc. (if appropriate).
	• Orient patient to location of bathroom.
	• Increase patient's physical activity by planning ambulation periods if possible.
	• Assist with mobility.
	• Provide a regular time for elimination (e.g., after breakfast or at patient's usual time).
	• Offer a warm bedpan to bedridden patient. Assist patient to assume a high Fowler's position with knees flexed. *This position best utilizes gravity and allows for effective Valsalva maneuver.* Curtain off the area; allow patient time to relax.
	• Initiate occupational/physical therapy consultation as needed.
	• Assist with passive/active ROM exercises.
	• Instruct in isometric abdominal and gluteal exercises *to strengthen muscles needed for evacuation* unless contraindicated.
	• Encourage as much patient self-help as possible.
	• Utilize pharmacologic agents as appropriate:
	  Metamucil: *increases fluid, gaseous, and solid bulk of intestinal contents*
	  Stool softeners (e.g., Colace)
	  Chemical irritants (e.g., castor oil, cascara, Milk of Magnesia). *These irritate the bowel mucosa and cause rapid propulsion of contents of small intestines.*
	  Suppositories: *aid in softening stools and stimulate rectal mucosa; best results occur when given 30 min before usual defecation time or after breakfast.*
	  Oil: retention enema *to soften stool*
	• Digitally remove fecal impaction.
	• Minimize rectal discomfort:
	  Warm sitz bath
	  Hemorrhoidal preparations
	
	PATIENT EDUCATION
	Explain to patient/significant others the importance of the following:
	• Balanced diet that contains adequate bulk, fresh fruits, vegetables
	• Adequate fluid intake (8 glasses/day)
	• Regular meals
	• Regular time for evacuation and adequate time for defecation
	• Regular exercise
	• Privacy for defecation
	• Administration of rectal suppositories, enemas, or laxatives when necessary	

Originated by: Marian D. Cachero-Salavrakos, RN, BSN
         Connie Powell, RN, MSN

Coping, ineffective family

The stress response seen in family members of a hospitalized patient.

RELATED FACTORS / DEFINING CHARACTERISTICS	NURSING INTERVENTIONS / *RATIONALES*	EXPECTED OUTCOMES

RELATED FACTORS

Unfamiliar environment
Loss of role as primary caretaker
Separation of family members
Knowledge deficit regarding illness prognosis
Inaccurate/incomplete/conflicting information
Loss of dominant figure in family structure

DEFINING CHARACTERISTICS

Expressed concern inappropriate to need
Distortion of reality
Restlessness
Verbalization of problem
Disregard for patient's needs
Inappropriate behavior
Limited interaction with patient
Statement of misconception
Intolerance
Agitation/depression
Abandonment

ONGOING ASSESSMENT

- Assess family's knowledge and understanding of the need for hospitalization and treatment plan.
- Assess level of family's anxiety.
- Assess normal coping patterns in family.
- Assess support systems available to family.
- Assess role of hospitalized patient in family structure.

THERAPEUTIC INTERVENTIONS

- Approach in calm, reassuring manner.
- Encourage questions or expressions of concern. *The amount of coping difficulties vary depending on developmental level, extent of social contacts outside the family, and former experience with separation.*
- Relay pertinent questions to physician.
- Schedule care conferences to maintain ongoing communication.
- Provide honest, appropriate answers to family members' questions.
- Encourage frequent visitation if the patient's condition permits *to decrease separation anxiety and increase sense of security.*
- Discuss ways families can continue to be involved in daily care.
- Maintain flexible visiting hours.
- Offer assistance in notifying clergy, other family members, etc., of patient's status.
- Refer family to social service, pastoral care, etc.

PATIENT TEACHING

- Orient to:
  Surroundings (cafeteria, parking, telephone, etc).
  Patient's room (call light, TV, etc.)
  Equipment
  Health professionals
- Discuss patient's condition and needed care with the patient and the family. *Distorted ideas, if not clarified, may be more frightening than realistic preparation.*

Effective family coping is demonstrated.

Originated by: Nedra Skale, RN, MS, CNA.

Coping, ineffective individual

Impaired ability to meet life's demands and role expectations caused by maladaptive behaviors or lack of knowledge, support, or problem-solving skills

RELATED FACTORS / DEFINING CHARACTERISTICS	NURSING INTERVENTIONS / *RATIONALES*	EXPECTED OUTCOMES

RELATED FACTORS

Change in or loss of body part

Diagnosis of serious illness

Unsatisfactory support system

Inadequate psychological resources (poor self-esteem; lack of motivation)

Work overload

Unrealistic perceptions

Inadequate coping method

Recent change in health status

Unmet expectations

Inadequate relaxation

Multiple life changes

Situational crises

Maturational crises

Anxiety/fear

DEFINING CHARACTERISTICS

Verbalization of inability to cope

Inability to make decisions

Inability to ask for help

Destructive behavior toward self

Inappropriate use of defense mechanisms

Physical symptoms such as:

　Overeating; lack of appetite

　Overuse of tranquilizers

　Excessive smoking/drinking

　Chronic fatigue

　Headaches

　Irritable bowel

Chronic depression

Emotional tension

High illness rate

Insomnia

General irritability

ONGOING ASSESSMENT

- Assess for presence of defining characteristics.
- Assess for contributing factors (see related factors).
- Assess specific stressors.
- Assess available/useful past and present coping mechanisms.
- Evaluate resources/support systems available to patient while in hospital and at discharge.
- Assess level of understanding and readiness to learn needed life-style changes.
- Assess decision-making/problem-solving ability.
　What is problem?
　Who or what is responsible for problem?
　What are options?
　What are pros and cons?
　What are possible alternatives?

THERAPEUTIC INTERVENTIONS

- Provide calm, supportive environment *to reduce stress.*
- Provide opportunities to express concerns, fears, feelings, expectations.
- Convey feelings of acceptance and understanding. Avoid false reassurances.
- Assist patient to evaluate situation and own accomplishments accurately.
- Establish a working relationship with patient through continuity of care. *An ongoing relationship establishes trust.*
- Explore attitudes and feelings about required life-style changes.
- Encourage patient to set realistic goals *to help gain control over situation.*
- Assist patient to develop appropriate strategies based upon personal strengths and previous experience. *It is more difficult to learn new behaviors in stressful times.*
- Provide information that patient wants and needs. *Do not provide more than patient can handle. Patients who are coping ineffectively have reduced ability to assimilate information.*
- Meet with medical team to discuss treatment plan *to facilitate consistent care.*
- Implement physical care routines that enable patient to function at optimum level.
- Provide outlets that foster feelings of personal achievement and self-esteem.
- Point out signs of positive progress or change. *Patients who are coping ineffectively may not be able to assess progress.*
- Encourage the patient to communicate feelings with significant others. *Unexpressed feelings can increase stress.*
- Involve social services, psychiatric liaison, pastoral care for additional and ongoing support resources.
- Administer tranquilizer, sedative as needed.
- Assist in development of alternative support system.
- Encourage participation in self-help groups as available.

PATIENT EDUCATION

- Instruct in need for adequate rest and balanced diet *to facilitate coping strengths. Inadequate diet and fatigue can themselves be stressors.*
- Teach use of relaxation, exercise, and diversional activities as methods to cope with stress.

Effective coping behaviors will be demonstrated.

Originated by: Meg Gulanick, RN, PhD

Diarrhea

A change in normal bowel habits characterized by frequent passage of loose, fluid, or unformed stools.

RELATED FACTORS / DEFINING CHARACTERISTICS	NURSING INTERVENTIONS / *RATIONALES*	EXPECTED OUTCOMES

RELATED FACTORS

Stress
Anxiety
Medication use
Bowel disorders:
  Inflammation
  Malabsorption
Enteric infections
Dietary intake
Tube feedings
Radiation
Chemotherapy
Bowel resection
Short bowel syndrome

DEFINING CHARACTERISTICS

Abdominal pain
Cramping
Frequency of stools
Loose/liquid stools
Urgency
Hyperactive bowel
  sounds/sensations

ONGOING ASSESSMENT

- Assess for abdominal pain, cramping, frequency, urgency, loose/liquid stools, and hyperactive bowel sensations.
- Inquire regarding:
  Drugs patient is or has been taking
  Idiosyncratic food intolerances
  Method of food preparation
  Osmolality of tube feedings
  Change in eating schedule
  Level of activity
  Adequacy or privacy for elimination
  Current stressors
- Check for history of:
  Previous GI surgery
  GI diseases
  Abdominal radiation
- Assess impact of therapeutic or diagnostic regimes on diarrhea. *Preparation for radiograph or surgery, and radiation or chemotherapy predisposes to diarrhea by altering mucosal surface and transit time through bowel.*
- Assess hydration status:
  I & O
  Skin turgor
  Moisture of mucous membrane
- Assess condition of perianal skin.

THERAPEUTIC INTERVENTIONS

- Give antidiarrheal drugs as ordered.
- Provide dietary alterations as allowed:
  Bulk (cereal, grains, Metamucil)
  "Natural" antidiarrheals (e.g., pretzels, matzos, cheese)
  Avoidance of stimulants (e.g., caffeine, carbonated beverages)
- Check for fecal impaction by digital examination. *Liquid stool (apparent diarrhea) may seep past a fecal impaction.*
- Minimize emotional impact of illness, hospitalization, and soiling accidents by providing:
  Privacy
  Opportunity for verbalization
- Compensate for malabsorption (i.e., provide fluids, consider nutritional support).
- Evaluate appropriateness of physician's radiograph protocols for bowel preparation on basis of age, weight, condition, disease, and other therapies.
- Assist with/administer perianal care after each BM.
- See Skin integrity, impaired, p. 48.

PATIENT EDUCATION

- Teach patient those etiologic factors that can be controlled.
- Teach patient importance of good perianal hygiene after each BM.

Diarrhea will be resolved.

Originated by: Audrey Klopp, RN, PhD, ET
      Virginia M. Storey, RN, ET

Diversional activity deficit

Lack of physical and mental exercise caused by confinement in the hospital.

RELATED FACTORS / DEFINING CHARACTERISTICS	NURSING INTERVENTIONS / *RATIONALES*	EXPECTED OUTCOMES

RELATED FACTORS
Prolonged hospitalization
Environmental lack of diversional activity
• Usual hobbies cannot be undertaken in hospital
Lack of usual level of socialization
Physical inability to perform tasks
 	
DEFINING CHARACTERISTICS
Verbal expression of boredom
Preoccupation with illness
Frequent use of call light in absence of physical need
Excessive complaints
Withdrawal
Depression
	ONGOING ASSESSMENT
	• Assess developmental level, attention span.
	• Assess for physical limitations.
	• Inquire about patient's interest and hobbies prior to hospitalization:
	    Art
	    Reading
	    Writing
	• Observe and document response to activities.
	
	THERAPEUTIC INTERVENTIONS
	• Provide frequent patient contact.
	• Be certain that patient is aware of your presence.
	• Set up a schedule with the patient *so he will know when to expect contact/activities.*
	• Provide materials for hobby/interests if possible.
	• Suggest new interests (crafts, puzzles, etc.).
	• Encourage family/friends to visit and bring diversional materials.
	• Provide dietary changes if possible. *Most hospital menus rotate weekly or biweekly and soon become repetitive for the long-term patient.*
	• Obtain consultants as needed: dietary, social work, psychiatric liaison, volunteers, etc..
	• Spend time with patient without providing physical care. *Engaging the patient in conversation without focusing on illness will divert the patient's attention and help pass the time.*
	
	PATIENT EDUCATION
	• Instruct patient/family concerning necessity for continued hospitalization.
	• Obtain instructional materials for new hobbies/interests.
	• Encourage continuation of formal education while hospitalized.
		Patient's attention will be diverted to interests other than illness and hospitalization.

Originated by: Sherry Adams, RN, ADN

Family processes, altered

(INEFFECTIVE FAMILY COPING)

A situation or event that causes a change in family members' roles or expectations. The inability of one or more members to adjust or perform, resulting in family dysfunction and prevention of the growth and development of the family and members.

RELATED FACTORS / DEFINING CHARACTERISTICS	NURSING INTERVENTIONS / *RATIONALES*	EXPECTED OUTCOMES
RELATED FACTORS Illness of family member Change in socioeconomic status Births and deaths Conflict between family members	**ONGOING ASSESSMENT** • Assess for precipitating events (divorce, illness, etc.). • Elicit past attempts at problem solving. • Assess members' perceptions of problem. • Evaluate strengths, coping skills, and current support systems.	Dysfunctioning family process will be reduced.

Continued.

Family processes, altered—cont'd

RELATED FACTORS / DEFINING CHARACTERISTICS	NURSING INTERVENTIONS / *RATIONALES*	EXPECTED OUTCOMES
Developmental needs of children **DEFINING CHARACTERISTICS** Inability to meet physical needs of family members Inability to function in larger society; no job, no community activity Inability to meet emotional needs of family members (grief, anxiety, conflict) Inability to meet developmental needs or foster growth and maturation of children Ineffective family decision-making process Rigidity in roles, behavior, and beliefs	**THERAPEUTIC INTERVENTIONS** • Explore feelings. Identify loneliness, anger, and aggression, *as the feelings of one family member impact on others in the family system.* • Phrase problems as "family" problems, *so they are owned and dealt with by the family.* • Encourage members to empathize or act out the parts of other family members. *Role playing allows members to see how they look to others, as well as increasing understanding of others' feelings.* **PATIENT EDUCATION** • Provide information regarding stressful situation. • Provide social work/psyche consults as needed. • Identify community resources that may be helpful in dealing with particular situations, i.e., hotlines, self-help groups, educational opportunities.	

Originated by: Mary O'Leary, RN, BSN

Fear

A strong and unpleasant emotion caused by the awareness or anticipation of pain or danger. This emotion is primarily externally motivated, and its source is specific. The person, place, or thing precipitating this feeling can be identified by the individual experiencing the fear.

RELATED FACTORS / DEFINING CHARACTERISTICS	NURSING INTERVENTIONS / *RATIONALES*	EXPECTED OUTCOMES

RELATED FACTORS
Anticipation of pain
Anticipation or perceived threat of danger
Unfamiliarity with environment
Impairment in comprehension and communication:
  Language barrier
  Knowledge deficit
  Sensory impairment
Specific phobias
See Anxiety, p. 4 for other related factors
	ONGOING ASSESSMENT
	• Assess the degree of the patient's fear and the measures he uses to cope with that fear. This can be done by interviewing the patient and significant others. *This assessment helps determine the effectiveness of coping strategies used currently by the patient.*
	• Document behavioral and verbal expressions of fear. *Symptoms will provide information regarding the degree of fear. Physiologic symptoms and/or complaints will intensify as the level of fear increases. Note that fear differs from anxiety in that it is a response to a recognized and usually external threat. Manifestations of fear are similar to those of anxiety.*
	
	THERAPEUTIC INTERVENTIONS
	• Acknowledge your awareness of the patient's fear. *This will validate the feelings the patient is having and communicate an acceptance of those feelings.*
	• Reassure the patient that he/she is safe. Stay with the patient if necessary. *The presence of a trusted person assures the patient of security and safety during a period of fear.*
		Fear will be managed or relieved.

RELATED FACTORS / DEFINING CHARACTERISTICS	NURSING INTERVENTIONS / *RATIONALES*	EXPECTED OUTCOMES

DEFINING CHARACTERISTICS

Increased respirations, heart rate, and respiratory rate

Dilated pupils

Diaphoresis

Tremors

Crying

Expression of extreme fearfulness

Denial

Physical or emotional paralysis

See Anxiety, p. 4

- Maintain a calm and tolerant manner while interacting with the patient. *The patient's feeling of stability increases in a calm and nonthreatening atmosphere.*
- Establish a working relationship with the patient through continuity of care. *An ongoing relationship establishes trust and a basis for communicating fearful feelings.*
- Orient to the environment as needed. *This promotes comfort and a decrease in fear.*
- When possible, adjust the patient's treatment and care to his routines. Reduce requests made of the patient. *Adjustments in care based on the patient's needs reflect awareness of him as an individual with special needs. They also reinforce the degree of control the patient has over his treatment and care. The patient's fear will lessen as he perceives that he has more control over his surroundings.*
- Use simple language and brief statements when instructing the patient regarding diagnostic and surgical procedures. *When experiencing excessive fear or dread, the patient may be unable to comprehend more than simple, clear, and brief instructions.*
- Reduce sensory stimulation by maintaining a quiet environment. *Fear may escalate with excessive conversation, noise, and equipment around the patient.*
- Encourage the patient to notify staff when he experiences fear. *Staff availability will reinforce a feeling of security for the patient.*
- Encourage patient to verbalize fearfulness and examine the fear-provoking situation.
- Avoid false reassurances. As the patient's fear subsides, encourage him to explore specific events preceding the onset of the fear. *Recognition and explanation of factors leading to fear are significant in developing alternative responses.*
- Assist the patient in developing his problem-solving abilities. *Learning to identify a problem and evaluate alternatives in resolving the problem aid the patient in coping.*
- Emphasize the logical strategies the patient can use when experiencing fear. *Solutions resulting from the desire to escape fear may be chaotic and counterproductive.*

PATIENT EDUCATION

- Reinforce the idea that fear is a normal and appropriate response to situations when pain, danger, or loss of control is anticipated or experienced
- Instruct patient in the performance of self-calming measures that may reduce fear or make it more manageable:
    Breathing modifications *to reduce the physiologic response to fear (i.e., increased BP, pulse, respiration)*
    Exercises in relaxation
    Exercises in guided imaging

Originated by: Ursula Brozek, RN, MSN
        Meg Gulanick, RN, PhD
        Janice Borman, RN, MSN, PhD Candidate
        Leona Dempsey, RN, MSN, CS

Fluid volume deficit
A state of vascular, cellular, or intracellular dehydration.

RELATED FACTORS / DEFINING CHARACTERISTICS	NURSING INTERVENTION / *RATIONALES*	EXPECTED OUTCOMES

RELATED FACTORS

Inadequate fluid intake
Active fluid loss (diuresis, abnormal drainage/bleeding, diarrhea)
Electrolyte/acid-base imbalances
Increased metabolic rate (fever, infection)
Fluid shifts (edema/effusions)

DEFINING CHARACTERISTICS

Decreased urine output
Concentrated urine
Dilute urine
Output greater than intake
Sudden weight loss
Decreased venous filling
Hemoconcentration
Increased serum sodium
Hypotension
Thirst
Increased pulse rate
Decreased skin turgor
Dry mucous membranes
Weakness
Sunken fontanels
Possible weight gain
Edema
Changes in mental status

ONGOING ASSESSMENT

- Assess turgor and mucous membranes for signs of dehydration.
- Assess color and amount of urine. Report urine output <30 ml/hr for 2 consecutive hours. *Concentrated urine denotes fluid deficit.*
- Weigh daily with same scale, preferably at the same time of day, *to evaluate true fluid status.*
- Monitor temperature. *Febrile states decrease body fluids through perspiration and increased respiration.*
- Monitor active fluid loss from wound drainage, tubes, diarrhea, bleeding, and vomiting; maintain accurate I & O.
- Evaluate specific etiology for fluid deficit *to guide intervention* (fever, diarrhea, fatigue at meals, GI bleeding). Refer to Diarrhea, p. 16; Nutrition, altered: less than body requirements, p. 37; Gastrointestinal bleeding, p. 284; Diabetes, p. 372.
- Determine patient's fluid preferences: type, temperature (hot/cold).
- Monitor serum electrolytes/urine osmolality and report abnormal values.
- Document baseline mental status and record during each nursing shift. *Dehydration can alter mental status.*
- Monitor and document vital signs.
- Evaluate whether patient has any related heart problem prior to initiating parenteral therapy. *Cardiac patients often have precarious fluid balance and are prone to develop pulmonary edema.*
- Observe for signs of orthostatic hypotension (drop of greater than 15 mm when changing from supine to sitting position). *This indicates reduced circulating fluids.*
- Monitor closely for signs of circulatory overload (headache, flushed skin, tachycardia, venous distention, elevated CVP, shortness of breath, increased BP, tachypnea, cough).

THERAPEUTIC INTERVENTIONS

- Encourage patient to drink prescribed fluid amounts.
- Be creative in selecting fluid sources (Jell-O, Popsicles, Gatorade)
- Assist patient if unable to feed self.
- Maintain daily activities *so patient is not too tired at mealtime.*
- Provide oral hygiene *to promote interest in drinking.*
- Administer parenteral fluids as ordered, monitoring IV flow rate evenly. *Infants and elderly patients are especially susceptible to fluid overload.*
- Should signs of fluid overload occur, stop infusion and sit patient up or dangle *to decrease venous return and optimize breathing.*

PATIENT EDUCATION

- Inform patient/significant others of importance of maintaining prescribed fluid intake and special diet considerations involved.

Adequate fluid volume and electrolyte balance will be maintained.

Originated by: Jackie Suprenant, RN, BSN
Carol Burkhart, RN, BSN, CCRN
Maureen T. Linehan, RN

Gas exchange, impaired

A state in which the individual experiences an imbalance between oxygen uptake and carbon dioxide elimination at alveolar-capillary membrane gas exchange area.

RELATED FACTORS / DEFINING CHARACTERISTICS	NURSING INTERVENTIONS / *RATIONALES*	EXPECTED OUTCOMES

RELATED FACTORS

Altered O_2 supply
Alveolar capillary membrane changes
Altered blood flow
Altered oxygen-carrying capacity of blood

DEFINING CHARACTERISTICS

Confusion
Somnolence
Restlessness
Irritability
Inability to move secretions
Hypercapnia
Hypoxia

ONGOING ASSESSMENT

- Assess respirations: note quality, rate, pattern, depth, flaring of nostrils, dyspnea on exertion, evidence of splinting, use of accessory muscles, position assumed for easy breathing.
- Assess breath sounds every shift.
- Monitor vital signs, noting any changes. *With initial hypoxia and hypercapnia, BP, heart rate, and respiratory rate all rise. As the hypoxia and/or hypercapnia becomes more severe, BP may drop, heart rate tends to continue to be rapid with arrhythmias, and respiratory failure may ensue, with the patient unable to maintain the rapid respiratory rate.*
- Assess for changes in orientation and behavior.
- Assess patient's ability to cough effectively to clear secretions. Note quantity, color, and consistency of sputum.
- Monitor arterial blood gases (ABGs) and note changes.
- Assess for presence of central cyanosis.

THERAPEUTIC INTERVENTIONS

- Maintain the prescribed oxygen delivery system at appropriate levels *so that the patient does not desaturate*. Note: If the patient is allowed to eat, O_2 still must be given to the patient, but perhaps in a different manner, e.g., from mask to a nasal cannula. *Eating is an activity and more O_2 will be consumed than when the patient is at rest.* Immediately after the meal, the original oxygen delivery system should be returned.
- Utilize pulse oximetry, as available, *to monitor O_2 saturation and pulse rate continuously*. Keep alarms on at all times. *Pulse oximetry has been found to be a useful tool in the clinical setting to detect changes in oxygenation.*
- Position patient with proper body alignment for optimal respiratory excursion (if tolerated, head of bed at >45 degrees). *This promotes good lung expansion and improves air exchange.*
- Pace activities and schedule rest periods *to prevent fatigue. Even simple activities (such as bathing) during bed rest can cause fatigue and increase in oxygen consumption.*
- Change patient's position every 2 hours. *This will facilitate secretion movement and drainage.*
- Suction as needed *to clear secretions*.
- *Provide reassurance and allay anxiety:*
  Have an agreed-upon method for the patient to call for assistance (e.g., call light, bell).
  Stay with the patient during episodes of respiratory distress.
- Anticipate need for intubation and mechanical ventilation if patient is unable to maintain adequate gas exchange.

PATIENT EDUCATION

- Explain the need to restrict and pace activities *to decrease oxygen consumption during the acute episode.*
- Explain the type of oxygen therapy being utilized and why its maintenance is important.
- Teach the patient appropriate deep breathing and coughing techniques *to facilitate adequate air exchange and secretion clearance.*

Optimal gas exchange will be maintained.

Originated by: Susan Galanes, RN, MS, CCRN

Grieving, anticipatory

A state in which an individual grieves before an actual loss. It may apply to individuals who suffer a perinatal loss or loss of a body part or to patients who have received a terminal diagnosis for themselves or a loved one.

RELATED FACTORS / DEFINING CHARACTERISTICS	NURSING INTERVENTIONS / *RATIONALES*	EXPECTED OUTCOMES

RELATED FACTORS
Perceived potential loss of significant other
Perceived potential loss of physiopsychosocial well-being
Perceived potential loss of personal possession
Situational crisis
Maturational crisis
Family crisis
Temporary disorganization
 	
DEFINING CHARACTERISTICS
Client shows distress at prospect of loss
Denial of potential loss
Sorrow
Crying
Guilt
Anger/hostility
Bargaining
Depression
Acceptance
Changes in eating habits
Alteration in activity level
Altered libido
Altered communication patterns
Fear
Hopelessness
Distortion of reality
	ONGOING ASSESSMENT
	• Identify behaviors that are suggestive of the grieving process (see defining characteristics).
	• Assess stage of grieving being experienced by client or significant others:
	    Denial
	    Anger
	    Bargaining
	    Depression
	    Acceptance
	• Assess the influence of the following factors on coping:
	    Past problem-solving abilities
	    Socioeconomic background
	    Educational preparation
	    Cultural beliefs
	    Spiritual beliefs
	• Assess whether the client and significant others differ in their stage of grieving.
	• Identify support systems available:
	    Family
	    Peer support
	    Primary physician
	    Consulting physician
	    Nursing staff
	    Clergy
	    Therapist/counselor
	    Professional/lay support group
	• Identify potential for pathologic grieving response (see Grieving, dysfunctional, p. 23).
	• Evaluate need for referral to social security representatives, legal consultants, or support groups.
	• Observe nonverbal communication. *Body language may communicate a great deal of information.*
	
	THERAPEUTIC INTERVENTIONS
	• Establish a good rapport with client/couple and significant others. Listen and encourage client/couple/significant others to verbalize feelings. *This opens lines of communication and facilitates successful resolution of grief.*
	• During the stage of shock and disbelief:
	    Provide as much privacy as possible.
	    Allow use of denial and other defense mechanisms.
	    Avoid reinforcing denial.
	    Avoid judgmental and defensive responses to criticisms of health care providers.
	    Do not encourage use of pharmacologic interventions.
	    Do not force client/couple to make decisions.
	• During the stage of developing awareness of potential loss:
	    Provide client/couple with ongoing information, diagnosis, prognosis, progress, and plan of care.
	    Encourage significant others to assist with patient's physical care.
	    Facilitate flexible visiting hours and include younger children and extended family when appropriate.
	    Help patient and significant others to share mutual fears and concerns, plans and hopes for each other.
	    Help significant others to understand that patient's verbalizations of anger should not be perceived as personal attacks.
	    Encourage significant others to maintain their own self-care needs for rest, sleep, nutrition, leisure activities, and time away from patient.
		The couple/client will verbalize their feelings and will establish and maintain functional support for themselves.

RELATED FACTORS / DEFINING CHARACTERISTICS	NURSING INTERVENTIONS / *RATIONALES*	EXPECTED OUTCOMES

Facilitate discussion with patient and significant other on "final arrangements," (e.g., burial, autopsy, organ donation, funeral).

Provide information about support groups. *Participation in group activities with others who have experienced similar circumstances may help couple successfully work through grief process.*

- If the grief is the result of an imminent death:

    Promote discussion on what to expect when death occurs.

    Encourage significant others and client/patient to share their wishes about which family members should be present at time of death.

    Help significant others to accept that not being present at time of death does not indicate lack of love or caring.

- Utilize a visual method to identify the client/patient's critical status, i.e., color-coded door marker. *This will inform all hospital personnel of the client/patient's status in an effort to ensure that staff do not act or respond inappropriately to crisis situation.*
- Initiate process that provides additional support and resources.
- Refer to other resources: counseling, pastoral support, group therapy, etc. *Client/couple may need additional help to deal with individual concerns.*
- Provide anticipatory guidance and follow-up as condition continues.

PATIENT EDUCATION

- Involve significant others in discussions. *This helps to reinforce understanding of all individuals involved.*
- Orient client/family to hospital procedures (cafeteria, local restaurants, rest facilities/lounges, etc.).

Originated by: Mary Leslie Caldwell, RN
                Charlotte Razvi, RN, MSN, PhD

Grieving, dysfunctional

(FAILURE TO GRIEVE)

A state in which an individual is unable or unwilling to acknowledge or mourn an actual or perceived loss. This subsequently may impair further growth, development, or functioning.

RELATED FACTORS / DEFINING CHARACTERISTICS	NURSING INTERVENTIONS / *RATIONALES*	EXPECTED OUTCOMES

RELATED FACTORS
 	
Ambivalence toward lost object
Inability to participate in socially sanctioned mourning process and rituals
Concurrent overwhelming stress
Absence of support
 	
DEFINING CHARACTERISTICS
 	
Mild to moderate decrease in mood
Constricted affect
Avoidance of affectively charged topics
	ONGOING ASSESSMENT
	
	- Identify actual/potential loss(es).
	- Explore nature of individual's past attitudes/relationship with lost object or person.
	- Assess past coping style and mechanisms used in stressful situations.
	- Assess current affective state.
	    Observe for presence/absence of emotional distress.
	    Observe quality/quantity of communication (verbal and nonverbal).
	- Assess degree of relatedness to others.
	- Determine degree of insight in present situation.
	- Identify disturbing topics of conversation or experiences.
	- Estimate degree of stress currently experienced.
	
	THERAPEUTIC INTERVENTIONS
	
	- Approach individual in an unhurried manner.
	- Provide atmosphere of acceptance:
	    Listen attentively.
	    Encourage verbalization of feelings and expressions of affect (such as crying).
		The experience of grieving will be initiated in a supportive environment.

Continued.

Grieving, dysfunctional—cont'd

RELATED FACTORS / DEFINING CHARACTERISTICS	NURSING INTERVENTIONS / *RATIONALES*	EXPECTED OUTCOMES

Somatic complaints
Regression
Guilt or rumination
Withdrawal from others and/or normal activities
Marked change or deviation from usual behavior pattern
"Acting out" behavior
Patient/significant others report failure to grieve
	• Communicate comfort in patient's discussion of loss and grief.
	• Offer feedback regarding patient's expressed feelings.
	• Encourage/facilitate expressions of acceptance or offers of emotional support by significant others to patient.
	• Recognize variation and need for individual adjustment to loss and change.
	• Recognize the need for the use of defense mechanisms. Do not personalize negative expressions or affect or unduly challenge some use of denial.
	• Reassure patient and significant others that some negative thoughts and feelings are normal. *Concern about how others may view one's full range of feelings may lead to further impediments in grieving process and increase a sense of isolation and loss.*
	• Support the use of adaptive coping mechanisms.
	• Discuss the actual loss with patient:
	    Support a realistic assessment of the event/situation.
	    Explore with the patient individual strengths and available resources.
	    Explore reasons for avoidance of feeling or acknowledging loss.
	    Review common changes in behavior associated with normal grieving (e.g., change in appetite and sleep patterns) with patient and significant others. Explain that although intensity and frequency decrease with time, the mourning period may continue longer.
	    Discuss normal coping behaviors in grief recovery (e.g., need for contact with others).
	• Encourage sharing of common problems with others.
	• Initiate referrals to others as appropriate.
	
	PATIENT EDUCATION
	• Explain that emotional response to loss is appropriate and commonly experienced:
	    Describe the "normal" stages of grief and mourning (denial, anger, bargaining, depression, acceptance).
	    Offer hope that emotional pain will decrease with time. *Many view the overt expression of feelings as a "weakness" or fear that they may lose control if they begin to acknowledge the depth of their emotions.*	

Originated by: Ann Filipski, RN, MSN, CS, Psy D Candidate
Jean L. Burke, RN,C, BSN

Growth and development, altered

Altered growth refers to a disturbance in physical growth. Physical growth can be retarded or accelerated, depending upon the source of the disorder. Altered development refers to differences in the usual patterns of mental and emotional maturation. Although accelerated development can be problematic, altered development usually refers to slower than average mental and/or emotional maturation.

RELATED FACTORS / DEFINING CHARACTERISTICS	NURSING INTERVENTIONS / *RATIONALES*	EXPECTED OUTCOMES

RELATED FACTORS
Genetic disorder:
Physical defects
Brain function defect
Hormonal dysfunction
Trauma:
Birth or prenatal
	ONGOING ASSESSMENT
	• Interview and elicit information concerning:
	    Family profile
	    Support systems
	    Individual profile:
	        Past medical history
	        Medications
		Potential abilities will be maximized.

RELATED FACTORS / DEFINING CHARACTERISTICS	NURSING INTERVENTIONS / *RATIONALES*	EXPECTED OUTCOMES

Accidental

Environmental

Disease:

Any that cause lasting debilitation.

Chronic illness that affects normal growth and development

DEFINING CHARACTERISTICS

Physical/biologic:

Small stature

Stunted limbs

Malformed extremities

Delayed growth milestones

Motor/self-care:

Poor gross motor

Poor fine motor

Lack of coordination

Delayed achievement of skills/competencies

Hyper- or hypoactive

Sensory:

Sight/hearing deficits

Perceptual deficits

Cognitive/intellectual

Short attention span

Poor impulse control

Thought/reasoning deficits

Perceptive deficit

Language:

Poor comprehension of spoken words

Inability to express self adequately

Learning difficulties

Psychosocial:

Delayed achievement of social skills

Learning difficulties

Aberrant behaviors

Psychosexual:

Sexual expression aberrant for age/social situation

Spiritual/moral:

Poor impulse control

Lack of understanding of right and wrong

Perceived current physical status

Personality as perceived by self and primary caretaker

Development:

Language

Fine and gross motor

School performance

- Perform a physical exam and note deviations from expected norms for age. *Abnormalities found in the newborn indicate a need for further investigation as some life-threatening disorders are associated with outward physical abnormalities; i.e., cardiac function can be impaired in the infant born with signs of trisomy 21 (Down's syndrome).*
- Obtain lab specimens pursuant to physical findings. *The lack of development or precocious development of secondary sex characteristics indicates need for hormone studies.*
- Perform a neuromuscular exam and note deviations. *The Denver Developmental Screening Test for children is a standardized screening tool that may be useful in determining developmental age.*
- Assess for potential learning disabilities with vision and hearing tests as well as other screening tools such as the Illinois Test of Psycholinguistic Abilities. *Educational testing is available and should be performed in an educational setting where strengths and weaknesses can be identified and appropriately addressed.*
- Evaluate socioeconomic status and environment for adverse conditions that affect growth, development, and behavior. Assess for signs of abuse and neglect, as well as psychiatric or aberrant behaviors in other family members. *Changes in behavior and development, especially in children, are sometimes symptoms of a problem in another close family member.*
- Assess behavior, coping strategies, and family interaction.

THERAPEUTIC INTERVENTIONS

- Listen carefully to the comments and concerns of the mother/caretaker. *Especially when caring for infants and children, the primary caretaker is usually able to identify changes or lack of change in growth and development.*
- Maintain a safe, structured environment individualized to patient needs.
- Use a form of communication best suited to individual needs:
  Word board, signing, personal language, electronic talking box
- Provide assistive devices as needed:
  Wheelchair, utensil grips, reach extenders
- Assist with ADL as needed but allow as much self-care as possible *to foster self-confidence, independence, and success.*
- Arrange referrals:
  Social worker, Occupational Therapist/Physical Therapist, Eye, Ear, Nose, Throat Specialist, Psychiatrist, Neurologist, Orthopedist
  Clergy: *religious/cultural beliefs may have to be addressed to facilitate/accomplish acceptable outcomes.*
- Contact educational system/teacher to facilitate testing, adaptation to school setting, and identification of level of learning capabilities. *The highly intelligent and capable child also needs appropriate challenges to stimulate learning and prevent boredom, lack of interest, and behavior problems.*
- Refer for genetic screening/testing if a genetic abnormality is suspected.
- Refer for psychologic or psychiatric counseling if necessary.

PATIENT EDUCATION

- Explain the necessity for well newborn care and serial follow-up evaluations.
- Explain all tests/procedures, including why and how they will be performed.
- Explain results of exams, including normal development.
- Provide information concerning disorders or deficits, their treatment and prognosis.
- Reinforce the need for continual involvement in special education or physical development programs.

Originated by: Michele Knoll Puzas, RN,C, MHPE

Health maintenance, altered

Altered health maintenance reflects a change in an individual's ability to perform the functions necessary to maintain health or wellness. That individual may already manifest symptoms of existing/impending physical ailment or display behaviors that are strongly or certainly linked to disease. In all cases, the ability to control these health maintenance behaviors is within the control of the client/patient. The nurses' role is to identify factors that contribute to an individual's ability to maintain healthy behavior and implement measures that will result in improved health maintenance activities.

RELATED FACTORS / DEFINING CHARACTERISTICS	NURSING INTERVENTIONS / *RATIONALES*	EXPECTED OUTCOMES

RELATED FACTORS

Presence of mental retardation, illness, organic brain syndrome

Presence of physical disabilities/challenges

Presence of adverse personal habits:
  Smoking
  Poor diet selection
  Morbid obesity
  Alcohol abuse
  Drug abuse
  Poor hygiene
  Lack of exercise

Evidence of impaired perception

Inherited physical and emotional diseases

Lack of material resources

Lack of knowledge

Unavailability of services

Poor housing conditions

Inability to communicate needs adequately (e.g., deafness, speech impediment)

Dramatic change in health status

Lack of support systems

Denial of need to change current habits

DEFINING CHARACTERISTICS

Demonstrated lack of knowledge

Failure to keep appointments

Expressed interest in improving behaviors

ONGOING ASSESSMENT

- Assess for physical defining characteristics.
- Assess patient's knowledge of health maintenance behaviors.
- Assess health history over past 5 years.
- Assess to what degree environmental, social, interfamilial disruptions/changes have correlated with poor health behaviors.
- Assess appointment schedule to determine whether changed/skipped appointments can be associated with other symptoms of an altered ability to maintain health.
- Determine patient's specific questions related to health maintenance.
- Determine patient's motives for failing to report symptoms reflecting changes in health status.
- Discuss noncompliance with instructions/programs with patient *to determine rationale for failure*.
- Assess patient's educational preparation and ability to integrate and relate information.
- Assess history of substance abuse.
- Assess history of other adverse personal habits, including:
  Smoking
  Obesity
  Lack of exercise
- Determine whether the patient's manual dexterity or lack of mobility is a factor in patient's altered capacity for health maintenance.
- Determine to what degree patient's cultural beliefs and personality contribute to altered health habits.
- Determine whether the required health maintenance facilities/equipment is available to patient.
- Assess whether economic problems present a barrier to maintaining health behaviors.
- Assess hearing, orientation to time, place, and person to determine the patient's perceptual abilities.
- Assess patient's relationship with family and supportive others.
- Obtain home assessment from visiting nurse to determine accessibility and quality of living conditions.
- Assess patient's experience of stress/disruptors as they relate to health habits.

THERAPEUTIC INTERVENTIONS

- Follow up clinic visits with telephone/home visits *to develop ongoing relationship with patient and to vocalize support for client*.
- Provide patient with a means of contacting *health care providers who will be available for questions/problem solution*.
- Compliment patient on positive accomplishments *to reinforce behaviors*.
- Involve family and friends in health planning conferences.
- Ensure that other agencies (Department of Children and Family Services [DCFS], Social Services, Visiting Nurse Association [VNA], Meals on Wheels, etc.) are following through with plans.
- Provide assistive devices (i.e., walker, cane, wheelchair) as necessary.

Health maintenance will be improved.

RELATED FACTORS / DEFINING CHARACTERISTICS	NURSING INTERVENTIONS / *RATIONALES*	EXPECTED OUTCOMES

Failure to recognize/ respond to important symptoms reflective of changing health state
Inability to follow instructions/programs for health mainte-nance
Physical characteris-tics may include:
  Body/mouth order
  Unusual skin color, pallor
  Physical dirtiness
  Clothing soiled
  Frequent infections (e.g., upper respi-ratory infection [URI], urinary tract infection [UTI])
  Frequent toothaches
  Obesity/anorexia
  Anemia
  Chronic fatigue
  Apathetic attitude
  Substance abuse
	PATIENT EDUCATION
	- Provide patient with rationales for importance of behaviors such as:
	  Balanced diet low in cholesterol *to prevent vascular disease*
	  Smoking cessation: *smoking behaviors have been directly linked to can-cer and heart disease*
	  Cessation of alcohol and drug abuse. *In addition to physical addictions, the physical consequences of substance abuse mitigate against abuse*
	  Regular exercise/rest *to promote weight loss and increase agility and stamina*
	  Proper hygiene *to decrease risk of infection and promote maintenance and integrity of skin and teeth*
	  Regular physical and dental checkups *to identify and treat problems early*
	  Reporting of unusual symptoms to a health professional *to initiate early treatment*
	  Proper nutrition
	  Regular inoculations	

Originated by: Deidra Gradishar, RNC, BS

Home maintenance / management, impaired

Individuals within a home establish a normative pattern of operation. A vast number of factors can negatively impact upon that operational baseline. When this happens, an indi-vidual or an entire family may experience a disruption that is significant enough to impair the management of the envi-ronment. One, or the collective's health or safety may be threatened. There may be a threat to relationships or to physical mobility within the home.

RELATED FACTORS / DEFINING CHARACTERISTICS	NURSING INTERVENTIONS / *RATIONALES*	EXPECTED OUTCOMES
RELATED FACTORS Illness or injury of the client or a family member Poor planning and organization Lack of material re-sources Lack of familiarity with community re-sources Lack of knowledge Inadequate/absent sup-port systems	**ONGOING ASSESSMENT** - Determine what areas of home management represent the greatest problems for the patient or family. - Assess patient for poor personal habits. - Assess whether lack of money is a cause for not maintaining a clean, safe home. - Assess history of substance abuse and determine its impact upon ability to maintain home. - Refer to visiting nurse for home assessment. Evaluate home for accessibil-ity, physical barriers. - Evaluate each member of family to determine whether basic physical and emotional needs are being met. - Assess patient's knowledge of the rationale for personal and environmental hygiene and safety.	A safe home environ-ment will be main-tained.

Continued.

RELATED FACTORS / DEFINING CHARACTERISTICS	NURSING INTERVENTIONS / *RATIONALES*	EXPECTED OUTCOMES

Prolonged recuperative time

Death of a significant other

Substance abuse

Cognitive, perceptual, or emotional disturbance

Inability to express needs

DEFINING CHARACTERISTICS

Patient or family expresses difficulty in maintaining home environment

Poor personal habits including:
    Soiled clothing
    Frequent illness
    Weight loss
    Body odor
    Substance abuse
    Depressed affect

Mental confusion

Poor fiscal management

Vulnerable individuals (i.e., infants, children, elderly, infirm) in the home are neglected

Patient/family members report frequent home injuries

Home visits reveal unsafe home environment or lack of basic hygiene measures

Patient describes lack of knowledge regarding a particular aspect of home management

Presence of vermin in home

Accumulation of waste in home

Inappropriate environmental temperature

- Assess facilities for bathing.
- Assess facilities for trash disposal.
- Assess patient's physical ability to perform home maintenance.
- Assess the thermal appropriateness of the home. Determine whether windows close and have screens.
- Assess impact of death of relative who may have been a significant provider of care.
- Assess patient's emotional/intellectual preparedness to maintain a home.
- Enlist assessments by social worker or community resources that may help family/individual.
- Assess whether patient has all assistive devices necessary to perform home maintenance.

THERAPEUTIC INTERVENTIONS

- Begin discharge planning immediately after admission *to assure that discharge is organized to meet individual needs of family.*
- Coordinate home assessment by visiting nurse and social services.
- Integrate family and patient into the discharge planning process. *This will ensure patient-centered objectives and promote compliance.*
- Arrange for ongoing home therapy (i.e., physical and speech therapy).
- Assist family in arranging for even distribution of workload. Build in relief for caretakers *to prevent fatigue during performance of physically/ emotionally exhausting tasks.*
- Arrange for alternate placement when family is unable to provide care.
- Plan a home visit *to test the efficacy of discharge plans.*
- Provide telephone support or support in the form of home visits.

PATIENT EDUCATION

- Ensure that family/patient has been instructed in the use of all assistive devices:
    Begin care instruction/demonstrations early enough during hospital stay *to enable patient time to learn tasks.*
    Teach care measures to as many family members as possible *to provide multiple competent providers and intrafamilial support.*

Originated by: Deidra Gradishar, RNC, BS

Hopelessness

A sustained subjective emotional and cognitive state in which the person does not see alternatives or choices available to solve problems or to achieve what is desired. In addition, the person cannot mobilize his/her own energy to accomplish goals.

RELATED FACTORS / DEFINING CHARACTERISTICS	NURSING INTERVENTIONS / *RATIONALES*	EXPECTED OUTCOMES

RELATED FACTORS

Chronic and/or terminal illness

Deteriorating physical condition

Impaired body image

New and/or unexpected signs or symptoms of a previous disease

Prolonged pain, discomfort, weakness

Impaired functional abilities

Prolonged treatments that cause discomfort

Prolonged treatments with no positive results

Treatments that alter body image

Prolonged diagnostic studies that are inconclusive

Prolonged dependence on life support equipment

Prolonged dependence on monitoring equipment

Prolonged restricted activity

Prolonged isolation secondary to disease processes

Loss of social support networks

Multiple stressful life events

DEFINING CHARACTERISTICS

Feels that life has no meaning or purpose

Feels empty and/or has a sense of loss or deprivation

Expresses sustained apathy in response to a situation perceived as impossible with no solutions

ONGOING ASSESSMENT

- Assess role the illness plays in patient's hopelessness (i.e., level of physical functioning, endurance for activities, duration and course of illness, prognosis and treatments involved).
- Assess physical appearance (i.e., grooming, posture, hygiene).
- Assess appetite, exercise, and sleep patterns.
- Evaluate patient's ability to set goals.
- Note whether patient perceives unachieved outcomes as failures.
- Note whether patient emphasizes failures instead of accomplishments.
- Assess for feelings of hopelessness, lack of self-worth, giving up, suicidal ideas.
- Assess for potential source of hope (i.e., self, significant others, religion).
- Assess person's expectations for the future.
- Assess person's social support network.
- Assess meaning of the illness and treatments to the individual and family.
- Assess patient's perception and need for control in the situation.
- Assess previous coping strategies used and their effectiveness.
- Identify patterns of coping related to illness that enhance problem-solving skills and enable the patient to achieve goals.
- Assess patient's belief in self and own abilities.
- Assess patient's values and satisfaction with role/purpose in life.
- Assess ability for solving problems.

THERAPEUTIC INTERVENTIONS

- Provide physical care the patient is unable to provide for self in a manner that communicates warmth, respect, and acceptance of the patient's abilities.
- Implement individualized strategies to resolve difficulties with diet, sleep, activity, endurance.
- Implement physical care routine that enables patient to function at optimum level and is compatible with patient/family resources.
- Assist patient to evaluate situations and accomplishments accurately.
- Help the patient set realistic goals by identifying short-term goals and revising them as needed.
- Provide opportunity for the patient to express feelings of pessimism.
- Express hope for the patient who feels hopeless.
- Encourage hopes that are active and reality-based.
- Support patient's relationships with significant others; involve them in patient's care as appropriate.
- Provide opportunities for patient to control environment.
- Promote ego integrity by:
    Encouraging the person to reminisce about past life (self-validation)
    Showing the person that he/she gives something to you as a clinician
- Encourage patient to set realistic goals and to acknowledge all accomplishments no matter how small.
- Facilitate problem solving by identifying the problem and appropriate steps.

PATIENT EDUCATION

- Provide accurate and ongoing information about illness, treatment effects, and care needed.
- Educate patient/family on using a combination of problem-solving and emotive coping.
- Help patient/family to learn and use effective coping strategies.

Alternatives and choices are recognized by the patient.

Continued.

Nursing Diagnosis Care Plans

RELATED FACTORS / DEFINING CHARACTERISTICS	NURSING INTERVENTIONS / *RATIONALES*	EXPECTED OUTCOMES
Lacks ambition, initiative, interest; is passive; shows decreased verbalization		
Has difficulty solving problems and making decisions		
Thought processes may be inflexible, slowed, and/or negative; may be unable to integrate information		
Unable to identify and/or accomplish desired goals and objectives		
Cannot recognize sources of hope		
May have weight changes, anorexia, and sleep disturbances		
May feel incompetent, vulnerable, discouraged with self and others and helpless and overwhelmed		
Withdrawn socially, poor eye contact, apathetic		
Uninvolved with self-care		
May feel resigned, depressed, angry, destructive		
Decreased ability to recall the past; lost ability to perceive time.		
Distorted thought perceptions and associations		
Possibly impaired judgment		
Suicidal thoughts		
Unrealistic perceptions about hope		
Confusion		
Overall sense of sadness		

Originated by: Judith Popovich, RN, MS, CCRN

Hyperthermia

A state in which an individual's temperature is elevated above normal. Normal temperatures vary from person to person and also within the individual. Variations occur after meals and exercise, after sleep, and as hormonal responses. Hyperthermia is a sustained temperature above the normal variance; usually greater than 38° C.

RELATED FACTORS / DEFINING CHARACTERISTICS	NURSING INTERVENTIONS / *RATIONALES*	EXPECTED OUTCOMES
RELATED FACTORS Exposure to hot environment Vigorous activity Medications Anesthesia Increased metabolic rate Illness/trauma Dehydration Inability to perspire **DEFINING CHARACTERISTICS** Body temperature >38° C Hot, flushed skin Diaphoresis Increased heart rate Increased respiratory rate Irritability Fluid/electrolyte imbalance Convulsions	**ONGOING ASSESSMENT** · Obtain age and weight. *Extremes of age or weight increase the risk for inability to control body temperature.* · Assess vital signs. · Measure I & O. · Monitor serum electrolytes. · Determine precipitating factors. **THERAPEUTIC INTERVENTIONS** · Control environmental temperature. · Remove excess clothing and covers. · Provide antipyretic medications as ordered. · Cool with tepid bath. *Do not use alcohol, as it cools the skin too rapidly, causing shivering. Shivering increases metabolic rate and body temperature.* · Provide ample fluids, PO or IV. · Provide cooling mattress. · Adjust cooling measures on the basis of physical response. · Notify physician of significant changes. **PATIENT EDUCATION** · Explain temperature measurement and all treatments. · Provide information regarding normal temperature and control. · Provide instruction regarding home care and temperature measurement.	Body temperature will be maintained below 38° C.

Originated by: Michele Knoll Puzas, RN,C, MHPE

Hypothermia

The state in which an individual's body temperature is sustained at a significantly lower level than normal; usually lower than 35° C.

RELATED FACTORS / DEFINING CHARACTERISTICS	NURSING INTERVENTIONS / *RATIONALES*	EXPECTED OUTCOMES
RELATED FACTORS Exposure to cold environment Illness/trauma Inability to shiver Poor nutrition Inadequate clothing Alcohol consumption Medications: vasodilators Excessive evaporative heat loss from skin	**ONGOING ASSESSMENT** · Assess for extremes in age and weight. · Assess vital signs. · Monitor electrolytes. · Evaluate for drug or alcohol consumption. · Determine precipitating event and risk factors. · Evaluate peripheral perfusion at frequent intervals. **THERAPEUTIC INTERVENTIONS** · Provide extra covering: Clothing, including head covering. *Heat loss tends to be greatest from the top of the head.*	Body temperature will be maintained above 36° C.

Continued.

Hypothermia—cont'd

RELATED FACTORS / DEFINING CHARACTERISTICS	NURSING INTERVENTIONS / *RATIONALES*	EXPECTED OUTCOMES

Decreased metabolic rate
Inactivity
Advanced age
 	
DEFINING CHARACTERISTICS
Body temperature <36° C
Cool, pale skin
Decreased heart rate
Decreased respiratory rate
Hypoxemia
Hypoglycemia
Fluid/electrolyte imbalance
Irritability
Mental confusion
Convulsions
Respiratory arrest
	Blankets
	• Keep patient's linen dry. *Moisture facilitates evaporative heat loss.*
	• Control environmental temperature.
	• Provide extra heat source:
	   Heat lamp, radiant warmer
	   Heated moisturized O_2
	   Warming mattress, pads, or blankets
	   Warmed IV fluids/lavage fluids
	• Regulate heat source according to physical response.
	
	PATIENT EDUCATION
	• Explain all procedures and treatments.
	• Provide information regarding normal temperature.
	• Enlist support services as appropriate.	

Originated by: Michele Knoll Puzas, RN,C, MHPE

Injury, potential for

(HIGH-RISK FALL STATUS)

A state in which a person is at increased risk for injury because of falling.

RISK FACTORS / DEFINING CHARACTERISTICS	NURSING INTERVENTIONS / *RATIONALES*	EXPECTED OUTCOMES

RISK FACTORS
Altered mental/emotional state
Medications that place patient at risk (sedative, narcotics, tranquilizer, laxative, analgesic)
Poor judgment
Limited ability to perform ADL
Altered mobility requiring assistance/assistive devices
Use of mechanical restraints
Visual or sensory impairment
 	
DEFINING CHARACTERISTICS
Previous history of falls/accidents
Lack of knowledge regarding safety procedures
	ONGOING ASSESSMENT
	• Assess mental status every shift or as needed. *Even previously alert patients may experience changes secondary to medications and electrolyte or fluid imbalance.*
	• Assess for prior history of falls.
	• Assess ability to ambulate and carry out ADL.
	• Assess need for assistive devices: walker, cane, etc.
	• Assess for physical and sensory impairment.
	• Assess need for restraints and, if they are indicated, evaluate any resistance to restraints.
	
	THERAPEUTIC INTERVENTIONS
	Institute and document appropriate safety precautions *to prevent injury and maintain safety.*
	• Environmental:
	   Place bed in low position.
	   Place side rails up.
	   Place bed brakes on.
	   Place call light within reach (instruct patient to call for assistance).
	   Assure adequate lighting.
	   Assure unobstructed walkway.
	   Assure that patient is able to reach bedside stand. Keep belongings at a level *so patient does not have to reach or bend over.*
	   Provide hand grips in bathroom, shower, toilet, and railings in hallways.
	• Physical needs
	   Utilize assistive devices (walkers, canes, wheelchairs) as appropriate.
		High-risk patient will be identified and risk of injury reduced.

RELATED FACTORS / DEFINING CHARACTERISTICS	NURSING INTERVENTIONS / *RATIONALES*	EXPECTED OUTCOMES
Unsteady gait Disorientation Lethargy Agitation Combativeness Sundown syndrome Poor eyesight Old age (over 65 years)	Ensure that patient is strong enough to use them and has been taught correct techniques. Use patient restraints as documented in policy manual. Establish regular schedule of elimination assistance. Monitor patient closely if having radiographic testing, etc., and receiving bowel prep. *Previously stable patient may develop unsteady gait when "hurrying" to bathroom.* If patient is receiving diuretics, assess need for bedside commode. Assist patient in ADL and ambulation when necessary. Ensure that appropriate footwear is used (shoes that fit and are secured tightly; *avoid floppy slippers, which can be hazardous*). Use hearing aid and corrective lenses while ambulating as necessary. Schedule safety check for high risk patients every shift or as needed. If applicable, remind patient to remain in bed while taking medications with sedative effect. • Psychological/social needs Orient patient to time, place, and person p.r.n. *to decrease confusion.* **PATIENT EDUCATION** • Teach patient/significant others how to minimize potential hazards in the environment. • Teach patient to observe activity restrictions as ordered by physician.	

Originated by: Yvonne Evans-Wordell, RN, MSN
Urakay Campbell, RN,
Barbara J. Hobbs, RN, MSN

Knowledge deficit

(PATIENT TEACHING; HEALTH EDUCATION)

A state in which cognitive information or psychomotor skills are lacking.

RELATED FACTORS / DEFINING CHARACTERISTICS	NURSING INTERVENTIONS / *RATIONALES*	EXPECTED OUTCOMES
RELATED FACTORS New condition, procedure, treatment Cognitive limitation Misinterpretation of information Decreased motivation to learn Emotional state affecting learning (anxiety, denial, or depression) **DEFINING CHARACTERISTICS** Questioning members of health care team Verbalizes inaccurate information Noncompliance	**ONGOING ASSESSMENT** • Assess orientation to person, place, environment. • Assess intellectual ability to learn. • Assess ability to see, hear, and read. • Assess physical ability to perform tasks. • Identify priority of learning need within the overall plan of care. • Assess motivation and willingness of patient/significant others to learn. • Question patient regarding previous experience and health teaching. • Identify any existing misconceptions regarding material to be taught. • Determine cultural influences on health teaching. **THERAPEUTIC INTERVENTIONS** • Provide physical comfort for learner *to reduce the stress of handling new information. This allows the patient to concentrate on what is being discussed or demonstrated.* • Provide a quiet atmosphere without interruption *to allow the patient to concentrate more completely.* • Establish objectives and goals for learning at the beginning of the session. *This allows the learner to know what will be discussed and expected during the session. This intervention helps to reduce patient fear and anxiety.*	Patient/significant others will be able to demonstrate or verbalize desired content.

Continued.

RELATED FACTORS / DEFINING CHARACTERISTICS	NURSING INTERVENTIONS / *RATIONALES*	EXPECTED OUTCOMES
Denial of need to learn Anger/hostility Depression Withdrawal from environment Altered orientation to environment Inability to read, hear, see Physical inability to perform task Incorrect task performance Expression of frustration or confusion when performing task Multiple hospitalizations for same problem Frequent exacerbations of illness Development of complications	• Allow learner to identify what is most important to him/her. *This clarifies learner expectations and helps the nurse match the information to be presented to the individual's needs.* • Explore attitudes and feelings about changes. *This assists the nurse in understanding how the learner may respond to the information and possibly how compliant the patient may be with the expected changes.* • Allow for and support self-directed, self-designed learning. *This enhances individual learning styles and allows learning to occur at the learner's pace.* • Assist the learner in integrating information into daily life. *This helps the learner make adjustments in daily life that will result in the desired change in behavior (or learning).* • Allow adequate time for integration that is in direct conflict with existing values or beliefs. • Provide explanation at the level of understanding of patient/significant other • Give clear, thorough explanations and demonstrations. • Provide information using various mediums (e.g., explanations, discussion, demonstration, pictures, written instructions, videotapes) *since different people take in information in different ways.* • When presenting material, move from familiar, concrete information to less familiar or more abstract concepts. *This provides the patient with the opportunity to understand new material in relation to familiar material.* • Focus teaching sessions on a single concept or idea. *This allows the learner to concentrate more completely on material being discussed.* • Keep sessions short *to prevent fatigue.* • Encourage questions from patient/significant other. *Learners often feel shy or embarrassed about asking questions and often want permission to ask them.* • Allow learner to practice new skills; provide immediate feedback on performance. *This allows patient to use new information immediately, thus enhancing retention. Immediate feedback allows learner to make corrections rather than practicing the skill incorrectly.* • Encourage repetition of information or new skill *to assist in remembering.* • Provide positive, constructive reinforcement of learning. *A positive approach allows the learner to feel good about learning accomplishments and maintain self-esteem while correcting mistakes.* • Document progress of teaching/learning. *This allows additional teaching to be based on what learner has completed, thus enhancing learner self-esteem and encouraging most cost-effective teaching.* • Refer patient to support groups as needed *to allow the patient to interact with others who have similar problems or learning needs.* • Include significant others whenever possible *to encourage ongoing support for patient.*	

Originated by: Martha Dickerson, RN, MS, CCRN

Mobility, impaired physical

A state in which a person has limitations of independent physical movement.

(IMMOBILITY)

RELATED FACTORS / DEFINING CHARACTERISTICS	NURSING INTERVENTIONS / *RATIONALES*	EXPECTED OUTCOMES

RELATED FACTORS

Musculoskeletal impairment
Neuromuscular impairment
Medical restrictions
Prolonged bed rest
Limited strength
Pain

DEFINING CHARACTERISTICS

Inability to move purposefully within physical environment, including bed mobility, transfer, and ambulation
Reluctance to attempt movement
Limited ROM
Decreased muscle strength, control, or mass
Imposed restrictions of movement, including mechanical, medical protocol, and impaired coordination
Inability to perform action as instructed

ONGOING ASSESSMENT

- Assess patient's ability to carry out ADL on daily basis.
- Assess patient/significant others' knowledge of immobility (what they know, need to know, or misunderstand).
- Assess for developing thrombophlebitis (calf pain, Homans' sign, redness, localized swelling, and rise in temperature).
- Assess skin integrity. Check for signs of redness, tissue ischemia (especially over ears, shoulders, elbows, sacrum, hips, heels, ankles, and toes).
- Monitor I & O record as needed; monitor daily consumption. Assess nutritional needs as they relate to immobility (possible hypocalcemia, negative nitrogen balance). *Pressure sores develop more quickly in patients with a nutritional deficit.*
- Assess elimination status (usual pattern, present patterns, signs of constipation).
- Assess emotional response to disability/limitation.
- Evaluate need for home assistance (physical therapy, visiting nurse, assistive device).

THERAPEUTIC INTERVENTIONS

- Encourage and facilitate early ambulation and other ADL when possible. Assist with each initial change: dangling, sitting in chair, ambulation.
- Obtain adequate assistance of people/Hoyer lift when transferring patient to bed, chair, or stretcher.
- Encourage appropriate use of assisting devices.
- Provide positive reinforcement during activity.
- Keep side rails up and bed in low position *to promote safe environment.*
- Consult rehabilitation medicine personnel as appropriate.
- Turn and position every 2 hours or as needed *to optimize circulation to all tissues and to relieve pressure.*
- Maintain limbs in functional alignment (e.g., with pillows, sandbags, or wedges).
    Support feet in dorsiflexed position *to prevent footdrop.*
    Use bed cradle *to keep heavy bed linens off feet.*
- Assist with passive/active ROM exercise *to increase venous return, prevent stiffness, and maintain muscle strength and endurance.*
- Turn to prone or semiprone position once daily unless contraindicated *to drain bronchial tree.*
- Use prophylactic antipressure devices as appropriate *to prevent tissue breakdown.*
- Clean, dry, and moisturize skin as needed.
- Encourage coughing and deep breathing exercises. Use suction as needed *to prevent buildup of secretions.* Use incentive spirometer *to increase lung expansion.*
- Encourage liquid intake of 2000-3000 ml/day unless contraindicated *to optimize hydration status and prevent hardening of stool.*
- Initiate supplemental high-protein feedings as appropriate.
- Set up a bowel program (adequate fluid, foods high in bulk, physical activity, stool softeners, laxatives) as needed. Record bowel activity level.
- Assist patient in accepting limitations. Emphasize abilities.
- See also: Self-care deficit, p. 44; Activity intolerance, p. 2; Constipation/ impaction, p. 12.

Optimal physical mobility will be maintained.

Continued.

Mobility, impaired physical—cont'd

RELATED FACTORS / DEFINING CHARACTERISTICS	NURSING INTERVENTIONS / *RATIONALES*	EXPECTED OUTCOMES

PATIENT EDUCATION
- Explain progressive physical activity to patient. Help patient/significant others to establish reasonable and obtainable goals.
- Instruct patient/significant others regarding hazards of immobility. Emphasize importance of position change, ROM, coughing exercises, etc.
- Reinforce principles of exercise, emphasizing that joints are to be exercised to the point of pain, not beyond.
- Instruct patient/family regarding need to make home environment safe.
- Encourage verbalization of feelings, strengths, and weaknesses.

Originated by: Linda Arsenault, RN, MSN, CNRN
     Marilyn Magafas, RN,C, BSN, MBA
     Karen Moyer, RN, MS, CCRN, CNA

Noncompliance

(COMPLIANCE; ADHERENCE)

Failure to follow prescribed treatment plan. If therapy is ineffective or based on a faulty diagnosis, even perfect compliance will not result in the expected therapeutic effect.

RELATED FACTORS / DEFINING CHARACTERISTICS	NURSING INTERVENTIONS / *RATIONALES*	EXPECTED OUTCOMES
RELATED FACTORS Denial Lack of knowledge Fear Conflicting instructions Cultural beliefs Lack of resources (financial, social, personal) Physical limitations Mental disability Side effects of treatment Dissatisfaction with outcomes Inconvenience Failure to recognize severity of problem/need for treatment **DEFINING CHARACTERISTICS** Therapeutic effect not achieved or maintained Missed appointments "Revolving door" hospital admissions Improper pill counts or missed prescription refills Body fluid analysis inconsistent with compliance	**ONGOING ASSESSMENT** • Compare actual therapeutic effect with expected effect. • Plot patient's pattern of hospitalizations and clinic appointments. • Ask patient to bring prescription drugs to appointment; count remaining pills. • Assess urine or serum drug level. • Conduct compliance-oriented history. Assess beliefs about current illness: "What do you think causes your (diagnosis or symptom)?" "How likely do you think it is that (symptom) will return?" "What worries you most about (diagnosis or symptom)?" • Assess beliefs about treatment plan: "Is there anything that worries you about this treatment plan?" "Are you worried about any possible side effects of this treatment? "Can you think of any problems you might have carrying out this treatment?" "Do you think that this treatment will help you?" **THERAPEUTIC INTERVENTIONS** • Involve patient in planning care. *Compliance problems are usually not solved by traditional patient teaching methods.* • Concentrate first on the compliance behavior that will make the greatest contribution to the therapeutic effect. • Increase the amount of supervision provided: *home health nurses and frequent return visits/appointments can provide increased supervision.* • Simplify therapy *to maximize potential for compliance.* • Provide social support through the patient's family and self-help groups. • Tailor the therapy to the patient's life-style. • Engage the patient in joint problem solving. • Develop a system for the patient to monitor his own progress. • Develop a behavioral contact. *This helps the patient understand/accept his or her role in the plan of care and clarifies what the patient can expect from the health care worker/system.* • Develop with the patient a system of rewards that follow successful compliance. Rewards can be administered by the patient or family at home.	Compliance behaviors will be evident.

Noncompliance—cont'd

RELATED FACTORS / DEFINING CHARACTERISTICS	NURSING INTERVENTIONS / *RATIONALES*	EXPECTED OUTCOMES
Patient admission of noncompliance Third-party report of noncompliance Health professional's impression of non-compliance (greatly underestimates incidence of noncompliance)	• Role play scenarios when noncompliance may easily occur. Demonstrate appropriate behaviors and help the patient to expand his repertoire of responses to difficult situations. • Role play scenarios when the patient is temporarily noncompliant. Demonstrate ways to return quickly to the treatment plan. • As compliance improves, gradually reduce the amount of professional supervision and reinforcement. **PATIENT EDUCATION** • Tailor the information in terms of what the patient feels is the cause of his health problem and his concerns about therapy. • Introduce complicated therapy one step at a time. • Include family members and significant others in the teaching. • Explore with significant others the effects of patient therapy on them. • Teach significant others to eliminate disincentives to the patient for compliance. • Teach significant others to increase rewards to the patient for compliance.	

Originated by: Jeff Zurlinden, RN, MS

Nutrition, altered: less than body requirements

The state in which an individual experiences an intake of nutrients insufficient to meet metabolic needs.

(STARVATION; WEIGHT LOSS; ANOREXIA)

RELATED FACTORS / DEFINING CHARACTERISTICS	NURSING INTERVENTIONS / *RATIONALES*	EXPECTED OUTCOMES
RELATED FACTORS Inability to ingest foods Inability to digest foods Inability to absorb/metabolize foods Inability to procure adequate amounts of food Knowledge deficit Pica Unwillingness to eat Increased metabolic needs caused by disease process or therapy **DEFINING CHARACTERISTICS** Loss of weight with or without adequate caloric intake >10-20% below ideal body weight Documented inadequate caloric intake	**ONGOING ASSESSMENT** • Document patient's actual weight on admission (do not estimate); weigh weekly. • Obtain nutritional history as appropriate. • Monitor urine/serum electrolytes, CBC, glucose, and urine sugar/acetone as needed. **THERAPEUTIC INTERVENTIONS** • Consult dietitian when appropriate. • Document appetite. Record exact I & O (do not estimate). • Encourage patient participation (daily log). *Determination of type, amount, and pattern of food/fluid intake is facilitated by accurate documentation by patient/nurse as the intake occurs; memory is insufficient.* • Assist patient with meals as needed. • Encourage frequent oral ingestion of high-calorie/high-protein foods and fluids. • Encourage use of high-fiber foods; give stool softeners as ordered to promote regular elimination patterns. • Encourage exercise. *Metabolism and utilization of nutrients are enhanced by activity.* • If nutritional deficit severe, see Enteral tube feeding p. 308. • Encourage family to bring food from home as appropriate. **PATIENT EDUCATION** • Review and reinforce the following to patient/significant others: Importance of maintaining adequate caloric intake	Optimal caloric intake will be maintained.

Continued.

37

RELATED FACTORS / DEFINING CHARACTERISTICS	NURSING INTERVENTIONS / *RATIONALES*	EXPECTED OUTCOMES
Caloric intake inadequate to keep pace with abnormal disease/metabolic state	Foods high in calories/protein that will promote weight gain and nitrogen balance (e.g., small frequent meals of foods high in calories and protein) • Assist patient/significant others in recognizing regular eating patterns. • Educate family about necessity of emotional support.	

Originated by: Jackie Suprenant, RN, BSN
                Maureen T. Linehan, RN
                Carol Burkhart, RN, BSN, CCRN

Nutrition, altered: more than body requirements

The state in which an individual is experiencing an intake of nutrients that exceeds metabolic demands.

(OBESITY; OVERWEIGHT)

RELATED FACTORS / DEFINING CHARACTERISTICS	NURSING INTERVENTIONS / *RATIONALES*	EXPECTED OUTCOMES

RELATED FACTORS
 Lack of knowledge of nutritional needs, food intake, and/or food preparation
 Poor dietary habits
 Use of food as coping mechanism
 Metabolic disorders
 Diabetes
 Sedentary activity level
 	
 DEFINING CHARACTERISTICS
 Weight 10-20% over ideal for height and frame
 Reported or observed dysfunctional eating patterns
	ONGOING ASSESSMENT
	 • Perform nutritional assessment as appropriate.
	 • Document patient's actual weight on admission (do not estimate).
	 • Monitor urine/serum electrolytes, CBC, glucose, and urine sugar/acetone as needed.
	
	 THERAPEUTIC INTERVENTION
	 • Consult dietitian when appropriate.
	 • Assist patient with selection of appropriate foods from each food group.
	 • Encourage patient to keep a daily log of food/liquid ingestion and caloric intake *as memory is inadequate for quantification of intake. A visual record may also help patient to make more appropriate food choices and serving sizes.*
	 • Encourage water intake.
	 • Encourage patient to be more aware of nutritional habits:
	     To realize the time needed for eating (encourage putting fork down between bites).
	     To focus on eating and to avoid other diversional activities (e.g., reading, television viewing, telephoning).
	     To observe for cues that lead to eating (e.g., odor, time, depression, and boredom).
	     To eat in the same place as often as possible.
	     To identify actual need for food.
	 • Encourage exercise.
	 • See Obesity, simple, p. 296.
	
	 PATIENT EDUCATION
	 • Review and reinforce dietitian's teaching regarding:
	     Four food groups and proper serving sizes
	     Caloric content of food
	     Methods of preparation
	 • Provide family counseling as needed, being sure to identify and include the person primarily responsible for grocery shopping and food preparation.
	 • Encourage diabetic patients to attend diabetic classes. Review and reinforce principles of dietary management of diabetes.
		Nutritional intake will be appropriate to meet metabolic needs.

Originated by: Jackie Suprenant, RN, BSN
                Carol Burkhart, RN, BSN, CCRN
                Maureen T. Linehan, RN

Pain

A highly subjective state in which a variety of unpleasant sensations and a wide range of distressing factors may be experienced by the sufferer. Pain may be acute, a symptom of injury or illness such as a myocardial infarction, or chronic, lasting longer than 6 months, the result of a long-term illness such as arthritis.

RELATED FACTORS / DEFINING CHARACTERISTICS	NURSING INTERVENTIONS / *RATIONALES*	EXPECTED OUTCOMES

RELATED FACTORS

Childbirth pain
Operative pain
Cardiovascular pain
Pain resulting from medical problems
Musculoskeletal pain
Pain resulting from diagnostic procedures or medical treatments
Pain resulting from trauma

DEFINING CHARACTERISTICS

Patient/significant others report pain
Guarding behavior, protectiveness
Self-focusing, narrowed focus (altered time perception, withdrawal from social or physical contact), depression, loss of appetite
Relief/distraction behavior (e.g., moaning, crying, pacing, seeking out other people or activities, restlessness, irritability, alteration in sleep pattern)
Facial mask of pain
Alteration in muscle tone: listlessness/flaccidness; rigidity/tension)
Autonomic responses not seen in chronic, stable pain (e.g., diaphoresis; change in BP, pulse rate; pupillary movements; decreased respiratory rate; pallor; nausea)

ONGOING ASSESSMENT

- Assess pain characteristics:
    Quality (e.g., sharp, burning, shooting)
    Severity (scale 1-10, 10 most severe)
    Location (anatomic description)
    Onset (gradual or sudden)
    Duration (how long, intermittent/continuous)
    Precipitating/relieving factors
- Assess for probable cause of pain. Whether pain is the result of:
    Childbirth pain
    Operative Pain: see specific operative procedure
    Cardiovascular pain: see specific diagnosis (e.g., Myocardial infarction, p. 103, Angina, pp. 67 and 69)
    Pain resulting from medical problems: see specific diagnosis (e.g., Urinary tract infection, p. 361, Peptic ulcer, p. 300)
    Musculoskeletal pain: see Extremity fracture, p. 430 or specific orthopaedic problem
    Pain resulting from diagnostic procedure or medical intervention
- Evaluate patient's response to pain and medications or therapeutics aimed at abolishing/relieving pain.
- Assess to what degree cultural, environmental, intrapersonal, intrapsychic factors may contribute to pain.
- Evaluate what the pain means to the individual. *The meaning of the pain will directly influence the patient's response. Pain will influence work, family role, self-concept, etc.*
- Assess patient's past coping mechanisms *to determine what measures worked best in the past.*
- Assess patient's expectations for pain relief. *Some patients may be content to have pain decreased; others will expect complete elimination of pain. This will impact on their perception of the effectiveness of the treatment modality and their willingness to participate in further treatments.*
- Assess patient's willingness/ability to explore a range of techniques aimed at controlling pain.
- Assess for effects of chronic pain:
    Depression
    Guilt
    Hopelessness
    Sleep, sexual, and nutritional disturbances
    Alterations in interpersonal relationships

THERAPEUTIC INTERVENTION

- Anticipate need for analgesics or additional methods of pain relief. *One can most effectively deal with pain by preventing it. Early intervention may decrease the total amount of analgesic required.*
- Respond immediately to complaint of pain. *In the midst of painful experiences patient's perception of time may become distorted. Prompt responses to complaints may result in decreased anxiety in patient. Demonstrated concern for patient's welfare and comfort fosters the development of a trusting relationship.*
- Eliminate additional stressors or sources of discomfort whenever possible. *Patients may experience an exaggeration in pain or a decreased ability to tolerate painful stimuli if environmental, intrapersonal, or intrapsychic factors are further stressing them.*

Pain will be relieved or reduced or patient will begin to show signs of adaptation.

Continued.

RELATED FACTORS / DEFINING CHARACTERISTICS	NURSING INTERVENTIONS / *RATIONALES*	EXPECTED OUTCOMES

- Give analgesics as ordered, evaluating effectiveness and observing for any signs and symptoms of untoward effects. *Pain medications are absorbed and metabolized differently by patients, so their effectiveness must be evaluated from patient to patient. Analgesics may cause side effects that range from mild to life-threatening.*
- Notify physician if interventions are unsuccessful or if current complaint is a significant change from patient's past experience of pain. *Patients who request pain medications at intervals more frequent then prescribed may actually require higher doses of analgesia or more potent analgesia.*
- Provide rest periods to facilitate comfort, sleep, and relaxation. *The patient's experiences of pain may become exaggerated as the result of fatigue. In a cyclic fashion, pain may result in fatigue, which may result in exaggerated pain and exhaustion. A quiet environment, a darkened room, and a disconnected phone are all measures geared toward facilitating rest.*
- Whenever possible reassure patient that:
    Pain is time-limited
    There is more than one approach to easing pain. *When pain is perceived as everlasting and unresolvable, the patient may give up trying to cope with it or experience a sense of hopelessness and loss of control*
- Perform range of motion (active or passive) and promote mobility through:
    Position changes
    Proper body alignment
    Support of extremities during movement and at rest
    Appropriate exercise
    Self-care whenever possible
    Daily ambulation when appropriate *Self-care enhances the patient's sense of autonomy while encouraging movement and mobility. Mobility will counteract the adverse consequences of disuse. Pain during exercise is an indication to modify the exercise to a more gentle activity.*
    Application of:
      Hot moist compresses. *Hot moist compresses have a penetrating effect. The warmth rushes blood to the affected area to promote healing.*
      Cold compresses to affected area when ordered. *Cold compresses may reduce local edema and promote some numbing, thereby promoting comfort.*
- Instruct the patient in use of one or a combination of the following techniques:
    Imagery: *The use of a mental picture or an imagined event that involves use of the five senses to distract oneself from painful stimuli.*
    Distraction techniques: *Heightening one's concentration upon nonpainful stimuli to decrease one's awareness and experience of pain.*
      Breathing modifications
      Nerve stimulation
    Relaxation exercises: *Techniques used to bring about a state of physical and mental awareness and tranquility. The goal of these techniques is to reduce tensions, subsequently reducing pain.*
    Massage of affected area when appropriate. *Massage decreases muscle tension and can promote comfort.*

PATIENT EDUCATION

- Provide anticipatory instruction on pain causes, appropriate prevention, and relief measures.
- Explain cause of pain/discomfort, if known.
- Instruct patient to report pain *so that relief measures may be instituted.*
- Instruct patient to evaluate and report effectiveness of measures used.

Originated by: Deidra Gradishar, RNC, BS
　　　　　　Linda Muzio, RN, MSN
　　　　　　Ann Filipski, RN, MSN, CS, PsyD Candidate
　　　　　　Janice Borman, RN, MSN, PhD Candidate
　　　　　　Susan R. Laub, RN, MEd, CS

Parenting, altered (actual/potential)

(INEFFECTIVE BONDING; CHILD ABUSE)

The state in which the ability of the nurturing figure(s) is at risk or the individual is unable to create an environment that promotes the optimum growth and development of another human being from infancy through adolescence.

RELATED FACTORS / DEFINING CHARACTERISTICS	NURSING INTERVENTIONS / *RATIONALES*	EXPECTED OUTCOMES

RELATED FACTORS

Lack of available role model

Ineffective role model

Physical and psychosocial abuse of nurturing figure

Lack of support

Unmet social, emotional, and maturational needs of parenting figures

Unrealistic expectations of self and/or partner

Limited cognitive functioning

Extremes of age

Past experiences

Culture

Fatigue

Physical discomforts/impairment

Social isolation

Mental or physical illness

Family or personal stress (financial, legal, recent crisis)

DEFINING CHARACTERISTICS

Lack of parental attachment behaviors

Inappropriate visual, tactile, auditory stimulation

Negative identification with characteristics of infant/child

Negative attachment of meanings to characteristics of infant/child

Verbalization of resentment toward infant/child

Verbalization of role inadequacy

Inattention to infant/child needs

Verbal disgust at body functions of infant/child

ONGOING ASSESSMENT

- Assess strengths, weakness, age, marital status, available sources of support, cultural background, and individual response to child-rearing and parenting role.
- Evaluate nature of emotional and physical parenting that parents received during their own childhood. *Parenting is learned, and individuals use their own parents as role models.*
- Assess parent(s) interpersonal communication skills and their relationship to each other, friends, and other family members.
- Assess motivation to learn.
- Determine degree of insight.
- Evaluate the significance of nonverbal communication.
- Identify disturbing conversational topics.
- Identify inappropriate emotional responses.
- Identify parent's significant life values.
- Identify appropriate use of defense mechanisms.
- Observe patient/partner for excessive stress level.
- Observe for evidence that patient/partner is reaching out for emotional support.

THERAPEUTIC INTERVENTIONS

- Provide an atmosphere of acceptance.
- Express warmth and friendliness to patient/partner. *This will facilitate patient/partner communication of concerns.*
- Encourage acceptance of responsibility for infant/child.
- Encourage awareness of positive responses from others.
- Encourage expression of feelings.
- Listen attentively and talk with patient. *This will promote trust between caregiver and patient/parent.*
- Encourage recognition of one's various roles in life.
- Encourage use of normal coping mechanisms.
- Explore with the patient/parents evidence of recurring problems.
- Explore with parents the effects of their behavior on their children.
- Introduce to groups/persons who have and are successfully dealing with similar parenting problems. *This will provide group support.*
- Refrain from negatively criticizing patient/parent.
- Maintain and support realistic assessment of the situation.
- Refer patient/parent to other support services as indicated.
- Recommend early correction of problem.
- Emphasize importance of recognition of tension within oneself.

PATIENT EDUCATION

- Explain the importance of maintaining a positive self-attitude.
- Explain that parental attitudes affect child development.
- Explain that undesirable thoughts and feelings are normal.
- Explain the causes of the health problems that may be present.

More effective parenting behaviors will be demonstrated.

Continued.

41

Parenting, altered—cont'd

RELATED FACTORS / DEFINING CHARACTERISTICS	NURSING INTERVENTIONS / RATIONALES	EXPECTED OUTCOMES
Noncompliance with health appointments for infant/child		
Inappropriate or inconsistent discipline practices		
Frequent childhood accidents		
Frequent illness of infant/child		
Growth and developmental lag		
Verbalization of desire for child to call parent by first name versus traditional name		
Child care from multiple caretakers without consideration of infant/child needs		
Compulsive seeking of role approval from others		
Abandonment of infant/child		
Running away by child		

Originated by: Caroline Sarmiento, RN, BSN

Powerlessness

The state in which a person perceives an inability to influence others to think, act, or feel a certain way; one perceives a loss of personal control over events or situations.

RELATED FACTORS / DEFINING CHARACTERISTICS	NURSING INTERVENTIONS / RATIONALES	EXPECTED OUTCOMES
RELATED FACTORS Acute or chronic illness Inability to communicate Dependence on others for activities of daily living Inability to perform role responsibilities Progressive debilitating disease Mental illness Substance abuse Obesity Disfigurement Lack of knowledge	**ONGOING ASSESSMENT** • Assess the role the illness plays in patient's powerlessness (i.e., uncertainty about events, duration and course of illness, prognosis, dependence on others for help and treatments involved). • Assess impact of powerlessness on patient's physical condition (i.e., appearance, oral intake, hygiene, sleep habits). • Note whether patient demonstrates need for information about illness, treatment plan, procedures. • Evaluate the effects of information provided on patient's behavior and feelings. • Assess for feelings of anger, frustration, withdrawal, submissiveness, anxiety, powerlessness. • Identify situations and/or interactions that may cause the patient to feel powerless. • Assess patient's power needs. • Assess patient's need for control of situations/events. • Assess for feelings of hopelessness, depression, apathy.	Feeling of powerlessness will be reduced.

RELATED FACTORS / DEFINING CHARACTERISTICS	NURSING INTERVENTIONS / *RATIONALES*	EXPECTED OUTCOMES

Personal characteristics that value control highly

Necessity to relinquish control to others

Lack of privacy

Altered personal territory

Social isolation

Lack of explanations from caregivers

No consultation regarding decisions

Social displacement

Relocation

Insufficient finances

Sexual harassment

DEFINING CHARACTERISTICS

Expression of dissatisfaction over being unable to control situation

Verbalization of feelings of giving up

Refusal or reluctance to participate in decision making when opportunities are provided

Apparent lack of motivation to learn

Diminished patient-initiated interaction

Anxiety

Uneasiness

Submissiveness; apathy

Withdrawal; depression

Expression of undifferentiated anger

Aggressive and/or violent behavior

Display of acting-out behavior

Feeling of hopelessness and resignation described

Possible withholding of information about self

Decreased participation in activities of daily living (i.e., personal hygiene, refusal of food or fluids, indifference to treatments)

- Assess patient's decision-making ability.
- Assess impact of illness and hospitalization on patient's sense of control.
- Assess patient's ability to set realistic goals.
- Assess patient's desires/abilities to be an active participant in self-care.

THERAPEUTIC INTERVENTIONS

- Provide physical care the patient is unable to provide for self in a manner that communicates warmth, respect, acceptance of the patient's abilities.
- Implement individualized strategies to resolve difficulties with hygiene, diet, sleep.
- Provide appropriate information to patient about illness, treatment plan, and procedures.
- Provide patient with opportunities for expressing feelings of anger, anxiety, powerlessness.
- Acknowledge patient's knowledge of self and personal situation.
- Enhance patient's power resources by fostering patient involvement in decision making, by giving information, and by enabling the patient to control environment as appropriate.
- Avoid using coercive power when approaching the patient *as this may intensify patient's feelings of powerlessness and result in decreased self-esteem.*
- Acknowledge the nurse's ability for "expert" and "reward" power; *these types of power in patient/nurse interaction may enable the patient to mobilize own power resources.*
- Assist patient with setting and achieving goals.
- Point out patient's accomplishments to foster hope.

Originated by: Judith Popovich, RN, MS, CCRN

Self-care deficit

(ACTIVITIES OF DAILY LIVING [ADLs])

State in which a person experiences difficulty in performing tasks of daily living, such as feeding self, dressing, bathing, toileting, transferring from bed, walking

RELATED FACTORS / DEFINING CHARACTERISTICS	NURSING INTERVENTIONS / *RATIONALES*	EXPECTED OUTCOMES

RELATED FACTORS
 	
Neuromuscular impairment, secondary to CVA, rheumatoid arthritis
Musculoskeletal disorder
Cognitive impairment
 	
DEFINING CHARACTERISTICS
 	
Inability to feed self independently
Inability to dress self independently
Inability to bathe and groom self independently
Inability to perform toileting tasks independently
Inability to transfer from bed to wheelchair
Inability to ambulate independently
Inability to perform miscellaneous common tasks:
  Telephoning
  Writing
	ONGOING ASSESSMENT
	
	• Assess ability to carry out ADLs (feed, dress, bathe, toilet, transfer, ambulate) on regular basis.
	• Assess specific cause of each deficit (e.g., weakness, visual problems, cognitive impairment). *Different etiologies may require more specific interventions.*
	• Assess patient's need for assistive devices to increase independence in ADL performance.
	• Assess for need of home health care after discharge.
	
	THERAPEUTIC INTERVENTIONS
	
	• Set short-range goals with patient *to facilitate learning and decrease frustration.*
	Feeding:
	• Encourage patient to feed self as soon as possible (using unaffected hand, if appropriate). Assist with setup as needed.
	• Ensure that patient wears dentures and eyeglasses if needed and available
	• Assure that consistency of diet is appropriate for patient's level of chewing and swallowing, as assessed by speech therapist.
	• Provide patient with appropriate utensils (straw, food guard, rocking knife) to aid in self-feeding.
	• Place patient in optimal position for feeding, preferably sitting up in chair.
	• Consider appropriate setting for feeding task where patient has supportive assistance yet is not embarrassed.
	• If patient has visual problems, carefully assess placement of food on plate.
	Dressing/Grooming:
	• Encourage use of clothing one size larger *to assure easier dressing and comfort.*
	• Suggest brassiere that opens in front and half slips *which may be easier to manage.*
	• Suggest elastic shoelaces *to eliminate tying.*
	• Place patient in wheelchair or stationary chair *to assist with support when dressing. Dressing can be very fatiguing.*
	• Provide frequent encouragement and assistance as needed with dressing *to reduce energy expenditure and frustration.*
	• Provide appropriate assistive devices for dressing as assessed by nurse and occupational therapist.
	• Provide privacy during dressing.
	• Plan daily activities so patient is rested prior to activity.
	Bathing/Hygiene:
	• Encourage patient to perform minimum of oral-facial hygiene as soon as possible.
	• Provide patient with appropriate assistive devices (long-handled bath sponge *to aid in bed bathing;* shower chair; safety mats for floor; grab bars for bath/shower).
	• Maintain privacy during bathing as appropriate.
	• Ensure that needed utensils are close by *to conserve energy and optimize safety.*
	• Encourage patient to comb own hair (a one-handed task).
	• Instruct patient to select bath time when rested and unhurried.
	• Offer frequent encouragement. *Patients often have difficulty seeing progress.*
	• Document increased independence in bathing.
		Optimal level of independence in self-care tasks is achieved in safe manner.

RELATED FACTORS / DEFINING CHARACTERISTICS	NURSING INTERVENTIONS / *RATIONALES*	EXPECTED OUTCOMES

Toileting:
- Evaluate/document previous and current patterns for toileting.
- Offer bedpan or place patient on toilet every 1 to 1½ hours during day and 3 times during night *to eliminate incontinence. Time intervals can be lengthened as patient begins to indicate needs to void and have bowel movements.*
- Encourage use of commode/toilet as soon as possible.
- Keep call light within reach and instruct patient to call as early as possible *so staff have time to assist with transfer to commode/toilet.*
- Provide privacy while patient is toileting.
- Keep toilet paper within easy reach but closely monitor patient for loss of balance/fall.

Transferring/Ambulation:
- Plan teaching session for transferring/walking when patient is rested.
  Tasks require energy. Fatigued patients may have more difficulty, become unnecessarily frustrated.
- Assist with bed mobility:
  Encourage to utilize strong side (if appropriate) as best as possible.
  Allow patient to work at own rate of speed.
  When patient is sitting up at side of bed, instruct him/her not to pull on staff.
- When transferring to w/c, always place chair on patient's strong side at slight angle to bed and lock brakes.
- When minimal assistance is needed, stand on patient's weak side, place nurse's hand under patient's weak arm. (Nurse: Keep your feet well apart; lift with legs, not back, to prevent back strain).
- For moderate assistance, place nurse's arms under both armpits with nurse's hands on patient's back. (This forces patient to keep weight forward).
- For maximum assistance, place right knee against patient's strong knee, grasp patient around waist with both arms, and pull him forward; encourage patient to put weight on strong side.
- Assist with ambulation (if appropriate).
  Stand on patient's weak side to assist with balance and support.
  If using cane, place cane in patient's strong hand and assure proper foot-cane sequence.
  See also Mobility, impaired physical p. 35.

Common miscellaneous skills:
- *Telephone:* Evaluate need for adaptive equipment through therapy department (pushbutton phone, larger numbers, increased volume).
- *Writing:* Encourage family to supply patient with felt-tip pens. They mark with little pressure and are easier to use). Evaluate need for splint on writing hand *to assist with holding.*

- Provide supervision for each activity until patient is no longer at risk.
- Encourage maximum independence.
- Institute care plans for related problems as appropriate: Self-concept disturbance p. 46; Activity intolerance, p. 2; Mobility, impaired physical, p. 35.

PATIENT EDUCATION
- Plan teaching sessions so patient has time to practice tasks.
- Instruct patient in use of assistive devices as appropriate.

Originated by: Margaret Gleason, RN, BSN

Self-concept disturbance

(PERSONAL IDENTITY DISTURBANCE;
SELF-ESTEEM DISTURBANCE)

Mild to marked alteration in an individual's view of himself or herself. One's self-concept is affected by (and may also affect) ability to function in the larger world and relate to others within it.

RELATED FACTORS / DEFINING CHARACTERISTICS	NURSING INTERVENTIONS / *RATIONALES*	EXPECTED OUTCOMES

RELATED FACTORS
Bodily injury
Actual or anticipated loss
Change in relationships with others
Change in social roles (e.g., hospitalization, assumption of the "sick role")
 	
DEFINING CHARACTERISTICS
Report by patient/ significant other(s) of change in self-concept
Change in affect and/ or appearance (sadness, anger, irritability, decreased attention to grooming)
Change in behavior (e.g., severe or prolonged denial, refusal to participate in care or treatment withdrawal, decrease in functioning, disproportionate sense of capability)
Change in cognitive/ intellectual functioning (impaired judgment/thinking, inability to make decisions, poor reality testing)
	ONGOING ASSESSMENT
	· Document past level of functioning:
	   Emotional
	   Social
	   Interpersonal
	   Intellectual
	   Vocational
	   Physical
	· Note quality/quantity of verbalizations regarding self.
	· Note report by patient/significant others of changes in self-concept.
	· Assess for evidence of change in behavior (see Defining Characteristics).
	
	THERAPEUTIC INTERVENTIONS
	· Provide environment conducive to expression of feelings:
	   Make frequent contact in unhurried manner.
	   Avoid excessive focus on physical tasks.
	   Listen in supportive manner.
	   Provide privacy.
	   Allow patient to personalize environment with own belongings and/or familiar persons as appropriate.
	· Convey sense of respect for abilities/strengths in addition to recognizing problems/concerns. *Assistance with problem solving and reality testing is best provided within the context of a trusting relationship.*
	· Serve as role model for patient/significant others in healthy expression of feelings/concerns.
	· Discuss "normal" impact of alteration in health status (temporary or permanent) on self-concept.
	· Reassure patient that such changes frequently result in a variety of emotional/behavioral responses.
	· Advise of realistic need for additional support in coping with change and stress.
	· Provide anticipatory guidance to minimize anxiety and fear of the unknown:
	   Explain routines and procedures in plan of treatment.
	   Orient patient/significant others to environment.
	   Use language and terminology patient/significant others can understand.
	   Provide opportunities for questions and verbalization of feelings.
	   Include patient/significant others in planning care whenever possible.
	   Observe response to information, caretakers, and environment. *Anxiety (if excessive) may interfere with ability to function and test reality.*
	· Assist in efforts to obtain understanding and mastery of new experiences:
	   Support efforts to maintain independence, reality, positive self-image, sense of capability, problem solving.
	   Provide realistic appraisal of progress.
	   Reinforce efforts at constructive change.
	   Recognize variations in manner and pace at which each individual attempts to adjust to illness.
	   Encourage involvement in varied activities and interaction with others.
	   Use referral sources (other professional or lay persons) as appropriate to support coping efforts.
	
	PATIENT EDUCATION
	· Teach patient the importance of an intact self-concept as it relates to physical and emotional well-being.
	· Teach patient to seek and/or plan activities likely to result in a healthy self-concept.
		Self-concept will be fostered and maximized.

Originated by: Ann Filipski, RN, MSN, CS, PsyD Candidate
               Susan R. Laub, RN, MEd, CS

Sexuality patterns, altered

(IMPOTENCE; INTIMACY)

The patient or significant other expresses concern regarding the patient's manner of expressing physical intimacy. Alteration in human sexual response may be related to physiologic, emotional, cognitive, and sociocultural factors (or some combination thereof).

RELATED FACTORS / DEFINING CHARACTERISTICS	NURSING INTERVENTIONS / *RATIONALES*	EXPECTED OUTCOMES

RELATED FACTORS

Physical limitation (chronic or time-limited), e.g., pain, surgery, trauma, acute illness, pregnancy, delivery, exercise intolerance, drug side effects, or decreased mobility or ROM

Fear, e.g., fear of pregnancy, AIDS, or other STDs

Knowledge deficit, e.g., birth control methods, "safe" sex

Altered self-concept, e.g., loss of significant other, social isolation, or incomplete socialization to sexual orientation

Emotional disorders, e.g., psychosis, depression

Situational factors (unavailability of partner, cultural taboo, lack of appropriate environment, etc.)

Past traumatic experience, e.g., rape

DEFINING CHARACTERISTICS

Verbalization of concern(s) regarding sexual functions

Questions regarding "normal" sexual function

Noncompliance with medications/treatments with known risk of impaired sexual function

Expressed decrease in sexual satisfaction

Reported change in relationship with partner(s)

ONGOING ASSESSMENT

- Assess patient's/couple's understanding of sexuality and physiology.
- Assess/explore patient's/couple's past sexual practices/attitudes and degree of satisfaction.
- Identify potential/actual difficulty as to:
  Nature
  Course
  Onset
  Duration
- Identify possible/actual causative factors or contributing situational variables (see Related Factors).
- Assess patient's and significant other's social skills and degree of comfort with sexual matters.

THERAPEUTIC INTERVENTIONS

- Use a relaxed, comfortable manner.
- Respect the sovereignty of the patient's body and define each patient in part as a sexual being.
- Provide atmosphere of acceptance and privacy when discussing sexuality. *Conveying a sense of "normalcy" regarding sexuality indicates acceptance of the holistic nature of human beings and helps decrease anxiety.*
- Encourage patient to share concerns/information with partner(s) or involve in sexual health counseling.
- Offer opportunities to ask questions and/or verbalize concerns.
- Discuss both physiologic and emotional influences on sexual functioning.
- Explore patient's/couple's awareness of and comfort with means of sexual satisfaction besides intercourse. *The highly complex and interactive nature of sexual functioning requires systemic assessment and intervention.*
- If environmental problem, provide appropriate degree of privacy. *In hospital and residential care facility, privacy allows expression of patient's physical intimacy.*
- Consider referral for further workup/treatment:
  Primary physician
  Specialized physician
  Psychiatric consultant
  Sexual dysfunction clinic
  Drug or alcohol rehabilitation program
  Clinical nurse specialist (ostomy, cardiac rehabilitation)
  Physical therapist
  Exercise conditioning program
- Consider referral to such self-help support groups as:
  Sexual Impotence Resolved
  Reach for Recovery
  United Ostomy Association
  Mended Hearts
  Huff & Puff
  HIV-Positive Support Group
  Rape Survivor Group
  Gay coming out groups
  Single/widowed/seniors group
  Self-help support groups are unique sources of empathy, information, and successful role models.

Optimal means of satisfying sexual needs will be achieved.

Continued.

RELATED FACTORS / DEFINING CHARACTERISTICS	NURSING INTERVENTIONS / *RATIONALES*	EXPECTED OUTCOMES
Actual/perceived limitation secondary to diagnosis or therapy Sexually inappropriate behavior within setting Frequent seeking of confirmation of sexual desirability	**PATIENT EDUCATION** • Provide health teaching regarding "normal" range of sexual functioning and practices through life cycle. • Explain birth control methods. • Explain methods of "safe sex" (use of condoms and other techniques that prevent the exchange of semen, vaginal secretions, or blood). • Explain, role model, and reward appropriate social skills. • If necessary, instruct the patient on how long after surgery, delivery, trauma, or MI to avoid sexual intercourse or orgasm. • Teach alternative positions for sexual intercourse that decrease effort or discomfort. • Explain forms of sexual expression other than intercourse, i.e., fellation, cunnilingus, or digital stimulation. • Teach and encourage other ways of expressing intimacy, including touching and speaking. • Explain the effects on sexual functioning of the patient's medication, disease process, surgery, or trauma.	

Revised by: Ann Filipski, RN, MSN, CS, PsyD Candidate
Jeff Zurlinden, RN, MS

Skin integrity, impaired (actual/potential)

A state in which an individual's skin is, or may become, adversely altered.

(PRESSURE SORES; BED SORES; DECUBITUS CARE)

RELATED FACTORS / DEFINING CHARACTERISTICS	NURSING INTERVENTIONS / *RATIONALES*	EXPECTED OUTCOMES

RELATED FACTORS
Mechanical forces (pressure, shear, friction)
Pronounced bony prominences
Extremes of age
Poor nutrition
Immobility
Incontinence
Environmental moisture
Altered cutaneous sensation
 	
DEFINING CHARACTERISTICS
No impairment:
Epidermis intact
No discoloration
Capillary refill <4 sec
Stage I:
Redness
Pallor
	ONGOING ASSESSMENT
	• Assess for presence of related factors.
	• Observe general condition of skin.
	• Specifically check intactness of skin over bony prominences, noting color, temperature.
	• Assess patient's ability to be involved in own care/movement.
	• Reassess whenever patient's condition or treatment plan results in an increased number of related factors. *The incidence of breakdown is directly related to the number of risk factors present.*
	• Stage any existing pressure sore(s), using defining characteristics.
	• Assess need for débridement. *Débridement must be accomplished to stage pressure sores accurately.*
	
	THERAPEUTIC INTERVENTION
	• Document findings of assessment.
	• If patient is restricted to bed:
	   Implement and post a turning schedule, restricting time in one position to 2 hr or less and customizing the schedule to patient's routine and to nursing care needs. *A schedule that does not interfere with the patient's and nurses' activities is likely to be followed.*
	• Implement pressure-relieving devices commensurate with degree of risk for skin impairment:
	   For low-risk patients: good-quality (dense, at least 3 inches thick) foam mattress overlay.
		Skin will remain intact *or* evidence of granulation will be present.

RELATED FACTORS / DEFINING CHARACTERISTICS	NURSING INTERVENTIONS / *RATIONALES*	EXPECTED OUTCOMES
Poor capillary refill or redness that persists after pressure is removed	For moderate risk patients: water mattress, static or dynamic air mattress For high-risk patients or those with existing Stage III or IV pressure sores (or with Stage II pressure sores *and* multiple risk factors): low-air-loss beds (Mediscus, Flexicare, Kinair) or air-fluidized ther-apy (Clinitron, Skytron). *Low-air-loss beds are constructed to allow ele-vated head of bed (HOB) and patient transfer. These should be used when pulmonary concerns necessitate elevating HOB or when getting patient up is feasible. Air-fluidized therapy supports patient's weight at well below capillary closing pressure but restricts getting patient out of bed.*	

Stage II:
Blisters (either intact or broken)
Painful, moist, super-ficial area, usually round or linear, with interrupted epidermis
	· Maintain functional body alignment.
	· Limit chair sitting to 2 hr at any one time.
	· Encourage ambulation if patient is able.
	· Increase tissue perfusion by massaging *around* affected area. *Massaging reddened area may damage skin further.*
	· Clean, dry, and moisturize skin, especially over bony prominences, b.i.d., or as indicated by incontinence or sweating. If powder is desirable *to re-duce friction,* use medical-grade cornstarch; avoid talc.
	· Encourage adequate nutrition and hydration:
	  2000-3000 calories/day (more if increased metabolic demands)
	  Fluid intake of 2000 ml/day unless medically restricted
	  Dietitian consultation as appropriate
	· Use lift sheets to move patient in bed and discourage patient from elevating HOB. *These measures reduce shearing forces on the skin.*
	· Leave blisters intact by wrapping in gauze or applying a hydrocolloid (Duoderm, Sween-Appeal), or a vaporpermeable membrane dressing (Op-Site, Tegaderm). *Blisters are sterile natural dressings.*
	· Consider options for débridement if eschar is present:
	  Wet-to-dry dressings
	  Collagenase ointments as ordered
	  Assistance with sharp surgical débridement if done at the bedside
	  Arrangement for whirlpool as indicated
	· *Promote granulation and epithelization* through use of principles of moist wound healing:
	  Wet-to-dry dressings
	  Hydrocolloid dressings
	  Vapor-permeable membrane dressings	

Stage III: Open lesion involving dermis and subcuta-neous tissue May have adherent necrotic material Drainage usually present		
Stage IV: Open lesion involving muscle, bone, joint, and/or body cavity Usually has adherent necrotic material Drainage usually present		
	PATIENT EDUCATION · Teach patient and family the cause(s) of pressure sore development. · Reinforce the importance of mobility/turning/ambulation in prevention and management of pressure sores. · Teach patient/family about need for increased calories and protein when pressure sores are present. · Teach patient/family proper use and maintenance of pressure-relieving de-vices to be used at home.	

Originated by: Audrey Klopp, RN, PhD, ET
              Virginia M. Storey, RN, ET
              Kathryn S. Bronstein, RN, PhD, CS

Sleep pattern disturbance

(INSOMNIA)

A disruption in the individual's usual diurnal pattern of sleep and wakefulness that may be temporary or chronic. Such disruptions may result in both subjective distress and apparent impairment in functional abilities.

RELATED FACTORS / DEFINING CHARACTERISTICS	NURSING INTERVENTIONS / *RATIONALES*	EXPECTED OUTCOMES

RELATED FACTORS
 	
Pain/discomfort
Environmental changes
Anxiety/fear
Depression
Medications
Excessive/inadequate stimulation
Abnormal physiologic status/symptoms (dyspnea, hypoxia, neurologic dysfunction, etc.)
Normal changes associated with aging
 	
DEFINING CHARACTERISTICS
 	
Patient/significant other report of alteration in "normal" sleep pattern
Difficulty in falling or remaining asleep
Complaints of not feeling rested
Early morning awakening
Restlessness
Lethargy/fatigue
Insomnia
Irritability
Dozing
Yawning
Altered mental status
Difficulty in arousal
Change in activity level
Altered facial expression (e.g., blank look, fatigued appearance)
Reddened eyes
	ONGOING ASSESSMENT
	
	• Assess past patterns of sleep in normal environment: amount, bedtime rituals, depth, length, positions, aids, and interfering agents. *Sleep patterns are unique to each individual.*
	• Assess patient's perception of cause of sleep difficulty and possible relief measures *to facilitate treatment.*
	• Document nursing observations of sleeping and wakeful behaviors
	• Identify factors that may facilitate or interfere with "normal patterns." *Considerable confusion and mythology about sleep exist. Knowledge of its role in health/wellness and the wide variation among individuals may allay anxiety, thereby promoting rest and sleep.*
	• Evaluate timing/effects of medications that disrupt sleep.
	
	THERAPEUTIC INTERVENTIONS
	
	• Maintain environment conducive to sleep/rest (e.g., quiet, comfortable temperature, ventilation, closed door).
	• Assist patient in observing any previous bedtime ritual *to promote relaxation.*
	• Provide nursing aids *to promote rest, relaxation* (e.g. back rub, bedtime care, pain relief, comfortable position, relaxation techniques).
	• Organize nursing care *to promote minimal interruption in sleep/rest.*
	  Eliminate nonessential nursing activities.
	  Prepare patient for necessary anticipated interruptions/disruptions.
	• Establish semblance of "normal" daily routine with periods of activity, rest. *Adherence to previously established patterns/routines minimizes energy required for adaptation and disruption in biologic rhythms.*
	• Provide soporifics (e.g., milk, avoidance of stimulants such as caffeine or cola beverages, and decreased exercise several hours before sleep) as needed.
	• Administer hypnotics as ordered and evaluate effectiveness. *Use of hypnotic medications should be thoughtful and avoided if less aggressive means are effective because of their potential for cumulative efforts and generally limited period of benefit.*
	• Discourage pattern of daytime naps unless deemed necessary or part of usual pattern. *Napping can disrupt normal sleep pattern.*
	• Increase daytime physical activities as indicated *to reduce stress and promote sleep.*
	• Limit fluids before bedtime *to reduce need for voiding during night.*
	
	PATIENT EDUCATION
	
	• Teach patient possible causes of sleeping difficulties and optimal ways to treat them.
		Optimal amounts of sleep will be achieved.

Originated by: Ann Filipski, RN, MSN, CS, PsyD Candidate
Janice Borman, RN, MSN, PhD Candidate
Marilyn Magafas, RN,C, BSN, MBA

Spiritual distress

An experience of profound disharmony in the client's belief or value system that threatens the meaning of the client's life. During spiritual distress the client loses hope, questions his belief system, or feels separated from his personal source of comfort and strength.

RELATED FACTORS / DEFINING CHARACTERISTICS	NURSING INTERVENTIONS / *RATIONALES*	EXPECTED OUTCOMES

RELATED FACTORS

Pain
Divorce
Loneliness
Abortion
Hospitalization
Surgery
Terminal illness
Chronic or debilitating illness
Separation from religious ties
Separation from loved ones
Loss or illness of a loved one
Birth of an unwanted, ill, or defective infant

DEFINING CHARACTERISTICS

Voices guilt, loss of hope, spiritual emptiness, feeling of being alone
Questions belief system
Appears anxious, depressed, discouraged, fearful, or angry

ONGOING ASSESSMENT

- Assess history of formal religious affiliation by asking:
  "What is your religion?"
  "What religious rituals or practices are important to you?"
  "What prayers or scriptures are important and helpful to you?"
  "What religious objects are important to you?"
  "Would talking with a clergy member help you?"
- Assess other significant beliefs by asking:
  "What beliefs are important to you?"
  "What gives you strength and inspiration?"
- Assess spiritual meaning of illness or treatment by asking:
  "What is the meaning of your illness?"
  "How does your illness or treatment affect your relationship with God, your beliefs, or other sources of strength?"
  "Does your illness or treatment interfere with expressing your spiritual beliefs?"
- Assess hope by asking:
  "At this time, what do you hope for?"
  "When you need hope, what helps you most?"
  "When you feel afraid or overwhelmed, what helps you most?"
- Assess unfinished business by asking:
  "Do you have unfinished business?"
  "What will bring you peace or harmony?"

THERAPEUTIC INTERVENTIONS

- Display an understanding and accepting attitude.
- Structure your interventions in terms of the patient's belief system. *The patients have a right to their beliefs, even if they conflict with the nurse's beliefs.*
- Develop an ongoing relationship with the patient.
- When requested by the patient or family, arrange for clergy or religious rituals.
- If requested, pray with the patient.
- Acknowledge and support the patient's hopes. *Hopes are different from denial or delusions. Supporting a hope for discharge does not mean supporting a denial of the seriousness of the patient's condition. Hope allows the patient to face the seriousness of the situation.*
- Do not provide logical solutions for spiritual dilemmas. *Spiritual beliefs are based on faith and are independent of logic.*
- See Hopelessness p. 29.

PATIENT EDUCATION

- Provide information in a way that does not interfere with the patient's beliefs, faith, or hopes.
- Inform the patient of how to obtain religious rites or seek spiritual guidance.

Patient expresses hope and values own belief system.

Originated by: Jeff Zurlinden, RN, MS

Thought processes, altered

(CONFUSION; DISORIENTATION; INAPPROPRIATE SOCIAL BEHAVIOR; ALTERED MOOD STATES; DELUSIONS; IMPAIRED COGNITIVE PROCESSES)

A condition in which an individual experiences a disruption in cognitive processes, defined as those mental processes by which knowledge is acquired. These mental processes include reality orientation, comprehension, awareness, and judgment. A disruption in these mental processes may lead to inaccurate interpretations of the environment and may also result in an inability to differentiate one's thoughts and feelings from the actualities and realities of the outside world (i.e., inability to evaluate reality accurately.) This diagnosis refers to those cognitive disruptions caused by thought and personality disorders.

RELATED FACTORS / DEFINING CHARACTERISTICS	NURSING INTERVENTIONS / *RATIONALES*	EXPECTED OUTCOMES

RELATED FACTORS

Organic mental disorders (non-substance-induced):
Dementia
Primary degenerative, e.g., Alzheimer disease, Pick disease
Multi-infarct, e.g., cerebral arteriosclerosis
Those organic mental disorders associated with other physical disorders
  Huntington chorea
  Multiple sclerosis
  Parkinson disease
  Cerebral hypoxia
  Hypertension
  Hepatic disease
  Epilepsy
Adrenal, thyroid, or parathyroid disorders
Head trauma
CNS infections (encephalitis, syphilis, meningitis)
Fear
Intracranial lesions (benign or malignant)
Sleep deprivation

Organic mental disorders (substance-induced):
Organic mental disorders attributed to the ingestion of alcohol (alcohol withdrawal, dementia associated with alcoholism)

For disorientation:

ONGOING ASSESSMENT

- Assess patient's degree of orientation to time, place, person, and situation regularly and frequently. *This will determine the amount of orientation the patient will need for his perception of reality and surroundings.*

THERAPEUTIC INTERVENTIONS

- Orient patient to surroundings and reality as needed.
  Use patient's name when speaking to him.
  Speak slowly and clearly. Present information in a matter-of-fact manner *to decrease chances for misinterpretation.*
  Refer to the time of day, date, and recent events in your interactions with the patient. Encourage patient to check calendar and clock frequently.
  Encourage patient to have familiar personal belongings in his environment.
  Be matter-of-fact and respectful when correcting patient's misperceptions of reality.
- Utilize words *you* and *I,* instead of *we,* to increase orientation and to encourage patient to maintain his sense of individuality. *Orientation to one's environment increases one's ability to trust others. Increased orientation assures a greater degree of safety for the patient. It also encourages the patient's cooperation in any necessary treatments or tests. Familiar personal possessions increase the patient's comfort level.*

For altered behavior patterns:

ONGOING ASSESSMENT

- Assess patient's behavior and social interactions for appropriateness regularly.
- Evaluate patient's ability and willingness to respond to verbal direction and limits regularly.
- Evaluate the potential for self-inflicted harm (intentional and nonintentional) regularly.
- Evaluate the potential for harm to others or damage to property (intentional and nonintentional) regularly. *Confusion, disorientation, impaired judgment, suspiciousness, and loss of social inhibitions all may result in socially inappropriate and/or harmful behavior to self or others. Patient's ability and/or willingness to respond to verbal direction and/or limits may vary with patient's mood, perceptions, degree of reality orientation, and environmental stressors.*
- Observe for statements reflecting a desire or fantasy to inflict harm on self or others.

THERAPEUTIC INTERVENTIONS

- Maintain routine interactions, activities, and close observation without increasing patient's suspiciousness. *Patients with impaired judgment and loss of social inhibitions require close observation to discourage inappropriate behavior and prevent harm or injury to self and others.*
- Develop an open and honest relationship in which expectations are respectfully and clearly verbalized. Make only those promises that can be kept.

Disorientation to time, place, person, and situation will be minimized, and the patient's ability to behave and interact with others in an appropriate manner will increase.

Socially appropriate behavior will increase.

RELATED FACTORS / DEFINING CHARACTERISTICS	NURSING INTERVENTIONS / *RATIONALES*	EXPECTED OUTCOMES
Organic mental disorders attributed to the ingestion of drugs/mood-altering substances (barbiturates), opoid substances, cocaine, amphetamines, phencyclidine, substances with hallucinogenic properties, substances with properties of cannabis plant) Organic mental disorders (substance-dependent) (A more severe form of the induced organic mental disorders in which there is evidence of physiologic dependence, involving tolerance and/or withdrawal): Schizophrenic disorders Thought disorder *not* due to an organic mental disorder Disorganized type Catatonic type Paranoid type Undifferentiated type Residual type Personality disorders in which there is evidence of altered thought processes Affective disorders in which there is evidence of actual thought processes	Verbalize acceptance of the patient despite the inappropriateness of his behavior. *Honesty, openness, and verbalized acceptance of the patient increase his self-respect and esteem. Keeping promises establishes a sense of trust and reliability between the patient and staff.* • Provide role modeling for the patient through appropriate social and professional interactions with other patients and staff. *Role modeling provides the patient an opportunity to observe socially appropriate behavior.* • Encourage patient to assume responsibility for his behavior; verbalize to patient staff's willingness to assist him in maintaining appropriate behavior when patient appears to need structure. *Encouraging patient to assume responsibility for own behavior will increase his sense of independence. Staff intervention will provide a feeling of security and reassurance.* • Provide situations for the patient in which group interactions with other patients allow him to obtain feedback regarding his behavior. *It is important for the patient to learn socially appropriate behavior through group interactions. This provides an opportunity for the patient to observe the impact his behavior has on those around him. It also facilitates the development of acceptable social skills.* • Provide positive reinforcement for efforts and appropriate behavior; confront patient when behavior is inappropriate and withdraw attention. *Attention drawn to the patient's inappropriate behavior may reinforce it.*	
DEFINING CHARACTERISTICS Disorientation to one or more of the following: time, person, place, situation Altered behavioral patterns (regression, inappropriate social behavior) Altered mood states (lability, hostility, irritability, inappropriate affect)	**For altered mood states:** ONGOING ASSESSMENT • Assess patient's mood and affect regularly. Affect *is defined as an emotion that is immediately expressed and observed. Affect is inappropriate when it is not in conjunction with the content of the patient's speech and/or ideation. Lability is described as repeated, abrupt, and rapid changes in affect. Mood is described as a pervasive and sustained emotion. Frequent and regular assessment of a patient's mood and affect will assist in determining the predominance of a particular affect or mood and any deviations. This assessment will also determine the presence of any lability or hostility.* • Assess for environmental and situational factors that may contribute to the patient's change in mood or affect. *It is important to remember that patients with thought disorders may also experience fluctuations in mood and affect based on external stimuli, including environmental and situational factors.* THERAPEUTIC INTERVENTIONS • Document observations of the patient's mood and affect regularly. *Documentation will provide a reliable data base.* • Demonstrate acceptance of the patient as an individual. *It is important to communicate to the patient one's acceptance of him regardless of his behavior.* • Demonstrate tolerance of the patient's fluctuations in affect and mood. Address inappropriate affect and mood in a calm, yet firm, manner. *Calmness communicates self-control and tolerance of the patient and his affect and mood. Addressing and setting limits for inappropriate behavior communicate clear expectations for the patient.* • Identify environmental stimuli that cause increased restlessness or agitation for the patient. Remove the patient when possible from external stimuli that appear to exacerbate irritable and hostile behavior. *The patient's ability to recognize irritating stimuli and remove himself from the source may be impaired. Removing the patient from external stimuli that exacerbate fluctuations in mood and affect encourage a sense of protection and security for the patient.* • Encourage the patient's involvement in group activities as tolerated. *Involvement in group activities is determined by various factors, including the group size, activity level, and patient's tolerance level. Remain aware that the patient's fluctuations in mood and affect will affect his ability to respond appropriately to others and his capacity to handle complex and multiple stimuli.*	The frequency and intensity of mood swings will be reduced.

Continued.

RELATED FACTORS / DEFINING CHARACTERISTICS	NURSING INTERVENTIONS / *RATIONALES*	EXPECTED OUTCOMES

Impaired ability to perform self-maintenance activities, i.e., grooming, hygiene, food and fluid intake
Altered sleep patterns
Altered perceptions of surrounding stimuli caused by impairment in the following cognitive processes:
  Memory
  Judgment
  Comprehension
  Concentration
  Ability to reason problem solve, calculate, and conceptualize
	For impaired ability to perform ADLs:
	
	ONGOING ASSESSMENT
	
	• Assess the patient's ability to initiate, perform and maintain self-care activities regularly.
	• Assess the patient's motivation to initiate, perform, and maintain self-care activities regularly. *Assessment of motivation to initiate, perform, and maintain self-care activities will identify areas of physical care in which the patient needs assistance. These areas of physical care include nutrition, elimination, sleep and rest, exercise, bathing, grooming, and dressing. It is important to distinguish between ability and motivation in the initiation, performance, and maintenance of self-care activities. Patients may present with ability and minimal motivation or motivation and minimal ability.*
	• Obtain history from patient, family, and friends regarding patient's dietary habits. *Information about the patient's dietary habits is important in determining the presence of food allergies. It will also determine the patient's personal food preferences, cultural dietary restrictions, and ability to verbalize hunger.*
	• Obtain accurate weight on admission and maintain ongoing records through the patient's length of treatment. Weigh the patient on a scheduled basis (daily, twice weekly, for example). *Accurate records of the patient's body weight help determine significant fluctuations.*
	• Maintain adequate records of the patient's intake and output, elimination patterns, and any associated concerns verbalized by the patient. *The patient with impaired thought processes is unable to self-monitor intake, output, and elimination patterns.*
	• Monitor laboratory values and report any significant changes. *Laboratory data provide objective information regarding the patient's nutritional intake and metabolism.*
	• Obtain information from the patient's family regarding personal grooming and hygiene habits. *This information will assist in developing a specific plan of grooming and hygiene activities.*
	
	THERAPEUTIC INTERVENTIONS
	
	• Obtain dietary consultation and determine the number of calories the patient will require to maintain adequate nutritional intake based on body weight and structure. *The patient with an altered thought process is impaired in maintaining adequate nutritional intake independently.*
	• Encourage adequate fluid intake and physical exercise. *Both ongoing exercise and adequate fluid intake help prevent constipation.*
	• Assist the patient with bathing, grooming, and dressing as needed. *The patient with impaired thought processes is unable to self-monitor personal grooming and hygiene adequately.*
	• Provide the patient with positive reinforcement for his efforts in maintaining self-care activities. *Positive reinforcement is perceived by the patient as support.*
	
	For altered sleep:
	
	ONGOING ASSESSMENT
	
	• Assess which particular sleep pattern is altered. Establish whether the patient has difficulty falling asleep, awakens during the night, early in the morning, or is experiencing insomnia. It is important to determine an accurate baseline in order to effectively assist the patient with the disturbed sleep pattern.
	• Maintain accurate records of the patient's sleep patterns.
	
	THERAPEUTIC INTERVENTIONS
	
	• Decrease stimuli before patient goes to bed:
	  Suggest a warm bath.
		Initiation and performance of self-maintenance activities will improve.
		
		The patient will experience a decrease in sleep pattern disturbances. Sleep will be optimized.

RELATED FACTORS / DEFINING CHARACTERISTICS	NURSING INTERVENTIONS / *RATIONALES*	EXPECTED OUTCOMES

Turn down TV/radio.
Dim the lights.
Sleep and rest will be encouraged when loud stimuli are minimized.

- Decrease patient's intake of caffeinated substances (tea, colas, coffee). *Caffeine stimulates CNS and may interfere with patient's ability to rest and sleep.*
- Administer medication with sedative effects late in evening. *This will discourage sleeping during day and promote restful night sleep.*
- Discourage long periods of nurse/patient contact at night. *Brief and frequent contacts as needed are less disruptive and communicate the importance of night sleep.*
- If the patient is experiencing hypersomnia, discourage sleep during the day. Limit the time patient spends in his room and provide stimulating activities. *Structured expectations will provide a focus for activities, and contact will also provide opportunity to examine feelings the patient may be avoiding through excessive sleep.*

For altered perceptions of surrounding stimuli:

ONGOING ASSESSMENT

- Assess and observe the patient's ability to verbalize his needs and trust those around him.
- Assess the patient's memory (recent and remote).
- Assess and observe the patient's judgment and awareness of safety.
- Assess the patient's ability to concentrate, follow instructions, and problem solve on an ongoing basis.
- Assess the patient's communication patterns. *Observe for the presence of delusions and/or hallucinations. Delusions are false beliefs that have no basis in reality. They may be fixed (persistent) or transient (episodic).* Hallucinations *are perceptions of external stimuli without the actual presence of those stimuli in the external world. Hallucinations may be visual, auditory, olfactory, tactile, and gustatory and are perceived by the patient as real.*

THERAPEUTIC INTERVENTIONS

- Encourage the patient to communicate his thoughts and perceptions with significant others in his environment. *Validation of the patient's needs, thoughts, and perceptions will encourage trust and openness.*
- Clarify the patient's misperceptions of events and situations that may result from memory impairment. *Clarification is necessary and more easily accepted when offered in a respectful manner.*
- Orient the patient to time, place, person, and situation as needed. *The patient's ability to orient himself may be impaired by memory loss.*
- Minimize situations that provoke anxiety. *Anxiety may impair the patient's ability to communicate, problem solve, and reason.*
- Provide protective supervision for the patient. *The patient's safety is a priority. The patient may be unable to accurately assess potentially dangerous items and situations such as wet floors, electrical appliances, verbal threats from other patients as a result of severe impairment in judgment.*
- Observe for cues indicating the patient may be experiencing delusional thinking. Assist the patient in recognizing the delusions. Acknowledge the patient's delusions without agreeing to the content of the delusions. *Delusions can be anxiety-provoking and distressing for the patient. It is important to acknowledge this distress but to convey that one does not accept the delusions as real.*

The patient's perceptions of surrounding stimuli will become more reality-based.

Continued.

Thought processes, altered—cont'd

RELATED FACTORS / DEFINING CHARACTERISTICS	NURSING INTERVENTIONS / *RATIONALES*	EXPECTED OUTCOMES
	• Observe for cues indicating the patient may be experiencing hallucinations, such as inappropriate gestures, laughter, talking to oneself without the presence of others. Communicate verbally with the patient by using concrete and direct words and avoiding gesturing. Encourage the patient to inform staff when he is experiencing hallucinations. Determine whether the patient's hallucinations are resulting in thoughts and/or plans to harm himself or others. *Early detection of behavior reflecting active hallucinations will encourage early response to the patient's behavior. This will decrease the likelihood of agitated and unpredictable behavior. It is important to acknowledge the presence of the hallucinations without accepting them as real.*	

Originated by: Ursula Brozek, RN, MSN

Tissue perfusion, altered (peripheral)

(PERIPHERAL VASCULAR DISEASE; INTERMITTENT CLAUDICATION; ARTERIAL INSUFFICIENCY)

Reduced arterial blood flow to peripheral tissues causing decreased nutrition and oxygenation at cellular level. Management is directed at removing vasoconstricting factors, improving peripheral blood flow, and reducing metabolic demands on the body.

RELATED FACTORS / DEFINING CHARACTERISTICS	NURSING INTERVENTIONS / *RATIONALES*	EXPECTED OUTCOMES
RELATED FACTORS Reduced cardiac output Hypovolemia Arterial spasm Embolism/thrombus Vasoconstriction secondary to medications, tobacco, etc. Local or generalized hypothermia Atherosclerosis Circumferential burns Indwelling arterial catheters (e.g., intra-aortic balloon pump) Rotating tourniquets Constricting casts Malpositioning/immobility Compartment syndrome **DEFINING CHARACTERISTICS** Pain, cramping, ache in extremity Intermittent claudication (pain or weakness in one or both legs relieved by rest)	**ONGOING ASSESSMENT** • Assess extremities for color, temperature, and texture. • Assess extremities for swelling, edema, ulceration. • Assess quality of peripheral pulses, noting capillary refill and dependent changes. • If no pulses are noted, assess arterial blood flow using Doppler ultrasonic instrumentation (if available). • Assess pain/numbness/tingling as to causative factors, time of onset, quality, severity, relieving factors. • Assess for bilateral involvement of extremities. • Assess for possible causative factors related to temporary/chronic impaired arterial blood flow. **THERAPEUTIC INTERVENTIONS** *For acute changes:* • Evaluate causative factors, initiating corrective measures (e.g., reposition extremity, deflate tourniquets, proper use of cooling blanket) as appropriate. *Early detection of cause facilitates prompt, effective treatment.* • Notify physician of signs of decreased perfusion. • Administer analgesic as ordered. • Anticipate need for possible embolectomy, heparinization, vasodilator therapy, thrombolytic therapy. *For chronic condition:* • Elevate head of bed and maintain affected extremity in a dependent position *to increase peripheral blood flow.* • Keep extremity warm (socks/blankets) *to prevent vasoconstriction and promote comfort.* • Administer analgesics as ordered. • Bathe in warm bath water—never hot. *Heat increases tissue metabolism at already compromised site and can lead to further tissue impairment.* • Change position at least every hour. Suggest sleeping with legs down.	Optimal peripheral tissue perfusion will be maintained.

RELATED FACTORS / DEFINING CHARACTERISTICS	NURSING INTERVENTIONS / *RATIONALES*	EXPECTED OUTCOMES

Numbness of toes on walking, relieved by rest
Foot pain at rest
Tenderness, especially at toes
Cool extremities
Pallor of toes/foot when leg is elevated for 30 sec
Dependent rubor (20 sec to 2 min after leg is lowered)
Decreased capillary refill
Diminished or absent arterial pulses
Shiny skin
Loss of hair
Thickened, discolored nails
Ulcerated areas/ gangrene
Edema
Change in skin texture
	• Remove all vasoconstricting apparel/appliances, e.g., clothing, shoes, bandages.
	• Do not elevate bed at the knee gatch.
	• Assist with progressive activity program, noting claudication and signs of overexertion.
	• Evaluate coping responses (e.g., depression, body image, problem, fear) and initiate appropriate interventions and consultations as needed.
	• Provide prophylactic pressure-relieving devices as appropriate.
	• See Skin integrity, impaired, p. 48.
	
	PATIENT EDUCATION
	• Instruct patient on appropriate diagnostic tests: Doppler studies, arteriography.
	• Instruct patient on how to prevent progression of disease and complications.
	Effects of temperature:
	  Keep extremities warm. Wear stockings to bed.
	  Keep house/apartment as warm as possible.
	  Wear enough clothes during winter.
	  Never apply hot water bottles or electric pads to feet/legs. *Burns may occur secondary to impaired nerve function.*
	  Avoid local cold applications.
	Foot care *to prevent ulceration and infection:*
	  Wash feet daily with warm soap/water. Dry thoroughly by gentle patting. Never rub dry.
	  Trim toenails carefully and only after soaking in warm water. Trim straight across. See podiatrist as needed.
	  Lubricate skin to *prevent cracking*.
	  Wear clean stockings.
	  Do not walk barefoot.
	  Wear correctly fitting shoes.
	  Inspect feet frequently for signs of ingrown toenails, sores, blisters, etc.
	Exercise/activity:
	  Do not cross legs or keep pillows behind knees.
	  Do not sit for extended intervals.
	  Begin a daily exercise program *to promote collateral circulation*.
	  Walk on flat surface.
	  Walk about half a block after intermittent claudication is experienced, unless otherwise ordered by the physician.
	  Stop and rest until all discomfort subsides.
	  Repeat same procedure for total of 30 min, 2 to 3 times/day.
	Smoking:
	  Avoid all tobacco, *which further decreases an already compromised circulation. Nicotine is a vasoconstrictor.*
	  Consider referral to stop smoking clinics as needed.
	Diet:
	  If atherosclerotic problem exists, provide diet counseling on need for reduction in fats.
	  If overweight, provide diet counseling regarding attainment of ideal body weight.
	Medications:
	  Take prescribed medications (vasodilators, anticoagulants), observing for reaction and side effects.	

Originated by: Meg Gulanick, RN, PhD

Urinary elimination, altered patterns of (incontinence)

(STRESS INCONTINENCE; URGE INCONTINENCE; OVERFLOW INCONTINENCE; REFLEX INCONTINENCE; CONSTANT INCONTINENCE)

There are several types of urinary incontinence; all are characterized by the involuntary passage of urine. Urinary incontinence is not a disease but rather a symptom. Incontinence occurs more frequently among women, and incidence increases with age. An estimated 10 million people are incontinent. This care plan addresses five types: stress, urge, overflow, reflex, and constant.

RELATED FACTORS / DEFINING CHARACTERISTICS	NURSING INTERVENTIONS / *RATIONALES*	EXPECTED OUTCOMES

STRESS INCONTINENCE

RELATED FACTORS

Multiple vaginal deliveries
Pelvic surgery
Hypoestrogenism (aging, menopause)
Diabetic neuropathy
Trauma to pelvic area
Obesity
Radial prostatectomy
Myelomeningocele
Infection

DEFINING CHARACTERISTICS

Leakage of urine during exercise
Leakage of urine during coughing, sneezing, laughing, or lifting

ONGOING ASSESSMENT

- Ask whether urine is lost involuntarily during:
  Coughing
  Laughing
  Sneezing
  Lifting
  Exercising
- Examine perineal area for evidence of pelvic relaxation:
  Cystourethrocele
  Rectocele
  Uterine prolapse
- Determine parity.
- Explore menstrual history.
- Ask about previous surgical procedures.
- Weigh patient.
- Culture urine.

THERAPEUTIC INTERVENTIONS

- Teach patient to perform Kegel exercises *to strengthen the pelvic floor musculature.*
- Administer symphathomimetics and estrogens as ordered *to increase sphincter tone and improve muscle tone.*
- Teach patient to use transcutaneous electrical nerve stimulator as indicated *to improve pelvic floor tone.*
- Teach female patient use of vaginal pessary, *a device reserved for poor surgical candidates that works by elevating the bladder neck, thereby increasing urethral resistance.*
- Prepare patient for surgery as indicated. *Many types of procedures are used to control stress incontinence; the most commonly performed are Marshall-Marchetti, Burch's colposuspension, and sling procedures.*
- Prepare patient for the implantation of an artificial urinary sphincter, *which uses a subcutaneous pumping device to deflate/inflate a cuff that controls micturation.*
- Encourage weight loss if obese.

Urinary continence or management of incontinence will be achieved.

RELATED FACTORS / DEFINING CHARACTERISTICS	NURSING INTERVENTIONS / *RATIONALES*	EXPECTED OUTCOMES

URGE INCONTINENCE

RELATED FACTORS

Uninhibited bladder contraction
CVA
Spinal cord injury
Parkinsonism
Multiple sclerosis
Benign prostatic hypertrophy
Infections
Psychogenic

DEFINING CHARACTERISTICS

Sudden, "unannounced" need to void
Frequent urinary accidents associated with "not getting there in time"
Inability to delay voiding

ONGOING ASSESSMENT

- Ask to describe episodes of incontinence; note descriptions of "feeling the need suddenly but being unable to get to the bathroom in time".
- Consider age; *this type of urinary incontinence is the most frequent type among the elderly.*
- Culture urine.

THERAPEUTIC INTERVENTIONS

- Administer medications that reduce or block detrusor contractions (anticholinergics); *these inhibit smooth muscle contractions and may reduce episodes of incontinence.*
- Prepare patient for surgical correction (sphincterotomy) as indicated; denervation, resulting in complete incontinence, may be undertaken (rhizotomy). Urinary diversion (ileal conduit) may be performed as a last resort.
- Educate patient in the use of biofeedback techniques *for control of pelvic floor musculature.*
- Facilitate access to toilet.

Urinary continence or management of incontinence will be achieved.

OVERFLOW INCONTINENCE

RELATED FACTORS

Bladder outlet obstruction
Prostatic hypertrophy
Extensive pelvic surgery
Myelomeningocele
Trauma
Multiple sclerosis
Diabetes mellitus
Infrequent voiding patterns
Fecal impaction
Drugs that lead to urinary retention:
Anticholinergic
Antispasmodics
Tricyclic antidepressants
Seizure medications

DEFINING CHARACTERISTICS

Frequency
Urgency
Dribbling
Bladder distention

ONGOING ASSESSMENT

- Assess for presence/history of related factors.
- Assess for frequency, urgency, or dribbling.
- Palpate bladder to determine distention; *overflow incontinence occurs when the bladder is overfilled but the outlet is obstructed. Pressures force out small amounts of urine.*

THERAPEUTIC INTERVENTIONS

- *Relieve urinary retention by:*
  Intermittent catheterization
  Indwelling catheterization
- Prepare patient for surgery *aimed at definitive repair of outlet obstruction.*
- Assist in management of systemic medical diseases.
- Teach and encourage routine voiding.
- Remove fecal impaction and normalize bowel evacuation.
- Notify physician if ordered drugs are possible causes of this type of urinary incontinence; adjust dosage and/or schedule according to order.

Urinary continence or management of incontinence will be achieved.

Continued.

Nursing Diagnosis Care Plans

RELATED FACTORS / DEFINING CHARACTERISTICS	NURSING INTERVENTIONS / *RATIONALES*	EXPECTED OUTCOMES

REFLEX INCONTINENCE

RELATED FACTORS

Spinal cord injury
Stimulation of perineum in presence of spinal cord injury

DEFINING CHARACTERISTICS

Loss of urine without warning

ONGOING ASSESSMENT

- Ask whether he/she feels:
  Urgency
  Sensation of voiding
- Document history of spinal cord injury, including level.

THERAPEUTIC INTERVENTIONS

- Teach patient (or perform for patient) intermittent (self-) catheterization.
- Consider use of external catheter.
- Use indwelling catheter as last resort; *although risk of infection is considerable with both external and indwelling catheters, indwelling catheters interfere with clothing, movement, and sexual activity and may result in odor or other embarrassing sensory phenomena.*

Urinary continence or management of incontinence will be achieved.

CONSTANT (OR CONTINUAL) INCONTINENCE

RELATED FACTORS

Pelvic surgery
Fistulas:
  Iatrogenic
  Postoperative
  Postradiation
Trauma
Exstrophy of bladder

DEFINING CHARACTERISTICS

Continual involuntary loss of urine

ONGOING ASSESSMENT

- Assess pattern of urine loss.

THERAPEUTIC INTERVENTIONS

- Use diapers or external collection devices. *Most of these patients are women with fistulas; indwelling catheters are useless in the presence of vesicovaginal or urethrovaginal fistulae.*
- Prepare patient for surgical correction as indicated.

PATIENT EDUCATION (ALL TYPES OF INCONTINENCE)

- Teach patient:
  Normal anatomy of GU tract
  Factors that normally control micturation and maintain continence
- Assist patient in recognizing that any episode(s) of incontinence that poses a social or hygienic problem deserves investigation *so that appropriate therapy can be implemented.*
- Inform patient of the high incidence of urinary incontinence. *This information may decrease feelings of hopelessness and isolation that frequently accompany urinary incontinence.*
- Assist patients, through careful interview, to identify possible causes for urinary incontinence.
- Teach patients the necessity, purpose, and expected results of urodynamic diagnostic evaluation. *Urodynamic studies evaluate bladder filling and sphincter activity and are particularly useful in differentiating stress and urge incontinence.*
- Provide information regarding all available methods of managing urinary incontinence *so that patient can make an informed decision.* Methods include:
  Use of absorbent pads or undergarments that accommodate absorbent pads
  Diapers
  Linen protectors for bedridden patient
  External collection devices:
    Male external catheters
    Female external catheters
  Indwelling catheters
  Intermittent catheterization
  Surgical procedures
  Electrical nerve stimulators
  Pharmacotherapeutic agents. *Patients need information on drugs used to treat urinary incontinence as well as those used for other problems that may precipitate or worsen incontinence.*

Urinary continence or management of incontinence will be achieved.

Urinary elimination altered patterns of—cont'd

RELATED FACTORS / DEFINING CHARACTERISTICS	NURSING INTERVENTIONS / *RATIONALES*	EXPECTED OUTCOMES
	Drugs that may precipitate or worsen incontinence: diuretics, sedatives, hypnotics, anticholinergics, alcohol.	

Drugs that may be used to treat urinary incontinence: α-blockers *(increase bladder pressures and decrease outlet pressures)*, β-blockers *(increase outlet resistance)*, cholinergics *(increase bladder pressures)*, anticholinergics *(depresses smooth muscle activity in hypertonic bladder)*, and α-adrenergics *(increase sphincter tone)*.
- Provide information on odor control. *Vinegar and commercially prepared solutions are useful in neutralizing urinary odor.*
- Familiarize patient with potential risk of skin breakdown. *Urea contained in urine metabolizes to ammonia within minutes and is responsible for "urine burns" or "scalding."* Spray or wipe preparations, such as Skin Prep and Bard Barrier Film, *protect skin from urine.*
- Refer to Help for Incontinent People (HIP), PO Box 544, Union, SC 29379.

Originated by: Audrey Klopp, RN, PhD, ET

Urinary retention

The state in which an individual experiences incomplete emptying of the bladder.

RELATED FACTORS / DEFINING CHARACTERISTICS	NURSING INTERVENTIONS / *RATIONALES*	EXPECTED OUTCOMES

RELATED FACTORS
General anesthesia
Regional anesthesia
High ureteral pressures caused by disease, injury, or edema
Pain
Infection
Inadequate intake
Ureteral blockage
 	
DEFINING CHARACTERISTICS
Decreased (<30 ml/hr) or absent urinary output for 2 consecutive hrs
Frequency
Hesitancy
Urgency
Lower abdominal distention
Abdominal discomfort
Dribbling
	ONGOING ASSESSMENT
	- Evaluate previous patterns of voiding.
	- Visually inspect lower abdomen for distention.
	- Palpate over bladder for distention.
	- Evaluate time intervals between voidings.
	- Assess amount, frequency, character (color, odor, specific gravity).
	- Determine balance between I & O.
	- Monitor urinalysis, urine culture, and sensitivity.
	- If indwelling catheter is in situ, assess for patency, kinking.
	- Monitor BUN and creatinine.
	
	THERAPEUTIC INTERVENTIONS
	- Initiate methods to facilitate voiding:
	  Encourage fluids
	  Offer cranberry juice daily *to keep urine acidic. This helps prevent infection.*
	  Position patient in upright position on toilet if possible.
	  Place bedpan/urinal or bedside commode within reach.
	  Provide privacy.
	  Encourage patient to void every 4 hr.
	  Have patient listen to sound of running water or place hands in warm water and/or pour warm water over perineum.
	  Offer fluids before voiding.
	  Perform Credé over bladder.
	- Administer bethanechol (Urecholine) as ordered *to stimulate parasympathetic nervous system to release acetylcholine at nerve endings and to increase tone and amplitude of contractions of smooth muscles of urinary bladder.*
	  Side effects: rare, after oral administration of therapeutic dose. In small subcutaneous doses: abdominal cramps, sweating, and flushing. In larger doses: malaise, headaches, diarrhea, nausea, vomiting, asthmatic attacks, bradycardia, lowered BP, atrioventricular block, and cardiac arrest.
	- Institute intermittent catheterization.
		Adequate urinary elimination patterns will be established.

Continued.

RELATED FACTORS / DEFINING CHARACTERISTICS	NURSING INTERVENTIONS / *RATIONALES*	EXPECTED OUTCOMES

	• Insert retention (Foley) catheter as ordered:
	  Tape catheter to abdomen (male) *to prevent ureteral fistula.*
	  Tape catheter to thigh (female).
	  Cleanse insertion site every shift with soap and water and dry thoroughly.	

PATIENT EDUCATION
- Educate patient/significant others about the importance of adequate intake, i.e., 8 to 10 glasses of fluids daily.
- Instruct patient/significant others on measures to help voiding (as described).
- Instruct patient/significant others on signs and symptoms of overdistended bladder (e.g., decreased or absent urine, frequency, hesitancy, urgency, lower abdominal distention, or discomfort).
- Instruct patient/significant others on signs and symptoms of urinary tract infection (e.g., chills and fever, frequent urination or concentrated urine, abdominal or back pain).
- See Urinary tract infection, p. 361.

Originated by: Doris M. McNear, RN, BSN

Cardiovascular Care Plans

DISORDERS

Anaphylactic shock
Angina pectoris: stable
Angina pectoris: unstable acute phase
Aortic aneurysm
Cardiac dysrhythmias
Cardiac tamponade
Cardiogenic shock
Chronic heart failure
Digitalis toxicity
Endocarditis
Hypertension
Hypertensive crisis

Mitral valve prolapse
Myocardial infarction: acute phase
Myocardial infarction: intermediate phase
Pulmonary edema, acute
Septic shock
Thrombophlebitis

THERAPEUTIC INTERVENTIONS

Cardiac catheterization
Cardiac surgery: immediate postoperative
 care
Cardiac surgery: intermediate postoperative
 care

Cardiac transplantation
Carotid endarterectomy
Femoral-popliteal bypass: immediate
 postoperative care
Intra-aortic balloon pump
Percutaneous balloon valvuloplasty
Percutaneous transluminal coronary
 angioplasty
Swan Ganz catheterization
Thrombolytic therapy in myocardial
 infarction
Transvenous pacemaker, permanent
Transvenous pacemaker, temporary
Ventricular assist device

Anaphylactic shock

(ALLERGIC REACTION)

An exaggerated form of hypersensitivity (antigen-antibody interaction) that occurs within 1-2 minutes after contact with an antigenic substance and progresses rapidly to respiratory distress, vascular collapse, systemic shock, and possibly death.

NURSING DIAGNOSES / DEFINING CHARACTERISTICS	NURSING INTERVENTIONS / *RATIONALES*	EXPECTED OUTCOMES

Decreased cardiac output *Related to:* Severe reactions to drugs, insect bites, diagnostic agents, or food
 	
DEFINING CHARACTERISTICS Hypotension Tachycardia Decreased CVP Decreased pulmonary pressures Decreased cardiac output Oliguria Decreased peripheral pulses
	ONGOING ASSESSMENT
	• Assess physical status and document changes. Report significant changes in the following to physician:
	    Vital signs, including temperature, pulse rate, BP, cardiac rhythm, respiratory rate
	    Lung sounds (rales, wheezing, stridor)
	    Jugular vein distention, pulmonary pressures
	    Skin color, rashes, temperature, moisture
	    Changes in level of consciousness or mentation
	    Patient's level of anxiety (mild or severe)
	
	THERAPEUTIC INTERVENTIONS
	• If ingested drugs or foods are the cause of the reaction, assist with forced emesis to delay absorption of the drug. If injected agents or insect bites are the cause of the reaction, apply a tourniquet above injection site or insect bite followed by infiltration of the site with epinephrine as ordered per physician.
	• Administer medications per physician order noting responses:
	    Epinephrine: *An endogenous catecholamine with both α- and β-receptor stimulating actions that provides rapid relief of hypersensitivity reactions. It is unknown whether epinephrine prevents mediator release or whether it reverses the action of mediators on target tissues, but its early administration is critical.*
	    Aminophylline: *A bronchodilator, pulmonary vasodilator, and smooth muscle relaxant that inhibits bronchospasm.*
	    Benadryl: *An antihistamine with anticholinergic and sedative side effects that is a useful therapeutic adjunct to epinephrine after the acute episode is controlled.*
	    Vasopressors: *Useful to reverse vasodilation in the acute state.*
	• Maintain hemodynamic parameters at prescribed levels:
	    Heart rate
	    BP
	    CVP
	    Pulmonary capillary wedge pressure/pulmonary artery
	    Urine output
		Shock state will be reduced.

Ineffective breathing pattern *Related to:* Facial angioedema Bronchospasm Laryngeal edema **DEFINING CHARACTERISTICS** Dyspnea Wheezing Tachypnea Stridor Tightness of chest Cyanosis	**ONGOING ASSESSMENT** • Monitor respiratory status and observe for changes (e.g., increased shortness of breath, tachypnea, dyspnea, wheezing, stridor). • Monitor ABGs and note changes. • Check breath sounds and report changes. • Monitor chest x-ray reports. **THERAPEUTIC INTERVENTIONS** • Position patient *for optimal lung expansion and ease of breathing.* • Administer O$_2$ per orders. • Instruct patient to breathe deeply and slow down respiratory rate. *Focusing on breathing may help to calm patient and facilitate improved gas exchange.* • Give medications (e.g., steroids, antihistamines, aminophylline, 1:1000 aqueous epinephrine) as ordered *to reverse bronchospasm* and record effects. • Maintain patent airway. Anticipate emergency intubation or tracheostomy. *Respiratory distress may progress rapidly.*	Normal breathing will be restored.

NURSING DIAGNOSES / DEFINING CHARACTERISTICS	NURSING INTERVENTIONS / *RATIONALES*	EXPECTED OUTCOMES

Fluid volume deficit *Related to:* Failure of hormonal and renal regulatory mechanisms
 	
Defining Characteristics
Decreased urine output
Concentrated urine
Decreased venous filling
Hypotension
Thirst
Tachycardia
	Ongoing Assessment
	• Assess fluid balance (I & O) every hour.
	• Obtain daily weights.
	• Assess for edema.
	
	Therapeutic Interventions
	• Maintain optimal fluid balance:
	    Administer parenteral fluid *to reverse hypovolemia,* as ordered.
	    Give fluid challenges as ordered and closely monitor and record effects.
	• Refer to Fluid volume deficit, p. 20.
		Adequate fluid volume will be maintained.

Altered renal perfusion *Related to:* Shock Hypovolemia **Defining Characteristics** Decreased urine output Decreased venous filling Hemoconcentration from third spacing Increased heart rate Increased BUN and creatinine levels	**Ongoing Assessment** • Monitor serum and urine electrolytes and osmolarity. Document changes and notify physician. • Monitor urine output every hour; document changes and notify physician. • Monitor daily weights. • Monitor I & O q1h. • Monitor laboratory data for elevation in BUN and creatinine levels, acid-base imbalances, particularly Na^+ and K^+. **Therapeutic Interventions** • Administer parenteral fluids as ordered *to prevent acute tubular necrosis secondary to decreased renal perfusion.* • See Renal failure, acute, p. 343.	Tissue perfusion to the kidneys will be maintained.
Potential altered level of consciousness *Related to:* Shock Hypovolemia **Defining Characteristics** Changes in alertness Changes in orientation Inappropriate responses (verbal) Agitation Decreased cerebral perfusion **Defining Characteristics** Agitation Lethargy Pupillary changes	**Ongoing Assessment** • Obtain neurologic checks. Report and record any changes. • Observe for seizure activity. • Monitor vital signs. **Therapeutic Interventions** • Protect patient from possible injuries (seizures, decreased gag reflex). • Maintain BP in prescribed range *to increase cerebral perfusion.* • Give fluids as ordered *to maintain BP.* • See Consciousness, alteration in level of, p. 234.	Cerebral perfusion will be maintained.

Continued.

■ Anaphylactic shock—cont'd

NURSING DIAGNOSES / DEFINING CHARACTERISTICS	NURSING INTERVENTIONS / *RATIONALES*	EXPECTED OUTCOMES

Potential impaired skin integrity *Related to:* Manifestations of allergic reaction
 	
 DEFINING CHARACTERISTICS Uticaria Pruritus Edema
	ONGOING ASSESSMENT
	 · Observe for signs of flushing (localized or generalized).
	 · Watch for development of rashes; note character: macules, papules, pustules, petechia.
	 · Assess for swelling/edema.
	
	 THERAPEUTIC INTERVENTIONS
	 · Give medications (e.g., Benadryl) as ordered.
	 · Prevent patient from excessive scratching. *Scratching can cause further skin damage.*
	    Instruct patient not to scratch.
	    Clip nails if patient is scratching in sleep.
	    Mitten hands if necessary.
	 · Be prepared for intubation or tracheostomy. *If facial edema is present, upper respiratory edema may also occur.*
		Urticaria will be resolved, and skin condition will return to normal.

Potential anxiety/fear *Related to:* Alteration in breathing Shock state Another allergic reaction Other possible allergens **DEFINING CHARACTERISTICS** Restlessness Withdrawal Indifference Demanding behavior Uncooperative behavior Tachycardia Tachypnea Diarrhea	**ONGOING ASSESSMENT** · Recognize patient's level of anxiety and note signs and symptoms. · Assess patient's coping mechanisms. **THERAPEUTIC INTERVENTIONS** · See Anxiety, p. 4; Fear, p. 18.	Anxiety and fear will be allayed.
Knowledge deficit: allergens *Related to:* No previous experience **DEFINING CHARACTERISTICS** Recurrent allergic reactions Inability to identify allergens	**ONGOING ASSESSMENT** · Assess patient's knowledge of his/her condition and allergens. **THERAPEUTIC INTERVENTIONS** · Explain symptoms and interventions to help prevent anaphylactic shock. · Instruct patient/significant others about factors that can precipitate a recurrence of shock and ways to prevent or avoid these precipitating factors. *The patient is at high risk for developing anaphylactic shock in the future if exposed to the same antigenic substance.* · Explain environmental factors that may increase risk of anaphylaxis (i.e., certain drugs, bee stings, food). · Instruct patient on use of insect sting kits (containing a chewable antihistamine, epinephrine in prefilled syringe, and instructions for use), if they are to be used, and how they are to be obtained. · Instruct patient with known allergies to wear Medic-Alert tags. *In case of emergency, persons providing care will then be aware of this significant history.* · Patient/significant others should be made aware that when giving past medical history they should include allergies to certain foods.	Patient/significant others will verbalize understanding of condition, prevention, and treatment.

Originated by: Chris Loftus, RN, BS
               Pat Anderson, RN

Angina pectoris, stable

(CHEST PAIN)

A clinical syndrome characterized by the abrupt or gradual onset of substernal discomfort caused by insufficient coronary blood flow and/or inadequate O_2 supply to the myocardial muscle. The characteristics of angina are usually constant for a given patient. The pain is precipitated by effort or emotional stress or both. Conditions such as fever, anemia, tachyarrhythmias, hypothyroidism, and polycythemia may also provoke angina. Stable angina usually persists only 3-5 minutes and subsides with cessation of the precipitating factor, rest, or use of nitroglycerin (NTG). Patients do not require hospitalization, though anginal episodes may occur during hospitalization for other medical problems.

NURSING DIAGNOSES / DEFINING CHARACTERISTICS	NURSING INTERVENTIONS / *RATIONALES*	EXPECTED OUTCOMES
Chest pain (myocardial ischemia) *Related to:* Atherosclerosis and/or coronary spasm Less common causes: severe aortic stenosis, cardiomyopathy, mitral valve prolapse, lupus erythematosus **DEFINING CHARACTERISTICS** No change in the frequency, duration, time of appearance, or precipitating factors during the previous 60 days Pain characteristics: Quality: choking, strangling, pressure, burning, tightness, ache, heaviness Location: substernal, may radiate to arms and shoulders, neck, back, jaw Severity: scale 1-10 (usually not at top of scale) Duration: typically 3-5 min Onset: episodic and usually precipitated by physical exertion, emotional stress, heavy meal, exposures to temperature extremes such as cold, smoking	**ONGOING ASSESSMENT** • Assess patient's description of pain, any exacerbating factors and measures used to relieve the pain. • Evaluate whether this is a chronic problem (stable angina) or a new presentation (see Angina pectoris, unstable, p. 69). • Monitor effectiveness of interventions. • Assess for the appropriateness of performing an ECG to evaluate ST-T wave changes *(to assist in differentiating between angina and myocardial infarction).* **THERAPEUTIC INTERVENTIONS** • At first signs of pain, instruct patient to relax and/or rest *to decrease myocardial O_2 demands.* • Instruct patient to take sublingual nitroglycerine (NTG SL). • If pain continues after taking 2-3 NTG SL, notify physician. *Chest pain unrelieved by NTG may represent unstable angina or myocardial infarction and should be evaluated immediately.* • Administer O_2 as ordered. • Offer assurance and emotional support, clarifying the difference between angina and "a heart attack".	Discomfort will be relieved.

Continued.

NURSING DIAGNOSES / DEFINING CHARACTERISTICS	NURSING INTERVENTIONS / *RATIONALES*	EXPECTED OUTCOMES

Knowledge deficit
Related to:
Unfamiliarity with disease process and treatment
 	
DEFINING CHARACTERISTICS
Overanxiousness
Multiple questions or lack of questioning
	ONGOING ASSESSMENT
	- Assess knowledge of patient/significant others.
	- Assess readiness, motivation, and interest in health/illness status.
	- Evaluate compliance with previously prescribed life-style changes.
	
	THERAPEUTIC INTERVENTIONS
	- Plan teaching sessions *so patient is not overwhelmed at one time.*
	- Consult cardiac rehab clinical nurse specialist about appropriate teaching materials (hospital television, brochures, group class).
	- Provide information regarding:
	Anatomy and physiology of coronary circulation
	Need to reduce identified risk factors for atherosclerosis
	  Hypertension: lower weight, reduced salt intake, exercise programs, and medications as prescribed
	  Smoking: *doubles risk of heart attack.* If patient can't quit alone, refer to American Heart Association, Lung Association, Cancer Society for support group and interventions
	  High blood cholesterol: emphasis on need to reduce intake of foods high in saturated fat, cholesterol, or both (fatty meats, organ meats, lard, butter, egg yolks, whole dairy products). Arrange for evaluation by dietitian as needed. Include spouse/significant others in meal planning
	  Diabetes: emphasis on control through diet and medication
	  Obesity: *affects hypertension, diabetes, and cholesterol levels*
	  Stress: reference to programs for stress management as appropriate
	  Sedentary existence: emphasis on benefits of exercise in reducing risks of heart attack. *Lack of exercise contributes to elevated cholesterol and overweight.* Refer to cardiac rehab program as needed. Keep exercise intensity below angina threshold.
	Risk factors that can't be modified: family history, age, sex
	Differentiating angina from noncardiac pain
	Need to avoid angina-provoking situations (heavy meals, extreme temperatures, emotional stress, stimulants)
	Use of sublingual NTG to relieve attacks:
	  Carry pills at all times.
	  Keep pills in dark, dry container, away from heat. *NTG is volatile and inactivated by heat, moisture, light.*
	  Replace pills every 3-4 mo. *Once bottle is opened, NTG begins to lose its strength. Tablets that are effective should sting in the mouth.*
	  Sit or lie down when taking NTG. *NTG causes vasodilation, which can lower blood pressure and cause dizziness.*
	  For chest pain, put pill under tongue and let dissolve. If not relieved in 5 min, take another. If still not relieved, take a third. If this doesn't relieve pain, call physician or go to emergency room.
	  Emphasize that NTG is a safe and nonaddicting drug. Use as needed
	  Headache is a common side effect and can be treated with acetaminophen (Tylenol).
	Use of prophylactic NTG to prevent pain
	Use of other medications for long-term management:
	  Long-lasting nitrates: *to increase coronary blood flow and decrease work of heart*
	  β-blockers: *to decrease myocardial oxygen demand.*
	  Calcium channel blockers: *increase coronary blood flow and reduce oxygen demands of heart.*
	Diagnostic tests for evaluating coronary artery disease:
	  ECG
	  Exercise stress test (with thallium)
	  Myocardial scans
	  Cardiac catheterization and coronary angiography
	Therapeutic procedures to relieve angina unresponsive to medications and life-style changes:
		Patient/significant others will be able to verbalize understanding of angina pectoris, its causes, and appropriate relief measures for pain.

NURSING DIAGNOSES / DEFINING CHARACTERISTICS	NURSING INTERVENTIONS / *RATIONALES*	EXPECTED OUTCOMES
	Percutaneous transluminal coronary angioplasty Coronary artery bypass graft surgery Comparisons of stable vs. unstable angina and myocardial infarction	
Decreased activity intolerance *Related to:* Occurrence of, or fear of chest pain Side effects of prescribed medications **DEFINING CHARACTERISTICS** Chest pain or dyspnea during activity Fatigue Abnormal heart rate or BP response to activity Dizziness during activity Change in skin temperature from warm to cool during activity ECG changes reflecting ischemia or arrhythmias	**ONGOING ASSESSMENT** · Assess patient's level of physical activity prior to experiencing angina. · Assess for defining characteristics before, during, and after activity. · Evaluate factors that may precipitate fatigue/discomfort. **THERAPEUTIC INTERVENTIONS** While in hospital: · Encourage adequate rest periods in between activities *to reduce oxygen demands.* · Assist with ADL as indicated. · Instruct in prophylactic use of NTG prior to physical exertion as needed. · Reinforce the need to "pace activities" (phone calls, visitors, daily hygiene). Discharge planning: · Assist patient in reviewing required home activities and developing an appropriate plan for accomplishing them (what to do in morning vs. afternoon; how to pace household chores throughout the week). · Remind patient not to work with arms above shoulders for long time *for this increases myocardial demands.* · Remind patient to continue taking medications (i.e., β-blockers), despite side effects of fatigue. *Often the body does adjust to the medications after several weeks.* · Evaluate need for additional support at home (housekeeper, neighbor to shop, family assistance). · Encourage a program of progressive aerobic exercise *to increase functional capacity.* Refer to cardiac rehab as appropriate.	Activity level will be maintained within limits of patient's capabilities.

Originated by: Beth Manglal-Lan, RN, BSN
                 Meg Gulanick, RN, PhD

Angina pectoris, unstable: acute phase (CCU)

(PREINFARCTION ANGINA; ACUTE CORONARY INSUFFICIENCY; CRESCENDO ANGINA)

Unstable (preinfarction) angina is a clinical syndrome characterized by a changing pattern of previously stable angina, new onset of severe angina, or occurrence of angina at rest. It is intermediate between death of some heart muscle (infarction) and transient muscle ischemia, which is often caused by a combination of arterial spasm and obstruction. Patients with unstable angina have an increased risk of arrhythmia, myocardial infarction, and sudden death and should be hospitalized in CCU.

NURSING DIAGNOSES / DEFINING CHARACTERISTICS	NURSING INTERVENTIONS / *RATIONALES*	EXPECTED OUTCOMES

Chest pain
Related to:
Myocardial ischemia
 	
DEFINING CHARACTERISTICS
New onset (<60 days) angina; or
	ONGOING ASSESSMENT
	· Solicit patient's description of or absence of pain.
	· Assess pain characteristics:
	    Quality: as with stable angina (squeezing, tightening, choking, pressing, burning)
	    Location: substernal area. May radiate to extremities (e.g., arms, shoulders)
		Discomfort will be relieved or reduced.

Continued.

NURSING DIAGNOSES / DEFINING CHARACTERISTICS	NURSING INTERVENTIONS / *RATIONALES*	EXPECTED OUTCOMES

Changing pattern of previously stable angina; or
Angina occurring at rest or with minimal exertion; or
Angina occurring during sleep
ECG changes:
  Normal or depressed ST segment
  ST segment elevation during pain with variant Prinzmetal's angina
	Severity: more intense than classic angina pectoris
	Duration: persists longer than 20 min
	Onset: minimal exertion or during rest or sleep
	Relief: usually does not respond to sublingual NTG or rest
	
	THERAPEUTIC INTERVENTIONS
	· Maintain strict bed rest *to decrease O$_2$ demands.*
	· Provide therapeutic environment conducive to rest and sleep.
	· Instruct patient to report pain as soon as it starts. *Important for diagnosis and easier to treat.*
	· Respond immediately to complaint of pain.
	· Administer O$_2$ as ordered.
	· Perform ECG immediately during and after episode of pain *to evaluate ST changes (to assist in diagnosing cardiac origin of pain and site of coronary artery involvement).*
	· Give medications as ordered, evaluating effectiveness and observing signs/symptoms of untoward reactions:
	  Nitrates: *Relax smooth muscles in vascular system, causing vasodilation that results in lower blood pressure, lower vascular resistance, and decreased work of the heart.*
	  Anticipate IV nitroglycerin drip.
	  Anticipate large doses to control pain (100-600 mg/min).
	  Monitor BP closely q15-30min, until stable.
	  Anticipate fluid challenge to treat hypotension. *Nitrates cause venous pooling, which lowers blood pressure).*
	  β-Blockers: *Are used to decrease myocardial oxygen demand.* Anticipate IV administration; Observe for side effects: hypotension, bradycardia, and heart failure. *β-blockers reduce pumping/contractility of heart muscle and decrease heart rate.*
	  Thrombolytic therapy: *Used to dissolve thrombus that may be partially occluding vessel.*
	· Anticipate intra-aortic balloon pump management if pain and ischemic changes persist despite maximal medical therapy. *It increases coronary blood flow while reducing work by left ventricle during contraction*
	· Anticipate cardiac catheterization and, depending on results, anticipate percutaneous transluminal coronary angioplasty or coronary artery bypass surgery.	

Potential decreased cardiac output
Related to:
Prolonged episodes of myocardial ischemia affecting contractility
 	
DEFINING CHARACTERISTICS
Variations in hemodynamic parameters (increased/decreased BP, increased heart rate, increased systemic vascular resistance, increased pulmonary artery pressures, abnormal heart sounds [S$_3$ or S$_4$], increased jugular venous distention, pulmonary congestion)
	ONGOING ASSESSMENT
	· Assess hemodynamic status every hour and especially during episode of pain.
	· Assess for myocardial ischemia (ST changes) on ECG.
	· Monitor ECG continuously for arrhythmias, especially during episode of pain.
	
	THERAPEUTIC INTERVENTIONS
	· Anticipate possible progression to myocardial infarction:
	  Monitor results of cardiac isoenzymes q8h as ordered.
	  Monitor frequency, duration, severity, and occurrence of pain.
	· If symptoms develop, institute SCP, Cardiac output, decreased, p. 9.
	· Maintain bed rest *to prevent increased O$_2$ demands.*
	· Anticipate development of life-threatening arrhythmias. *Ischemic muscle is electrically unstable and produces arrhythmias. Tachyarrhythmias or bradyarrhythmias may occur.*
	  Anticipate/administer lidocaine for ventricular arrhythmias per protocol.
	  If high-degree atrioventricular block develops, anticipate atropine/isoproterenol IV and insertion of temporary pacemaker *to increase heart rate.*
		Optimal cardiac output will be maintained.

NURSING DIAGNOSES / DEFINING CHARACTERISTICS	NURSING INTERVENTIONS / *RATIONALES*	EXPECTED OUTCOMES
Arrhythmias, ECG changes (depressed or elevated ST segment) Restlessness, mentation changes		

Anxiety/Fear
Related to:
Recurrent anginal attacks
Incomplete relief from pain by usual means (nitroglycerin and rest)
Fear of impending doom and death
Alteration in activity level precipitating chest pain (decreased activity level)
 	
DEFINING CHARACTERISTICS
Mild:
  Restlessness
  Increased awareness
  Increased questioning
Moderate/severe:
  Glancing about/ increased alertness
  Facial tension/wide-eyed
  Focus on self
  Poor eye contact
  Increased perspiration
  Anorexia/GI problems
  Overexcitement, jitteriness
  Expressed concern
  Trembling
  Constant demands
	ONGOING ASSESSMENT
	• Assess level of anxiety (mild to severe) and patient's coping pattern.
	
	THERAPEUTIC INTERVENTIONS
	• Institute SCP, Anxiety, p. 4.
	• Encourage patient to call for nurse when pain or anxiety develops. *Anxiety and fear increase heart rate and blood pressure and cause release of epinephrine, which may produce an arrhythmia).*
	• Immediately respond to any complaint of pain. *Prompt treatment may decrease myocardial ischemia and prevent damage.*
	• Make every effort to remain at bedside throughout episode of pain.
	• Check on patient frequently *to provide reassurance*.
		Anxiety level will be reduced.

Knowledge deficit
Related to:
Unfamiliarity with disease process, treatment, recovery
 	
DEFINING CHARACTERISTICS
Multiple questions or lack of questioning
Verbalized misconceptions
	ONGOING ASSESSMENT
	• Assess present level of understanding by patient/significant others.
	• Assess physical/emotional readiness for learning by patient/significant others.
	
	THERAPEUTIC INTERVENTIONS
	• Instruct patient to report pain *so that relief measures may be instituted.*
	• Instruct patient to evaluate and report effectiveness of measures used.
	• Teach patient/significant others:
	  Anatomy and physiology of the coronary condition
	  Atherosclerotic process and implications of angina pectoris
	  Special emphasis on the use of nitroglycerin and its side effects when chest pain occurs
	• Remind patient that further teaching will take place after transfer from unit.
		Patient/significant others will be able to verbalize understanding of anatomy/ physiology of unstable angina, causes, and appropriate relief measures for pain.

Originated by: Teodorina M. Saez, RN, BSN

Aortic aneurysm

(DISSECTING ANEURYSM)

Aortic aneurysms are localized dilated areas of the thoracic or abdominal arterial segments that result from the atrophy of the medial layer. Dissecting aneurysms (dissecting hematomas) occur when the layers of the media are dissected, resulting in the formation of a false channel between the intimal and the adventitial arterial layers. Dissection of the aorta is commonly classified according to location. Type I and type II involve the ascending aorta; type III involves the descending aorta. Dissecting aortic aneurysm is the most common catastrophe involving the aorta and has a high mortality rate if not detected early and treated appropriately. It can be treated through surgical intervention or with medical therapy.

NURSING DIAGNOSES / DEFINING CHARACTERISTICS	NURSING INTERVENTIONS / *RATIONALES*	EXPECTED OUTCOMES
Potential for injury: further dissection *Related to:* Conditions that increase stress on the arterial wall: Hypertension Pregnancy with hypervolemia Coarctation of the aorta Defect in the vessel wall: Marfan's syndrome Cystic degeneration in the media Iatrogenic causes **DEFINING CHARACTERISTICS** Pain: Characteristics: excruciating, ripping, tearing, sudden onset Location: Anterior chest, radiating to the back Pulse deficits: Difference in BP in both arms, change in pulse status in the femoral artery Change in lower extremities; cool temperature, numbness Aortic murmur (diastolic) Neurologic deficits: Decreased level of consciousness Mediastinal widening and pleural effusions on chest x-ray Decreased urinary output	**ONGOING ASSESSMENT** • Assess and monitor for signs and symptoms indicating progressive dissection (see Defining Characteristics). *A high index of suspicion is key to the treatment to reduce mortality. Clinical signs and symptoms indicate the site and progression of dissection:* *Type I dissection may affect brachiocephalic vessel, resulting in ischemia of brain and arm.* *Dissection extending proximally to the aortic annulus may produce direct loss of the support of the aortic cusps and acute aortic regurgitation (type II).* *Types I and III dissection may cause ischemia of intestines, kidneys, or legs.* **THERAPEUTIC INTERVENTIONS** • Administer pain medicines as ordered: Document location, intensity, and duration of pain. Document effect of pain medicines. • Provide nursing measures that alleviate pain: Position of comfort: Side lying may be more comfortable for patients exhibiting back pain Elevate head of bed for patients who are short of breath *to promote maximum lung expansion.* Physical comfort: *hand holding provides emotional support* Physiologic intervention: application of cold towel to forehead Relaxation techniques • Administer potent vasodilator (Nipride) medication. *Goal is to maintain systolic BP <130 mm Hg* Use infusion pump. Infuse the drug in a separate line, preferably a central line, *to minimize infiltration and prevent tissue damage, as well as prevent inaccurate absorption of the drug.* • Administer β-blockers *to decrease heart rate and decrease myocardial contractility, thus reducing the stress applied to the arterial walls during each heart beat. The goal is to maintain heart rate <70 beats per minute.* • For type I and II dissections, anticipate surgical treatment and prepare patient. • For type III dissection, chronic medical treatment is usually indicated and consists of the following long-term measures: Decrease or eliminate identified factors that will increase blood pressure, heart rate: Anxiety, stress, fear, pain all elicit sympathetic responses that potentiate further dissection. Provide a quiet environment as much as possible. Regulate staff rounds to provide patient rest periods. Pace activities (eating, personal hygiene, visitors) appropriately. Limit visitors and phone calls. Provide continuity of nursing staff if possible. Administer sedatives as ordered.	Progression of dissection will be detected and appropriate treatment will be instituted.

NURSING DIAGNOSES / DEFINING CHARACTERISTICS	NURSING INTERVENTIONS / *RATIONALES*	EXPECTED OUTCOMES

Potential decreased cardiac output
 Related to:
 Drug-induced
 Progressive dissection
 Rupture of the aorta
 	
 DEFINING CHARACTERISTICS
 Tachycardia
 Decreasing BP
 Decreasing urinary output
 Restlessness
	ONGOING ASSESSMENT
	 • Observe for and document clinical signs and symptoms of decreasing cardiac output (see Defining Characteristics).
	 • Assess all potential causes of decreased cardiac output.
	
	 THERAPEUTIC INTERVENTIONS
	 • If decreased cardiac output is drug-induced, anticipate the following:
	 For Sodium Nitroprusside (Nipride):
	   Stop the drug.
	   Administer isotonic solution (0.9 NSS) or plasma expanders *to maintain increased intravascular volume.*
	 For β-Blocker:
	   May stop the drug or reduce dose. *β-blocker has a negative inotropic effect, which can potentiate heart failure. Presence of rales and S_3 indicates heart failure.*
	 • If decreased cardiac output is related to further dissection (severe aortic insufficiency) or ruptured aorta, anticipate emergency angiography and surgery:
	   Send blood specimen for type and cross match, and other routine preop blood work.
	   Stay with patient to provide emotional support.
	   Assist primary physician in discussing surgery with both patient and family.
	   Administer medications, IV fluids, and blood as ordered *to maintain adequate cardiac output prior to surgery.*
	   Prepare patient for surgery per hospital policy and procedure.
	 • For immediate postop course, see Cardiac surgery, adult: immediate postoperative care, p. 125
		Adequate cardiac output is maintained.

Anxiety/fear *Related to:* Sudden onset Impending surgery Close monitoring by medical/nursing staff Fear of death Multiple tests and procedures **DEFINING CHARACTERISTICS** Verbalization of fear Tense, anxious appearance Request to have family at bedside all the time Restlessness Increased questioning Constant demands Glancing about/ increased alertness	**ONGOING ASSESSMENT** • Assess level of anxiety. • Assess usual coping strategies. **THERAPEUTIC INTERVENTIONS** • Encourage verbalization of fear/anxiety. *Identifying patient's fear/anxiety will facilitate staff's planning of strategies to reinforce patient's usual coping mechanisms.* • Provide emotional support and reassurance that he/she is being observed carefully and help is available when needed. • Ensure that call light is within reach at all times. • Explain tests and procedures being done. Emphasize their importance in diagnosing and treating the problem. • Update patient with test results. • Assist primary physician in explaining the treatment regime. • Inform patient of planned tests and procedures. • Provide adequate time for rest and some quiet time *to allow patient to sort out feelings.* • Allow family to stay with patient as much as possible. • Allocate time to discuss treatment regime with family alone.	Anxiety will be reduced or relieved.
Knowledge deficit: follow-up care *Related to:* New medical problem Unfamiliarity with surgical procedure	**ONGOING ASSESSMENT** • Assess patient's knowledge and understanding of the disease. • Assess patient's understanding of medical versus surgical treatment. • Assess patient's ability to learn. • Monitor progress of learning.	Patient/family will verbalize understanding of disease process, treatment options, and goals of therapy.

Continued.

Aortic aneurysm—cont'd

NURSING DIAGNOSES / DEFINING CHARACTERISTICS	NURSING INTERVENTIONS / *RATIONALES*	EXPECTED OUTCOMES

DEFINING CHARACTERISTICS
Frequent questioning
Verbalization of need to learn
	THERAPEUTIC INTERVENTIONS
	• Utilize teaching tools/methods appropriate for the patient and family *to facilitate learning process:*
	  Individualized teaching
	  Group teaching with other patients
	  Pamphlets and other appropriate reading materials
	  Follow-up calls post discharge
	• Instruct patient about the following:
	  Cause of aneurysm
	  Medical vs. surgical treatment
	  Preoperative preparation
	  Goals of the therapy (avoid excess blood pressure and strain to the diseased thoracic arterial wall or over the graft site)
	  Use of antihypertensive medications as ordered
	  Importance of compliance
	  Effects of meds
	  Dietary restrictions. *Low-salt diet usually indicated for maintaining normotensive blood pressure*
	  Relationship of obesity and high blood pressure
	  Avoiding activities that are isometric or abruptly raise blood pressure (e.g., lifting and carrying of heavy objects, constipation)
	  Methods for coping with stress and recommend appropriate life-style changes	

Originated by: Lumie Perez, RN, BSN, CCRN

Cardiac dysrhythmias

(ARRHYTHMIAS; TACHYCARDIA; BRADYCARDIA; FLUTTER; FIBRILLATION)

Any disturbance in rhythm, rate, or conduction of the heart beat. Dysrhythmia may be categorized in many ways: by origin (atrial, junctional, ventricular, etc.), by rate (tachyarrhythmias, bradyarrhythmias), by chronicity (acute, chronic). In this care plan, dysrhythmias are categorized by rate.

NURSING DIAGNOSES / DEFINING CHARACTERISTICS	NURSING INTERVENTIONS / *RATIONALES*	EXPECTED OUTCOMES
Potential decreased cardiac output *Related to:* Rapid heart rate/ rhythm: atrial tachycardia, atrial flutter/ fibrillation with fast ventricular response, junctional tachycardia, ventricular tachycardia, paroxysmal supraventricular tachycardia (PSVT) Etiology: Ischemia	**ONGOING ASSESSMENT** • Monitor heart for rate and rhythm. • If ECG monitored, note dysrhythmia continuously, observing for *changes* in rate, rhythm, ectopy. • Evaluate monitor leads that show the most prominent ''p'' waves, such as lead II, V_1, or MCL_1. *These leads aid in differentiating atrial from ventricular dysrhythmias.* • Assess for signs of reduced cardiac output that may accompany tachycardia (see Defining Characteristics). *Not all patients are symptomatic with each episode. Several factors can influence response to the tachycardia: actual heart rate, duration, associate medical problems, etc.).* • Assess for causative factors (see Etiology). *Dysrhythmias are best suppressed when precipitating factors are eliminated or corrected.* • Evaluate patient's emotional response to acute/chronic episodes of tachycardia.	Optimal cardiac output is maintained.

NURSING DIAGNOSES / DEFINING CHARACTERISTICS	NURSING INTERVENTIONS / *RATIONALES*	EXPECTED OUTCOMES

Electrolyte imbalance (especially hypokalemia)
Anxiety/emotional factors
Drug induced (e.g., aminophylline, isoproterenol, dopamine, digoxin toxicity)
Substance abuse (e.g., cocaine, alcohol)
Physical activity
Heart failure
Pulmonary embolism
Hypoxemia
Stimulant intake (coffee, alcohol)
Chronic lung disease

DEFINING CHARACTERISTICS

Rapid pulse
Decreased blood pressure
Dizziness, lightheadedness, syncope
Changes in mental status
Shortness of breath, rales
Cool, clammy skin
Chest pain
Pallor
Fatigue, weakness
Increased jugular venous distention (JVD)

THERAPEUTIC INTERVENTIONS

- If patient is asymptomatic, provide reassurance that this is not a life-threatening dysrhythmia.
- Provide oxygen therapy as ordered *to decrease tissue irritability.*
- Anticipate need for Holter monitoring for transient dysrhythmia.
- If *acute arrhythmia, order stat ECG as appropriate to document.*
- Determine specific type of dysrhythmia *to anticipate appropriate treatment.*
    For atrial or junctional dysrhythmias:
        Anticipate use of vasotonic measures such as carotid sinus massage (compression) or Valsalva maneuver. *These stimulate the vagus nerve, which may slow the heart. They may also be used to help diagnose the underlying dysrhythmia.*
        By physician's order, the nurse may assist with submerging the patient's face in ice water for a few seconds *to help terminate the dysrhythmias. This treatment should not be used with patients at risk for coronary spasm.*
        Anticipate/prepare medications *given to reduce ventricular response: digoxin, calcium channel blockers, β-blockers.*
        After ventricular response is reduced, anticipate use of quinidine *to reduce atrial irritability. This is not recommended for patients with sick sinus syndrome, tachy-brady syndrome.*
        Instruct patient to avoid intake of stimulants: caffeine, alcohol, tobacco, amphetamines.
        Anticipate electrical cardioversion if dysrhythmia is chronic and unresponsive to medical therapy. *During cardioversion, low levels of energy are used to reset the natural cardiac cycle by electrically interfering with existing dysrhythmia. In nonemergencies, the patient should be sedated prior to the procedure.*
    For ventricular tachycardia:
        Recognize that this is a potentially life-threatening dysrhythmia.
        Administer medications as ordered, noting effectiveness. Lidocaine (IV), procainamide (IV or oral), and quinidine (oral) may be used, depending on the clinical setting.
        If the patient has not lost consciousness, have the patient cough very hard every few seconds. *"Cough CPR" procedures mechanically cardiovert dysrhythmia. A backup defibrillator should be ready in case the patient converts to ventricular fibrillation.*
        Anticipate use of adjunct therapies (precordial thump, defibrillation, overdrive pacing) by trained personnel
        For torsades de pointes (*a specific type of multidirectional ventricular tachycardia that alternates in amplitude and direction of electrical activity; the dysrhythmia often requires no immediate intervention but may be life-threatening. Generally this dysrhythmia is associated with a prolonged QT interval on the ECG*):
        Anticipate medical therapies assistive to the treatment of torsades de pointes:
            Isoproterenol: *helps to shorten the QT interval. A prolonged QT interval is a precursor to torsades de pointes, though not exclusively.*
            Magnesium sulfate
            Lidocaine
        Evaluate QT interval on 12-lead ECG. Be especially alert for a 25% or greater increase from the normal QT adjusted for heart rate and sex.
        Anticipate the need to obtain serum antiarrhythmic drug levels and/or electrolyte levels (potassium, calcium, magnesium).
        Anticipate/prepare for emergency cardioversion/defibrillation or overdrive pacing.For ventricular fibrillation:
        Initiate basic CPR.
        Notify physician.
        Assist with further advanced life support measures as ordered (defibrillation, medications).

Continued.

NURSING DIAGNOSES / DEFINING CHARACTERISTICS	NURSING INTERVENTIONS / *RATIONALES*	EXPECTED OUTCOMES
Potential decreased cardiac output *Related to:* Slow heart rate/ rhythm (e.g., sinus bradycardia, atrial fibrillation/flutter with slow ventricular response, second- and third-degree heart block) *Etiology:* Ischemia Drug-induced (e.g., digoxin toxicity, β-blockers) Excessive parasympathetic stimulation (e.g., sensitive carotid sinus artery, inferior MI) Diseases of the conduction system Cardiomyopathy	**ONGOING ASSESSMENT** · Monitor heart for rate and rhythm. · If ECG monitored, note dysrhythmia continuously, observing for *changes in rate rhythm, ectopy.* · Evaluate monitor leads that show most prominent "p" waves, such as lead II, V_1, or MCL_1 *These leads aid in differentiating atrial from ventricular dysrhythmias.* · Assess for signs of reduced cardiac output that may accompany bradycardia (see Defining Characteristics). *Not all patients are symptomatic with each episode. Several factors can influence patient's response to the bradycardia: actual heart rate, duration, associated medical problems, etc.).* · Assess for causative factors (see Etiology). *Dysrhythmias are best suppressed when precipitating factors are eliminated or corrected.* · Evaluate patient's emotional response to acute/chronic episodes of bradycardia. · Assess need for parenteral IV line, *in case IV medications are subsequently ordered.* · Carefully monitor patient's response to activity. *It may increase or further decrease heart rate.* · Monitor for side effects of medication therapy: *Atropine may cause tachycardia; low doses may actually decrease heart rate. Isoproterenol may cause tachycardia, especially VT, VF; also may decrease blood pressure. Do not administer with epinephrine. Isoproterenol is not recommended for routine use in cardiac arrest.*	Optimal cardiac output is maintained.
DEFINING CHARACTERISTICS Reduced blood pressure Slow, weak pulse Dizziness, lightheadedness, syncope (Stokes-Adams disease) Changes in mental status Shortness of breath, cough, rales Cool, clammy skin Chest pain Pallor	**THERAPEUTIC INTERVENTIONS** · If patient is asymptomatic, consult physician about further medical treatment. *No treatment may be indicated. Many patients have heart rates below 50-60 secondary to medication therapy. Current medications may simply be discontinued. Serum potassium and digoxin levels should be ordered to screen for digoxin toxicity.* · Instruct patient to avoid Valsalva maneuver (e.g., straining for stool) and vagal stimulating activities (e.g., vomiting). · Be cautious when performing nasotracheal suctioning *to prevent vagal stimulation.* · Anticipate need for Holter monitoring *to document transient dysrhythmias.* · If patient is symptomatic, administer atropine IV push, as per protocol. *Atropine decreases vagal tone and increases conduction through the AV node.* · If unresponsive to atropine, administer isoproterenol, as per protocol. *Isoproterenol increases cardiac output and increases myocardial workload and thus is not indicated for patients with ischemic heart disease.* · Anticipate temporary pacemaker insertion. *Pacemakers supplement the body's natural pacemaker to maintain a preset heart rate.* See Transvenous pacemaker, temporary, p. 177. · If bradyarrhythmia is unresponsive to medical therapy and deteriorates to asystole: Initiate basic CPR. Notify physician. Assist with further advanced life support measures as ordered (e.g., medication, pacemaker).	
Knowledge deficit: cause and treatment of dysrhythmia *Related to:* Anxiety Educational level/ background	**ONGOING ASSESSMENT** · Assess for defining characteristics. · Assess patient's current knowledge level about dysrhythmia, medications, treatments, procedures. **THERAPEUTIC INTERVENTIONS** · Explain patient's dysrhythmia and/or treatment regimen in language and terms patient and family are able to understand.	Patient verbalizes cause and treatment regimen for dysrhythmia.

Cardiac tamponade—cont'd

NURSING DIAGNOSES / DEFINING CHARACTERISTICS	NURSING INTERVENTIONS / *RATIONALES*	EXPECTED OUTCOMES

Knowledge deficit
Related to:
New procedures/ equipment
Unfamiliarity with disease process
 	
DEFINING CHARACTERISTICS
Questioning
Verbalized misconceptions
Lack of questions
	ONGOING ASSESSMENT
	▪ Assess patient's/significant others' knowledge of cardiac anatomy and physiology.
	▪ Assess patient's/significant others' physical/emotional readiness to learn. *During the acute stages family or significant others may require most teaching. This will minimize their feelings of helplessness and assist them in providing support to patient.*
	
	THERAPEUTIC INTERVENTIONS
	▪ When appropriate, provide information about:
	  Disease process and rationale for prescribed therapy. *This will help allay anxiety*
	  Follow-up care
	▪ Structure teaching to allow for answering questions.
	▪ Use teaching aids (pamphlets, visual aids, etc.) *to facilitate learning.*
		Patient/significant others will verbalize a basic understanding of disease process and therapy.

Originated by: Donna Creachbaum, RN, BS, CCRN
            Carol Ruback, RN, MSN, CCRN

Cardiogenic shock

(PUMP FAILURE; CONGESTIVE HEART FAILURE)

An acute state of decreased cardiac output tissue perfusion usually associated with myocardial infarction, massive pulmonary embolism, cardiac surgery or cardiac tamponade. It is a self-perpetuating condition because coronary blood flow to the myocardium is compromised, causing further ischemia and ventricular dysfunction. This care plan focuses on the care of an unstable patient in a shock state. As patient's condition improves, see chronic heart failure, p. 84

NURSING DIAGNOSES / DEFINING CHARACTERISTICS	NURSING INTERVENTIONS / *RATIONALES*	EXPECTED OUTCOMES

Decreased cardiac output
Related to:
Mechanical:
  Alteration in preload
  Alteration in afterload
  Inotropic changes in heart
Electrical:
  Alterations in cardiac rate
  Alterations in cardiac rhythm
  Alterations in conduction
Structural:
  Valvular dysfunction
  Septal defects
	ONGOING ASSESSMENT
	▪ Assess mental status.
	▪ Assess hemodynamic parameters (BP, heart rate, CVP, pulmonary artery pressures, cardiac output, neck veins).
	▪ Assess skin color, temperature, moisture.
	▪ Assess I & O.
	▪ Assess respiratory rate, rhythm, breath sounds.
	▪ Assess ABGs.
	
	THERAPEUTIC INTERVENTIONS
	▪ See Cardiac output, decreased, p. 9.
	▪ Place patient in optimal position, usually supine with head of bed slightly elevated *to promote venous return and facilitate ventilation.*
	▪ Initiate and titrate drug therapy as ordered. *Therapy can be more effective when initiated early.*
	  Dopamine: *Positive inotropic and chronotropic effect on the heart that improves stroke volume and cardiac output. High dose, however, can cause peripheral vasoconstriction and can be arrhythmiogenic.*
	  Dobutamine: *Positive inotropic effect increases cardiac output. Reduces afterload by decreasing peripheral vasoconstriction, also resulting in higher cardiac output.*
		Adequate cardiac output will be maintained.

Continued.

NURSING DIAGNOSES / DEFINING CHARACTERISTICS	NURSING INTERVENTIONS / *RATIONALES*	EXPECTED OUTCOMES
DEFINING CHARACTERISTICS Mental status changes: confusion, restlessness, apathy Variations in hemodynamic parameters (BP, heart rate, CVP, pulmonary artery pressures, cardiac output, neck veins) Pale, cool, clammy skin Cyanosis, mottling of extremities Oliguria, anuria Sustained hypotension with narrowing of pulse pressure Pulmonary congestion, rales Respiratory alkalosis or metabolic acidosis	Nipride: *Increases cardiac output by decreasing afterload. Produces peripheral and systemic vasodilation by direct action to smooth muscles of blood vessels.* Nitroglycerin IV: *May be used to reduce excess preload, if contributing to pump failure, and to reduce afterload.* Diuretics: *Used when volume overload is contributing to pump failure.* • If intra-aortic balloon pump (IABP) is indicated, institute intra-aortic balloon pump, p 151.	

Impaired gas exchange
Related to:
Altered blood flow
Alveolar capillary membrane changes
 	
DEFINING CHARACTERISTICS
Fast, labored breathing
May have Cheyne-Stokes respirations
Rales
Tachycardia
Hypoxia
Restlessness
Confusion
	ONGOING ASSESSMENT
	• Assess rate, rhythm, depth of respiration.
	• Assess for abnormal breath sounds.
	• Assess vital signs.
	• Assess skin, nailbeds, and mucous membranes for pallor or cyanosis.
	• Assess ABGs with changes in respiratory status and 15-20 min after each adjustment in O_2 therapy *to evaluate effectiveness of O_2 therapy.*
	
	THERAPEUTIC INTERVENTIONS
	• Place patient in optimal position for ventilation. *Slightly elevated head of bed (HOB) facilitates diaphragmatic movement.*
	• Initiate O_2 therapy as prescribed.
	• See Pulmonary edema, p. 113.
	• Prepare patient for mechanical ventilation if noninvasive O_2 therapy ineffective:
	    Explain need for mechanical ventilation *to allay anxiety and gain compliance.*
	    Assist in intubation procedure.
	    Institute Mechanical ventilation, p. 213.
		Gas exchange and adequate oxygenation of body tissues will be achieved.

Fear/anxiety *Related to:* Guarded prognosis; mortality rate 80% Unfamiliar environment Dyspnea Dependence on IABP or mechanical ventilation Fear of death	**ONGOING ASSESSMENT** • Assess patient's level of anxiety. **THERAPEUTIC INTERVENTIONS** • Institute Anxiety, p. 4. *Controlling anxiety will help decrease physiologic reactions that can aggravate condition.* • Assure patient and significant others of close, continuous monitoring that will ensure prompt interventions. • Avoid unnecessary conversations between team members in front of patient. *This will reduce patient's misconceptions and fear/anxiety.* • Contact religious representative/counselor *to provide spiritual care and support, if appropriate.* • See also Spiritual distress, p. 51 and Hopelessness, p. 29.	Fear and anxiety will be reduce.

NURSING DIAGNOSES / DEFINING CHARACTERISTICS	NURSING INTERVENTIONS / *RATIONALES*	EXPECTED OUTCOMES
DEFINING CHARACTERISTICS Sympathetic stimulation Restlessness Increased awareness Increased questioning Uncooperative behavior Avoids looking at equipment or vigilant watch over equipment		
Knowledge deficit *Related to:* Disease process Prescribed therapy **DEFINING CHARACTERISTICS** Verbalization of lack of knowledge or misconceptions Questions Lack of questions	**ONGOING ASSESSMENT** • Assess patient's/significant others' level of understanding of disease process and prescribed therapy. • Assess patient's/significant others' readiness for learning. *Teaching in the acute stage may be limited to family or significant others. This will minimize their feelings of helplessness and assist them in providing support to patient.* **THERAPEUTIC INTERVENTIONS** • When appropriate, provide information about: 　Disease process and rationale for prescribed therapy. *This will help allay anxiety* 　Follow-up care • Structure teaching to allow for answering questions. • Utilize teaching aids (pamphlets, visual aids, etc.) *to facilitate learning.*	Patient/significant others will verbalize understanding of disease process and treatment.

Originated by: Salvacion P. Sulit, RN, BSN, CCRN

Chronic heart failure (class 2 and 3)

(CONGESTIVE HEART FAILURE [CHF]; CARDIOMYOPATHY; LEFT SIDED FAILURE; RIGHT SIDED FAILURE)

Heart failure is the inability of the heart to pump sufficient blood to meet the oxygen demands of the tissues. This care plan focuses on patients with chronic heart failure in New York Heart Association (NYHA) classes 2 and 3. Class 2 patients experience slight limitations in their physical activity. They can usually perform most ordinary physical activities without problem; however, they may experience fatigue, palpitations, dyspnea, or angina. Class 3 patients experience marked limitations of their activity. They are usually fairly comfortable at rest, but less than ordinary activity can cause fatigue, palpitations, dyspnea, or anginal pain. The goals of therapy for heart failure are to improve cardiac output, reduce cardiac workload, prevent complications, assess for signs of decompensation, and provide patient education.

NURSING DIAGNOSES / DEFINING CHARACTERISTICS	NURSING INTERVENTIONS / *RATIONALES*	EXPECTED OUTCOMES
Fluid volume excess *Related to:* Decreased cardiac output causing: Decreased renal perfusion, which stimulates the renin-angiotensin-aldosterone system and causes release of ADH Altered renal hemodynamics (diminished medullary blood flow), which results in decreased capacity of nephron to excrete water **DEFINING CHARACTERISTICS** Weight gain Edema Rales Jugular venous distention (JVD) Ascites Decreased urine output Development of S_3 or S_4, or murmur of tricuspid or mitral regurgitation Elevated CVP and PCWP Decreased serum albumin and serum sodium	**ONGOING ASSESSMENT** • Assess weight daily and consistently: before breakfast on the same scale, after voiding, in the same amount of clothing, without shoes. *This facilitates accurate measurement.* • Monitor for a significant (>2 lb) weight change in 1 day. • Evaluate weight in relation to nutritional status. *In some heart failure patients weight may be a poor indicator of fluid volume status. Poor nutrition and decreased appetite over time result in a decrease in weight, which may be accompanied by fluid retention though the net weight remains unchanged.* • Evaluate appropriate route of administration of medications. *Fluid volume excess in abdomen may interfere with absorption of oral medications. Oral medications may need to be given IV.* • Monitor for potential side effects of diuretics: hypokalemia, hyponatremia, hyperuricemia. *Long-term administration of spironolactone (Aldactone) may cause endocrine dysfunction. Carbohydrate intolerance may occur in patients with latent diabetes mellitus, especially if they are receiving thiazides.* • Assess for presence of edema by palpating area over tibia, ankles, feet, and sacrum. *Pitting edema is manifested by a depression that remains after one's finger is pressed over an edematous area and then removed. Grade edema 1+, indicating barely perceptible, to 4+, indicating severe. Measurement of the extremity with a measuring tape is another method of following edema.* • Auscultate breath sounds and assess for labored breathing. • Assess for JVD and ascites. Monitor abdominal girth *to follow ascites accurately.* • Monitor intake. Include items that are liquid at room temperature such as Jello, sherbet, and Popsicles. **THERAPEUTIC INTERVENTIONS** • Restrict fluid and sodium as ordered. *This will help to decrease extracellular volume.* • Give diuretics as ordered. *Weight should decline no faster than 2 lb in 1 day.* Monitor for excessive response to diuretics (>2 lb loss in 1 day) and BUN elevated out of proportion to serum creatinine level. • Instruct patient to avoid medications that may cause fluid retention, such as nonsteroidal anti-inflammatory agents, certain vasodilators, and steroids. • In preparation for discharge, instruct patient in how to weigh self and monitor intake and output at home (if indicated); emphasize that significant change in weight or fit of clothing should be reported.	Optimal fluid balance will be maintained.

Chronic heart failure—cont'd

NURSING DIAGNOSES / DEFINING CHARACTERISTICS	NURSING INTERVENTIONS / *RATIONALES*	EXPECTED OUTCOMES

Decreased cardiac output
Related to:
Increased or decreased preload
Increased afterload
Decreased contractility
Tachy- or bradyar-rhythmia
 	
DEFINING CHARACTERISTICS
Variations in hemodynamic parameters (BP, HR, neck veins, urine output)
Dizziness
Weakness/fatigue
Arrhythmias/ECG changes
Weight gain, edema, ascites
Abnormal heart sounds
Nausea, vomiting
Mental confusion
Cyanosis
Exertional dyspnea
Orthopnea
Paroxysmal nocturnal dyspnea (PND)
Decreased activity tolerance
	ONGOING ASSESSMENT
	• Assess for signs and symptoms of decreased cardiac output (see Defining Characteristics).
	• Monitor serum electrolytes *as possible causative factor for arrhythmias.*
	
	THERAPEUTIC INTERVENTIONS
	• Weigh daily and keep record of I & O. *This provides evidence of fluid retention.*
	• If increased preload is a problem, restrict fluids as ordered *to decrease extracellular fluid volume.*
	• If decreased preload is a problem, increase IV fluids and closely monitor *to increase extracellular fluid volume.*
	• Administer the following medication as ordered:
	    Diuretics *to reduce volume and enhance sodium H_2O excretion*
	    Inotropes *to improve myocardial contractility*
	    Vasodilators *to reduce preload and afterload*
	    Ace inhibitors *to decrease peripheral vascular resistance and venous tone and suppress aldosterone output*
	    Antiarrhythmics *to correct tachy- or bradyarrhythmias. Note: Frequently patients with heart failure have arrhythmias that don't respond to medical therapy. This may be a chronic problem. Some antiarrhythmics have a negative inotropic effect, which may exacerbate heart failure.*
	• If the condition becomes acute or does not respond to therapy, anticipate the need for:
	    Invasive hemodynamic monitoring
	    Intra-aortic balloon pump
	    Right or left ventricular assist device
	    Investigational medications
	    Intermittent infusions of IV inotropic medications
	    Heart transplant
		Optimal cardiac output within limits of cardiac condition is achieved.

Alteration in electrolyte balance
Related to:
Increased total body fluid (dilutes electrolyte concentration)
Decreased renal perfusion (results in greater reabsorption of sodium)
Diuretic therapy (enhances renal excretion of total body water and sodium)
Low-sodium diet
 	
DEFINING CHARACTERISTICS
Hyponatremia: Na < 136 mEq/L: may be accompanied by headache, apathy, tachycardia, and generalized weakness
	ONGOING ASSESSMENT
	• Monitor serum electrolytes per unit routine and especially in the event of large weight gain or loss.
	• Monitor fluid losses and gains.
	• Assess for presence of symptoms of electrolyte imbalance (see Defining Characteristics).
	• Assess for ECG changes.
	• Monitor digoxin level and effects in presence of hypokalemia.
	
	THERAPEUTIC INTERVENTIONS
	• For hyponatremia:
	    Encourage sodium restriction as ordered. Provide dietary instruction. *In chronic heart failure hyponatremia is dilutional; it is caused by a greater concentration of water than sodium.*
	    Administer diuretics as ordered and monitor response. *This will help restore water/sodium balance.* Monitor effectiveness of diuretics.
	    Encourage fluid restriction as ordered. Utilize ice chips, hard candy, or frozen juice sticks to quench thirst. *Restriction of intake will help maintain fragile fluid-electrolyte balance.*
	    Instruct patient to avoid salt contained in over-the-counter preparations such as antacids (Alka-Seltzer).
	• For hypokalemia (commonly caused by prolonged use of thiazide or loop diuretics):
	    Administer oral or IV supplement as ordered. Oral supplements should be given directly after meals or with food *to minimize GI irritation.*
		Electrolyte balance will be maintained.

Continued.

Chronic heart failure—cont'd

NURSING DIAGNOSES / DEFINING CHARACTERISTICS	NURSING INTERVENTIONS / *RATIONALES*	EXPECTED OUTCOMES

Hypokalemia: K < 3.8 mEq/L: may have fatigue; GI distress; increased sensitivity to digoxin; atrial and ventricular arrhythmia; ST segment depression; broad, sometimes inverted, progressively flatter T wave and enlarging U wave
 	
Hypernatremia: Na > 147 mEq/L: may be accompanied by thirst, dry mucous membranes, fever, and neurologic changes if severe
 	
Hyperkalemia: K > 5.1 mEq/L: may be accompanied by muscular weakness, diarrhea, and the following ECG changes: tall, peaked T waves; widened QRS; prolonged PR interval; decreased amplitude and disappearance of P wave; or ventricular arrhythmia
	Encourage daily intake of potassium-rich foods (raisins, bananas, cantaloupe, dates, and potatoes).
	• For hypernatremia:
	  Carefully replace water orally or IV. *Hypernatremia is commonly caused by large loss of water. Heart failure patients have a precarious fluid balance status.*
	  Anticipate reduction in diuretic dosage.
	• For nonacute *hyperkalemia:*
	  Anticipate reduction in potassium supplement.
	  Provide diet with potassium restriction as ordered.
	  Discontinue potassium sparing diuretics as ordered.
	  Instruct patient to avoid salt substitutes containing potassium.
	• In emergency situations (serum K > 6.0 mEq/L):
	  Place patient on ECG monitor.
	  Administer the following temporary measures as ordered:
	    Regular insulin and hypertonic dextrose IV: *This causes a shift of K^+ into the cells. Onset of action is 30 min and duration is several hours*
	    $NaHCO_3$: *This causes rapid movement of potassium (K^+) into the cells. The onset is within 15 min and the duration of action is 1-2 hr.*
	    Cation-exchange resins: *These reduce the serum K^+ slowly but have the advantage of actually removing K^+ from the body. Frequently they are given with one of the other measures.*
	    CaCl given IV: *Duration of action is 1 hr; immediately antagonizes the cardiac and neuromuscular toxicity of hyperkalemia.*
	    Dialysis: *An effective method of removing potassium but is reserved for situations in which more conservative measures fail.*	

Decreased activity tolerance
Related to:
Decreased cardiac output
Deconditioning
 	
DEFINING CHARACTERISTICS
Patient verbalizes feeling weak and fatigued with activity
Patient verbalizes uncertainty of ability to perform daily living activities
Abnormal HR, BP, and respiratory response to activity
	ONGOING ASSESSMENT
	• Assess patient's current level of activity.
	• Assess potential for physical injury with activity.
	• Evaluate need for O_2 during increased activity. *This may help compensate for the increased O_2 demand.*
	
	THERAPEUTIC INTERVENTIONS
	• Establish guidelines and goals of activity with patient and significant others. *Motivation is enhanced if the patient participates in goal setting.*
	• Use slow progression of patient activity *to prevent sudden increase in cardiac workload:*
	  Dangling 10-15 min tid
	  Deep breathing exercises tid
	  Active ROM exercise tid
	  Walking in room 1-2 min tid
	  Walking in hall 25 ft, then progressively increasing distances, saving energy for return trip
	• Teach appropriate use of environmental aides (e.g., bed rails, bedside commode, chair in bathroom, hall rails). *Appropriate aides will enable the patient to achieve optimal independence for self-care.*
	• Consult cardiac rehabilitation or physical therapy for assistance in increasing activity tolerance. *Specialized therapy or cardiac monitoring may be necessary when initially increasing activity.*
	• Adjust medication schedule to provide optimal times for activity. *Timing nitrate and vasodilator therapy may allow exercise without development of symptoms.*
		Optimal activity level is achieved.

Chronic heart failure—cont'd

NURSING DIAGNOSES / DEFINING CHARACTERISTICS	NURSING INTERVENTIONS / *RATIONALES*	EXPECTED OUTCOMES

	▪ Instruct patient to stop activity that causes:
	  Chest pain
	  Increased dyspnea
	  Excessive fatigue and weakness
	  Diaphoresis
	  Dizziness or syncope
	  This will minimize the potential for physical injury.
	▪ Provide emotional support while increasing activity levels *to minimize feelings of fear and anxiety.*	

Altered nutrition: less than body requirements
Related to:
Decreased appetite, nausea, GI irritability, and decreased absorption associated with:
  Decreased perfusion of GI organs
  Hepatic venous congestion
  Medication side effects
  Depression, fatigue, and dyspnea
  Dietary restrictions
 	
DEFINING CHARACTERISTICS
Calorie count less than minimal daily requirement
Observed or expressed lack of appetite or dissatisfaction with dietary restrictions
Dry weight loss (below ideal for body build and age)
Decreased serum albumin
Nausea, vomiting, diarrhea
	ONGOING ASSESSMENT
	▪ Assess eating habits and caloric intake (count).
	▪ Assess compliance with diet restrictions:
	  Knowledge level about Na, cholesterol, and fluid restrictions and dietary substitutes.
	  Ability to adhere to restrictions. *Financial resources and food shopping, storage, and preparation can affect compliance.*
	▪ Monitor weight and skin turgor.
	▪ Assess GI status:
	  Nausea and vomiting
	  Bowel activity
	  Liver function, size
	▪ Monitor serum albumin.
	▪ Assess emotional status.
	▪ Assess activity tolerance.
	
	THERAPEUTIC INTERVENTIONS
	▪ Collaborate with dietitian *to provide complete assessment and consistent teaching.*
	▪ If patient is experiencing decreased appetite and nausea, alter medication schedule when possible *to decrease gastric irritation and promote absorption (e.g., some medications better tolerated with food).*
	▪ If dietary intake is inadequate because of symptoms related to low cardiac output:
	  Administer medications ordered for decreased or increased GI motility and irritation *to provide symptomatic relief.*
	  Suggest small frequent meals with rest periods before and after *to decrease feeling of fullness (hepatic venous congestion) and to minimize fatigue associated with eating and digestion.*
	  See other interventions *to improve cardiac output and decrease fluid excess.*
	▪ Assist the patient/family in adjustment to dietary restrictions.
	▪ Provide simple written as well as verbal instructions. *Visual aids improve comprehension and retention and are a readily available reference.*
	  Include in diet teaching:
	  Reason for sodium restriction. *Increased knowledge may improve compliance.*
	  Alternate seasonings *to improve palatability of food prepared without salt. Lack of food intake may be related to absence of accustomed flavor.*
	  Foods to avoid generally (e.g., canned soup and vegetables, prepared frozen dinners, fast-food restaurant meals) and ways to recognize hidden sodium (preservatives, labels, consumer information service).
	  Knowledge may improve compliance.
	▪ Provide emotional support and understanding to patient and family. *Response to the multiple stressors of chronic illness may include depression, lack of appetite, noncompliance.*
		Optimal nutritional status will be achieved.

Continued.

NURSING DIAGNOSES / DEFINING CHARACTERISTICS	NURSING INTERVENTIONS/ *RATIONALES*	EXPECTED OUTCOMES

Anxiety/fear
Related to:
Dyspnea
Role change, loss of control, dependency caused by change in health status
Threat of death
Knowledge deficit related to diagnosis and treatment plan
 	
DEFINING CHARACTERISTICS
Restlessness
Insomnia
Increased awareness
Inability to concentrate
Poor appetite
Expressed feelings of uneasiness or fear
Tense appearance (ranges from facial expression to tremors)
Symptoms of sympathetic NS stimulation (palpitations, increased dyspnea, peripheral vasoconstriction)
	ONGOING ASSESSMENT
	• Assess for signs and symptoms of anxiety:
	  Behavioral clues: irritable, unable to sleep, unable to concentrate, poor appetite
	  Visual clues: tense facial muscles, tremors, jittery movements
	• Assess causative factors (e.g., changes in physical status, knowledge deficit, fear of death or permanent disability, loss of control).
	• Identify support systems available to patient and patient's usual coping mechanisms.
	• Evaluate response to interventions aimed at alleviating fear/anxiety.
	• Assess knowledge level and readiness to learn.
	
	THERAPEUTIC INTERVENTIONS
	• Establish relationship of trust by providing continuity of care and conveying attitude of acceptance, respect, and interest *to encourage verbalization of fears, which in itself may relieve anxiety and assist in identification of appropriate interventions.*
	• Provide calm, quiet atmosphere. *Excess stimuli increase anxiety.*
	• If dyspnea or fear of dyspnea is the problem:
	  Administer O_2 as indicated *to decrease work of breathing and sensation of increased breathlessness.*
	  Review other measures patient can take to treat or prevent occurrences.
	  Review ways patient can seek help.
	• If change in health status or role, or fear of death is identified problem, assist the patient to utilize usual coping mechanisms or explore alternate ones, enlisting support systems (social service, psychiatry, chaplain, significant other) as needed *to assist with adjustments to illness.*
	• If lack of knowledge is a cause of anxiety, offer information at level the individual is able and ready to accept. *Anxious persons may be reassured with basic information and may not be ready to concentrate on details.*
	• See also Anxiety, p. 4.
		Anxiety/fear will be reduced or relieved.

Sleep pattern disturbance
Related to:
Anxiety/fear
Physical discomfort
Medical schedule and effects
 	
DEFINING CHARACTERISTICS
Fatigue
Difficulty remaining asleep
Frequent daytime dozing
Irritability
Inability to concentrate
	ONGOING ASSESSMENT
	• Assess current sleep pattern and sleep history.
	• Assess for possible deterrents to sleep:
	  Nocturia
	  Discomfort
	  Fear of paroxysmal nocturnal dyspnea (PND)
	
	THERAPEUTIC INTERVENTIONS
	• Discourage daytime napping and increase daytime activity. *This will help the patient be tired enough to sleep at bedtime.*
	• Decrease fluid intake before bedtime *to decrease need to awaken to void.*
	• Avoid evening or bedtime diuretic. If needed, diuretic should be given early morning and afternoon.
	• Adjust medication schedule *to provide for undisturbed night, if possible.*
	• Adhere to patient's bedtime rituals *to promote relaxation.*
	• Encourage verbalization of fears.
	• Review measures patient can take in the event of chest pain, palpitations, or PND.
	• Review how patient can summon help in nighttime. *This will help relieve anxiety.*
		Adequate sleep/rest will be achieved.

Self concept disturbance *Related to:* Chronic illness that brings many losses: health, usual role, self-esteem, ability to care for self	**ONGOING ASSESSMENT** • Assess meaning of illness, hospitalization, and medical care for patient. • Note and document quality and quantity of verbalizations regarding self. • Assess and document significant others' behavior toward patient. Determine whether the behavior has changed since illness. • Assess patient's level of involvement in care. • Assess patient's short- and long-term goals.	Positive expression of continued self-worth is verbalized.

NURSING DIAGNOSES / DEFINING CHARACTERISTICS	NURSING INTERVENTIONS / *RATIONALES*	EXPECTED OUTCOMES
DEFINING CHARACTERISTICS Change in affect, appearance, and physical ability Verbalization of fear, despair, and ambivalence Decreased social activities leading to isolation	**THERAPEUTIC INTERVENTIONS** • Provide a private, nonhurried environment conducive to expression of feelings. • Assist the patient to identify changes illness has made in his/her life. • Foster independence by identifying factors patient can change and control. • Maintain patient's dignity. Do not infantilize, judge, or overlook preferences. *This will help protect self-concept.* • Encourage activities that may help the patient reach goals. • Encourage interaction with others in similar situation. *A reference group will help to establish and reinforce new role.*	

Knowledge deficit
Related to:
Unfamiliarity with pathology and treatment
Information misinterpretation
New medications
Chronicity of disease
Ineffective teaching/ learning in past
Cognitive limitation
 	
DEFINING CHARACTERISTICS
Questioning members of health care team
Denial of need to learn
Verbalizes incorrect/ inaccurate information
Development of avoidable complications
	ONGOING ASSESSMENT
	• Assess ability to learn.
	• Assess motivation and willingness of patient/significant others to learn.
	• Identify existing misconceptions regarding care.
	
	THERAPEUTIC INTERVENTIONS
	• Educate patient/significant others about the following:
	  Normal heart and circulation: *This is helpful in understanding the disease process.*
	  CHF disease process: *Knowledge of disease and disease process will promote adherence to suggested medical therapy.*
	  Factors that increase risk of progression of disease process: *Identification of risk factors enables patient to prevent or minimize their effects.*
	  Importance of adhering to therapy. *This will point out possible consequences of noncompliance and promote adherence.*
	  Symptoms to be aware of and when to report to physician. *When the patient can identify symptoms that require prompt medical attention, complications can be minimized or possibly prevented.*
	  Dietary modification to limit sodium ingestion. *Understanding rationale behind dietary restrictions may establish motivation necessary for making this adjustment in life-style.* (See previous nutrition intervention, p. 87).
	  Activity guidelines (see specific information in decreased activity tolerance guidelines, p. 86). *Providing specific information lessens uncertainty and promotes adjustment to recommended activity levels.*
	  Medications: instruct on action, use, side effects, and administration. *Prompt reporting of side effects can prevent drug-related complications*
	  Psychological aspects of chronic illness. *This will encourage patient to verbalize fears and anxiety.*
	  Overall goals of medical therapy. *This will help clarify misconceptions and may promote compliance.*
	  Community resources. *Referral may be helpful for financial and emotional support.*
	• Encourage questions from patient/significant others. *Allows verification of understanding of information given.*
	• Allow patient to maintain self-esteem. *This will promote a sense of control and self-reliance.*
	• Document progress of teaching/learning. *This will give the patient a feeling of continuity of care when being seen by other caregivers.*
		Patient/significant others will understand and verbalize causes, treatment, and follow-up care related to chronic heart failure.

Continued.

Cardiovascular Care Plans

NURSING DIAGNOSES / DEFINING CHARACTERISTICS	NURSING INTERVENTIONS/ *RATIONALES*	EXPECTED OUTCOMES
Noncompliance *Related to:* Financial (expensive therapy) Difficulty in making major life changes Complexity of treatment regimen Lack of knowledge Negative side effects of prescribed treatment Increased amount of symptoms despite previous adherence Nonsupportive family Health beliefs that conflict **DEFINING CHARACTERISTICS** Verbalization of noncompliance Multiple hospitalizations for same problem Frequent exacerbations of illness Noncompliance with medications and diet; missed appointments	**ONGOING ASSESSMENT** · Assess patient's life-style and habits. · Assess patient's willingness to be compliant. · Evaluate extent and results of previous noncompliant behavior. **THERAPEUTIC INTERVENTIONS** · Determine cause of noncompliance. Differentiate knowledge deficit or misconceptions from nonadherence for other reasons. *This will determine the appropriate method of intervention.* · Reinforce patient's need to take responsibility for managing own care. *This will encourage the patient to participate in the suggested medical regimen.* · Explore with patient alternate coping strategies. *This will help alleviate the patient's feelings of loss of control.* · Monitor and reinforce compliant behavior *to promote future compliance* · Provide written instructions whenever possible. *This will minimize the patient's feelings of being overwhelmed.* See also Knowledge deficit, p. 33. · Refer to social services department for resolution of family problems, financial difficulties, disability insurance, and coping difficulties.	Optimal compliance with treatment is achieved.

Originated by: Lorraine M. Heaney, RN
Jean M. Hughes, RN
Carol Keeler, RN, MSN

Digitalis toxicity

A condition wherein the serum digitalis level is two to three times higher than therapeutic level. The margin between therapeutic and toxic doses is relatively narrow. Patients with therapeutic levels may develop digitalis toxicity and patients with toxic levels (digoxin level over 2.5 ng/ml or digitoxin level over 20 ng/ml) may not demonstrate any manifestations of digitalis toxicity. The margin is further reduced in elderly patients and in conditions such as hypokalemia, myxedema, electrolyte imbalance, hypoxia, CHF, renal failure, and pulmonary disease.

NURSING DIAGNOSES / DEFINING CHARACTERISTICS	NURSING INTERVENTIONS / *RATIONALES*	EXPECTED OUTCOMES
Altered nutrition: less than body requirements *Related to:* GI side effects of digitalis toxicity: anorexia, nausea, vomiting, diarrhea **DEFINING CHARACTERISTICS** Complaints of nausea/ vomiting Retching Straining Vomiting Loss of appetite Documented inadequate caloric intake Weight loss	**ONGOING ASSESSMENT** - Assess for signs and symptoms of epigastric distress. - Monitor actual food intake. - Assess hydration status: skin turgor, mucous membranes, I & O, weight. - Record and report contents, color, and amount of emesis. **THERAPEUTIC INTERVENTIONS** - Administer antiemetics as ordered. - Offer small but frequent meals as tolerated. - Offer general liquid to soft diet as tolerated. - Anticipate parenteral fluid replacement if nausea and vomiting persist. - See Nutrition, altered: less than body requirements, p. 37.	Adequate nutritional intake will be maintained.
Potential decreased cardiac output *Related to:* Cardiac arrhythmia: Ventricular arrhythmia: PVCs, particularly ventricular bigeminy Ventricular tachycardia Atrial arrhythmias: Atrial tachycardia Atrial fibrillation or flutter PACs A-V conduction disturbances: First-degree A-V block Second-degree A-V block (Wenckebach phenomenon, Mobitz type II) Disturbances of sinus impulse formation: Sinus bradycardia Sinus arrest Sinoatrial block	**ONGOING ASSESSMENT** - Evaluate ECG. Determine baseline rhythm. Note and document any change in rate, rhythm, ectopy. - Provide continuous ECG monitoring as appropriate *to ensure early detection of arrhythmias.* - If arrhythmia occurs, determine hemodynamic response of patient and notify physician immediately if significant or symptomatic. - Observe for abnormalities in electrolytes. *Hypokalemia, hypomagnesia, and hypercalcemia can predispose to digitalis toxicity.* **THERAPEUTIC INTERVENTIONS** - Ensure that digitalis has been discontinued. - If arrhythmia occurs, anticipate use of any of the following medications: Diphenylhydantoin (Dilantin): useful for ventricular arrhythmias. *May improve sinoatrial and AV conduction.* Lidocaine (Xylocaine): used for ventricular ectopy. *Does not slow conduction through the A-V node or cause significant depression of myocardial function. Not effective for junctional tachycardias.* Propranolol (Inderal): *its antiadrenergic activity is useful for decreasing automaticity, such as atrial tachycardia and some ventricular arrhythmias.* Quinidine and procainamide: *useful for decreasing ventricular automaticity.* Digibind: Digoxin immune Fab (OVINE) indicated for life-threatening arrhythmias, such as ventricular tachycardia or ventricular fibrillation, or bradyarrhythmias such as severe sinus bradycardia or second- or third-degree heart block not responsive to atropine.	Optimal cardiac rhythm and hemodynamic status will be maintained.

Continued.

Digitalis toxicity—cont'd

NURSING DIAGNOSES / DEFINING CHARACTERISTICS	NURSING INTERVENTIONS / *RATIONALES*	EXPECTED OUTCOMES
DEFINING CHARACTERISTICS Signs of hemodynamic compromise (hypotension, syncope, pallor, sweating, cold clammy skin, fatigue, weakness, confusion, restlessness, decrease in urine output)	• Anticipate use of external pacemaker. *In rare cases of high-degree or complete A-V block, especially when the underlying rhythm is atrial fibrillation, a temporary pacer may be required.*	

Knowledge deficit
Related to:
Unfamiliarity with therapeutic regimen
 	
DEFINING CHARACTERISTICS
Inability to describe therapeutic regimen
Verbalization of misconceptions
Noncompliance
	ONGOING ASSESSMENT
	• Assess current knowledge base of patient/significant others.
	• Assess readiness, motivation, and interest in health/illness status.
	
	THERAPEUTIC INTERVENTIONS
	• Instruct patient/significant others about:
	    Purpose of digitalis therapy
	    Dosage, frequency, administration, actions
	    Side effects and toxic manifestations of digitalis:
	        GI symptoms: anorexia, nausea, vomiting, diarrhea
	        CNS symptoms: drowsiness, mental confusion, color vision (green or yellow) with halos
	        Cardiac effects: skipped heart beats, irregular pulse, increased or decreased heart beat
	    Pulse taking
	• Utilize informational sources such as pamphlets, time schedule of medications, or medication charts.
		Patient and significant others will verbalize/demonstrate understanding of digitalis therapy.

Originated by: Beth Manglal-Lan, RN, BSN

Endocarditis

(INFECTIVE ENDOCARDITIS, SUBACUTE
BACTERIAL ENDOCARDITIS [SBE],
PROSTHETIC VALVE ENDOCARDITIS [PVE])

An inflammatory process that affects the heart's inner lining and usually the valves. Ineffective endocarditis usually is caused by direct invasion of bacteria such as streptococci, pneumococci, and staphylococci. However, gram-negative bacilli and fungi may also be the causative agent. Persons at risk for developing endocarditis include patients with history of valve disease who undergo dental, genitourinary, surgical, or other invasive procedure; patients with prosthetic valves; immunosuppressed patients; IV drug users; patients with mitral valve prolapse or dialysis shunts. Common complications include congestive heart failure and arterial embolization of endocardial vegetations.

NURSING DIAGNOSES / DEFINING CHARACTERISTICS	NURSING INTERVENTIONS / *RATIONALES*	EXPECTED OUTCOMES

Hyperthermia
Related to:
Bacteremia
 	
DEFINING CHARACTERISTICS
Increase in body temperature >98.6° F
Tachycardia
Malaise
Chills
Positive blood cultures
Elevated WBC
	ONGOING ASSESSMENT
	• Assess patient's description of illness, including:
	  Possible port of entry (i.e., dental work, genitourinary instrumentation, cardiac surgery, prosthetic valve, IV drug use)
	  Chills
	  Night sweats
	• Assess vital signs.
	• Monitor blood culture reports *to evaluate adequacy of antibiotic therapy.* Obtain three sets of blood cultures at least 1 hr apart as ordered *to determine etiology of infection.*
	• Monitor WBC.
	• Continue to monitor temperature q4h. *Continued fever may be caused by: drug allergy, drug-resistant bacteria, superinfection.*
	
	THERAPEUTIC INTERVENTIONS
	• Use appropriate therapy for elevated temperature: antipyretics, cold therapy.
	• Administer prescribed antibiotic agent(s) as ordered *to suppress invading organisms.*
	• See Hyperthermia, p. 31.
		Normal body temperature will be maintained.

Potential decreased cardiac output *Related to:* Damage to valve leaflets resulting in valvular insufficiency **DEFINING CHARACTERISTICS** Rales Dyspnea New onset or change in heart murmur Low urine output Decreased BP Slow capillary refill Jugular venous distention Change in mental status	**ONGOING ASSESSMENT** • Assess respirations every shift and prn. for rate, depth, quality, and use of accessory muscles. • Auscultate lungs every shift and prn for rales and wheezes; report/record changes. *Valvular damage resulting in signs of congestive heart failure may be a complication.* • Assess heart rate, rhythm, BP, presence of murmur. Record and report changes. • Monitor fluid balance closely (I & O, weight gain, jugular venous distention, edema). • Assess for restlessness, fatigue, change in mental status. • Monitor ABGs. **THERAPEUTIC INTERVENTIONS** If signs of valvular insufficiency occur: • Initiate O₂ therapy as needed. • See Cardiac output, decreased, p. 9. • Anticipate need for valve replacement if hemodynamic status does not improve.	Adequate cardiac output will be maintained.

Continued.

Endocarditis—cont'd

NURSING DIAGNOSES / DEFINING CHARACTERISTICS	NURSING INTERVENTIONS / *RATIONALES*	EXPECTED OUTCOMES
Potential for injury *Related to:* Long-term antibiotic therapy **DEFINING CHARACTERISTICS** Skin rash, urticaria Decreased urine output Elevated BUN and creatinine Hearing loss	**ONGOING ASSESSMENT** • Assess drug level. Obtain peak and trough levels as ordered and report *to ensure therapeutic levels and prevent potential negative outcomes.* • Observe for signs of hypersensitivity (i.e., skin rash). • Assess renal function (I & O, BUN, and creatinine). *Many antibiotics are nephrotoxic.* • Assess hearing changes. **THERAPEUTIC INTERVENTIONS** • If skin rash develops, stop use of drug and report immediately. • Assist patient to maintain a well-hydrated state. • Notify physician of any loss of hearing. *Ototoxicity is a risk of garamycin therapy.*	Complications of antibiotic therapy will be reduced.
Potential alteration in tissue perfusion *Related to:* Emboli from infective vegetations in the heart **DEFINING CHARACTERISTICS** Arthralgia Myalgia Petechiae Splinter hemorrhages Osler nodes Abdominal pain Decreased urine output Change in mental status Shortness of breath (SOB)	**ONGOING ASSESSMENT** • Assess for pulmonary embolus: rate, depth, quality, use of accessory muscles, and change in breath sounds. • Assess for mesenteric ischemia: auscultate bowel sounds and evaluate for abdominal tenderness. • Assess for renal ischemia: I & O, hematest urine every shift, urine specific gravity q4h. • Assess for peripheral embolization: petechiae, splinter hemorrhages in nail beds, Osler nodes (painful red nodes on pads of fingers and toes). • Assess for embolization to joints: ROM, joint tenderness. *Vegetations frequently migrate to other organs and tissues.* **THERAPEUTIC INTERVENTIONS** • If signs and symptoms of embolization and decreased tissue perfusion occur, record and report to physician. • See (as indicated): Thromboembolism, p. 188.	Optimal perfusion to tissues will be maintained.

Knowledge deficit
Related to:
Requires information for self-management secondary to new condition
 	
DEFINING CHARACTERISTICS
Questioning
Verbalized misconceptions
Lack of questions
	ONGOING ASSESSMENT
	• Assess level of understanding of disease.
	• Assess physical/emotional readiness for learning by patient/significant others.
	
	THERAPEUTIC INTERVENTIONS
	• Establish good rapport with patient/significant others.
	• Encourage patient/significant others to ask questions and verbalize concerns
	• Provide information on the following:
	    Basic cardiac anatomy and physiology with attention to valve structure and function
	    Sources and prevention of infection/bacteremia
	    Signs and symptoms of infection/bacteremia
	• Discuss the purpose and method of administration of antibiotic agent(s).
	• Provide information on the side effects of antibiotic agent(s). Encourage patient to seek prompt medical attention if side effects occur.
	• Educate patient to inform all physicians and dentists of history of infective endocarditis. *Previous episode of infective endocarditis increases risk of subsequent episodes.*
	• Provide wallet card from American Heart Association outlining recommended prophylaxis. Refer to cardiac clinical nurse specialist or cardiologist for assistance.
	• Document teaching.
		Patient will understand causes, treatment, and follow-up care.

Originated by: Carol Ruback, RN, MSN, CCRN

Hypertension

(HIGH BLOOD PRESSURE, INCREASED SYSTEMIC PRESSURE)

Sustained elevation of arterial blood pressure above the normal upper limit of 140/90 or 20 points above that considered normal for one's age. This care plan focuses on patients with mild to moderate hypertension.

NURSING DIAGNOSES / DEFINING CHARACTERISTICS	NURSING INTERVENTIONS / *RATIONALES*	EXPECTED OUTCOMES
Decreased cardiopulmonary, renal, cerebral, or peripheral tissue perfusion *Related to:* Diminished blood flow caused by increased vascular resistance Hypervolemia **DEFINING CHARACTERISTICS** Tachypnea Labored respiration Adventitious breath sounds Angina, palpitation Urine output less than 30 ml/hr Increasing BUN/creatinine Hematuria or proteinuria Mental status changes Restlessness/agitation/apathy Cool, clammy skin Pallor, cyanosis Mottled skin Decreased/absent peripheral pulse	**ONGOING ASSESSMENT** · Assess for evidence of decreased tissue perfusion as outlined in defining characteristics every 2-4 hr or more often as appropriate. · Assess vital signs every 2-4 hr or more often as appropriate. Use proper BP equipment with cuff bladder that is two–thirds limb diameter *to ensure accurate measurements.* · Assess breath sounds and heart sounds every 4 hr to detect changes from baseline that indicate changes in cardiopulmonary status. · Assess and record I & O and daily weight. · Document findings and notify physician of untoward change(s). · Monitor and document effectiveness of medications. · Monitor for side effects of medications (e.g., hypokalemia, hypovolemia). **THERAPEUTIC INTERVENTIONS** · Implement measures to reduce vascular resistance and improve tissue perfusion: Give antihypertensive drugs, diuretics as ordered. Discourage intake of coffee, tea, colas, and chocolate, which are high in caffeine. *Caffeine stimulates sympathetic nervous system.* Discourage smoking, *which causes vasoconstriction and contributes to decreased tissue oxygenation by reducing oxygen availability.* Maintain physical and emotional rest. *Administer sedative prn to reduce stress and associated vasoconstriction.* Maintain fluid and dietary sodium restrictions *to reduce fluid retention, which contributes to hypertension.* · Assure adequate fluid intake unless contraindicated. *Volume depletion enhances potency of antihypertensive drugs and also reduces perfusion to kidneys.*	Adequate tissue perfusion will be maintained or attained.
Knowledge deficit: Nature of and complications of hypertension; management regimen *Related to:* Cognitive limitation Lack of interest Lack of information **DEFINING CHARACTERISTICS** Statement of misconceptions, knowledge gaps Request for information	**ONGOING ASSESSMENT** · Assess patient's and family's level of knowledge of disease and prescribed management. · Assess readiness for learning. **THERAPEUTIC INTERVENTIONS** · Encourage questions about disease and prescribed treatments. · Involve family or significant others *so they can effectively provide support upon discharge.* · Plan teaching in stages, considering patient/family readiness. Provide information in terms that patient and family can understand by using appropriate teaching aids in the following areas: Nature of disease and its effect on target organs (i.e., renal damage, visual impairment, heart failure, stroke) Risk factors (obesity, diet high in unsaturated fat and cholesterol, smoking, stress) Rationale for weight reduction (if overweight) and low-salt diet Possible side effects of medications Interaction with over-the-counter drugs such as cough and cold medicines and aspirin compounds, *which have vasoconstricting effect*	Verbalizes understanding of the disease and its long-term effects on target organs.

Continued.

Hypertension—cont'd

NURSING DIAGNOSES / DEFINING CHARACTERISTICS	NURSING INTERVENTIONS / *RATIONALES*	EXPECTED OUTCOMES
	Avoidance of alcoholic drinks within 3 hr of medication *because of vasodilating effect, possible contribution to orthostatic hypotension*	

Encourage potassium-rich foods (e.g., fruit juices, bananas) as appropriate. *Most diuretics are potassium wasting.*

Teach relaxation techniques to combat stress, *which can influence physiologic responses that aggregate hypertension.*

Role of physical exercise in weight reduction

Safety measures to observe:

    Avoid sudden changes in position to *reduce severity of orthostatic hypotension.*

    Avoid hot tubs and saunas *which cause vasodilation and potential hypotension.*

    Avoid prolonged standing *which can cause venous pooling.*

Signs and symptoms to report to physician:

    Chest pain

    Shortness of breath

    Edema

    Weight gain

    Nose bleeds

    Changes in vision

    Headaches, dizziness

- Instruct patient to take own blood pressure, *to provide patient with sense of control and ability to seek prompt medical attention.*
- Assist in establishing medication routine considering his/her work and sleep habits. *This will minimize the chance of error and potentiate better compliance with therapy.*
- Instruct patient on use of sedatives and tranquilizers if prescribed *to assist patient in coping with situational stress.*
- Provide information about community resources and support groups *that can assist and support patient in changing life-style* (e.g., American Heart Association, weight loss programs, stop smoking programs).

NURSING DIAGNOSES / DEFINING CHARACTERISTICS	NURSING INTERVENTIONS / *RATIONALES*	EXPECTED OUTCOMES
Altered nutrition: more than body requirement *Related to:* Excessive intake in relation to metabolic needs resulting in overweight or obesity High sodium intake which promotes fluid retention, weight gain, and hypertension	**ONGOING ASSESSMENT** • Assess patient and family attitudes toward food and salt. • Assess patient's need for psychological support in his/her effort to reduce weight and/or sodium intake. • Weigh daily and record. Notify physician of weight gain. **THERAPEUTIC INTERVENTIONS** • Implement prescribed reducing, no-added-salt diet. *Excess caloric intake and sodium intake result in obesity and fluid retention, respectively: both predispose to hypertension and subsequent complications.* • Communicate with dietitian regarding patient's likes and dislikes and cultural preferences. • Support and reinforce patient effort to adhere to prescribed diet.	Ideal body weight and nutritional status will be attained or maintained.
DEFINING CHARACTERISTICS Overweight (10% over ideal weight for height and frame) Obesity (20% over ideal weight for height and frame) Edema Weight gain		

NURSING DIAGNOSES / DEFINING CHARACTERISTICS	NURSING INTERVENTIONS / *RATIONALES*	EXPECTED OUTCOMES
Potential discomfort: headache and dizziness *Related to:* Headache caused by increased arterial vascular pressure, which causes arterioles to dilate and exert pressure on surrounding tissues Dizziness caused by hypotensive state related to drug therapy **DEFINING CHARACTERISTICS** Complaints of occipital headache, usually on waking Restlessness or irritability Facial mask of discomfort Complaints of dizziness or lightheadedness	**ONGOING ASSESSMENT** · Assess for nonverbal signs of discomfort. · Assess occurrence, quality, severity, and location of headache. · Assess precipitating and relieving factors. **THERAPEUTIC INTERVENTIONS** · Administer analgesics as ordered. Patient may also need sedative or tranquilizer as adjunct *to reduce stress and discomfort.* · Minimize environmental stimuli. Restrict visitors if necessary. *Stress and anxiety can increase perception of pain and discomfort.* · Encourage relaxation techniques (deep breathing exercise, imagery, etc.). · Assist with ambulation if necessary *to prevent patient from falling if dizziness occurs. Dizziness is associated with both hypertension, and hypotension secondary to drug therapy.* · Elevate head of bed 30 degrees to minimize changes in position *that can trigger dizziness or lightheadedness.* · Change position slowly. Sit before standing up from a lying position *to allow the body to adapt to redistribution of blood.*	Maximum level of comfort will be maintained.
Noncompliance *Related to:* Financial constraints Difficulty in making life-style changes Lack of knowledge Negative side effects of prescribed treatment **DEFINING CHARACTERISTICS** Verbalized noncompliance Elevated blood pressure Evidence of development of complications (i.e., renal failure, visual impairment, heart failure, stroke) Evidence of exacerbation of symptoms (i.e., hypertensive crisis) Failure to keep appointments	**ONGOING ASSESSMENT** · Assess patient's life-style and habits. · Assess patient's willingness to be compliant. · Assess previous patterns of compliant/noncompliant behavior. **THERAPEUTIC INTERVENTIONS** · If noncompliance is a problem, determine the cause, *for this will dictate the appropriate method of intervention.* If knowledge deficit, see Knowledge deficit, p. 33. If financial constraints, refer to social services department. If negative side effects of prescribed treatment, explain that many side effects can be controlled or eliminated. If lack of adequate support in changing life-style, initiate referral to support group (e.g., American Heart Association, weight loss programs, stop smoking programs, stress management classes, social services). · Instruct patient to take own blood pressure, *which will provide patient with immediate feedback and a sense of control.* · Reinforce compliant behavior *to promote future compliance.* · Include significant others in explanations and teaching *to encourage their support and assistance in patient's compliance.*	Optimal compliance with treatment is achieved.

Originated by: Salvacion P. Sulit, RN, BSN, CCRN

Hypertensive crisis

(ACCELERATED HYPERTENSION; MALIGNANT
HYPERTENSION; PHEOCHROMOCYTOMA)

A systolic blood pressure >200 mm Hg and/or a diastolic blood pressure >120 mm Hg, associated with signs and symptoms of end-organ damage such as renal failure, retinal hemorrhage, intracranial bleed, and/or encephalopathy. Common treatment uses nitroprusside (Nipride) drug therapy because of its short half-life and fast response.

NURSING DIAGNOSES / DEFINING CHARACTERISTICS	NURSING INTERVENTIONS / *RATIONALES*	EXPECTED OUTCOMES

Potential injury
Related to:
Complication of nitroprusside therapy
 	
DEFINING CHARACTERISTICS
Mild/severe hypotension
Thiocyanate accumulation: blurred vision, delirium, hypothyroidism, convulsions, metabolic acidosis
	ONGOING ASSESSMENT
	• Assess vital signs closely, continuously monitoring BP while titrating nitroprusside.
	• Monitor thiocyanate levels q72h as appropriate. Discontinue if level is increased to 10 mg/100 ml and notify physician. *Nitroprusside is converted to thiocyanate when it is metabolized.*
	
	THERAPEUTIC INTERVENTIONS
	• Administer an IV infusion of nitroprusside, using an infusion pump *for reliable dosing:*
	  Dose: 0.5 to 10 μg/kg/min.
	  Change solution every 24 hr.
	  Maintain separate IV line for nitroprusside *because of incompatibility with other medications.*
	  Cover infusion container with opaque material *because nitroprusside is light-sensitive.*
	• Maintain a constant infusion rate of main IV line while nitroprusside via piggyback is infusing *to prevent patient from receiving bolus of nitroprusside.*
	• Titrate nitroprusside to maintain prescribed BP range. If hypotension occurs, stop nitroprusside immediately, notify physician, and lower head of bed to flat or Trendelenburg's position *to increase venous return.*
		Complications of nitroprusside therapy will be decreased.

Potential decreased cardiac output
Related to:
Increased afterload secondary to vasoconstriction
 	
DEFINING CHARACTERISTICS
Variations in hemodynamic parameters: heart rate, CVP, pulmonary wedge pressure, urine output
Rales, tachypnea, dyspnea, cough, abnormal ABGs, frothy sputum
Weight gain, edema
Anxiety, restlessness
Syncope, dizziness
	ONGOING ASSESSMENT
	• Assess for signs of decreased cardiac output.
	• Monitor and record respiratory rate, heart rate, and BP every hour until stable.
	• Monitor and record I & O every hour.
	• Weigh daily and record *to monitor fluid status.*
	
	THERAPEUTIC INTERVENTIONS
	• See Cardiac output, decreased (as appropriate), p. 9.
	• Administer and adjust medications as ordered to maintain BP within prescribed parameters:
	  Systolic: _____
	  Diastolic: _____
	  Mean arterial pressure: _____
	  Note: Notify physician if BP is above or below these parameters.
		Optimal cardiac output will be maintained.

Altered level of consciousness *Related to:* Encephalopathy Cerebral vascular accident	**ONGOING ASSESSMENT** • Assess for signs and symptoms of alteration in level of consciousness/responsiveness. **THERAPEUTIC INTERVENTIONS** • Maintain head of bed at 30 degree elevation *to reduce intracranial pressure.* • Maintain on complete bed rest; instruct patient to change positions gradually.	Optimal state of consciousness will be maintained.

NURSING DIAGNOSES / DEFINING CHARACTERISTICS	NURSING INTERVENTIONS / *RATIONALES*	EXPECTED OUTCOMES

DEFINING CHARACTERISTICS
 	
Change in alertness, orientation, verbal response, eye opening, motor response, pupillary reaction
Memory impairment
Impaired judgment
Agitation
Inappropriate affect
Impaired thought process
Blurred vision
Focal motor weakness
	• Explain to patient the necessity of avoiding Valsalva maneuver *to prevent potential increases in intracranial pressure:*
	    Stress importance of exhaling when patient is being positioned.
	    Provide stool softener as ordered.
	• Keep oral airway at bedside; be prepared to protect patient if seizures occur.
	• Keep side rails up at all times, bed in low position, a functioning call light within reach.
	• Reorient patient to environment as needed.
	• If restraints are needed, position patient on side, never on back, *to prevent aspiration.*
	• If an alteration in level of consciousness is present, see Consciousness, alteration in level of, p. 216.	

Potential for injury: renal function alteration
Related to:
Increased systemic BP
Hypotension secondary to drug therapy
 	
DEFINING CHARACTERISTICS
Urine output <400-600 ml/24 hr
Elevated serum BUN, potassium, creatinine, phosphorus levels
Low serum calcium level
	ONGOING ASSESSMENT
	• Assess, monitor, and document:
	    I & O every hour
	    Daily weights
	    Serum BUN, creatinine, and uric acid levels
	    Urine specific gravity every 4 hr
	    Urinalysis
	• Notify physician of abnormal findings.
	
	THERAPEUTIC INTERVENTIONS
	• Administer diuretics/fluids as ordered.
	• See Renal failure, acute (as appropriate), p. 314.
		Absence of signs and symptoms of renal failure.

Discomfort
Related to:
Increased intracranial pressure
 	
DEFINING CHARACTERISTICS
Headache
Dizziness
Nausea, vomiting
Restlessness
	ONGOING ASSESSMENT
	• Solicit patient's description of discomfort factors, documenting in patient's own words.
	
	THERAPEUTIC INTERVENTIONS
	• Provide rest periods *to facilitate comfort, sleep, relaxation.*
	• Provide quiet environment. Keep lights low, noise minimal. Limit visitors.
	• Give medications (e.g., acetaminophen [Tylenol]), prochlorperazine [Compazine]) as ordered, evaluating effectiveness and observing for any untoward effects.
	• Use any additional comfort measures whenever appropriate:
	    Position of comfort
	    Positive suggestion
	    Reassurance and contact
	• Notify physician if interventions are unsuccessful or if current complaint is a significant change.
		Discomfort will be reduced.

Knowledge deficit
Related to
Unfamiliarity with disease process, treatment, and procedures
	ONGOING ASSESSMENT
	• Solicit patient's description and understanding of:
	    Precipitating events
	    Disease process
	    Treatment and procedures
		Patient/significant others will verbalize a basic understanding of the disease process, procedures, and treatment.

Continued.

■ **Hypertensive crisis—cont'd**

NURSING DIAGNOSES / DEFINING CHARACTERISTICS	NURSING INTERVENTIONS / *RATIONALES*	EXPECTED OUTCOMES

DEFINING CHARACTERISTICS
 Noncompliance with medications, diet, follow-up care, preventive measures
 Verbalizes lack of knowledge, asks questions about hypertension
	THERAPEUTIC INTERVENTIONS
	 • *To enhance compliance with therapy,* explain to patient/significant others:
	 Disease process:
	   Signs and symptoms of recurrence or progression (headache, diplopia, weakness, faintness, nausea)
	   Possible complications
	 Treatment and procedures:
	   Importance of decreasing or maintaining stable weight
	   Importance of low-fat, low-salt diet
	   Importance of maintaining proper fluid intake and observing limitations, such as caffeinated coffee, tea, and alcohol
	   Importance of knowing medications, dosages, and times
	   Importance of follow-up appointments	

Originated by: Nola D. Johnson, RN
                Carol Ruback, RN, MSN, CCRN

Mitral valve prolapse (MVP)

(BARLOW'S DISEASE; FLOPPY VALVE)

The mitral valve rests between the left atrium and ventricle. Prolapse of this valve refers to the upward movement of the mitral leaflets back into the left atrium during systole. Primary MVP usually results from abnormality in the connective tissue of the leaflets, annulus, or chordae tendinae and occurs in about 5% of the general population. Secondary causes of mitral valve prolapse include rheumatic fever, cardiomyopathy, and ischemic heart disease. Most persons with primary MVP are asymptomatic, though others may experience incapacitating symptoms: chest pain, palpitations, dizziness, fatigue, dyspnea, and anxiety. Diagnostic findings include midsystolic click, late systolic murmur, ECG and echocardiogram abnormalities, and angiographic findings.

NURSING DIAGNOSES / DEFINING CHARACTERISTICS	NURSING INTERVENTIONS / *RATIONALES*	EXPECTED OUTCOMES

Knowledge deficit
 Related to:
 Unfamiliarity with disease process, treatment, recovery
 	
 DEFINING CHARACTERISTICS
 Asking multiple questions
 Expressing fears
 Being overly anxious
 Asking no questions
 Verbalizing misconceptions
	ONGOING ASSESSMENT
	 • Assess patient's/significant others' knowledge of MVP.
	 • Assess readiness to learn.
	 • Assess emotional and psychological needs.
	
	 THERAPEUTIC INTERVENTIONS
	 • Teach patient about occurrence of disease: fairly common; large number of undiagnosed, asymptomatic people in general population. Common in women but also diagnosed in men.
	 • Teach patient about causative factors *to increase understanding of disease process:*
	   Etiology usually unknown
	   Can be primary or secondary to previous ischemic heart disease, rheumatic fever, cardiomyopathy, or ruptured chordae tendinae
	   Important to understand that serious heart disease is usually not present, that symptoms are more a nuisance than significant, and that prognosis for life is excellent
	 • Teach patient the physiology of the disease: prolapse of one or both valve leaflets into the left atrium.
		Patient/significant others will verbalize understanding of occurrence of disease, causative factors, physiology of disease, diagnostic procedure, treatment, and complications

NURSING DIAGNOSES / DEFINING CHARACTERISTICS	NURSING INTERVENTIONS / *RATIONALES*	EXPECTED OUTCOMES

	• Inform patient of usual diagnostic procedures *to prepare for testing and to decrease anxiety:*
	    Cardiac auscultation for murmur or click
	    Echocardiogram to evaluate valve motion
	• Teach patient about the treatment of the disease:
	    Usually no treatment is indicated. *Patients need reassurance that this is not a severe cardiac condition*
	    Avoidance of stimulation of catecholamine release if patient experiences chest pain or arrhythmias
	    Use of exercise *to reduce anxiety over condition and increase self-esteem*
	    β-blocker or calcium channel blocker medication *to reduce chest pain and control arrhythmias (if complication)*
	    Self-limitation of activities and stresses that precipitate symptoms
	• Teach patient about controversial use of prophylaxis for infective subacute bacterial endocarditis.
	    It is felt that many common invasive procedures will leave a pathway in which bacteria can travel to the heart.
	    Patient should contact physician for prophylactic antibiotics before any dental procedures (especially teeth cleaning), gynecologic procedures, or other invasive procedures).
	• Teach patient about possible, though often rare, complications of the disease:
	    Arrhythmia
	    Chest pain
	    Endocarditis
	    Progressive mitral regurgitation leading to congestive heart failure
	    Systemic emboli from platelets and fibrin deposits that collect on the leaflets	

Potential body image disturbance *Related to:* Knowledge of "cardiac" condition Fatigue secondary to beta blocker medication Need for prophylactic antibiotics **DEFINING CHARACTERISTICS** Verbalized feelings about "heart" and altered life-style Preoccupation with heart Inappropriate concerns over self and prognosis	**ONGOING ASSESSMENT** • Assess perception of change in body function and meaning of illness and medical care to patient. • Assess perceived impact of changes. • Note verbal references to heart and related discomfort and any change in life-style. **THERAPEUTIC INTERVENTIONS** • Provide accurate information about causes, prognosis, and treatment of condition. *Many patients have anxiety when diagnosed with a heart disease they and most people know little about.* • Provide reassurance that it is possible to lead a "normal life" with MVP. • For problems with fatigue, encourage patient to allow several weeks for adjustment to β-blocker side effects. • Encourage appropriate pacing of daily activities *to reduce fatigue*. • Provide emotional support when increasing activity. • Remind patient that though risk of bacterial endocarditis is small, appropriate prophylaxis may be warranted and should reduce further anxiety. • For female patients of childbearing years, instruct that pregnancy is usually not contraindicated. • See also Body image disturbance, p. 6.	Positive feelings about altered heart function will be acknowledged.

Continued.

■ **Mitral valve prolapse—cont'd**

NURSING DIAGNOSES / DEFINING CHARACTERISTICS	NURSING INTERVENTIONS / *RATIONALES*	EXPECTED OUTCOMES
Chest pain *Related to:* The etiology of pain is uncertain but may be related to excessive stretch of chordae tendinae and papillary muscles **DEFINING CHARACTERISTICS** Complaint of chest pain that is nonanginal in character May last seconds to several hours Typically left precordial, sharp, stabbing May be substernal or diffuse Usually not specifically related to exertion or stress Usually not relieved by nitroglycerin (NTG) May present with inverted T waves and ST depression associated with exercise Restlessness Irritability Facial mask of pain	**ONGOING ASSESSMENT** • Note, record, and report type, location, intensity, and length of occurrence of chest pain. Ascertain whether pain is related to exertion, eating, or stress conditions. *Patients with MPV can have a variety of types of chest pain, some of which can mimic angina. Primary MVP does not involve pathology of coronary arteries. However, some patients with MVP may also have unrelated but additional problem of coronary spasm causing angina.* • Assess cardiac status: Note pulse rate, rhythm, and volume. Note BP. Check skin color, temperature, moisture, perfusion. Obtain ECG if indicated. **THERAPEUTIC INTERVENTIONS** • Permit unrestricted activity if patient is asymptomatic. • Encourage rest if pain is exertionally induced. • Provide nonstressful environment. • Provide psychological and emotional support *to allay fears of the seriousness of this benign disease.* • Provide relief of atypical chest pain by administering medications as ordered: β-blockers Calcium channel blockers • Instruct patient about positions that may reduce chest pain *by increasing venous return and lessening prolapse:* Lying down Squatting	Chest pain will be reduced or resolved.
Potential decreased cardiac output *Related to:* Altered cardiac rate and rhythm, specifically paroxysmal tachycardia **DEFINING CHARACTERISTICS** Palpitations (sudden, rapid, regular fluttering sensation in the chest) Faintness, lightheadedness Weakness Shortness of breath Rapid pulse ECG abnormalities Decreased blood pressure	**ONGOING ASSESSMENT** • Assess reports of palpitations, noting precipitating and relieving factors. *Stimulants such as caffeine, cigarettes, stress, and activity may increase occurrence of arrhythmias.* • Evaluate hemodynamic response to arrhythmias: Pulse rate, rhythm and volume BP Respiratory rate, quality **THERAPEUTIC INTERVENTIONS** • Provide reassurance that arrhythmias are usually benign in nature. • Administer medications as ordered. β-*blockers are usually the drug of choice.* • Instruct patient in avoidance of catecholamine stimulants. • Encourage exercise program as appropriate *to decrease sympathetic tone.*	Optimal cardiac output will be maintained.

Originated by: Marilyn Rousseau, RN
              Barbara Gallagher, RN, BSN

Myocardial infarction: acute phase (1 to 3 days)

(CORONARY THROMBOSIS; "CORONARY" OR "HEART ATTACK;" MI)

Acute myocardial infarction is a destructive process that produces irreversible tissue damage to regions of the heart muscle. It is caused by profound and sustained ischemia related to atherosclerotic narrowing of the coronary artery, spasm to the artery, thrombus formation, or any combination of each. This care plan focuses on the acute phase during hospitalization in the coronary care unit.

NURSING DIAGNOSES / DEFINING CHARACTERISTICS	NURSING INTERVENTIONS / *RATIONALES*	EXPECTED OUTCOMES

Chest pain
Related to:
Myocardial ischemia/ myocardial infarction (MI)
Reduced coronary blood flow
Inadequate myocardial perfusion
 	
DEFINING CHARACTERISTICS
Patient report and verbalizations of pain
Restlessness, apprehension
Moaning, crying
Facial mask of pain
Diaphoresis
Change in vital signs: BP, heart rate, respiratory rate
Pallor, weakness
Nausea and vomiting
Fear and guarding behavior
	ONGOING ASSESSMENT
	Assess for characteristics of myocardial pain:
	• Quality
	  Choking, squeezing, aching, "viselike"
	  Intense pressure with heaviness
	  Burning
	  Other
	• Severity: scale 1-10 (10 most severe)
	• Onset: sudden/constant
	• Duration
	  At least 20 min; usually 1-2 hr
	  Residual soreness 1-3 days
	  Pain could be intermittent
	• Location
	  Anterior chest, usually substernal
	  May radiate to shoulder, arms, jaw, neck, and epigastrium
	• Precipitating factors:
	  Physical or emotional exertion
	  May occur at rest
	• Other characteristics:
	  Not relieved with rest or nitrates
	  Not affected by position change or breathing
	  May be associated with nausea and vomiting, dyspnea, anxiety, diaphoresis, fatigue
	
	THERAPEUTIC INTERVENTIONS
	General
	• Maintain bed rest, at least during periods of pain *to reduce workload of the heart.*
	• Position patient comfortably, preferably Fowler's position, *which allows for full lung expansion by lowering the diaphragm.*
	• Maintain a quiet, relaxed atmosphere; display confident manner. *Physical and emotional rest is promoted in such a setting.*
	• Allow rest periods for relaxation/sleep.
	• Offer emotional support in terms of positive reinforcements and encouragements *to help the patient cope and manage the emotional stress that accompanies an acute MI, thereby reducing risk of complications.*
	• If patient complains of pain:
	  Report immediately to physician *for prompt treatment.*
	  Assess ECG immediately *to note changes.*
	  Monitor vital signs.
	  Administer O$_2$ per order *to increase O$_2$ supply.*
	  Institute medical therapy per order (see specific interventions that follow).
	  Reassess response to interventions.
	Specific
	• Administer morphine sulfate as ordered per unit protocol. *Morphine sulfate is a narcotic analgesic that reduces the workload on the heart through vasodilation. It provides sedation and decreases patient's perception of pain.*
	  Monitor vital signs; note changes after morphine (hypotension; bradycardia).
	  Administer IV morphine at increments of 2-5 mg over 5 min.
		Prompt relief of chest pain.

Continued.

NURSING DIAGNOSES / DEFINING CHARACTERISTICS	NURSING INTERVENTIONS / *RATIONALES*	EXPECTED OUTCOMES

	Repeat dose until pain is relieved or a total of 10 mg has been given if vital signs are stable.
	Monitor closely for side effects of morphine:
	    Hypotension
	    Decreased respirations
	    Bradycardia
	    Nausea
	Have naloxone (Narcan) on standby *to reverse effect of morphine as needed.*
	• Initiate IV nitrates as ordered per unit protocol. *Nitrates cause vasodilation and reduce workload of heart by decreasing venous return. Nitrates also dilate the coronary vessels, thus increasing the blood flow and O_2 supply to the myocardium.*
	    Monitor BP and heart rate before beginning medication *to document baseline parameters.* BP should be at least 100/70 mm Hg.
	    Prepare in glass bottle with special tubing; note that nitroglycerin (Tridil) should not be infused with any parenteral medication *because it is incompatible with any other medications except heparin, which can only be piggybacked at the rubber hub of the IV tubing proximal to the angiocath.*
	    Start at low dose, usually 5-10 μ/min through an infusion pump to *regulate delivery of the drug.*
	    Titrate dose according to patient's pain and BP at small increments *to obtain optimum effect.*
	    Check vital signs every 5 min after change in dose and q 15 min thereafter until stable. *Nitrates (Tridil) are both coronary dilators and peripheral vasodilators causing hypotension.*
	    Report immediately a significant decrease in blood pressure.
	       Anticipate a fluid challenge *to correct hypotension.*
	    If patient complains of headache (common side effect), treat with acetaminophen (Tylenol).
	    Continually reassess patient's chest pain and response to medication. If no relief from optimal dose of medication, report to physician for evaluation for intra-aortic balloon pump, thrombolytic treatment, angioplasty, cardiac catheterization, or bypass surgery.
	• Initiate SCP for Thrombolytic therapy p. 168 if applicable or appropriate.	

Potential nausea/ vomiting *Related to:* Activation of a vagal reflex that occurs frequently with inferior site MIs and with severe pain Common side effects of opiates **DEFINING CHARACTERISTICS** Patient complains of nausea/vomiting Retching Straining Expelling gastric contents	**ONGOING ASSESSMENT** • Assess for signs and symptoms of epigastric distress. • Assess color, consistency, amount of emesis. • Note any vasovagal responses from suppositories and straining. *Bradycardia, hypotension, dizziness, and lightheadedness are common side effects.* **THERAPEUTIC INTERVENTIONS** • Position patient comfortably in Fowler's position. • Keep emesis basin at bedside. • Record and report contents, color, and amount of emesis. • Administer antiemetics as ordered; prochlorperazine (Compazine) or trimethobenzamide (Tigan) suppositories prn. Assess response. • If no response from antiemetics, report to physician for other remedies. • Offer ice chips as desired. • Offer small but frequent meals as tolerated. • Offer general liquid to soft diet as tolerated. • Provide mouth care/mouth wash as necessary.	Discomfort associated with nausea and vomiting will be relieved.

NURSING DIAGNOSES / DEFINING CHARACTERISTICS	NURSING INTERVENTIONS / *RATIONALES*	EXPECTED OUTCOMES

Chest pain
Related to:
Pericarditis secondary to acute MI
 	
DEFINING CHARACTERISTICS
Complaint of pain
Pericardial friction rub (transient)
ST-segment elevation in most limb and precordial ECG leads without reciprocal ST-segment depression
Fever
	ONGOING ASSESSMENT
	▪ Assess characteristics of pericardial pain. It is similar to MI pain, except that pericardial pain:
	    Increases with deep inspiration, turning of thorax, lying down
	    Relieved by sitting up or leaning forward
	    Quality:
	      Sharp, stabbing, knifelike, "pleuritic"
	      Moderate to severe or only an ache (deep or superficial)
	    Onset: sudden, 1-3 days after MI
	    Duration:
	      Intermittent or continuous
	      May last for days
	      Residual soreness
	  Accurate assessment facilitates appropriate treatment
	▪ Assess vital signs:
	    BP: check for pulsus paradoxus (abnormal decrease in systolic BP during inspiration)
	    Heart rate
	    Respirations
	    Temperature
	▪ Auscultate chest for heart sounds; document presence or change in pericardial rub.
	
	THERAPEUTIC INTERVENTIONS
	▪ Position patient comfortably, preferably sitting up in bed 90 degrees or leaning forward propped on a pillow on a side table *as these positions effectively relieve discomfort.*
	▪ Offer assurance and emotional support through explanations of pericarditis. *Patients fear that this pain is another "heart attack" and need reassurance.*
	▪ Give medications as ordered, usually aspirin q6h or indomethacin (Indocin) q8h *to reduce inflammation around the heart.* Give medications on full stomach *to prevent gastric irritation.*
	▪ Offer pillow *to support chest when coughing.*
		Discomfort will be reduced.

Potential decreased cardiac output
Related to:
Altered preload, afterload, and contractility secondary to:
  Acute MI (especially anterior site) affecting pumping ability of the heart
  Papillary muscle rupture, mitral insufficiency
  Ventricular aneurysm
 	
DEFINING CHARACTERISTICS
Low urine output
Decreased BP
Decreased or increased heart rate
Change in mental status
Rales
Dyspnea
	ONGOING ASSESSMENT
	▪ Assess respiration every shift and prn for rate, depth, quality, and use of accessory muscles.
	▪ Auscultate lungs every shift and prn for rales and wheezes; report/record changes.
	▪ Assess for heart rate, rhythm, BP, presence of S_3 or S_4, systolic murmur. Record and report changes.
	▪ Monitor fluid balance (I & O), weight gain, jugular venous distention, edema.
	▪ Assess for restlessness, fatigue, change in mental status.
	▪ Monitor ABGs.
	
	THERAPEUTIC INTERVENTIONS
	If signs of left ventricular failure occur:
	▪ Initiate O_2 as needed *to reduce hypoxia.*
	▪ Report to physician.
	▪ Initiate treatment for Decreased cardiac output, p. 9.
		Optimal cardiac output will be maintained.

Continued.

NURSING DIAGNOSES / DEFINING CHARACTERISTICS	NURSING INTERVENTIONS / *RATIONALES*	EXPECTED OUTCOMES

Potential decreased cardiac output
Related to:
Electrical instability/ irritability secondary to ischemia or necrosis:
  PVC
  Ventricular tachycardia
  Idioventricular rhythm
  Presence of acute ECG changes (increased ST segment)
Conduction system defects:
  With inferior ventricular MI:
    Sinus bradycardia
    First- and second-degree heart block
    Wenckebach
  With anterior ventricular MI:
    Second-degree heart block (Mobitz type II)
    Complete heart block
    Right bundle branch block
    With atrial infarct: Atrial arrhythmias
	ONGOING ASSESSMENT
	• Monitor patient's heart rate and rhythm continuously. Document and report arrhythmias noted. *Monitoring of appropriate leads facilitates prompt detection of conduction problem.*
	  Monitor in lead II, observing for left anterior hemiblock (S-wave deep).
	  If anterior MI with left anterior hemiblock is present, monitor in modified chest lead (MCL_1) for right bundle branch block.
	• Check vital signs during arrhythmias; note other associated signs and symptoms. Note rate and quality of pulses.
	• Assess ventilation and oxygenation; note change in consciousness.
	• Monitor PR, QRS, and QT intervals and note change *to reduce the potential for the occurrence of lethal arrhythmias. Many antiarrhythmia drugs also depress the conduction of normal impulses and can cause further arrhythmias.*
	• Assess response to treatment and management
	
	THERAPEUTIC INTERVENTIONS
	• Institute treatment as appropriate and as per protocol:
	  Lidocaine/procainamide (Pronestyl) for PVC, ventricular tachycardia
	  Atropine SO_4 for symptomatic bradycardia
	  Isoproterenol/temporary pacemaker for complete heart block
	  Temporary pacemaker for Mobitz type II, new bifascicular bundle branch block
	  Cardioversion for atrial arrhythmias, ventricular tachycardia
	  Defibrillation for ventricular fibrillation
	  Precordial thump or CPR as appropriate
		Risk of complications from arrhythmias will be reduced.

DEFINING CHARACTERISTICS Decreased or increased heart rate; decreased BP Change in mental status Weakness, dizziness Restlessness Loss of peripheral pulses Abnormal heart sounds Chest pain Seizure activity Hemodynamic compromise Cardiopulmonary arrest		

NURSING DIAGNOSES / DEFINING CHARACTERISTICS	NURSING INTERVENTIONS / *RATIONALES*	EXPECTED OUTCOMES
Anxiety/fear *Related to:* Threat to or change in health status Threat of death Threat to self-concept Change in environment Unmet needs **DEFINING CHARACTERISTICS** Tense appearance, apprehension; feelings of impending doom Fidgety/listless behavior Restless/unable to relax Repeatedly seeking assurance Signs of denial; indifference to surroundings Sad expression; crying Slow speech Expressed concern regarding changes in life-style	**ONGOING ASSESSMENT** • Assess patient's level of anxiety. Note all signs and symptoms, especially nonverbal communication. • Assess patient's normal coping patterns. **THERAPEUTIC INTERVENTIONS** • See Anxiety, p. 4. • After assessing readiness, explain in simple terms patient's illness (e.g., various aspects of MI, need for cardiac monitoring); identify and clarify misconceptions *to help patient adjust to emotional stress.* • Foster patient's optimism that recovery is fully anticipated. Offer realistic assurances. • Assist patient to understand that emotions felt are normal, anticipated responses to acute MI. • Establish rest periods between care and procedures *to help patient relax and regain emotional balance.* • Provide diversional materials (e.g., newspapers, magazines, music, and television), *which can be relaxing and prevent feelings of isolation.* • Administer mild tranquilizer/sedatives as ordered *to reduce stress.*	Anxiety/fear will be reduced/managed and coped with.

Activity intolerance
Related to:
Generalized weakness
Altered mobility
Imbalance between O_2 supply and demand
 	
DEFINING CHARACTERISTICS
Weakness/fatigue with ADL activity performance
Increased heart rate of >15 beats over resting rate during activity
Increased BP >20 mm Hg systolic during activity
Decreased BP of >10 mm Hg systolic during activity
Chest pain, dizziness
Skin color changes/diaphoresis
Dyspnea
	ONGOING ASSESSMENT
	• Assess patient's respiratory and cardiac status before initiating activity.
	• Observe and document response to activity. Report abnormal responses.
	
	THERAPEUTIC INTERVENTIONS
	• Encourage adequate rest periods, especially before activities (e.g., ADL, visitors, meals).
	• Provide emotional support when increasing activity *to reduce possible anxiety about "overexertion" of heart.*
	• Maintain progression of activity as ordered by physician and/or cardiac rehabilitation team by monitoring cardiac rehabilitation stages:
	Stage 1: Complete bed rest
	Stage 2:
	    Wash face, hands, personal areas (in bed). Nurse will wash back and legs.
	    Use bedside commode with assistance.
	    Perform active ROM exercises tid per protocol.
	Stage 3: Dangle 15-30 min tid
	Stage 4:
	    Have bath in chair
	    Shave at bedside
	    Sit in chair with legs elevated for 30-60 min tid
	    Perform ROM exercises while sitting in chair
	• Instruct patient not to hold breath while exercising or moving about in bed and not to strain for bowel movement. *These activities stimulate Valsalva maneuver, which leads to bradycardia and resultant change in cardiac output.*
	• Provide light meal (progress from liquids to regular diet as appropriate).
	• Instruct patient that further cardiac rehabilitation/activity progression will occur after transfer from intensive care setting.
		Responses/tolerance to activity will be optimal.

Continued.

Cardiovascular Care Plans

NURSING DIAGNOSES / DEFINING CHARACTERISTICS	NURSING INTERVENTIONS / *RATIONALES*	EXPECTED OUTCOMES

Knowledge deficit
Related to:
Unfamiliarity with disease process, treatment, recovery
 	
DEFINING CHARACTERISTICS
Multiple or no questions
Confusion over events
Expressed need for information
	ONGOING ASSESSMENT
	• Assess readiness of patient/significant others for teaching/counseling.
	• Note baseline knowledge.
	
	THERAPEUTIC INTERVENTIONS
	• Establish good rapport with patient/significant others *for effective communication.*
	• Encourage patient/significant others to ask questions and verbalize concerns.
	• Provide information on the following (as appropriate), limiting each session to 10-15 min *so patient is not overwhelmed.*
	    Positive aspects of the unit (CCU)
	    Diagnosing of MI in CCU (e.g., with ECG, blood tests)
	    Healing process and recovery
	    Cardiac anatomy
	    MI versus angina
	    Risk factors for MI
	• Use available teaching tools (e.g., anatomic heart model, brochures, cassette tapes for MI, flip charts).
	• Use appropriate resources (e.g., unit nurses, clinical specialists, physician).
	• Document teaching.
	• Inform patient that more extensive teaching sessions will be instituted after transfer to the medical floor.
		Patient/significant others will verbalize understanding of patient's condition, healing process of MI, need for observation in CCU, and diagnosis/treatment of MI.

Originated by: Cynthia Antonio, RN, BSN

Myocardial infarction: intermediate phase (days 4-10)

The intermediate phase of recovery begins with transfer from the critical care unit (CCU). During this period, the nurse's focus shifts to rehabilitation of the post-MI patient. Progressive low-level activities are used to prevent or reduce deleterious physiologic and psychological effects of bed rest. Education and counseling assist the patient in optimal return to physical and psychosocial functioning and needed lifestyle changes.

NURSING DIAGNOSES / DEFINING CHARACTERISTICS	NURSING INTERVENTIONS / *RATIONALES*	EXPECTED OUTCOMES

Knowledge deficit: myocardial infarction and follow-up care
Related to:
Unfamiliarity with disease process, treatment, recovery
 	
DEFINING CHARACTERISTICS
Questioning
Verbalizing misconceptions
Not verbalizing feelings
	ONGOING ASSESSMENT
	• Assess patient's physical and emotional readiness to learn.
	• Assess patient's/significant others' understanding of disease process, recovery process, diet, medications, activity progression, preventive care.
	
	THERAPEUTIC INTERVENTIONS
	• Plan teaching sessions *so patient is not overwhelmed at one time.*
	• Determine specific learning needs and patient goals. *Teaching standardized content that patient already knows wastes valuable time and hinders critical learning.*
	• Provide environment conducive to learning.
	• Consult cardiac rehabilitation clinical specialist about appropriate teaching materials (hospital television, heart model, group class, handouts).
	• Provide information as needed regarding:
	    Coronary artery disease
	    Angina versus myocardial infarction (MI) pain characteristics
	    Immediate treatment for MI
		Patient/significant others will verbalize understanding of disease state, recovery process, diet, medications, activity, and preventive care.

NURSING DIAGNOSES / DEFINING CHARACTERISTICS	NURSING INTERVENTIONS / *RATIONALES*	EXPECTED OUTCOMES

	Healing process from MI
	Resumption of activities of daily living
	Risk factor modification
	Dietary regime
	Medications
	Progressive activity/exercise plan:
	   Home walking program
	   Stair climbing
	   Lifting/household chores
	   Driving a car
	   Shopping/movies/restaurants/social visits
	   Sexual activity
	Coping mechanisms to help adjustment to new or altered life-style
	Immediate treatment for recurrence of chest pain	

Activity intolerance
Related to:
Imposed activity restriction
Generalized weakness; deconditioned state
Imbalance between O_2 supply and demand
Sedentary life-style
 	
DEFINING CHARACTERISTICS
Report of fatigue or weakness
Abnormal heart rate or BP response to activity
Exertional discomfort
Dyspnea
Chest pain
Dizziness
Diaphoresis
	ONGOING ASSESSMENT
	• Assess patient's respiratory/cardiac status before activity.
	• Observe and document response to activity. *Physical activities increase the demands placed on the healing myocardium. Close monitoring of patient's response serves as a guide for optimal progression of activity.*
	   Pulse >20 beats over resting or 120 beats/min
	   Palpitations
	   BP increases >20 mm Hg
	   BP decreases >10 mm Hg
	   Dyspnea, weakness
	   Chest pain, dizziness
	   Skin color changes, diaphoresis
	   If abnormal responses are noted, refer to physician and cardiac rehabilitation team.
	• Monitor the number of visitors and their length of stay *so patient obtains needed rest.*
	• Monitor active ROM exercise tid *to maintain muscle strength and decrease the risk of thromboembolism.*
	
	THERAPEUTIC INTERVENTIONS
	• Encourage adequate rest periods, especially before activities, *to reduce cardiac workload and facilitate myocardial healing.*
	• Assist with self-care activities as needed.
	• Provide emotional support when increasing activity. *Patients are frequently afraid of "overexerting" their heart.*
	• Maintain progression of activity as ordered by cardiac rehabilitation team, physician. *Note: Not everyone progresses at same rate. Some patients progress slowly because of complicated MI, lack of motivation, inadequate sleep, fear of "overexertion," related medical problems, and previous sedentary life-style. In contrast, others who experience small infarcts and who had high fitness and activity levels before hospitalization may progress very rapidly; therefore, the following cardiac rehabilitation walking distances are only meant to be a guide.*
	   Cardiac rehabilitation stages:
	     Stage 1: Date_____
	     Dangle 15-30 min tid. Feed self
	     Stage 2: Date_____
	       Partial bath in chair, shave self; sit in chair 30-60 min tid
	     Stage 3: Date_____
	       Partial bath at sink; bathroom privileges; up in chair whenever desired; walk in room
	     Stage 4: Date_____
	       Self morning care; walk in hall 150 ft tid
	     Stage 5: Date_____
	       Sit in hall; walk 300 ft tid
		Optimal activity tolerance will be maintained.

Continued.

NURSING DIAGNOSES / DEFINING CHARACTERISTICS	NURSING INTERVENTIONS / *RATIONALES*	EXPECTED OUTCOMES

	Stage 6: Date_____
	    Walk 600 ft tid
	Stage 7: Date_____
	    Stair climbing with cardiac rehabilitation nurse
	Stage 8: Date_____
	    Progressive walking as tolerated	

Potential body image disturbance/self-concept disturbance *Related to:* Actual/perceived changes in physiologic functioning Increased amount of disease-related symptoms Changes in health status Threat of death Perceived/actual change in role Possible change in life-style (job, physical activity) **DEFINING CHARACTERISTICS** Refusal to accept rehabilitative efforts Inappropriate attempts to direct own treatment Signs of grieving: crying, despair, anger Refusal to participate in self-care Self-destructive behavior Withdrawal from social contacts Focus on past strength, function Feelings of helplessness Preoccupation with change or loss Change in self-perception of role Change in usual patterns of responsibility	**ONGOING ASSESSMENT** • Assess contributing factors. • Assess usual coping methods. • Assess meaning of MI on patient and significant others. • Assess for common reaction, such as denial, anger, anxiety, and depression. **THERAPEUTIC INTERVENTIONS** • Encourage verbalization of feelings. *Allow time for patient to work through different stages of coping.* • Provide anticipatory guidance *to reduce anxiety and fear of the unknown.* Provide reliable information about future limitations (if any) on physical activity and role performance. • Assist person to accept help from others. Stress that this is just *temporary* state. • Identify outlets that foster feelings of personal achievement and self-esteem. • Explore strengths and resources with person. • Realistically point out positive changes in person's condition. *Patients frequently don't note progress they make during recovery.* • Encourage referral to cardiac rehabilitation program or "coronary club" *to increase self-confidence in physical abilities and provide mechanism for ongoing verbalization of feelings and clarification of misconceptions.*	Positive expressions of continued self-worth will be verbalized.
Potential chest pain *Related to:* Myocardial ischemia/infarction Pericarditis	**ONGOING ASSESSMENT** • Assess characteristics of pain, *differentiating between myocardial infarction and pericarditis* (see Myocardial infarction: acute phase, p. 103), *and between stable and unstable angina* (see Angina pectoris, unstable: acute phase, p. 69). *Not all chest pain requires "urgent" treatment. Accurate differentiation facilitates correct and aggressive treatment as indicated.* • Assess hemodynamic response to pain.	Pain will be alleviated or reduced.

NURSING DIAGNOSES / DEFINING CHARACTERISTICS	NURSING INTERVENTIONS / *RATIONALES*	EXPECTED OUTCOMES

DEFINING CHARACTERISTICS
 	
Patient report and verbalization of pain
Restlessness, apprehension
Facial mask of pain
Diaphoresis
Change in vital signs (BP, heart rate, respiratory rate)
Pallor, weakness
Fear and guarding behavior
	THERAPEUTIC INTERVENTIONS
	• Instruct patient to report pain *so relief measures can be instituted.*
	• Maintain bed rest, at least during periods of pain *to reduce cardiac workload.*
	• Position comfortably, preferably Fowler's position.
	• Maintain a quiet and relaxed atmosphere; display confident manner.
	• Administer medications as ordered, noting effectiveness and side effects.
	• If nonpericardial chest pain is not relieved within 15-30 min:
	  Report immediately to physician
	  Assess appropriateness of immediate ECG *to document ST changes.*
	  Maintain vital signs.
	  Administer O_2 per order *to increase myocardial oxygen supply.*
	  Institute medical therapy per order.
	  Stay with patient *to provide support and reassurance.*
	  Anticipate need for IV. *Analgesics are routinely administered intravenously since intramuscular injections raise serum creatinine phosphokinase (CPK) levels, which are used to assess extent of myocardial injury.*
	• If pericardial pain is noted:
	  Position patient comfortably, preferably sitting up in bed 90 degrees or leaning forward propped on a pillow set on a side table.
	  Offer assurance and emotional support.
	  Reinforce that this pain is not another "heart attack" *to reduce anxiety.*
	  Give medications as ordered, usually aspirin q6h or indomethacin (Indocin) q8h *to reduce inflammation around heart;* give medications on full stomach *to reduce gastric discomfort.*
	  Auscultate chest for heart sounds and document presence or change in pericardial rub.	

Potential decreased cardiac output
Related to:
Altered preload
Altered afterload
Altered contractility
 	
DEFINING CHARACTERISTICS
Low urine output
Decreasing BP, increasing or decreasing heart rate
Cutaneous sign of vasoconstriction
Change in mental status
Dizziness
Weakness, fatigue
Restlessness
Abnormal heart sounds
Abnormal lung sounds
Neck vein distention
Edema
Chest pain
	ONGOING ASSESSMENT
	• Assess physical status closely, document changes, report significant changes in parameters:
	  Arterial BP, orthostatic changes, pulsus paradoxus, heart rate
	  Apical/radial pulses, peripheral pulses (strength, equality)
	  Heart sounds
	  Lung sounds
	  Jugular venous distention
	  Mentation
	  Urine output
	  Skin color, temperature
	  Daily weights
	
	THERAPEUTIC INTERVENTIONS
	• Administer routine cardiac medications as ordered; observe for side effects and toxicity.
	• Maintain optimal fluid intake.
	• If signs of left ventricular failure are noted:
	  Initiate O_2 as needed.
	  Report to physician.
	  Initiate treatment for Decreased cardiac output, p. 9.
		Optimal hemodynamic status will be maintained.

Continued.

111

NURSING DIAGNOSES / DEFINING CHARACTERISTICS	NURSING INTERVENTIONS / *RATIONALES*	EXPECTED OUTCOMES
Potential decreased cardiac output *Related to:* Cardiac dysrhythmias (atrial, junctional, ventricular) secondary to ischemia, electrolyte imbalance, altered electrical conduction/ rhythm/rate **DEFINING CHARACTERISTICS** Irregular heart rate Tachycardia/ bradycardia Decreasing/increasing K$^+$ levels Hypoxia	**ONGOING ASSESSMENT** • Monitor heart for rate, rhythm, and ectopy every 4 hr as needed. • If telemetry ECG monitoring is available, continuously monitor ECG for rate, rhythm, abnormality, and change in PR, QRS, and QT intervals if appropriate. • Observe for abnormalities in electrolytes. **THERAPEUTIC INTERVENTIONS** • If arrhythmia occurs, determine patient response, document, and report if significant or symptomatic. *Both tachy- and bradyarrhythmias can reduce cardiac output and myocardial tissue perfusion.* • Have antiarrhythmic drugs readily available. • Treat arrhythmias according to medical orders or protocol and evaluate response. See Treatment, Myocardial infarction: acute phase, p. 103.	Optimal cardiac rhythm and cardiac output will be maintained.

Potential sexual dysfunction *Related to:* Anxiety/fear of sexual inadequacy and/or death during intercourse Altered self-concept Decreased activity tolerance Physiologic limitations secondary to MI (pain, shortness of breath, fatigue) Knowledge deficit/ misconceptions Effects of medication Partner's fear/ reluctance **DEFINING CHARACTERISTICS** Verbalization of concerns about sexual function Questions about "normal" sexual activity Decreased self-esteem Actual/perceived limitations imposed by disease and/or therapy Sexually inappropriate behavior within setting Inability to achieve desired satisfaction	**ONGOING ASSESSMENT**
	 • Assess for indication of potential sexual dysfunction.
	 • Assess patient's/significant others' understanding of resumption of sexual activity post MI.
	 • Assess sexual patterns *before* MI. *Some cardiac patients may have chronic sexual problems, which require more intensive treatment and referral.*
	
	 THERAPEUTIC INTERVENTIONS
	 • Provide counseling session with patient and significant other before discharge *to provide guidelines for resumption of sexual activity, to relieve anxieties, and to clear up common misconceptions:*
	   Convey normalcy of anxiety about resuming sex.
	   Assess any symptoms previously experienced during sexual activity.
	   Explain need to share concerns with partner.
	   Evaluate need for separate counseling sessions for patient and partner *to facilitate verbalization of personal fear/feelings.*
	 • Instruct patient on guidelines to follow when resuming sex:
	   Realistic schedule for resuming (when can climb two flights of stairs, walk three blocks briskly).
	   Times to avoid sex: 2-3 hr after eating or drinking alcohol, when tired from another activity.
	   Avoidance of extramarital or new partners at first *(increased anxiety places greater demands on heart).*
	   Resumption of usual comfortable positions.
	   Warning signs of overexertion.
	 • Encourage use of exercise tolerance testing *to document patient's functional capacity and provide objective information of physical stamina.*
	 • Encourage patient to develop a progressive exercise program. *The positive effects of physical training include improved activity tolerance and increased self-confidence and self-esteem.*
	 • Instruct patient that if angina, shortness of breath, or arrhythmias should consistently occur, prophylactic medication such as nitroglycerin may be prescribed.
	 • If patient has reduced exercise tolerance secondary to MI:
	   Teach techniques to reduce oxygen consumption (positioning, time of day when unhurried and rested, etc.).
	   Recommend nitroglycerin as needed before sexual activity.
	   Discuss alternative methods for sexual satisfaction.
	 • Refer to cardiac rehabilitation clinical nurse specialist or other appropriate health professional as needed.
		Optimal level of sexual activity is maintained.

Originated by: Meg Gulanick, RN, PhD

Pulmonary edema, acute

(PULMONARY CONGESTION)

Pulmonary edema is a pathologic state in which there is abnormal extravascular water accumulation in the lung.

NURSING DIAGNOSES / DEFINING CHARACTERISTICS	NURSING INTERVENTIONS / *RATIONALES*	EXPECTED OUTCOMES

Impaired gas exchange *Related to:* Pulmonary-venous congestion Alveolar-capillary membrane changes **DEFINING CHARACTERISTICS** Restlessness Irritability Inability to move secretions Pink, frothy sputum Hypercapnia Hypoxia Cough Rales Dyspnea Cyanosis	**ONGOING ASSESSMENT**
	• Assess respiratory rate, depth; presence of shortness of breath; use of accessory muscles.
	• Assess breath sounds in all lung fields, noting aerations, presence of rales, wheezes.
	• Assess sputum/tracheal secretions, noting color, consistency, quantity.
	• Obtain and monitor serial ABGs:
	    Routinely q8h as appropriate
	    20-30 min after a change in O_2 therapy
	
	THERAPEUTIC INTERVENTIONS
	• Provide O_2 as needed to maintain Po_2 at acceptable level. Anticipate possibility of mechanical ventilation. See Mechanical ventilation, p. 213.
	• If ABGs are expected to be drawn more frequently than at four 1-hr intervals, suggest appropriateness of an arterial line *for patient comfort and ease in obtaining necessary ABG's.*
	• Position patient for optimal breathing patterns (high Fowler's position; feet dangling at bedside).
	• Encourage slow, deep breaths as appropriate.
	• Assist with coughing or suctioning prn.
	• Assist with positioning *for optimal lung expansion for chest x-ray examination.*
	• Administer prescribed medication carefully:
	    If diuretics are used, monitor K^+ levels, I & O, need for Foley catheter.
	    If morphine sulfate is used, monitor respiratory rate; observe for bradycardia, nausea. Keep naloxone (Narcan) available: *in the event of morphine overdose, Narcan reverses effects of morphine.*
	    If aminophylline is used, monitor ventricular rate and frequency of ectopics closely: *aminophylline is a cardiac stimulant.* Monitor aminophylline levels prn.
		Improved ventilation and oxygenation.

Decreased cardiac output *Related to:* Increased preload Increased afterload Decreased contactility Combined etiologies **DEFINING CHARACTERISTICS** Variations in hemodynamic parameters (BP, heart rate, CVP, pulmonary artery pressure, cardiac output, neck veins, urine output, peripheral pulses) Arrhythmias/ECG changes Weight gain, edema, ascites Nausea, vomiting Abnormal heart sounds	**ONGOING ASSESSMENT**
	• Assess hemodynamic parameters (see Defining Characteristics). Monitor pulmonary artery (PA), pulmonary capillary wedge (PCW) waveforms closely. If pulmonary capillary wedge pressure (PCWP) correlates within 10% of pulmonary artery diastolic pressure (PADP), monitor PADP instead of PCWP *to prevent pulmonary infarction or balloon rupture from repeated readings.*
	• Assess skin color, temperature.
	• Assess fluid balance, weight gain.
	• Assess heart sounds, noting murmurs, gallops, S_3, S_4.
	• Assess heart rate rhythm (both apical and radial).
	• Assess mentation, noting restlessness, confusion.
	
	THERAPEUTIC INTERVENTIONS
	• Anticipate need for hemodynamic monitoring. If ordered:
	    Prepare patient for insertion of Swan-Ganz catheter.
	    Assemble equipment per unit routine.
	    Observe patient for hypotension *(nitrates cause vasodilation).* If this occurs, stop medication immediately, lower head of bed as appropriate *to increase venous return,* and notify physician. Anticipate need for pressor/fluid treatment.
	    Position patient for optimal reduction of preload (high Fowler's position, dangling feet at bedside).
	    If diuretics are used, monitor K^+ levels, I & O, need for Foley catheter.
		Optimal cardiac output will be maintained.

Continued.

NURSING DIAGNOSES / DEFINING CHARACTERISTICS	NURSING INTERVENTIONS / *RATIONALES*	EXPECTED OUTCOMES
Anxiety, restlessness Dizziness, weakness, fatigue	If rotating tourniquets are used: Apply per unit routine. Avoid using extremity with IV line. Monitor peripheral pulses every 15 min *to assess circulation to extremity.* Do not inflate cuff longer than 45 min, *to prevent ischemic damage to extremity.* At the end of use, remove one cuff at a time (every 15 min), *to prevent sudden venous return and potential cardiac overload.* • If increased afterload (systemic blood pressure) is the etiology, anticipate measures for afterload reduction: Use D₅W for peripheral lines. Use central ports for medication infusion. Use infusion pumps *to maintain patency of lines.* If PCWP readings change more than 10% from previous readings, recheck all lines and recalibrate system. Report to physician as needed. See Swan-Ganz catheterization, p. 165. • If increased preload is the etiology, anticipate use of rotating tourniquets, nitrates, or diuretics *to reduce venous return.* If nitrates are used: Prepare IV nitrate in glass bottle using special tubing *because IV nitroglycerin is absorbed into the plastic.* Evaluate need to prepare as a multiple concentration *to decrease total amount of IV fluids administered.* Initiate dose at_____. Titrate nitrate to PCWP of_____or until desired effect:_____. If nitroprusside (Nipride) is used: Make certain patient has a clear, audible BP by cuff. If not, evaluate need for arterial line *for continuous BP monitoring.* Prepare nitroprusside per unit routine. Administer via infusion pump *for reliable dosing.* Titrate dose 0.5-10 μg/kg/min. Do not infuse with any other medicines. Protect from sunlight *because nitroprusside is light-sensitive.* Anticipate potential side effects: hypotension, sweating, nausea, confusion. Confer with physician about the desired goals, e.g., heart rate_____. Monitor hemodynamic parameters every 5-10 min until stable. Monitor thiocyanate levels prn. *Nitroprusside is converted to cyanide when it is metabolized.* • If arrhythmia is the etiology: Monitor continuously for arrhythmias. Administer prescribed medication per unit protocol. Monitor patient's electrolytes, especially K⁺ levels. • If hypotension is a related problem: Evaluate need for hemodynamic monitoring/arterial line *for continuous BP monitoring.* Anticipate use of pressor agents. If dopamine or dobutamine (Dobutrex) is prescribed: Titrate dose 0.5-20 μg/kg/min for dopamine. Titrate dose 0.5-10 μg/kg/min for dobutamine. Keep phentolamine (Regitine) on standby *in the event of extravasation of dopamine.* Anticipate potential side effects: tachycardia, decreased urine output (with high doses of dopamine). If necessary, dopamine and dobutamine may be infused through the same line.	

Pulmonary edema, acute—cont'd

NURSING DIAGNOSES / DEFINING CHARACTERISTICS	NURSING INTERVENTIONS / *RATIONALES*	EXPECTED OUTCOMES
Anxiety/fear *Related to:* Dyspnea Excessive monitoring equipment Increased staff attention **DEFINING CHARACTERISTICS** Sympathetic stimulation Restlessness Increased awareness Increased questioning Avoidance of looking at equipment Constant demands, complaints Uncooperative behavior	**ONGOING ASSESSMENT** • Assess patient's level of anxiety and normal coping pattern **THERAPEUTIC INTERVENTIONS** • Remain with patient during periods of acute respiratory distress. • Promote an environment of confidence and reassurance. • Anticipate need and use of morphine sulfate *to reduce anxiety and fear associated with shortness of breath.* • Institute treatment for Anxiety, p. 4.	Anxiety will be reduced.
Discomfort *Related to:* Dyspnea Prolonged bed rest Fatigue Uncomfortable therapeutic interventions **DEFINING CHARACTERISTICS** Complaints of thirst Diaphoresis Pain; dyspnea Restlessness Uncomfortable feeling from mask or Foley catheter	**ONGOING ASSESSMENT** • Assess patient's level of comfort, noting both verbal and nonverbal communication. • Assess characteristics of patient's discomfort. • Monitor ABGs closely, *so that most comfortable mode of O_2 delivery is used without compromising oxygenation.* **THERAPEUTIC INTERVENTIONS** • Position patient in preferred position. • Offer frequent back rubs and massages. • Turn patient from side to side q2h as tolerated by respiratory status. • Keep extra pillows available; use pillows to help prop patient upright. • Obtain egg crate mattress/flotation pad as needed. • Keep patient's linens dry. • Provide frequent oral hygiene. • Provide ice chips *to lessen complaints of thirst and dry mouth.* Maintain accurate I & O records.	Comfort will be maximized.
Potential infection *Related to:* Increased pulmonary congestion Increased use of invasive equipment **DEFINING CHARACTERISTICS** Elevated temperature WBC count increased Foul-smelling sputum or urine Phlebitic area about IV site Redness, swelling, tenderness at catheter insertion site	**ONGOING ASSESSMENT** • Assess patient's IV sites, noting any incidence of redness, soreness, drainage. • Assess all indwelling catheters for patency, cleanliness. For central lines, examine IV site more frequently, q8h. • Assess patient's temperature per unit protocol. If temperature is >38.5° C, notify physician immediately; prepare for possible blood culture and repeat temperature q 2-4h. • Assess respiratory secretions for color and odor. • Assess patient's WBC. • If infection is suspected, send tip of catheter for culture. **THERAPEUTIC INTERVENTIONS** • Change tubing, bottles, site per unit protocol. • Remove unnecessary IV lines as soon as possible *to reduce potential for introduction of bacteria.* • If patient has Swan-Ganz catheter or arterial line, encourage physician to change line q72-96h. • Encourage patient to cough and breathe deeply every hour while awake *to reduce occurrence of pneumonia.*	Occurrence of infection will be reduced.

Continued.

NURSING DIAGNOSES / DEFINING CHARACTERISTICS	NURSING INTERVENTIONS/ *RATIONALES*	EXPECTED OUTCOMES
	· If suctioning is needed, use aseptic technique. · Administer antibiotics as prescribed, remembering to check for possible allergies and incompatibility with other medicines. · Administer antipyretics as prescribed.	
Knowledge deficit *Related to:* New equipment New environment New medications/ treatments **DEFINING CHARACTERISTICS** Questioning Verbalized misconceptions Lack of questions	**ONGOING ASSESSMENT** · Assess understanding of patient/significant others of need for increased monitoring, invasive equipment, and of treatment of pulmonary edema in acute phase. · Assess physical and emotional readiness for learning of patient/significant others. **THERAPEUTIC INTERVENTIONS** · During acute phase of illness, explain only necessary treatments and procedures *to prevent sensory overload.* · Keep all information simple and brief. · Include significant others in explanations, reassuring them that more information will be given once patient is through the acute phase. · Document all areas of explanations in nursing notes, including patient's/significant others' response to explanations.	Patient/significant others will verbalize and understand need for increased monitoring equipment in the unit; rationale regarding treatment of pulmonary edema.

Originated by: Nancy J. Cooney, RN, BSN, MBA
                 Laurie VadeBoncouer, RN, BSN

Septic shock

(SEPSIS; BACTEREMIA; WARM SHOCK; COLD SHOCK)

Septic shock occurs after bacteremia of gram-negative bacilli (most common) or gram-positive cocci that results in a systolic BP <90 mm Hg (or a drop >25%), urine output <30 cc/hr, and metabolic acidosis. The circulatory insufficiency is initiated by endotoxin, which causes an increase in capillary permeability and a decrease in systemic vascular resistance (SVR). Hyperdynamic, warm shock is present in 30 to 50% of patients in early septic shock and is characterized by strong beta-adrenergic stimulation of the heart, with tachycardia and increased cardiac output if adequate blood volume is available. Hypodynamic, cold septic shock tends to occur relatively late in septic shock as a result of hypovolemia and release of myocardial depressant factors, causing a fall in cardiac output.

NURSING DIAGNOSES / DEFINING CHARACTERISTICS	NURSING INTERVENTIONS / *RATIONALES*	EXPECTED OUTCOMES

Actual infection
Related to:
An infectious process of either gram-negative or gram-positive bacteria
	ONGOING ASSESSMENT
	· Assess general status; document and report significant changes:
	  Assess level of consciousness/mentation.
	  Utilize neurologic checklist, using Glascow Coma Scale.
	  Assess skin turgor, color, temperature, and peripheral pulses.
	  Monitor temperature q4h.
	  Assess related factors thoroughly *to identify a source for the sepsis.*
		Cause of infection will be determined and appropriate treatment initiated.

NURSING DIAGNOSES / DEFINING CHARACTERISTICS	NURSING INTERVENTIONS / *RATIONALES*	EXPECTED OUTCOMES

The most common causative organisms and their related factors are:
Escherichia coli: commonly occurs in GU tract, biliary tract, IV catheter, colon or intra-abdominal abscesses
Klebsiella: from the lungs, GI tract, intravenous catheter, urinary tract, or surgical wounds
Proteus: GU tract, respiratory tract, abscesses, or biliary tract
Bacteroides fragilis: female genital tract, colon, liver abscesses, decubitus ulcers
Pseudomonas aeruginosa: lungs, urinary tract, skin, and IV catheter
Candidemia-line-related infection, especially hyperalimentation infusion, pulmonary and urinary abscesses
 	
DEFINING CHARACTERISTICS
Changes in LOC: lethargy, confusion
Fever/chills may or may not be present
Ruddy appearance with warm, dry skin
Leucocytosis
	• Monitor for toxicity from antibiotic therapy, especially with hepatic and/or renal insufficiency/failure patients:
	   Aminoglycocides should be followed with urinalysis and serum creatinine levels at least three times/week.
	   Chloramphenicol should be restricted from patients with liver disease.
	
	THERAPEUTIC INTERVENTIONS
	• Initiate appropriate antibiotics as ordered.
	• Remove any possible source of infection, e.g., urinary catheter, IV catheter.
	• Manage the cause of infection and anticipate surgical consult as necessary:
	   To drain pus/abscess
	   To resolve obstruction
	   To repair perforated organ
	• Maintain temperature in adequate range *to prevent stress on the cardiovascular system:*
	   Administer antipyretics as ordered.
	   Apply cooling mattress.
	   Administer tepid sponge baths.
	   Limit number of blankets/linens used to cover patients.
	• Initiate appropriate isolation measures *to prevent the spread of infection.*	

Fluid volume deficit
Related to:
Early septic shock (warm shock)
Decrease in systemic vascular resistance (SVR)
Increased capillary permeability
 	
DEFINING CHARACTERISTICS
Hypotension
Tachycardia
Decreased urine output <30 ml/hr
Concentrated urine
	ONGOING ASSESSMENT
	• Assess for presence of hypotension and tachycardia.
	• Closely monitor I & O, assessing urine for concentration.
	• Obtain daily weights and record.
	• When initiating fluid challenges, closely monitor patient *to prevent iatrogenic volume overload.*
	
	THERAPEUTIC INTERVENTIONS
	• Notify physician of signs of fluid volume deficit.
	• Perform fluid resuscitation aggressively, starting with 300 to 500 cc of crystalloid, followed by an additional 500 cc over 15-20 min. Continue with further fluid resuscitation as ordered. *The fluid needs in septic patients may exceed 8-20 L in the first 24 hr.*
	   Use caution in the elderly patient, *who may be more prone to congestive heart failure.*
	   Adjust fluid as ordered *to obtain an optimal PCWP of 12 mm Hg in absence of MI and PCWP of 14-18 mm Hg if MI has occurred.*
		Fluid volume deficit will be reduced.

Continued.

NURSING DIAGNOSES / DEFINING CHARACTERISTICS	NURSING INTERVENTIONS / *RATIONALES*	EXPECTED OUTCOMES
	• Notify physician of response to fluid challenge. • Administer vasoactive substances, such as dopamine, neosynephrine, or Levophed, as ordered, if poor or no response to fluid resuscitation. *In early septic shock the cardiac output is high or normal. At this point, the vasoactive agents are administered for their alpha effect.*	

Decreased cardiac output
Related to:
Late septic shock: a decrease in tissue perfusion leads to increased lactic acid production and systemic acidosis, which causes a decrease in myocardial contractility
Gram-negative infections may cause a direct myocardial toxic effect
 	
DEFINING CHARACTERISTICS
Decreased peripheral pulses
Cold and clammy skin
Hypotension
Agitation/confusion
Decreased urinary output <30 ml/hr
Abnormal ABGs:
  Acidosis
  Hypoxemia
	ONGOING ASSESSMENT
	• Monitor vital signs and hemodynamic parameters every hour, and report to physician if out of the following ranges:
	  BP mean <60, >110
	  Pulse <50, >130
	  Respiration <10, >30
	  Temperature <36°, >38.5°
	  CVP_____
	  PCWP_____
	  CO _____
	• Monitor for arrhythmias.
	• Assess skin warmth and peripheral pulses every hour.
	• Assess level of consciousness every hour.
	• Monitor urine output every hour and maintain accurate record.
	• Monitor ABG results.
	• Monitor blood lactate levels.
	
	THERAPEUTIC INTERVENTIONS
	• Place patient in the physiologic position for shock: head of bed flat with the trunk horizontal and lower extremities elevated 20-30 degrees with knees straight. Do not use Trendelenburg's (head down) position because *it causes pressure against the diaphragm. A reflex vasoconstrictive action that decreases blood supply to brain after the initial increase in blood flow can occur.*
	• Administer inotropic agents (Dobutrex, Dopamine, Digoxin, or Inocor) *to improve myocardial contractility.* Continuously monitor their effectiveness.
	• *Treat acidosis* with sodium bicarbonate.
		Cardiac output will be increased.

Altered breathing pattern
Related to:
Lactic acidosis
 	
DEFINING CHARACTERISTICS
Tachypnea
Change in depth of breathing
Complaint of shortness of breath
Use of accessory muscles
	ONGOING ASSESSMENT
	• Assess respiratory rate, rhythm, and depth every hour.
	• Assess for any increase in work of breathing:
	  Shortness of breath
	  Use of accessory muscles
	
	THERAPEUTIC INTERVENTIONS
	• Position patient with proper body alignment *for optimal lung expansion.*
	• Provide reassurance and allay anxiety by staying with patient during acute episodes of respiratory distress. *Air hunger can produce an extremely anxious state.*
	• Maintain O₂ delivery system *so that the appropriate amount of oxygen is applied continuously and the patient does not desaturate*
	• Anticipate the need for intubation and mechanical ventilation. See Mechanical ventilation, p. 198.
		Optimal breathing pattern will be maintained.

Potential impaired gas exchange *Related to:* ARDS Pneumonia Pulmonary edema	**ONGOING ASSESSMENT** • Assess respirations every hour, noting quality, rate, pattern, depth, and use of accessory muscles. • Assess breath sounds every hour. • Assess for changes in orientation and behavior. • Monitor ABGs and note changes. • Utilize pulse oximetry, as available, *to monitor O₂ saturation and pulse rate continuously.*	Optimal gas exchange will be maintained.

NURSING DIAGNOSES / DEFINING CHARACTERISTICS	NURSING INTERVENTIONS / *RATIONALES*	EXPECTED OUTCOMES
DEFINING CHARACTERISTICS Hypercapnia Hypoxia Rales Use of accessory muscles Tachypnea Irritability Restlessness	**THERAPEUTIC INTERVENTIONS** • Maintain prescribed oxygen delivery system or ventilator setting *so that patient does not desaturate.* • Change position q2h *to facilitate movement and drainage of secretions.* Be sure to position patient with proper body alignment *for optimal respiratory excursion.* • Suction as needed *to clear secretions.* • See ARDs, p. 186 Pneumonia, p. 196 or Gas exchange, impaired, p. 21 as appropriate.	

Altered level of consciousness
Related to:
Hypotension
Hypoxemia
Sepsis
 	
DEFINING CHARACTERISTICS
Confusion
Lethargy
Agitation
Impaired judgement
Glasgow Coma Score <11
	ONGOING ASSESSMENT
	• Assess LOC/responsiveness every hour, using Glasgow Coma Scale.
	• Assess for confusion/impaired judgment
	
	THERAPEUTIC INTERVENTIONS
	• Reorient to environment as needed.
	• Report change in LOC.
	• Utilize preventive measures for patient with impaired judgement:
	    Keep side rails up at all times and bed in low position.
	    If restraints are used, position patient on side. Never restrain on back *to lessen possibility of aspiration.*
		Optimal state of consciousness will be maintained.

Urinary retention *Related to:* Hypotension Nephrotoxic drugs (antibiotics) **DEFINING CHARACTERISTICS** Urine output <30 cc/ hour Elevated BUN and creatinine Hematuria, proteinuria Tubular casts in urine Fixed specific gravity	**ONGOING ASSESSMENT** • Monitor and record I & O every hour. • Assess for patency of Foley catheter. • Monitor blood and urine: BUN, creatinine, electrolytes, urinalysis. • Monitor urine specific gravity and check for blood and protein every 4 hr. **THERAPEUTIC INTERVENTIONS** • Maintain IV fluids and inotropic agents at prescribed rates *to maintain BP, cardiac output, and, ultimately, renal perfusion.* • Notify physician of any abnormalities. • See Renal failure, acute, p. 343 as appropriate.	Optimal urine elimination will be maintained.

Potential for injury: bleeding
Related to:
Sepsis:
    Deficiency in clotting factors
    DIC
 	
DEFINING CHARACTERISTICS
Oozing of blood from drains, wounds, IV sites
	ONGOING ASSESSMENT
	• Assess for signs of bleeding:
	    Petechiae, purpura, hematomas
	    Blood oozing from IV sites, drains, or wounds
	    Bleeding from mucous membranes:
	        Hemoptysis
	        Blood obtained during suctioning
	    Bleeding from GI/GU tract
	• Determine blood loss and report to physician.
	• Monitor PT, PTT, FSP, bleeding time, and hemoglobin/hematocrit.
	
	THERAPEUTIC INTERVENTIONS
	• If bleeding is present, refer to Disseminated intravascular coagulation, p. 459.
		Potential for injury from bleeding will be reduced.

Continued.

Septic shock—cont'd

NURSING DIAGNOSES / DEFINING CHARACTERISTICS	NURSING INTERVENTIONS / *RATIONALES*	EXPECTED OUTCOMES
Bleeding from mucous membranes PT >25 sec PTT >60-90 sec Thrombocytopenia Elevated fibrin split products Prolonged bleeding time		
Knowledge deficit *Related to:* New condition **DEFINING CHARACTERISTICS** Increased frequency of questions posed by patient and significant others Inability to respond correctly to questions asked Family's/significant others' avoidance of patient's condition	**ONGOING ASSESSMENT** • Assess readiness of patient/significant others to learn. • Evaluate patient/significant others, understanding of patient's overall condition. **THERAPEUTIC INTERVENTIONS** • Explain all procedures before performing them. *This will help to decrease the patient's fear of the unknown.* • Orient patient and significant others to ICU surroundings, routines, equipment alarms, and noises. *The ICU is a busy and noisy environment, which can be very upsetting to both patient and significant others.* • Keep the patient/significant other's informed of disease process and present status of patient.	Patient/significant others will demonstrate understanding of disease process and treatment utilized.

Originated by: Sue Galanes, RN, MS, CCRN
                Revelyn Manabot, RN, BSN

Thrombophlebitis   *Inflammation of the wall of veins.*

(DEEP VEIN THROMBOSIS [DVT]; PHLEBITIS; PHLEBOTHROMBOSIS)

NURSING DIAGNOSES / DEFINING CHARACTERISTICS	NURSING INTERVENTIONS / *RATIONALES*	EXPECTED OUTCOMES
Altered peripheral tissue perfusion *Related to:* Venous stasis Injury to vein Hypercoagulability **DEFINING CHARACTERISTICS** Deep vein (most often involved): may be asymptomatic; severe pain, fever, chills, malaise, possible swelling, cyanosis of affected part, loss of sensation	**ONGOING ASSESSMENT** • Assess patient q4h for signs and symptoms of superficial and deep vein thrombosis. • Assess pain for causative factors, time of onset, quality, radiation, severity • Check laboratory values reflecting coagulation profile (e.g., PT, PTT). • Be aware of results of blood flow studies. • Report abnormalities in assessment to physician. • Observe for side effects of anticoagulant therapy (see Potential for injury, p. 121). **THERAPEUTIC INTERVENTIONS** • Encourage and maintain bed rest, with affected extremity elevated *to minimize possibility of embolus.* • Apply elastic stockings or bandage wraps as ordered *to improve venous blood flow and decrease venous stagnation.* • Apply warm soaks *to relieve pain and inflammation as ordered.* • Administer analgesics as ordered/indicated by assessment *to relieve pain and promote physical comfort.*	Incidence of embolization will be reduced.

NURSING DIAGNOSES / DEFINING CHARACTERISTICS	NURSING INTERVENTIONS / *RATIONALES*	EXPECTED OUTCOMES

Superficial (rarely involved): heat, pain, swelling, tenderness on palpation of posterior calf (Pratt's sign), induration along length of affected vein	• Administer and monitor anticoagulant therapy as ordered (heparin/warfarin [Coumadin]) *to prevent further clot formation by decreasing normal activity of clotting mechanism.*
	• Make sure heparin is administered via mechanical infusion device.
	• Maintain adequate hydration *to prevent increased viscosity of blood:*
	   Encourage oral fluids.
	   Regulate IV infusions as scheduled.
	   Document patient's I & O.	

Impaired gas exchange: acute, potential
Related to:
Dislodgement of thrombus (embolus)
 	
DEFINING CHARACTERISTICS
Cyanosis
Dyspnea
Tachypnea
Substernal, sharp chest pain
Palpitations
Tachycardia
Hemoptysis
Diaphoresis
Engorged neck veins
Anxiety
Restlessness
Sense of impending-doom
	ONGOING ASSESSMENT
	• Assess patient for signs and symptoms of pulmonary embolus. See Thromboembolism, p. 200.
	• Monitor vital signs q4h.
	• Check laboratory values, i.e. ABGs, chest X-ray, PT, and PTT.
	• Auscultate breath sounds q4h.
	• Document observations.
	
	THERAPEUTIC INTERVENTIONS
	• Elevate HOB.
	• Administer O_2 as ordered.
	• Provide emotional support *to reduce stress and O_2 consumption:*
	   Create nonstressful environment.
	   Administer sedatives as ordered.
	• Prepare the patient for transfer to ICU (if transfer is impending):
	   Explain transfer to patient/significant others.
	   Offer reassurance.
	   Accompany patient to unit.
		Incidence of recurrence or extension of thromboembolism will be reduced, and gas exchange will be maximized.

Potential for injury *Related to:* Heparin therapy **DEFINING CHARACTERISTICS** *Too much heparin:* Bleeding from IV sites, drains, wounds Petechiae, purpura, hematoma Bleeding from mucous membranes GI, GU bleeding Bleeding from respiratory tract PTT 2 ½ times normal *Too little heparin:* Continued evidence of further clot formation (newly developed signs of pulmonary embolus or peripheral thromboemboli) PTT not at desired level	**ONGOING ASSESSMENT** Note adverse effects of heparin therapy. Too much heparin: • Note any increase in bleeding from sites (e.g., GI and GU tracts, IV sites, respiratory tract, wounds). • Observe for development of new purpura, petechiae, or hematomas • Inquire about bone and joint pain. • Observe for mental status changes indicating an intracranial bleed. • Check PTT *to monitor therapeutic effect of heparin and reduce risk of bleeding.* Notify physician. Too little heparin: • Ensure that infusion is not interrupted (e.g., infiltrated IV, malfunctioning infusion device). • Check PTT *to monitor therapeutic effect of heparin and reduce risk of bleeding.* Notify physician. **THERAPEUTIC INTERVENTIONS** • Reevaluate heparin dose and administer as ordered.	Risk of injury will be reduced.

Continued.

Thrombophlebitis—cont'd

NURSING DIAGNOSES / DEFINING CHARACTERISTICS	NURSING INTERVENTIONS / *RATIONALES*	EXPECTED OUTCOMES
Knowledge deficit *Related to:* Unfamiliarity with pathology, treatment and prevention **DEFINING CHARACTERISTICS** Multiple questions Lack of questions Misconceptions	**ONGOING ASSESSMENT** · Assess patient's understanding. · Assess patient's readiness for learning. **THERAPEUTIC INTERVENTIONS** · Instruct patient to avoid rubbing or massaging calf *to prevent breaking off clot, which may circulate as embolus.* · Recommend properly applied elastic stockings and instruct patient of importance of wearing them *to increase venous return.* · Encourage early ambulation of surgical patients; encourage leg exercise for bedridden patients, if not contraindicated, *to prevent stasis.* · Instruct patient to avoid long periods of sitting with legs crossed. · Inform patient of signs and symptoms of thrombophlebitis. · Instruct patient to report promptly to physician any symptoms of abnormal bleeding *for prompt intervention.*	Patient and/or significant others will verbalize understanding of disease and management.

Originated by: Gloria Young, RN, BS

Cardiac catheterization

(CORONARY ANGIOGRAPHY)

Cardiac catheterization and coronary angiography are specialized diagnostic procedures in which the internal structure of the heart and coronary arteries can be viewed to determine myocardial function, valvular competency, presence or absence of coronary artery disease, location and severity of coronary artery disease and to assess the effects of percutaneous transluminal coronary angioplasty (PTCA) and coronary artery bypass surgery (CABG).

NURSING DIAGNOSES / DEFINING CHARACTERISTICS	NURSING INTERVENTIONS / *RATIONALES*	EXPECTED OUTCOMES

Knowledge deficit
Related to:
Precatheterization:
  Unfamiliarity with cardiac catheterization
 	
DEFINING CHARACTERISTICS
Expressed need for information
Multiple questions
Lack of questions
Increase in anxiety level
Statements revealing misconceptions
	ONGOING ASSESSMENT
	· Assess patient's knowledge of heart anatomy, disease, and catheterization.
	· Assess patient's/significant other's readiness to learn.
	
	THERAPEUTIC INTERVENTIONS
	· Use appropriate materials (e.g., booklets, television, film, heart model) for teaching patient *to facilitate learning and retention of information.*
	· Provide information about:
	  Heart anatomy and physiology
	  Patient's heart problem (valve disease, coronary artery disease)
	  Cardiac catheterization:
	    Indications
	    Precatheterization preparations
	    Procedure
	    Postcatheterization care
	· Include family in teaching plan as appropriate *to decrease feelings of helplessness and increase ability to provide support for patient.*
	· Be in room when catheterization team evaluates patient (as appropriate). Interpret physician's information (as appropriate) *to clarify and reinforce information as necessary and provide explanations of potential need for PTCA or CABG surgery.*
	· Encourage patient to verbalize questions and concerns *so that misunderstandings and misconceptions can be identified and clarified.*
	· Provide time to listen to and answer questions and concerns. Provide time for one-to-one interaction, if possible.
		The patient will verbalize a basic understanding of heart anatomy, disease, and cardiac catheterization procedure

NURSING DIAGNOSES / DEFINING CHARACTERISTICS	NURSING INTERVENTIONS / *RATIONALES*	EXPECTED OUTCOMES
Potential altered tissue perfusion *Related to:* Postcatheterization: Arterial vasospasm Thrombus formation Embolus **DEFINING CHARACTERISTICS** Decrease or absence of peripheral pulses Lessening in temperature of affected extremity Presence of mottling, pallor, rubor, or cyanosis in affected extremity Presence of pain, numbness, tingling in affected extremity Decrease or absence of motion in affected extremity	**ONGOING ASSESSMENT** Precatheterization: · Assess and record presence or absence and quality of peripheral pulses. · Mark pedal pulses with an *X*. · Assess and record skin color, temperature, capillary refill of all extremities. · Assess and record baseline sensation and motion of all extremities. Postcatheterization: · Assess and monitor affected extremity for occlusion q15min for 1 hr, then q30mins for 1 hr, then q1h until stable. · Assess and record presence and quality of pulses distal to catheter insertion site (radial pulse for brachial site, dorsalis pedis for femoral site). · If dorsalis pedis pulse is being monitored, mark site with *X*. · Assess and record color, temperature, and capillary refill of affected extremity. · Assess sensation and motion of affected extremity. · Check cannulation site for swelling. *Severe edema can hinder peripheral circulation by constricting the vessels.* **THERAPEUTIC INTERVENTIONS** · Instruct patient to report immediately presence of pain, numbness, or tingling; decrease or absence of sensation or motion in extremity distal to cannulation site *for quick assessment, diagnosis, and treatment.* · Report to physician immediately decreases or absence of pulse, change in skin color or temperature, presence of pain, numbness or tingling, decrease or absence of sensation or motion in affected extremity. · Obtain Doppler ultrasonic reading *to check for diminished or absent pulse.* · Prepare for possible thrombectomy or embolectomy *to remove blood clot that may be compromising or obstructing circulation in affected extremity.* · Prepare to heparinize if ordered.	Tissue perfusion of affected extremity will be maintained.
Potential for injury: bleeding *Related to:* Disruption of vessel integrity Heparin administration during cardiac catheterization **DEFINING CHARACTERISTICS** Significant bleeding noted on dressing Apprehension and restlessness Hematoma at site of insertion Increased heart rate, increased respiratory rate, decreased BP	**ONGOING ASSESSMENT** · Assess insertion site and dressing for evidence of bleeding q15min for 1 hr, then q30min for 1 hr, then q1h until stable. · Assess for restlessness, apprehension, and change in vital signs. · Monitor vital signs, Hb, and HCT. **THERAPEUTIC INTERVENTIONS** · Maintain bed rest with affected extremity straight for 6 hr *to minimize risk of bleeding.* Apply soft restraints to affected extremity *to remind patient not to move.* · If femoral site is used, do not elevate head of bed >30 degrees for 6 hr. · Maintain occlusive pressure dressing to cannulation site *to facilitate clot formation.* · Avoid sudden movements with affected extremity *to facilitate clot formation and wound closure at insertion site.* For bleeding: · Circle, date, and time amount of drainage or size of hematoma. · Estimate blood loss. · Reinforce dressing; apply pressure to site. · Apply sandbag (10 pounds) to bleeding site. · Notify physician if bleeding is significant.	Risk of bleeding will be reduced.
Fluid volume deficit *Related to:* Dye-induced diuresis Restricted intake before procedure	**ONGOING ASSESSMENT** · Assess and monitor hydration status, mental status, skin, and hemodynamic status. · Obtain urine specific gravity q. 4 hr until normal. *Concentrated urine with high specific gravity may indicate presence of dye in system and/or hypovolemia.* · If patient requires nitrates, monitor BP closely, anticipating drop in BP and need for additional fluids *secondary to hypovolemic state.*	Potential for dehydration will be reduced.

Continued.

NURSING DIAGNOSES / DEFINING CHARACTERISTICS	NURSING INTERVENTIONS / *RATIONALES*	EXPECTED OUTCOMES
DEFINING CHARACTERISTICS Nervousness and apprehension Poor skin turgor Dry, sticky mucous membranes Decrease in urine output Decrease in BP; increase in heart rate and respiratory rate Pale, cool, clammy skin	**THERAPEUTIC INTERVENTIONS** · Maintain strict I & O for several hours after catheterization. · Anticipate frequent use of urinal/bedpan for several hours after catheterization. Keep urinal within reach. · Give oral fluids as tolerated. · Keep water pitcher/juices at bedside. · Institute IV fluids as ordered, monitoring flow rate *to prevent accidental fluid overload.*	
Anxiety/fear *Related to:* Unknown outcome of cardiac catheterization **DEFINING CHARACTERISTICS** Increased questioning Increased irritability Restlessness Anger Withdrawal	**ONGOING ASSESSMENT** · Assess patient's level of anxiety. **THERAPEUTIC INTERVENTIONS** · Institute treatment, Anxiety, p. 4. · Be with patient when physician returns *to reinforce and explain information.* · Provide emotional support as needed.	Anxiety/fear will be relieved.
Pain/discomfort *Related to:* Incision Restricted movement Myocardial ischemia **DEFINING CHARACTERISTICS** Patient complains of discomfort Restlessness and increased anxiety Increased irritability Maintains rigid, nonmoving position Facial mask of pain Change in vital signs: Increased BP, heart rate, and respiratory rate	**ONGOING ASSESSMENT** · Solicit patient's description of pain. · Assess pain characteristics: Quality Severity Location Onset Duration Precipitating factors or relieving factors · Check incision for hematoma formation. **THERAPEUTIC INTERVENTIONS** For incisional pain: · Medicate as ordered and note response. · Use additional comfort measures whenever appropriate. · Assist patient in changing position (within limitations). · Use distraction when applicable. · Provide reassurance and emotional support. · Notify physician if interventions are unsuccessful *so that appropriate measures will be taken to relieve pain.* For restricted movement: · Assist patient in changing position within activity limitations at least q2h *to minimize discomfort and restlessness.* Position to maintain proper body alignment. Support dependent parts with pillows. · Offer back rubs *to help relieve or ease discomfort from lying on back for several hours.* · Apply antipressure devices to bed as appropriate. For anginal pain: · Notify physician of pain. · Give medications (nitroglycerin) as ordered. Monitor BP closely, anticipating drop in BP and need for additional fluids.	Discomfort will be reduced or relieved.

Cardiac catheterization—cont'd

NURSING DIAGNOSES / DEFINING CHARACTERISTICS	NURSING INTERVENTIONS / *RATIONALES*	EXPECTED OUTCOMES

	• If pain is unrelieved within 5 min:
	  Call physician immediately for further assessment and medical intervention.
	  Anticipate need for ECG.
	• See Angina pectoris: unstable, p. 69.	

Originated by: Patricia Farrell, RN,C
              Maureen Kangleon, RN

Cardiac surgery; adult: immediate postoperative care

(BYPASS (CABG); VALVE REPLACEMENT)

Coronary artery bypass grafting (CABG): The surgical approach to coronary artery disease is coronary artery bypass grafting. An artery from the chest wall (internal mammary) or a vein from the leg (saphenous) is used to supply blood distal to the area of stenosis. Bleeding and myocardial ischemia are potential postoperative complications.

Valvular heart surgery: Rheumatic fever, infection, calcification, or degeneration can cause the valve to become stenotic (incomplete opening) or regurgitant (incomplete closure). Whenever possible, the native valve is repaired. If the valve is beyond repair, it is replaced. Replacement valves can be tissue or mechanical. Tissue valves have a short longevity; mechanical valves last longer, but the patient must be continuously anticoagulated. Valve surgery involves intracardiac suture lines; therefore these patients are at high risk for conduction defects and postoperative bleeding.

Extracorporeal circulation (ECC): The heart–lung machine: A still heart and bloodless field are required for cardiac surgery. The heart-lung machine is used to divert blood from the heart and lungs, to oxygenate it, and to provide flow to the vital organs while the heart is stopped.

The major components of extracorporeal circulation are:

1. Anticoagulation: Heparin is used to prevent clots from forming.

2. Hemodilution: The blood is diluted to prevent sludging in the microcirculation.

3. Hypothermia: The entire body is cooled to decrease the metabolic demands during surgery. These factors facilitate extracorporeal circulation but also affect postoperative management. Fluid shifts, bleeding, and electrolyte shifts are common aftereffects of ECC.

NURSING DIAGNOSES / DEFINING CHARACTERISTICS	NURSING INTERVENTIONS / *RATIONALES*	EXPECTED OUTCOMES
Decreased cardiac output *Related to:* Low cardiac output syndrome occurs to some extent in all patients after ECC (see definition)	**ONGOING ASSESSMENT** • Continuously monitor cardiac rhythm, BP, CVP, PAD, LAP. • Assess pulses and capillary refill. • Assess and report changes in ABGs. • Assess hourly urine outputs. • Assess breath sounds and serial chest X-rays (CXRs).	Cardiac output will be sufficient to maintain vital organ perfusion.

Continued.

NURSING DIAGNOSES / DEFINING CHARACTERISTICS	NURSING INTERVENTIONS / *RATIONALES*	EXPECTED OUTCOMES
The more prolonged the pump run, the more profound the ventricular dysfunction Other factors include preoperative state of the heart and results of the surgical procedure **Defining Characteristics** Left ventricular failure: Increased LAP, increased PCWP, increased PAD Tachycardia Decreased BP, decreased CO Sluggish capillary refill Diminished peripheral pulses Changes in chest X-ray (CXR): Enlarged heart Increased pulmonary vascular markings Pulmonary edema Rales Decreased arterial and venous oxygen Acidosis Falling urine output Right ventricular failure: Increased RAP, increased CVP, increased HR Decreased LAP, decreased PCWP, decreased PAD (unless biventricular failure present) Jugular venous distention Decreased BP, decreased perfusion, decreased CO	**Therapeutic Interventions** ▪ Maintain hemodynamics within parameters set by surgeon: HR_____to _____ BP_____to_____ CVP-RAP_____to _____ Hemodynamic parameters may be maintained by titration of vasoactive drugs, most commonly: IV nitroglycerin: *dilates coronary vasculature, decreases spasm of mammary grafts, dilates venous system.* Nipride: *lowers systemic vascular resistance, decreases BP. Elevated pres sure on new grafts may cause bleeding.* Dopamine: *increased contractility, vasopressor effect, increases renal blood flow in low doses.* Dobutrex: *increased contractility without vasopressor effect. May slightly vasodilate.* Inocor: *increased contractility and vasodilation.* Isuprel: *increased HR, contractility; decreased pulmonary resistance for RV failure.* ▪ Maintain oxygen therapy as ordered. ▪ If unresponsive to usual treatment, anticipate use of mechanical assistance (IABP; ventricular assist device). ▪ See also Cardiac output, decreased, p. 9.	

Cardiac surgery; adult: immediate postoperative care—cont'd

NURSING DIAGNOSES / DEFINING CHARACTERISTICS	NURSING INTERVENTIONS / *RATIONALES*	EXPECTED OUTCOMES

Fluid volume deficit
Related to:
Total fluid volume may be normal or increased but because of ECC changes in membrane integrity causes fluid leaks into extravascular spaces
Diuresis
Blood loss
 	
DEFINING CHARACTERISTICS
Decreased filling pressures (CVP, RA, PAD, PCWP, LA)
Decreased BP; tachycardia
Decreased cardiac output/cardiac index
Decreased urine output with increased specific gravity
If blood loss occurs:
  Decreased Hb/Hct
  Increased chest tube drainage
  Alteration in coagulation factors
	ONGOING ASSESSMENT
	• Assess hemodynamics.
	• Monitor I & O.
	• Check urine specific gravity.
	• Assess chest tube drainage and report excess.
	• Check CBC and coagulation factors.
	• Repeat CBC (or spin hematocrit) if excess bleeding persists.
	
	THERAPEUTIC INTERVENTIONS
	• Administer volume as ordered *to maintain filling pressures within set parameters.*
	• Milk chest tubes *to maintain patency. Clotted tubes may precipitate cardiac tamponade; see p. 78.*
	• Administer coagulation factors (FFP, platelets, vitamin K, protamine, cryoprecipitate, vasopressin) as ordered *to correct deficiencies.*
	• Keep cross-matched blood available in case major bleeding occurs.
		Circulating blood volume will be sufficient to meet metabolic demands.

Potential decreased cardiac output
Related to:
Dysrhythmias that occur for many reasons in cardiac surgical patients:
  Ectopy usually results from irritability caused by ischemia, electrolyte imbalances, or mechanical irritation
  Bradyarrhythmias and *heart block* may be seen in valve surgery because of suture lines or edema in the area of specialized conduction tissue
	ONGOING ASSESSMENT
	• Continuously monitor cardiac rhythm.
	• Document rhythm strip once per shift or prn.
	• Monitor 12-lead ECG as ordered.
	• Assess electrolytes, especially potassium, magnesium, and calcium.
	• If heart block occurs in a patient who has been on digitalis before surgery, check serum digoxin level. *ECG may cause release of digoxin from tissues, transiently elevating digoxin level and depressing AV conduction.*
	
	THERAPEUTIC INTERVENTIONS
	• Maintain temporary pacemaker at bedside. *Temporary epicardial pacing wires are often placed prophylactically since dysrhythmias are common. During the first 24 hr the wires may be connected to a pulse generator kept on standby. See also Transvenous pacemaker, temporary, p. 177.*
	• Keep emergency medications readily available: lidocaine, atropine, Isuprel, epinephrine, calcium, verapamil.
	• Administer potassium as ordered *to keep serum level at 4-5 mEq.*
	• Administer magnesium as ordered *to keep level >2.0 mg.*
	• Administer calcium as ordered *to keep level at 8-10 mg.*
	• Reassess electrolyte levels if brisk diuresis occurs.
	• If arrhythmias are unresponsive to medical treatment, avoid *precordial thump. Use countershock instead to reduce risk of trauma to vascular suture lines.*
		Optimal cardiac rhythm and output will be maintained.

Continued.

NURSING DIAGNOSES / DEFINING CHARACTERISTICS	NURSING INTERVENTIONS / *RATIONALES*	EXPECTED OUTCOMES
Supraventricular tachyarrhythmias may be caused by atrial stretching, mechanical irritability secondary to cannulation, or rebound from preoperative β-blockers **DEFINING CHARACTERISTICS** Bradycardia (decreased <60) Tachycardia (increased >100) Ectopy (extra beats) Heart block Hypotension Dizziness Cool skin Decreased urine output Palpitations		

Potential for injury: cardiac tamponade
Related to:
Blood or fluid accumulation in pericardial sac or mediastinum
 	
DEFINING CHARACTERISTICS
Decreased BP
Narrowed pulse pressure
Pulsus paradoxus
Tachycardia
Electrical alternans
Equalization of pressures (CVP, PAP, PCWP)
Jugular venous distention
Widened mediastinum or enlarged heart on chest x-ray
	ONGOING ASSESSMENT
	- Assess for defining characteristics.
	- Evaluate status of chest tube drainage *to ensure patency of tubes* every hour. Notify physician if drainage is greater than 100 cc for consecutive 3 hr.
	- Monitor Hb and Hct.
	
	THERAPEUTIC INTERVENTIONS
	- Milk or strip chest tubes.
	- Keep chest tubes free of kinks.
	- If cardiac tamponade is rapidly developing with cardiovascular decompensation and collapse:
	    Assemble open chest tray for bedside intervention or prepare patient for transport to surgery.
	    Maintain aggressive fluid resuscitation, which may be required as tamponade is evacuated.
	    Administer vasopressor agents (dopamine, Levophed) as ordered *to maximize systemic perfusion pressure to vital organs.*
		Risk of injury is reduced.

NURSING DIAGNOSES / DEFINING CHARACTERISTICS	NURSING INTERVENTIONS / *RATIONALES*	EXPECTED OUTCOMES

Alteration in myocardial tissue perfusion
Related to:
Most often seen in coronary patients; may occur in any cardiac surgical patient. Causes include spasm of native coronary or of internal mammary artery graft, low flow or thrombosis of vein grafts, coronary embolus, perioperative ischemia (see Myocardial infarction, p. 103).
 	
DEFINING CHARACTERISTICS
T-wave inversion
ST elevation or depression
Ventricular irritability in the acute phase (patients will be under the effects of general anesthesia and, therefore, unable to verbalize/express chest pain)
	ONGOING ASSESSMENT
	• Continuously monitor ECG
	• Obtain 12 lead upon admission and prn. Compare to preop ECG. *Primary nurse must know which vessels were bypassed and carefully evaluate the corresponding areas on the 12-lead ECG.*
	   Right coronary artery (RCA): leads II, III, AVF
	   Posterior descending: R waves in V_1 and V_2
	   Left anterior descending: V_1 to V_4
	   Diagonals: V_5 to V_6
	   Circumflex, obtuse marginal: I, AVL, V_5
	• Monitor CPK, LDH, and isoenzymes.
	
	THERAPEUTIC INTERVENTIONS
	• Titrate IV nitroglycerin *for increased coronary perfusion and alleviation of coronary spasm.*
	• Maintain adequate diastolic BP with vasopressors. *Coronary artery flow occurs during diastole. Pressures of at least 40 mm Hg are needed to drive coronary flow and prevent graft thrombosis.*
	• Minimize intrathoracic pressures:
	   PEEP of less than 10 cm
	   TV 10-15 cc/kg. Use increased rates to increase minute volumes. *These measures will help prevent external graft compression.*
	• Maintain arterial saturation >95%.
	• Notify surgeon of any signs of ischemia.
		Risk of perioperative ischemia and/or infarction will be reduced.

Potential alteration in fluid composition, electrolyte imbalance *Related to:* Fluid shifts are often accompanied by changes in fluid composition Patients on diuretics before surgery generally have decreased potassium and magnesium **DEFINING CHARACTERISTICS** Na below 130 or above 142 K below 4.0 or above 5.0 Cl below 98 or above 115 Ca below 9.0 or above 11.0	**ONGOING ASSESSMENT** • Observe and document serial laboratory data. Monitor Na, K, Cl, glucose, Ca, BUN, and creatinine as ordered. Notify of abnormalities. *Diabetic patients or those on epinephrine infusions will have elevated serum glucose levels and may require more frequent assessment of glucose levels.* • Monitor ECG for changes; document; and notify physician. • Determine contributing factors (e.g., anesthesia, medications) to any change. **THERAPEUTIC INTERVENTIONS** • Maintain adequate electrolyte balance by administering desired electrolytes as ordered. *Hypertonic solutions may be used to correct Na and Cl deficiencies. K and Ca may be corrected by administration of K^+ or CaCl. (Note: K and CaCl are given via central IV over 1 hr to ensure accuracy).* • Maintain adequate glucose levels. Use chemstrips to determine serum glucose and document. • Administer IV insulin as ordered. *Subcutaneous insulin may be poorly absorbed because of hypothermia and decreased perfusion in early postop phases.*	Electrolyte balance will be maintained.

Continued.

NURSING DIAGNOSES / DEFINING CHARACTERISTICS	NURSING INTERVENTIONS / *RATIONALES*	EXPECTED OUTCOMES
Glucose below 90 or above 150 BUN above 20 Creatinine above 1.8 ECG changes: widening QRS, ST changes, and atrioventricular blocks		

NURSING DIAGNOSES / DEFINING CHARACTERISTICS	NURSING INTERVENTIONS / *RATIONALES*	EXPECTED OUTCOMES
Impaired gas exchange *Related to:* Initially the cardiac surgical patient will require mechanical ventilation because of use of general anesthesia. Weaning and extubation occur as soon as anesthetic agents wear off in most patients. Exceptions are any unstable patient, patients with LV failure, patients who require FiO$_2$'s >60% to maintain adequate O$_2$ saturations, x-ray evidence of pneumothorax or large effusions, patient with unstable sternum, cardiac assist device, or transthoracic IAB. Reasons for respiratory insufficiency include retraction and compression of lungs during surgery, secretions, and pulmonary vascular congestion Surgical incision may cause chest discomfort and inhibit deep breathing and coughing	**ONGOING ASSESSMENT** • Check rate and depth of ventilation. • Check chest expansion. • Evaluate breath sounds. • Monitor serial chest x-rays. • Check temperature q4h. • Obtain differential if WBC is elevated. • Evaluate color, consistency, and amount of sputum. *Discolored or foul-smelling secretions should be cultured.* • Check ABGs within 20 min whenever ventilator settings are changed. **THERAPEUTIC INTERVENTIONS** • Maintain ventilator settings as ordered. General guidelines: Tidal volume (TV) 10-15 cc/kg Rate 10-14/min FiO$_2$ to keep Po$_2$ greater than 80 PEEP + 5 cm. *Considered physiologically equal to upper airway resistance* • Change ventilator settings as ordered to maintain ABGs within accepted limits. (Note: Patients with preexisting pulmonary dysfunction will have lower Po$_2$ and higher Pco$_2$ values). • Suction PRN. *During surgery the lungs are kept deflated and atelectasis as well as mucous plugs may result.* • Hyperventilate and hyperoxygenate during suctioning *to prevent desaturation.* • Encourage coughing and deep breathing. Use pillow to splint incision. • Use pain medications *to decrease incisional discomfort so that patient will cough and deep breath.* • Consider chest physiotherapy. • See also Mechanical ventilation, p. 213.	Adequate ventilation will be maintained.
DEFINING CHARACTERISTICS *Ventilated patients:* Increasing FiO$_2$ required to maintain adequate oxygenation Evidence of pleural effusions, pulmonary edema, or infiltrates on CXR		

NURSING DIAGNOSES / DEFINING CHARACTERISTICS	NURSING INTERVENTIONS / *RATIONALES*	EXPECTED OUTCOMES
Extubated patients: Increased Pco_2 Decreased Po_2/O_2 saturation Rapid, shallow respirations Weak, ineffective cough Rales, rhonchi CXR as above		

Alteration in level of consciousness
Related to:
Although general anesthesia accounts for initial decrease in consciousness, thorough neurologic assessment is necessary to rule out postoperative neurologic complications
Reasons for potential neurologic complications:
  Atherosclerosis is not limited to coronary vessels; carotids may be involved. Nonpulsatile flow at lower perfusion pressures may cause cerebral ischemia
  Embolization of air, calcium, or thrombus may occur during aortic cannulation or decannulation
  Anticoagulation may lead to intravascular hemorrhage
 	
DEFINING CHARACTERISTICS
Unequal pupils
Failure to awaken from anesthesia
Focal deficit upon awakening
Confusion, memory loss
Agitation
	ONGOING ASSESSMENT
	• Check pupils.
	• Check ability to follow commands.
	• Assess hand grasps.
	• Determine factors contributing to any changes.
	
	THERAPEUTIC INTERVENTIONS
	• Reorient to surroundings as needed.
	• Record serial assessments.
	• Notify surgeon immediately of any changes in neurologic assessment.
	• See Consciousness, alteration in level of, p. 234.
		Optimal state of consciousness will be maintained.

Continued.

NURSING DIAGNOSES / DEFINING CHARACTERISTICS	NURSING INTERVENTIONS / *RATIONALES*	EXPECTED OUTCOMES
Potential for infection *Related to:* Surgical incisions Multiple lines and devices Frequent blood draws **DEFINING CHARACTERISTICS** Temperature >38.5°C Increased WBC Redness around wounds or IV sites Infiltrates on CXR Wound drainage	**ONGOING ASSESSMENT** · Check temperature q4h. · Monitor daily CBC. · If WBC increases, check differential. · Assess incisions for erythema or drainage. · Monitor IV site. **THERAPEUTIC INTERVENTIONS** · Remove IV lines after 72 hr; rotate sites. · Change IV bags/tubings per hospital protocol. · Cap open stopcock parts. Change if contaminated. · Maintain aseptic techniques when entering lines for blood draws or medication administration. · Discontinue all invasive lines and devices (IVs, Foley, pacing wires, central and arterial lines) as soon as possible. · Provide vigorous pulmonary toilet. · Cover wounds with sterile dressings until dry. · Draw blood cultures if temperature >38.5°C.	Nosocomial infections will be prevented.
Anxiety *Related to:* ICU environment Unfamiliarity with postoperative care Altered communication secondary to intubation Fear of pain related to major surgery Fear of death **DEFINING CHARACTERISTICS** Restlessness Increased awareness Glancing about Trembling/fidgety Constant demands Facial tension Insomnia Wide-eyed appearance Tense appearance Sad expression	**ONGOING ASSESSMENT** · Recognize patient's level of anxiety. Note signs and symptoms, especially nonverbal communication. · Assess patient's normal coping patterns by talking with family and significant others. **THERAPEUTIC INTERVENTIONS** · Orient to environment. · Display calm, confident manner *to increase feeling of security.* · Assist patient to understand that emotional responses are normal, anticipated responses to cardiac surgery. · Prepare for and explain common postoperative sensations (coldness, fatigue, discomfort, coughing, uncomfortable endotracheal tube). Clarify misconceptions *to allay fear.* · Explain each procedure before doing it, even if previously described. *High anxiety levels can reduce attention level and retention of information.* · Provide pain medication at first sign of discomfort *to minimize discomfort and reduce fear.* · Provide nonverbal means of communication (slate, paper and pencil, gestures). Be patient with attempts to communicate. Know and anticipate usual patient concerns. · Ensure continuity of staff *to facilitate communication efforts and provide stability in care.* · Encourage visiting by family or significant others *so patient doesn't feel alone.*	Anxiety will be reduced or relieved.
Pain *Related to:* Incisions Restricted mobility Presence of catheter and tubes **DEFINING CHARACTERISTICS** Complaint of pain Restlessness Facial mask of pain Guarding/protective behavior	**ONGOING ASSESSMENT** · Solicit description of pain, using nonverbal communication as appropriate. · Monitor effectiveness of pain medications. **THERAPEUTIC INTERVENTIONS** · See also Anxiety, p. 4. · Anticipate need for analgesics. · Respond immediately to complaint of pain. · Provide quiet environment as feasible *to foster relaxed state.* · Provide comfort measures (position changes, back rubs, ice chips), distraction techniques. · Facilitate removal of catheter/tubes as early as appropriate. · See also Pain, p. 39.	Comfort will be maximized.

NURSING DIAGNOSES / DEFINING CHARACTERISTICS	NURSING INTERVENTIONS/ *RATIONALES*	EXPECTED OUTCOMES
Sleep pattern disturbance *Related to:* Pain Fear/anxiety Unfamiliar/distracting environment Increased nursing care Inability to assume usual sleep position **DEFINING CHARACTERISTICS** Restlessness Insomnia Dozing Yawning Interrupted sleep Fatigued appearance Mental status changes (ICU psychosis)	**ONGOING ASSESSMENT** ▪ Assess sleep pattern, documenting amount of meaningful sleep. **THERAPEUTIC INTERVENTIONS** ▪ If lack of meaningful sleep is a problem, see Sleep pattern disturbance, p. 50.	Optimal sleep will be achieved.
Impaired physical mobility *Related to:* Bedrest/activity restriction Invasive catheters Critical physical condition **DEFINING CHARACTERISTICS** Inability to move purposefully within physical environment Limited ROM	**ONGOING ASSESSMENT** ▪ Assess for signs of respiratory problems. ▪ Assess skin integrity for signs of redness and tissue ischemia. **THERAPEUTIC INTERVENTIONS** ▪ Reposition patient q2h. Use pillow support *to maintain proper body alignment.* ▪ Perform ROM exercises. ▪ Institute antipressure devices as appropriate. ▪ See Mobility, impaired physical, p. 35.	Optimal physical mobility will be achieved.
Altered body temperature *Related to:* Hypothermia used in conjunction with ECC **DEFINING CHARACTERISTICS** Rectal temperature <37° C Skin cool with decreased perfusion Tachycardia or heart block	**ONGOING ASSESSMENT** ▪ Monitor and document changes in skin temperature, perfusion, and capillary refill every hour; notify physician of changes. ▪ Monitor rectal temperature continuously by rectal probe. Assure accuracy of rectal probe by checking manual temperature q. 4 hr. ▪ Continuously monitor ECG and maintain pacemaker on standby. **THERAPEUTIC INTERVENTIONS** ▪ Use extra blanket, mattress, or warm packs *to increase temperature slowly.* ▪ *Protect skin against burns by* providing layer of protection between patient's skin and warming apparatus.	Adequate body temperature will be maintained.

Originated by: Sonia Ortaliza, RN
Donna Creachbaum, RN, BS, CCRN

Cardiac surgery: intermediate postoperative care

The intermediate care phase (postop day 3 to hospital discharge, around postop day 7-9) focuses on progressive rehabilitation, patient teaching, and identification and prevention of postoperative complications.

(CORONARY ARTERY BYPASS SURGERY [CABG]; HEART SURGERY; CARDIAC REHABILITATION)

NURSING DIAGNOSES / DEFINING CHARACTERISTICS	NURSING INTERVENTIONS / *RATIONALES*	EXPECTED OUTCOMES
Ineffective breathing pattern/impaired gas exchange *Related to:* Adequate lung expansion Ineffective cough Retained pulmonary secretions Pleural effusion Fatigue Pain Altered oxygen-carrying capacity of blood **DEFINING CHARACTERISTICS** Dyspnea, shortness of breath Abnormal breath sounds Decreased oxygenation on serial ABGs (Po_2, saturation) Abnormal chest x-ray film Decreased Hct and Hb Changes in mental status Restlessness Tachypnea	**ONGOING ASSESSMENT** · Inspect chest for respiratory rate and rhythm. · Auscultate breath sounds for adventitious sounds. · Monitor ABGs and chest x-ray film as needed. · Monitor hemoglobin and hematocrit. **THERAPEUTIC INTERVENTIONS** · Encourage use of incentive spirometer 10 times each hour as tolerated *to prevent atelectasis and optimize lung expansion.* · Demonstrate and teach coughing, deep breathing, and splinting techniques. Encourage coughing and deep breathing 10 times per hour while patient is awake *to keep airway patent, prevent atelectasis, and improve lung function.* · Assist with splinting of chest for more effective coughing. *Postop patients may be reluctant to cough and deep breathe because of fear of pain and injury to sternotomy site. Use of splinting technique (e.g., pillow, hands across chest) decreases tension on incision and reduces pain, thus promoting improved coughing and deep breathing.* · Provide pain medication prn *to optimize effective cough and deep breathing. Postoperative pain/anxiety may decrease patient's willingness to cough/deep breathe.* · Provide fluids or vaporizer to *assist in loosening secretions.* · Provide rest periods between breathing/coughing exercises. · Provide O_2 therapy as ordered. Use nasal cannula during meals if necessary; use portable O_2 during patient ambulation. · Turn, reposition, ambulate patient per cardiac rehabilitation protocol (see guidelines under activity tolerance problem below). · Provide respiratory treatments if indicated.	Optimal gas exchange will be maintained.

Pain *Related to:* Surgical incisions Postextubation throat pain
 	
 DEFINING CHARACTERISTICS Patient or significant others verbalize pain Protective decreased physical activity Restlessness, irritability, altered sleep pattern, anxiety Facial mask of pain
	ONGOING ASSESSMENT
	 · Assess patient's subjective complaints of pain or discomfort.
	
	 THERAPEUTIC INTERVENTIONS
	 For incisional pain:
	 · Anticipate need for analgesics, especially before activities.
	 · Administer medications as ordered, evaluating effectiveness and observing for side effects.
	 · Reassure patient that incisional pain is to be expected. *Many patients think any pain in the sternal area represents ischemia.*
	 · Use additional comfort measures when appropriate.
	    Heat pad
	    Distraction techniques
	    Relaxation techniques
	 · Provide rest periods *to facilitate comfort and relaxation.*
	 · Instruct patient to report pain *so relief measures can be instituted promptly.*
	 For throat pain/discomfort, provide ice chips, throat lozenges, viscous lidocaine, if ordered.
	 Elevate graft leg *to improve circulation and reduce venous pooling.*
		Pain will be alleviated or reduced.

NURSING DIAGNOSES / DEFINING CHARACTERISTICS	NURSING INTERVENTIONS / *RATIONALES*	EXPECTED OUTCOMES
Alteration in muscle tone (listlessness, flaccidity/rigidity, tenseness) Reluctance to cough		

NURSING DIAGNOSES / DEFINING CHARACTERISTICS	NURSING INTERVENTIONS / *RATIONALES*	EXPECTED OUTCOMES
Activity intolerance *Related to:* Imposed activity restrictions Generalized weakness; deconditioned state Fatigue secondary to sleeping difficulty **DEFINING CHARACTERISTICS** Report of fatigue or weakness Abnormal heart rate or BP response to activity Exertional discomfort Dyspnea Dizziness Diaphoresis	**ONGOING ASSESSMENT** • Assess patient' respiratory/cardiac status before activity. • Observe and document response to activity. Report abnormal responses listed below. *Physical activities increase demands placed on the healing myocardium. Close monitoring of patient's response provides a guide for optimal progression of activity.* Pulse >20 beats over resting, or 120 BPM Palpitations BP increases >20 mm Hg BP decreases >10 mm Hg Dyspnea, weakness Chest pain, dizziness Skin color changes, diaphoresis • Monitor number of visitors and length of stay *so patient obtains needed rest.* **THERAPEUTIC INTERVENTIONS** • Encourage adequate rest periods, especially before activities *to reduce cardiac workload.* • Assist with self-care activities as needed. Evaluate need for chair in bathroom during morning care. • Provide emotional support when increasing activity. *Patients sometimes don't notice progress since rehabilitation is a slow process. Emphasize positive steps.* • Encourage active ROM exercise tid *to maintain muscle strength and decrease risk of thromboembolism.* • Provide portable oxygen as needed. • Maintain progression of activity as ordered by cardiac rehabilitation team or physician. *Gradual increase in activity under supervision promotes self-care and decreases patient anxiety.* Note: *Everyone does not progress at the same rate. Generally, uncomplicated bypass patients recover faster than valve patients. Other factors (e.g., related medical problems, previous sedentary life-style, lack of motivation, inadequate sleep, fear of "overexertion") can also affect progress. Therefore, the following cardiac rehabilitation walking distances are only meant to be a guide.* Cardiac rehabilitation stages: Stage 1: Date_____ Dangle 15-30 min tid. Feed self Stage 2: Date _____ Partial bath in chair, shave self; sit in chair 20-60 min tid Stage 3: Date_____ Partial bath at sink; bathroom privileges; in chair whenever desired; walk in room Stage 4: Date_____ Self morning care; walk in hall 150 ft tid Stage 5: Date_____ Sit in hall; walk 300 ft tid Stage 6: Date_____ Walk 600 feet tid Stage 7: Date _____ Stair climbing with cardiac rehabilitation nurse Stage 8: Progressive walking as tolerated	Optimal activity tolerance will be maintained.

Continued.

Cardiac surgery: intermediate postoperative care—cont'd

NURSING DIAGNOSES / DEFINING CHARACTERISTICS	NURSING INTERVENTIONS / *RATIONALES*	EXPECTED OUTCOMES
Sleep pattern disturbance *Related to:* Pain Anxiety/fear Decreased physical activity New surroundings Medical procedures **DEFINING CHARACTERISTICS** Inability to fall asleep Inability to stay asleep	**ONGOING ASSESSMENT** • Assess current pattern of sleep/rest. • Assess patient's perception of cause of sleep difficulty and possible relief measures *to facilitate treatment*. • Evaluate timing/effects of medications that disrupt sleep. **THERAPEUTIC INTERVENTIONS** • Provide comfort measures (e.g., back rubs, pillows, blankets). Adequate sleep/rest patterns will be maintained to aid postoperative recovery. • Assist patient in selecting position of optimal comfort. *The sternal incision prevents patients from sleeping on preferred side or stomach position. Remind patient that this is temporary problem. After the sternum heals, he/she can sleep in any position.* • Minimize interruptions in sleep during night. Organize care. • Provide pain medications as needed. *Reduction of pain facilitates relaxation and sleep.* • Assist patient in reducing anxiety. *Verbalization of feelings may decrease fear and facilitate sleep. Postoperative patients frequently need reassurance that recovery is possible and progressive.* • Minimize long napping during day when possible. *Napping may decrease sleep time at night.* • Encourage frequent ambulation and sitting in chair during day.	Adequate sleep/rest patterns will be maintained to aid postoperative recovery.

Altered nutrition: less than body requirements
Related to:
Decreased appetite secondary to weakness, pain, anxiety
Decreased GI motility secondary to anesthesia
 	
DEFINING CHARACTERISTICS
Nausea/vomiting
Poor intake of food
Refusal to eat
Expressed lack of appetite
Complaints of gastric upset/gas pain
	ONGOING ASSESSMENT
	• Assess intake of food at every meal.
	• Monitor fluid balance.
	• Assess for signs of dehydration (decreased urine output, dry mucous membranes, change in mental status, etc.).
	• Assess for GI function:
	    Auscultate for bowel sounds.
	    Monitor frequency of bowel movements/passing of flatus.
	• Evaluate patient's food preferences.
	
	THERAPEUTIC INTERVENTIONS
	• Get dietary consultation *to assist in planning meals/snacks.*
	• Encourage patient to report feelings of nausea.
	• Administer antiemetics and/or antacids as ordered *to decrease GI upset.*
	• Administer laxative as ordered to *facilitate passing of stool to decrease gastric compression.*
	• Encourage ambulation *since exercise increases appetite and facilitates return of GI function.*
		Nutrition will be adequate to meet body requirements.

Altered peripheral tissue perfusion
Related to:
Saphenous vein grafting causing loss of vasomotor tone and peripheral pooling of blood
Bed rest/immobility
 	
DEFINING CHARACTERISTICS
Edema, swelling of affected parts
Coolness, pallor of lower extremities
	ONGOING ASSESSMENT
	• Assess posterior, tibial, and pedal pulses daily.
	• Note color and temperature of extremities and presence of edema or pain at least q4h.
	• Check for calf tenderness.
	• Question patient about pain in legs and change in sensation.
	
	THERAPEUTIC INTERVENTIONS
	• Apply TED hose *to promote venous return, especially to graft leg, in bypass surgery patients:*
	    TED hose should be removed daily to *assess extremity adequately.*
	    As activity increases, TED hose can be removed at night.
	• Ambulate *to promote venous return.*
	• Assist patient with active ROM exercises two or three times daily per cardiac rehabilitation protocol *to prevent venous pooling.*
	• Instruct patient to avoid leg crossing and knee gatching.
		Adequate peripheral circulation will be maintained.

NURSING DIAGNOSES / DEFINING CHARACTERISTICS	NURSING INTERVENTIONS / *RATIONALES*	EXPECTED OUTCOMES
Tenderness of affected extremities Pain, tingling, numbness		
Potential for infection *Related to:* Surgical incision Central/peripheral IV lines Foley catheter External pacing wires **DEFINING CHARACTERISTICS** Febrile Increased WBC count Redness, swelling, drainage from incision site/IV site Excessive tenderness at incision site Burning on urination Cloudy, foul-smelling urine	**ONGOING ASSESSMENT** • Assess incisional sites daily (chest and donor leg) for signs and symptoms of infection/drainage. • Assess vital signs at least every shift for fever, tachycardia. • Assess for burning on urination; cloudy, foul-smelling urine. • If pacing wires (external) present, monitor for drainage from pacing wire site. • Obtain cultures if indicated for urine, blood, wound. **THERAPEUTIC INTERVENTIONS** • Maintain aseptic technique during procedures *to prevent infection.* • Keep incision dry and clean. Incision usually kept uncovered after third postoperative day unless drainage noted. • Instruct patient that some drainage from donor leg can be expected with increased activity. • Keep TED stockings clean. Alternate pairs of stockings as needed.	Occurrence of infection will be decreased.

Potential decreased cardiac output
Related to:
Altered preload
Altered afterload
Altered contractility
Altered heart rate
 	
DEFINING CHARACTERISTICS
Low urine output
Decreasing BP, increased/decreased heart rate
Decreasing or absent pulse
Change in mental status
Weight gain, edema
Dizziness
Weakness, fatigue
Restlessness
Abnormal heart sounds
Abnormal lung sounds
Neck vein distention
	ONGOING ASSESSMENT
	• Assess physical status closely, document changes, report significant changes in parameters:
	  Arterial BP, orthostatic changes. *Fluid restrictions and/or lack of appetite may result in decreased circulating blood volume, as noted by orthostatic blood pressure changes.*
	  Heart rate
	  Apical/radial pulses; peripheral pulses (strength, equality)
	  Heart sounds
	  Lung sounds
	  Jugular venous distention
	  Change in mental status
	  Urine output
	  Skin color, temperature
	• Monitor daily weight *to assess for fluid retention.*
	• Monitor cardiac rate and rhythm. *Change in rhythm (e.g., tachycardia, bradycardia, atrial fibrillation/flutter) may decrease cardiac output.*
	
	THERAPEUTIC INTERVENTIONS
	• Administer routine cardiac medications as ordered; observe for side effects and toxicity.
	• Maintain optimal fluid intake.
	• Administer O_2 as ordered.
	• Maintain output >30 cc/hr.
	• If signs of left ventricular failure are noted:
	  Initiate O_2 as needed.
	  Report to physician.
	  Initiate treatment for, Cardiac output, decreased, p. 9.
		Optimal hemodynamic status will be maintained.

Continued.

NURSING DIAGNOSES / DEFINING CHARACTERISTICS	NURSING INTERVENTIONS / *RATIONALES*	EXPECTED OUTCOMES
Potential alteration in cardiac rhythm (atrial, junctional, ventricular rhythms) *Related to:* Ischemia Irritability of cardiac muscle secondary to manipulation during surgery Hypoxia Electrolyte imbalance **DEFINING CHARACTERISTICS** Irregular heart rate Tachycardia/ bradycardia Decreasing/increasing K levels Hypoxia Palpitations Shortness of breath	**ONGOING ASSESSMENT** • Monitor heart rate, rhythm, and ectopy every shift. *Arrhythmias commonly occur 24-72 hr after surgery, but may occur at any time during hospitalization.* • If ECG monitoring is available, continuously monitor ECG for rate, rhythm, abnormality, and change in PR, QRS, and QT intervals if appropriate. • Observe for abnormalities in cardiac electrolytes. *Hypokalemia makes heart susceptible to ventricular arrhythmias.* **THERAPEUTIC INTERVENTIONS** • If arrhythmia occurs, determine whether acute or chronic. *Many valve patients have chronic atrial arrhythmias that persist postoperatively.* • Evaluate patient's response to arrhythmia; document; report if significant or symptomatic. • Have antiarrhythmics readily available. • Treat arrhythmias according to medical orders or protocol. • If patient has external pacing wires in place *(these are sometimes placed during surgery for emergency use postoperatively to treat bradycardia and override tachyarrhythmias):* Avoid putting extra tension on wires *to prevent dislodgment.* When not in use, wires should be secured in plastic syringe *to prevent ambient electrical current that could lead to arrhythmias.* • If bradyarrhythmias occur, anticipate use of pacemaker generator with connection to external pacing wires.	Baseline cardiac rhythm will be maintained.
Potential self-concept disturbance *Related to:* Actual/perceived changes in physiological functioning Increased amount of disease-related symptoms Change in health status Threat of death Perceived/actual change in role Possible change in life-style (job, physical activity) **DEFINING CHARACTERISTICS** Refusal to accept rehabilitation efforts Inappropriate attempts to direct own treatment Signs of grieving: crying, despair, anger Refusal to participate in self-care Self-destructive behavior Withdrawl from social contacts	**ONGOING ASSESSMENT** • Assess contributing factors. • Assess usual coping methods. • Assess meaning of heart surgery on patient and significant others *(reactions may vary from happiness that previous angina or shortness of breath will be relieved to fear of being "cardiac cripple").* • Assess feelings about incision. *Some cardiac patients are repulsed by the long sternal incision; others may regard it as a "status" symbol.* • Assess for common reactions, such as denial, anger, anxiety, and depression. **THERAPEUTIC INTERVENTIONS** • Encourage verbalization of feelings. *Allow patient time to work through different stages of coping.* • Provide anticipatory guidance *to minimize anxiety and fear of the unknown.* Provide reliable information about future limitations (if any) on physical activity and role performance. • Assist patient to accept help from others. Stress that state is *temporary.* • Identify outlets that foster feelings of personal achievement and self-esteem. • Explore strengths and resources with patient. • Realistically point out positive changes in person's condition. *Patients frequently don't see their own progress during recovery.* • Encourage referral to cardiac rehabilitation program or "coronary club" *to increase confidence in self and physical abilities; provide mechanism for ongoing verbalization of feelings and clarification of misconceptions.*	Patient will verbalize positive expressions of continued self-worth.

NURSING DIAGNOSES / DEFINING CHARACTERISTICS	NURSING INTERVENTIONS / *RATIONALES*	EXPECTED OUTCOMES
Focus on past strength, function Feelings of helplessness Preoccupation with change or loss Change in perception of self and role Change in usual patterns of responsibility		

Knowledge deficit: myocardial infarction and follow-up care
Related to:
Unfamiliarity with disease process, treatment, recovery
 	
DEFINING CHARACTERISTICS
Questioning
Verbalizing misconceptions
Not verbalizing feelings
	ONGOING ASSESSMENT
	• Assess patient's physical and emotional readiness to learn.
	• Assess patient's/significant others' understanding of surgical procedure, recovery process, diet, medications, activity progression, preventive care, wound care, pacing wires (if present).
	• Determine specific learning needs and patient goals. *Teaching standardized content patient already knows wastes valuable time and hinders critical learning.*
	
	THERAPEUTIC INTERVENTIONS
	• Plan teaching session *so patient is not overwhelmed at one time*.
	• Provide environment conducive to learning.
	• Consult cardiac rehabilitation clinical specialist about appropriate teaching materials (hospital television, heart model, group class, handouts).
	• Provide information *as needed* about:
	  Surgical procedures (bypass grafting; valve replacement)
	  Healing process post surgery
	  Epicardial pacing wires
	  Resuming activities of daily living
	  Dietary regime
	  Medications (especially anticoagulants for valve patients)
	  Progressive activity/exercise plan:
	    Home walking program
	    Climbing of stairs
	    Lifting/household chores
	    Driving car
	    Shopping/movies/restaurants/social visits
	    Sexual activity
	  Coping mechanisms to help adjustment to new or altered life-style.
	  Immediate treatment for recurrence of chest pain, shortness of breath, palpitations, etc.
	  Preventive care
	    Risk factors of heart disease
	    Effects of smoking and alcohol on heart
	    Incisional care and observation
	    Use of TED hose at home
	    Prophylactic antibiotics for dental and surgical procedures for valve patients
	  Follow-up medical care
	  Medic-Alert identification
		Patient/significant others will verbalize understanding of disease state, surgical procedure, recovery process, diet, medications, activity, and preventive care.

Originated by: Antoinette Harris-Hardy, RN, BSN
        Barbara Gallagher, RN, BSN

Cardiac transplantation

(HEART TRANSPLANT)

Cardiac transplantation is a treatment option for persons with end-stage cardiac disease for whom all possible modes of surgical and medical treatment have been exhausted. Transplant candidates must meet certain criteria, including age, other disease processes, renal function, social supports, and psychological stability, to maximize the potential for success. The surgical procedure entails the excision of both donor and recipient hearts and transplantation of the donor heart into the recipient (orthotopically transplanted). With ongoing compliance to medical therapy and adherence to life-style changes, the transplant patient can live an active and productive life.

NURSING DIAGNOSES / DEFINING CHARACTERISTICS	NURSING INTERVENTIONS / *RATIONALES*	EXPECTED OUTCOMES
Decreased cardiac output *Related to:* Arrhythmias induced by edema of conductive tissue in the donor heart secondary to manipulation of the nodal tissue at time of transplantation Ischemia occurring during transport of donor graft or secondary to surgical procedure Electrolyte/acid-base imbalance **DEFINING CHARACTERISTICS** Cardiac dysrhythmias: Junctional rhythms Symptomatic bradycardia Ventricular ectopy Rapid/slow pulse Shortness of breath Dizziness Change in mental status Decreased BP Cool, clammy skin	**ONGOING ASSESSMENT** • Monitor ECG continuously, documenting any signs of inadequate heart rate (sinus pause, sinus arrest, junctional rhythm, heart blocks, and bradycardias) or ventricular ectopy. *The rate and rhythm of the transplanted heart depend on the sinus node impulse in the donor heart. Remnant P waves from native heart are of no clinical significance because these electrical impulses do not cross the suture line. Junctional rhythms are secondary to suture line edema in the atrium and generally resolve within 2 weeks.* • Assess for signs of decreased cardiac output. *Transplanted hearts are denervated; therefore, heart rate changes gradually in response to altered metabolic needs via circulating catecholamines secreted from the adrenal medulla (i.e., there may be no compensatory tachycardia indicating hypovolemia or pump failure).* • Monitor electrolyte and acid-base balance. **THERAPEUTIC INTERVENTIONS** • Initiate and maintain isoproterenol hydrochloride (Isuprel) drip as ordered *to increase heart rate.* • Use temporary epicardial pacing wires *to maintain an adequate heart rate* as needed. Check rate, mA, mode, and connections frequently. Keep pacer wires wrapped in rubber gloves and taped securely to chest wall. • If ventricular ectopy occurs, administer lidocaine bolus followed by drip as ordered (1 mg/kg for initial bolus, rebolus 10 min later, followed with a lidocaine drip at 2-4 mg/min). • Give potassium replacement as ordered *to maintain serum K+ level greater than 4.0. Hypokalemia causes ventricular irritability.* • Correct uncompensated metabolic acidosis with $NaHCO_3$ as ordered. *Acidosis precipitates ventricular ectopy.* • See Cardiac output, decreased, p. 9; Cardiac dysrhythmias, p. 74.	Optimal cardiac output is maintained.
Potential decreased cardiac output *Related to:* Biventricular failure secondary to preexisting pulmonary hypertension Global ischemia of donor heart before transplantation Cardiac tamponade	**ONGOING ASSESSMENT** • Monitor cardiac output by thermodilution on admission and prn. • Assess right side of heart performance by documentation of central venous pressure (CVP). • Assess left side of heart performance by documentation of pulmonary artery pressure (PAP), pulmonary capillary wedge pressure (PCWP), left arterial pressure (LAP), SVR, and arterial BP. • Monitor intake and output hourly. • Assess for signs of cardiac tamponade. • Monitor MCT drainage. • Assess for signs of: Decreased systemic perfusion Pulmonary venous congestion Systemic venous congestion	Optimal cardiac output is maintained.

NURSING DIAGNOSES / DEFINING CHARACTERISTICS	NURSING INTERVENTIONS / *RATIONALES*	EXPECTED OUTCOMES
DEFINING CHARACTERISTICS Cool, pale skin; poor capillary refill; diminished pulses; diaphoresis; decreased urine output Dyspnea, tachypnea, increased pulmonary artery diastolic pressure (PAD), pulmonary edema Jugular neck vein distention, ascites, peripheral or sacral edema Development of S_3 or S_4 gallop Muffled heart sounds, pulsus paradoxus	**THERAPEUTIC INTERVENTIONS** • Administer parenteral fluids as ordered *to maintain adequate filling pressures and optimize cardiac output.* • Institute measures *to reduce workload of heart* by maintaining normothermia, quiet environment, and placing patient in semi-Fowler's position. • Administer inotropes as ordered *to increase myocardial contractility* (dopamine, dobutamine, calcium). • Administer vasodilators (Nipride, Tridil) as ordered *to control systemic vascular resistance, thereby reducing heart workload.* • Maintain adequate oxygenation *to optimize cardiac function and reduce pulmonary vascular resistance.* • Administer Isuprel as ordered *to reduce pulmonary vascular resistance and increase heart rate.* • See Cardiac output, decreased, p. 9.	
Potential for injury: bleeding/ hemorrhage *Related to:* Pericardial sac is larger than normal after transplant; therefore, a small new heart leaves an area that may conceal postoperative bleeding Nonsurgical bleeding may be enhanced by preoperative anticoagulation or intraoperative cardiopulmonary bypass and heparinization Surgical bleeding may be enhanced by elaborate suture lines and cannulation sites, as well as coagulopathy **DEFINING CHARACTERISTICS** Tachycardia Hypotension Narrowing pulse pressure Decreased cardiac output Decreased CVP, PAP, PCWP Skin cool, clammy Poor capillary refill, diminished pulses Decreased urine output	**ONGOING ASSESSMENT** • Assess pulse, BP, hemodynamic measurements. • Assess peripheral pulses, capillary refill. • Monitor I&O. • Assess MCT drainage for significant cessation (i.e., tamponade) and/or increase (i.e., hemorrhage). • Monitor Hct/Hb. • Monitor PT/PTT, platelet count; check ACT prn. • Observe amplitude of ECG configuration. • Assess heart tones. • Evaluate CXR for widening of mediastinal shadow. **THERAPEUTIC INTERVENTIONS** • Raise head of bed to 30 degrees and turn patient hourly *to prevent impedance of mediastinal drainage.* • Strip chest tubes q30min for 12h, then hourly. Note amount and type of drainage (with or without clots); document output. • Maintain 20 cm H_2O suction to MCT *to facilitate drainage.* • Keep sternotomy tray at bedside at all times. • Maintain current type and cross to keep 2 units packed red blood cells (PRBCs) available at all times during ICU stay. *(Washed and cytomegalovirus (CMV)-negative because of patient's suppressed immune system).* • Replace volume losses with colloids or crystalloids as ordered. May consider autotransfusion. If patient is bleeding rapidly, anticipate return to operating room.	Potential for bleeding/ hemorrhage is reduced.

Continued.

Cardiac transplantation—cont'd

NURSING DIAGNOSES / DEFINING CHARACTERISTICS	NURSING INTERVENTIONS / *RATIONALES*	EXPECTED OUTCOMES
Frank bleeding, >100 cc/hr for 4 hr from MCT Decreased Hct/Hgb Coagulopathy Decreased QRS voltage Muffled heart sounds Widened mediastinum		

Knowledge deficit
Related to:
Unfamiliarity with:
    Surgical procedure
    Long-term care
 	
DEFINING CHARACTERISTICS
Questioning
Verbalizing misconceptions
Lack of questioning
	ONGOING ASSESSMENT
	• Assess patient/significant others' knowledge.
	• Assess physical/emotional readiness of patient/significant others to learn:
	    Receptiveness
	    Eagerness
	    Asking questions
	    Not fatigued or in pain
	• Assess patient/significant others' understanding of surgical procedure, follow-up care, diet, medications, activity progression, special precautions for avoiding infections, and risk factor modification.
	
	THERAPEUTIC INTERVENTIONS
	• Describe surgical procedure, including ICU regimen and expected length of stay.
	• Provide opportunity for patient/family to ask questions and verbalize anxieties, fears about discharge planning.
	• Coordinate discharge teaching with cardiac rehab. program, diet, occupational and physical therapy, respiratory therapy, social work, and any other significant departments *to ensure adequate understanding of care.*
	• Inform patient and family that patient will have periodic endomyocardial biopsy by cardiologist in operating room suite *to assess for heart rejection. Biopsy is an outpatient procedure; frequency tapers significantly 6 months after surgery.*
	• Inform patient he/she will not experience exertional chest pain and cannot rely on pulse rate to reflect tolerance or effects of activity accurately *because transplanted heart is denervated.*
	• Instruct patient on low-salt and low-cholesterol diet. *Low-salt diet will help decrease amount of steroid-induced fluid retention. Low-cholesterol diet will decrease risk of future heart disease.* Instruct patient to avoid fresh fruits and vegetables *because of increased amount of bacteria in these foods.* All foods should be steamed or cooked *to reduce bacteria.*
	• Instruct patient in medication regimen by using a medication flow chart specific for medications to be taken at home:
	    Because cyclosporine A is in an oil base, administer in a glass *to prevent adherence to the container walls* and with orange juice or chocolate milk *to enhance palatability.*
	    Cyclosporine A should be given on an empty stomach *to facilitate absorption;* steroids should be given with food.
	• Caution patients of increased potential for bone "brittleness" related to steroids. Suggest wearing comfortable flat shoes *to decrease possible falls and injury.*
	• Discuss possibility of emotional lability and mood alteration, *partly related to steroids, cyclosporine A, and stress of surgery and postoperative phase.*
	• Instruct patient that chest movements associated with coughing, doing housework, climbing stairs, and driving may cause some discomfort for several weeks at home. No driving for at least 6-8 wk or as advised by physician. Depending on patient's occupation, return to work is not suggested for at least 3-6 mo; sometimes patient will need to change jobs.
	• Instruct on importance of practicing good hygiene measures *to decrease incidence of infection from skin irritations and sores.*
	• Instruct on need to wear a mask if going outside, when around large numbers of people or those with colds.
		Patient and significant others will be able to demonstrate and communicate understanding of disease state, surgical procedures, recovery phase, activities, medications, and preventive care by date of discharge.

Cardiac transplantation—cont'd

NURSING DIAGNOSES / DEFINING CHARACTERISTICS	NURSING INTERVENTIONS / *RATIONALES*	EXPECTED OUTCOMES
	• Review signs/symptoms of sternal wound complications, such as dehiscence, wound drainage, redness or swelling, or sternal instability, which may occur up to 1 mo postoperatively. • Discuss modification of risk factors *to decrease possibility of future heart disease.*	
Potential ineffective coping *Related to:* Fear of dying Stress of waiting for surgery Perceived body image changes Fear of possibility of heart rejection after transplantation **DEFINING CHARACTERISTICS** Nervous behaviorisms Verbalized fears of no longer "being whole" after heart transplant Anorexia Insomnia Withdrawn behavior Indifference to self and surroundings Lack of concentration; inability to concentrate or complete tasks Verbal cues, crying, hostility, and negative expectations	**ONGOING ASSESSMENT** • Assess patient's feelings about self, body, appearance. • Assess patient's usual coping mechanisms and their previous effectiveness. • Assess for signs of ineffective coping (see Defining Characteristics). *Ineffective coping mechanisms must be identified to promote constructive behaviors.* **THERAPEUTIC INTERVENTIONS** • Encourage patient and family to express feelings. *Verbalization of feelings and sharing of emotions facilitate effective coping.* • Establish open lines of communication: Initiate brief visits to patient. Define your role as patient informant and advocate. Understand the grieving process. • Involve social services and pastoral care for additional and ongoing support resources for patient and significant others. • Provide reading materials and resource persons as needed. Sometimes it *decreases anxiety* to have a person who has had a heart transplant talk with and answer questions of the patient or family. • Introduce new information, using simple terms, and reinforce instructions or repeat information as necessary. *Depending on degree of anxiety, patient and/or family may not be able to absorb all information at one time.*	Effective coping behaviors will be demonstrated.
Potential infection *Related to:* Immunosuppressive drug therapy Disruption of skin and iatrogenic sources of infection **DEFINING CHARACTERISTICS** Increased WBC Increased temperature Impaired wound healing Wound drainage Pulmonary infections	**ONGOING ASSESSMENT** • Observe wound healing process q8h., prn for drainage, wound edge approximation, edema, sensitivity, and temperature of surrounding tissue. • Monitor WBC and cyclosporine A (CSA) levels daily. Expect adjustments of CSA and steroids, depending on results. • Monitor vital signs routinely. Monitor temperature q2h if elevated. • Monitor cultures, sensitivities, and viral titers of blood, sputum, and urine three times a week for 3 weeks postoperatively, then prn at surgeon's discretion. • Culture any suspicious drainage from wound sites. **THERAPEUTIC INTERVENTIONS** • Keep patient in private room with high efficiency particulate air filter (HEPA) capability throughout hospitalization. • In ICU, enforce strict protective isolation because *during this period immunosuppression is greatest and ICU environment is classically known to harbor many bacteria and viruses in light of its patient population.* • When patient is transferred to step-down unit, enforce modified protective isolation. Patient is always to be in private room with HEPA filter capability *to prevent cross contamination and infection.* • Exclude personnel with infectious diseases (e.g., colds, flu) from patient care *because of patient's suppressed immune system.*	Incidence of infection is reduced.

Continued.

Cardiac transplantation—cont'd

NURSING DIAGNOSES / DEFINING CHARACTERISTICS	NURSING INTERVENTIONS / *RATIONALES*	EXPECTED OUTCOMES
	• Control environmental traffic (i.e., limit visitors and staff members into patient's room) *to protect patient from exposure to potential environmental organisms.* • Wash with germicidal detergent (Staphene/hexachlorophene) all equipment entering room. • Change all dressings, ECG patches, and taping (i.e., endotracheal tube) daily *to decrease skin irritation and assure close monitoring of invasive line sites. A primary cause of infection is directly related to interruption of skin barrier.* • Change all respiratory equipment q24h and encourage aggressive pulmonary toiletry because *pulmonary infections are second most common source of infection caused by effects of steroids and CSA.* • Change all tubings and IV solutions q24h *to decrease incidence of contamination from equipment.* Maintain aseptic technique. • Ensure adequate diet high in calories and protein. *Infection risk greater in patients with end-stage heart disease because of their pre-surgical debilitated state.*	

Potential for injury
Related to:
The effects of steroids and immunosuppressant drug therapy
 	
DEFINING CHARACTERISTICS
Steroid-induced diabetes
Increased hydrochloric acid causing development of gastric ulcers
Hypertension
Weight gain
Generalized edema
Cushing's syndrome
Calcium and phosphorus depletion
Dry skin
	ONGOING ASSESSMENT
	• Assess patient for signs and symptoms of diabetes:
	  Check urine dipsticks for glucose and ketones.
	  Observe for polyuria.
	  Note excessive thirst.
	  Check serum glucose prn until maintenance dose of steroid established.
	• Assess gastric pH.
	• Monitor I & O, daily weight, BP.
	• Assess for peripheral, sacral, periorbital, facial edema.
	• Assess skin integrity.
	• Assess for bruising, possible fractures, and vague complaints of bone pain.
	• Monitor renal functioning by checking BUN, creatinine, and CSA levels. *CSA is nephrotoxic.*
	
	THERAPEUTIC INTERVENTIONS
	• Administer antacids as ordered.
	• Place on low-sodium diet *to decrease fluid retention.*
	• Apply support hose and elevate extremities *to reduce edema.*
	• Keep skin well moistened with lotions *to prevent unnecessary itching from dry skin,* secondary to CSA, dryness of environment (HEPA filtering), and bed linens.
	• Reposition q2h *to minimize potential for skin breakdown.*
	• Pad bed rails *to decrease incidence of bruising from hitting rails.*
		Injury resulting from immunosuppressive therapy is reduced.

Potential for injury: allograft rejection
Related to:
Acute rejection:
  Characterized by perivascular and interstitial mononuclear cell infiltration; progresses to necrosis if untreated. Occurs 5-30 days from transplant
 	
DEFINING CHARACTERISTICS
Decreased QRS voltage
Atrial arrhythmias
	ONGOING ASSESSMENT
	• Assess overall status for increasing malaise, decreasing exercise tolerance.
	• Evaluate ECG daily for:
	  Decreased QRS voltage *(may be seen with conventional immunosuppressants)*
	  Atrial arrhythmias
	  Conduction defects
	• Monitor CSA trough level (drawn 1 hr before dose).
	• Monitor WBC and T-cell counts.
	• Assess peripheral circulation.
	• Assess hemodynamic measurements.
	• Assess vital signs.
	• Assess I&O hourly; weigh daily.
	• Assess for systemic venous congestion.
	
	THERAPEUTIC INTERVENTIONS
	• Administer immunosuppressive agents daily, as ordered.
		Early detection of rejection will be achieved.

Cardiac transplantation—cont'd

NURSING DIAGNOSES / DEFINING CHARACTERISTICS	NURSING INTERVENTIONS / *RATIONALES*	EXPECTED OUTCOMES
Conduction defects Nontherapeutic CSA levels Increasing T-cell count Signs and symptoms of biventricular pump failure: Cool, pale skin; poor capillary refill; diminished pulses; diaphoresis; decreased urine output; dyspnea; tachypnea; increased PAD; pulmonary edema; jugular neck vein distention; ascites; peripheral or sacral edema	• Keep right internal jugular site clean for future biopsies. (Note: Swan-Ganz catheters are in left internal jugular.) *Endomyocardial biopsy is definitive procedure to confirm rejection.* • Describe to patient procedure of the endocardial biopsy, including use of local anesthesia at biopsy catheter insertion site and use of operating room for procedure.	

Originated by: Laura Baratta, RN, MSN
    Carol Ruback, RN, MSN, CCRN
    Meg Gulanick, RN, PhD

Carotid endarterectomy
(VASCULAR SURGERY)

Surgical procedure to remove atherosclerotic plaque from the inner wall of the carotid artery.

NURSING DIAGNOSES / DEFINING CHARACTERISTICS	NURSING INTERVENTIONS / *RATIONALES*	EXPECTED OUTCOMES
Potential alteration in level of consciousness *Related to:* Cerebral ischemia **DEFINING CHARACTERISTICS** Change in alertness, orientation, speech, motor response Agitation or somnolence Weakness: paresis of an extremity Facial droop Pupillary signs	**ONGOING ASSESSMENT** • Assess responsiveness/level of consciousness (LOC) q1h or as indicated. • Assess continuity of thought processes. • Assess motor responses q2h. • Assess vital signs and pupillary reaction q2h. **THERAPEUTIC INTERVENTIONS** • Record assessment of neurologic status. • Report sudden or progressive deterioration in neurologic status *to minimize damage from inadequate cerebral blood flow.* • Keep side rails up and call light within reach. • Reorient as necessary. • Inform neurologic resource person of status.	Optimal LOC will be maintained.

Continued.

NURSING DIAGNOSES / DEFINING CHARACTERISTICS	NURSING INTERVENTIONS / *RATIONALES*	EXPECTED OUTCOMES
Altered cerebral tissue perfusion *Related to:* Edema from surgery Clot formation Hemorrhage **DEFINING CHARACTERISTICS** Hypertension Hypotension Headache Hematoma Altered LOC Incisional bleeding	**ONGOING ASSESSMENT** • Monitor BP q1h. • Assess LOC and motor responses q1-2h. • Check dressing and incision line for bleeding. • Check for symmetry of neck. Check behind neck of supine patient. *Blood may pool; hematoma formation posterior from incision line possible.* • Assess quality of pulse proximal and distal to incision. **THERAPEUTIC INTERVENTIONS** • Maintain bed rest. • Administer antihypertensives as ordered *to prevent extreme elevations in BP.* • Keep BP at 120-150 systolic and 70-90 diastolic or 86-110 mean arterial pressure (MAP). Notify physician if out of this range. • Change or reinforce dressing as needed. • Report excessive incisional drainage or sudden change in vital signs or neurologic status.	Maximum cerebral perfusion will be achieved.
Potential for infection *Related to:* Surgical incision as entry for pathogens **DEFINING CHARACTERISTICS** Redness, pain, swelling at incision site Purulent drainage Elevated temperature Elevated WBC	**ONGOING ASSESSMENT** • Identify high-risk population. • Assess incisional site. • Assess drainage on dressing. • Monitor temperature. • Obtain culture from incisional site, if signs of infection present. **THERAPEUTIC INTERVENTIONS** • Use aseptic technique with dressing changes *to minimize entry of pathogens into incision.* • Maintain occlusive dressing. • Notify physician of signs of infection.	Potential for infection is reduced.

Pain
 Related to:
 Surgical incision
 	
 DEFINING CHARACTERISTICS
 Patient verbalizes pain
 Decreased activity or guarding behavior
 Restlessness, irritability
 Altered sleep pattern
 Facial mask of pain
 Autonomic responses (diaphoresis, altered BP, pulse respiration rate, pallor, pupil dilation)
	ONGOING ASSESSMENT
	 • Assess patient's description of pain.
	 • Assess characteristics of pain:
	     Location
	     Severity
	     Quality
	 • Assess autonomic responses to pain.
	
	 THERAPEUTIC INTERVENTIONS
	 • Instruct patient to report pain.
	 • Anticipate need for analgesics *to prevent occurrence of severe, intractable pain.*
	 • Administer analgesics as needed.
	 • Encourage rest periods.
	 • Offer additional comfort measures.
		Pain will be relieved.

Knowledge deficit *Related to:* New procedure **DEFINING CHARACTERISTICS** Questions about surgical procedure	**ONGOING ASSESSMENT** • Assess intellectual ability. • Assess physical ability to perform tasks. • Identify need to learn and encourage patient to identify needs and set goals. • Assess cultural influences. **THERAPEUTIC INTERVENTIONS** • Ensure physical comfort and maintain quiet atmosphere *to provide environment conductive to learning.*	Patient or significant others will state or demonstrate new knowledge gained.

Carotid endarterectomy—cont'd

NURSING DIAGNOSES / DEFINING CHARACTERISTICS	NURSING INTERVENTIONS / *RATIONALES*	EXPECTED OUTCOMES

Physical inability to perform tasks
Questions about postop care
	• Establish rapport with patient and family.
	• Allow time for patient/significant others to verbalize questions.
	• Explain surgical procedure and postoperative care at level of understanding. Keep explanations brief and simple.
	• Use alternate forms of information *to increase attention and retention of information.*
	• Question patient on health teaching *to determine level of understanding and document progress.*
	• Identify outside support as needed:
	    Social worker
	    Support groups
	    Literature	

Originated by: Deborah Jezuit, RN, MS

Femoral-popliteal bypass: immediate postoperative care

(REVASCULARIZATION)

The repair of lesions in femoral popliteal area by surgical bypass graft.

NURSING DIAGNOSES / DEFINING CHARACTERISTICS	NURSING INTERVENTIONS / *RATIONALES*	EXPECTED OUTCOMES

Potential fluid volume deficit
Related to:
Surgical procedure
Hemorrhage
 	
DEFINING CHARACTERISTICS
Early:
  Visualized bleeding from incision/graft
  Increased heart rate
  Decreased BP
  Anxiety
  Restlessness
  Coolness, pallor, cyanosis
  Thirst
Late:
  Oliguria
  Clammy skin
  Venous collapse
	ONGOING ASSESSMENT
	• Check surgical site and donor site (if present) every hour for signs/symptoms of hemorrhage:
	    Increased edema
	    Increased pain
	    Change in color
	    Decreased pulses
	• Monitor vital signs every hour and prn.
	• Mark distal pulses with ink and check every hour. Use Doppler ultrasound if needed. Note pulse presence and strength; color, temperature, sensation, and movement of extremities.
	• Assess patient's level of consciousness (LOC). Note nonverbal signs.
	• Monitor I&O every hour.
	• Monitor central venous pressure (CVP) every hour.
	• Assure that packed red blood cells (PRBCs) and fresh frozen plasma (FFP) are available for patient in blood bank
	• Obtain hematocrit for suspected and/or active bleeding.
	• Obtain daily weights.
	• Monitor lab results as ordered: hemoglobin, hematocrit, PT, PTT, electrolytes.
	
	THERAPEUTIC INTERVENTIONS
	• Administer fluids as ordered.
	• Ensure that surgical site is easily visualized; instruct patient/family to notify staff if bleeding is noted.
	• Perform dressing changes per physician order. Document incision approximation, presence of sutures/staples, and overall appearance. Note presence, amount, and color of drainage.
		Potential for fluid volume deficit will be reduced.

Continued.

147

NURSING DIAGNOSES / DEFINING CHARACTERISTICS	NURSING INTERVENTIONS / *RATIONALES*	EXPECTED OUTCOMES
	• Keep adequate amounts of sterile gauze, Kerlix, gloves, and sutures in near proximity *in case of acute hemorrhage.* • Guard the patient from trauma *to prevent injury to surgical area.*	
Potential altered perfusion: peripheral circulation *Related to:* Graft occlusion Coagulopathy **DEFINING CHARACTERISTICS** Burning, itching, pain in tissues distal to site of occlusion Pain aggravated with passive/active movement of limb Numbness/coldness of limb Arterial pulsation weak/absent distal to the occlusion *Acute occlusion produces fall in mean and pulse pressures in distal arteries and decreases tissue Po_2*	**ONGOING ASSESSMENT** • Assess color and warmth of extremity. • Assess patient's level of pain at surgical site and distally. • Check for Homan's sign q4h. • Mark distal pulses with ink and check every hour for pulse rate, rhythm, and volume in extremity. Compare with the unoperated side. • Assess sites distal to graft for color, movement, and sensation. **THERAPEUTIC INTERVENTIONS** • Maintain lower extremities slightly higher than heart level *to aid in venous return and prevent edema formation.* • Instruct patient/family on importance of keeping affected extremity straight *to prevent kinking in graft, which may precipitate clot formation.* • Gently reposition patient every 1-2 hr with knee gatch flat *for optimal blood flow.* • Administer prophylactic heparin therapy as ordered.	Peripheral circulation will be optimized.
Potential for infection *Related to:* Surgery Invasive procedures **DEFINING CHARACTERISTICS** Reddened incisional site Drainage from incision Elevated temperature	**ONGOING ASSESSMENT** • Assess incisional sites for local symptoms of infection. • Monitor temperature q4h. • Monitor WBC, especially neutrophils/bands. Notify MD if temperature >38.5° C or if patient shows other signs/symptoms of infection. • Identify nosocomial pathogens in patient area (e.g., respiratory/urine bacteria). • Send cultures (wound, blood, etc.) as ordered. **THERAPEUTIC INTERVENTIONS** • Wash hands before, after contact with patient *to prevent nosocomial infection.* • Maintain aseptic technique during bedside procedures (e.g., catheter care, IV site care). • Use isolation procedures as appropriate. *Lack of physical structure in ICU mandates importance of following correct isolation procedure to prevent spread of disease.* • Limit visitors and discourage those with current or recent infection from visiting. • Ensure adequate IV/oral hydration. • Assist patient with selection of high-protein, high-vitamin, high-calorie diet or administer hyperalimentation as ordered *to promote healing.* • Initiate measures for control of fever (i.e., tepid water bath, alcohol bath for temperature >38.5° C). Avoid use of cooling mattress *(may decrease lower extremity perfusion).* • Administer medications as ordered for infection.	Risk of infection will be reduced.
Pain *Related to:* Incisional pain Occlusive pain	**ONGOING ASSESSMENT** • Solicit patient's description of pain, documenting in patient's own words. • Assess pain characteristics: quality, severity, location, onset, duration, precipitating/relieving factors.	Comfort will be maximized.

NURSING DIAGNOSES / DEFINING CHARACTERISTICS	NURSING INTERVENTIONS / *RATIONALES*	EXPECTED OUTCOMES
DEFINING CHARACTERISTICS Patient and/or significant others report pain Guarding behavior, protective self-focusing, narrowed focus Relief/distraction behavior Facial mask of pain Alteration in muscle tone (rigid, tense)	• Solicit techniques patient considers helpful in decreasing pain. • Observe effectiveness of analgesic and/or therapies used to reduce pain. **THERAPEUTIC INTERVENTIONS** • Anticipate need for analgesics and respond immediately to complaint of pain. • Use other comfort measures when appropriate (e.g., decrease the number of stressors in environment. • Use distraction techniques. *Patient then focuses less on pain and more on television, newspaper, games, etc.*	
Potential alteration in skin integrity *Related to:* Internal: Altered tissue perfusion Altered nutritional status Altered immunologic state Generalized edema Transparent skin Hypothermia or hyperthermia Altered skin turgor External: Mechanical factors Shearing Pressure Use of restraints Use of warm compresses Use of monitoring devices Chemical: Infiltrations Physical: Anesthesia Paralyzing drugs Barbiturates Irritations caused by excretions **DEFINING CHARACTERISTICS** Reddened skin Abrasions Change in skin color Change in skin temperature Edema Poor skin turgor (worsening) Pain	**ONGOING ASSESSMENT** • Assess skin appearance for: Color, temperature, turgor Moisture, edema Perfusion Presence/absence of breakdown • Assess nutritional status: Daily weight I&O every hour Total caloric intake over 24 hr • Establish medical and surgical risk factors; see Defining Characteristics. • Assess current skin care rendered. • Evaluate lab data as ordered (specifically hemoglobin/hematocrit (H/H), Chemstrip). • Check IV patency before administering drugs and blood products. • Monitor IV sites every hour and document. **THERAPEUTIC INTERVENTIONS** • Document signs/symptoms of tissue ischemia, redness, and change in skin color. • Administer adequate nutritional/hydration requirements as ordered. • Use skin barriers (i.e., Stomahesive, Duoderm) on skin areas where tape is frequently used and areas are exposed to irritating secretions/excretions. • Cover skin with protective barriers if areas are at risk. • Use paper tape for frequent dressing changes. • Provide prophylactic use of antipressure devices. • Use liquid film barriers on skin when securing endotracheal tube (ETT). *This prevents skin breakdown on face/neck caused by tape removal.* • Turn/reposition patient q1-2h gently and assess appearance of skin. Document any changes. *This allows for continuous monitoring of skin integrity and helps to prevent skin breakdown.*	Skin integrity will be maintained.

Continued.

NURSING DIAGNOSES / DEFINING CHARACTERISTICS	NURSING INTERVENTIONS / *RATIONALES*	EXPECTED OUTCOMES
Skin breakdown Decubitus ulcers Dry skin Cyanosis		
Altered nutrition: less than body requirements *Related to:* NPO post surgery Delay in starting oral diet, hyperalimentation, nasogastric tube feedings post op Poor appetite **DEFINING CHARACTERISTICS** Weight loss with adequate caloric intake 10-20% or greater under ideal body weight Documented inadequate caloric intake Caloric intake inadequate to keep pace with abnormal disease/metabolic state	**ONGOING ASSESSMENT** · Document patient's actual weight on admission. · Obtain nutritional history as appropriate. · Obtain weight as ordered: minimum, one weight/week. · Monitor urine/serum electrolytes, CBC, glucose, acetone *to ensure patient's nutritional intake is adequate. Frequent monitoring of these levels ensures therapeutic treatment by medical staff and dietitian.* **THERAPEUTIC INTERVENTIONS** · Consult dietitian when appropriate. · Document appetite and nutritive intake. · Assist patient with meals as necessary. · Encourage frequent oral ingestion of high-calorie protein foods/fluids.	Nutritional state will be maximized.
Knowledge deficit *Related to:* New surgical procedure **DEFINING CHARACTERISTICS** Multiple questions Lack of questions Misconceptions of health status Request for information Display of anxiety and/or fear Noncompliance Inability to verbalize health maintenance regimen Development of complications	**ONGOING ASSESSMENT** · Assess patient's/significant others' readiness for learning. · Assess knowledge regarding surgery and postoperative management. **THERAPEUTIC INTERVENTIONS** · Explain proper leg positioning and reasons for positioning. · Explain the need for frequent circulatory assessments. *This relieves patient's anxiety about the staff's need to be at the bedside often.* · Instruct patient to alert nurse of any change in sensation in lower extremities or any bleeding/swelling. *This prevents delay in detecting changes in circulation and allows prompt treatment.* · Discuss patient's surgery and its relation to signs/symptoms patient is experiencing. · Instruct on deep breathing exercises. · Encourage family to participate in patient's care and rehab. · Reinforce information given by physician to family.	Patient/significant others are able to verbalize understanding of surgical procedure and related care.

Originated by: Marie G. Mazurek, RN, BSN
Melissa Moline, RN, BA

Intra-aortic balloon pump
(COUNTERPULSATION DEVICE)

The intra-aortic balloon pump (IABP) is a mechanical assist device for the failing heart aimed at increasing coronary perfusion and decreasing myocardial workload and O_2 consumption. It is indicated for refractory angina, ischemia-associated ventricular arrhythmias, pump failure (cardiogenic shock), intraoperative myocardial infarction (MI), acute myocardial infarction, mechanical defects (ventricular septal defects, papillary muscle dysfunction), and perioperative support and stabilization.

NURSING DIAGNOSES / DEFINING CHARACTERISTICS	NURSING INTERVENTIONS / *RATIONALES*	EXPECTED OUTCOMES
Potential decreased cardiac output *Related to:* Balloon or pump malfunction, secondary to: Loss of or poor hemodynamic or ECG signals Arrhythmias/paced rhythms Inappropriate timing/inadequate diastolic augmentation Kinked catheter Low helium Balloon catheter leak/rupture/ malposition **DEFINING CHARACTERISTICS** Variations in hemodynamic parameters (BP, pulmonary artery pressure, cardiac output, heart rate, pulmonary artery wedge pressure, left atrial pressure) Arrhythmias, ECG changes Abnormal heart sounds Abnormal lung sounds Restlessness, mentation changes Decreased urine output Recurrent or persistent anginal pain	**ONGOING ASSESSMENT** • Assess hemodynamic status q30min for 2 hr, then gradually less often as patient stabilizes. • Assess for myocardial ischemia: chest pain, ST-T wave changes on ECG. • Assess and maintain clear ECG tracing with upright tall QRS segment to ensure proper balloon triggering. If paced rhythm, assess that triggering is from R wave, not paced spike. • Assess and maintain clear arterial pressure waveform. Balloon must inflate at dicrotic notch and deflate before systole. • Assess and maintain good pulmonary pressure tracings to ensure reliable hemodynamic measurements that determine therapy. • Monitor timing of inflation/deflation every hour *to ensure optimal afterload reduction and perfusion of coronary arteries.* **THERAPEUTIC INTERVENTIONS** • Observe for cardiac arrhythmias continuously. If tachycardia results in inadequate augmentation, pumping ratio may be adjusted to 1:2 as appropriate. • Keep alarms on at all times. • Document in chart arterial pressure tracing with balloon on and off: At insertion of balloon Routinely q4h For any change in tracing • Flush arterial lines after obtaining blood samples *to maintain patency.* • Keep catheter system visible at all times. Keep tubing connection tight and catheter free of kinks. • If technical problems resulting in hemodynamic compromise should occur: Institute IABP troubleshooting procedure per protocol. Notify medical and surgical physicians. Anticipate cardiovascular decompensation, titrate cardiotonic drugs, and maintain pressure. Reassure patient *to prevent untoward cardiovascular response to anxiety.*	Optimal cardiac output will be maintained.
Pain *Related to:* Insertion of balloon and subsequent restriction in movement	**ONGOING ASSESSMENT** • Assess quality, quantity, location of pain, associated manifestations, precipitating and relieving factors. **THERAPEUTIC INTERVENTIONS** • Anticipate need for comfort. • Provide comfort measures: position change, back rubs, distraction techniques, analgesics as ordered.	Optimum level of comfort will be maintained.

Continued.

Intra-aortic balloon pump—cont'd

NURSING DIAGNOSES / DEFINING CHARACTERISTICS	NURSING INTERVENTIONS / *RATIONALES*	EXPECTED OUTCOMES
DEFINING CHARACTERISTICS Complaint of pain and stiffness Restlessness, irritability Facial mask of pain	• Position to maintain correct body alignment; support dependent parts with pillows. • Provide passive ROM to joints without bending cannulated leg *to prevent joint stiffness and venous stasis.* • Provide rest periods *to facilitate comfort.* • Instruct patient to report both pain and effectiveness of intervention promptly *to optimize therapy.* • See Pain, p. 39.	

Potential altered peripheral tissue perfusion *Related to:* Presence of catheter, causing occlusion of femoral artery Catheter displacement Thrombus from platelet aggregation on balloon catheter Peripheral embolization Arterial spasm Presence of radial arterial line, causing occlusion of radial artery
 	
 DEFINING CHARACTERISTICS Extremity: Decrease or absence   of pulse   Cool/discolored   extremity   Tingling, numb-   ness, or pain Subclavian: Change in level of   consciousness   (LOC)   Loss of radial pulse   X-ray: catheter po-   sition too high Renal: Flank pain   Decrease in urine   output   X-ray: catheter posi-   tion too low Mesentery: Abdominal pain/   distention   GI bleeding   Acidosis   Catheter position too   low on x-ray film
	ONGOING ASSESSMENT
	 • Assess and record quality of peripheral pulses, and color and temperature of extremity to be cannulated before insertion of catheter *to establish baseline.*
	 • Perform Allen test before insertion of radial arterial line *to assess presence of adequate collateral flow through ulnar artery.*
	 • Monitor pulses, and color and temperature of cannulated extremity over four 30-min periods, then every 1 hr. Mark site of pedal pulses with *X.*
	 • Monitor for local pain, numbness, and tingling in cannulated extremity that may signify ischemia.
	 • Observe for signs and symptoms of obstruction of subclavian, renal, or mesenteric artery. If noted, call physician, document catheter position on x-ray examination, and anticipate repositioning.
	
	 THERAPEUTIC INTERVENTIONS
	 • *Ensure adequate anticoagulation* for duration of balloon pumping by monitoring clotting time and administering prescribed medication and fluids.
	 • Apply TED hose to unaffected leg.
	 • Perform ROM exercise to arms and unaffected leg q2-4h *to prevent venous stasis (may lead to thrombus formation).*
	 • Maintain safety measures *to prevent catheter displacement:*
	   Keep cannulated leg straight. Log roll patient when turning *to prevent catheter displacement.*
	   Do not raise head of bed more than 30 degrees.
	   Weigh carefully on portable bed scale.
	   Apply soft restraint to ankle when necessary *to prevent movement of extremity.*
	 • Do not decrease pumping rate lower than 1:4 and limit time to 30 min. *Deflated balloon encourages thrombus formation*
	 • Should balloon pumping cease longer than 10 min, manually inflate/deflate catheter several times q10 min *to prevent thrombus formation.*
		Adequate blood flow to affected extremity and general circulation will be maintained.

Intra-aortic balloon pump—cont'd

NURSING DIAGNOSES / DEFINING CHARACTERISTICS	NURSING INTERVENTIONS / *RATIONALES*	EXPECTED OUTCOMES
Potential for injury: aortic femoral dissection or injury *Related to:* Trauma during insertion Movement of balloon tip **DEFINING CHARACTERISTICS** Arterial injury Hypotension Tachycardia Pain or discomfort in lower back Hematoma at or near insertion site Decreased Hct/Hb Decreased urine output Abdominal pain or distension Change in acid-base balance	**ONGOING ASSESSMENT** • Assess for signs and symptoms of aortic dissection or injury and/or retroperitoneal bleeding. If this occurs, notify physician. **THERAPEUTIC INTERVENTIONS** • Maintain safety measures (see above problem regarding catheter displacement), *to prevent upward displacement of balloon.* • If injury or rupture occurs: Administer blood replacement as ordered. Anticipate cardiovascular decompensation: Prepare emergency medication. Anticipate emergency surgical repair of vessel. Provide emotional support to patient.	Risk for injury will be reduced.
Potential for injury: hematologic disturbance *Related to:* Thrombocytopenia resulting from disruption of platelet integrity caused by trauma from balloon pumping Anemia resulting from blood loss during insertion of balloon and frequent blood sampling Heparinization, used to decrease risk of thrombus formation **DEFINING CHARACTERISTICS** Abnormal coagulation studies Petechiae Hematuria Guaiac positive stool/ nasogastric drainage	**ONGOING ASSESSMENT** • Assess/monitor daily CBC, PTT, PT, platelets. Report any abnormalities to physician. • Observe for swelling/hematoma at insertion site. • Observe for other signs of bleeding: petechiae, hematuria, guaiac-positive stool/nasogastric drainage, and skin bruising. **THERAPEUTIC INTERVENTIONS** • Administer blood or platelets as necessary and as ordered by physician. • Minimize blood drawing *to prevent anemia.* • Titrate heparin to maintain PTT as prescribed (1½-2 times control) *to prevent overanticoagulation.*	Potential for thrombocytopenia and consequent bleeding tendency will be reduced.

Continued.

NURSING DIAGNOSES / DEFINING CHARACTERISTICS	NURSING INTERVENTIONS / *RATIONALES*	EXPECTED OUTCOMES
Potential for infection *Related to:* Invasive procedures and long-term catheter insertion in femoral area Debilitated condition predisposing to infection **DEFINING CHARACTERISTICS** Febrile Elevated WBC Redness, drainage, swelling, tenderness at catheter insertion site	**ONGOING ASSESSMENT** · Monitor temperature q4h. If patient febrile, take temperature q2h. Notify physician. Obtain cultures as ordered. · Monitor WBC daily. **THERAPEUTIC INTERVENTIONS** · Ensure sterile technique in insertion of all invasive lines and subsequent dressing changes. · Keep femoral dressing dry and intact *to reduce potential for bacterial growth*. · Change catheter insertion site dressing daily and prn. Monitor catheter site for redness, drainage, and tenderness. Send any drainage for culture. · Provide perineal and Foley catheter care every shift. · Maintain all other lines and dressings per unit protocol.	Risk for infection will be reduced.
Impaired physical mobility *Related to:* Bed rest Balloon insertion Leg catheter Critical physical condition Restricted movement because of other invasive lines **DEFINING CHARACTERISTICS** Inability to move purposefully within physical environment (patient on bed rest) Limited range of motion (ROM) (affected leg must be kept straight)	**ONGOING ASSESSMENT** · Assess for signs and symptoms of pulmonary complications, impaired skin integrity, decreased muscle strength, and foot drop, which can result from prolonged immobility. · Assess respiratory rate, rhythm, heart sounds. · Monitor altered blood gases (ABGs) and chest x-ray films as appropriate. **THERAPEUTIC INTERVENTIONS** · Position patient q2h to either side or back. Use pillow support to maintain proper leg alignment. · Perform ROM exercises to arms, unaffected leg, and ankle of affected leg q2-4h *to prevent joint stiffness and venous stasis*. · Use footboard, boot, or shoe *to prevent foot drop*. · Institute prophylactic antipressure devices *to help maintain skin integrity*. · Maintain dry skin. · Apply lotion and massage around pressure areas q4h. · Encourage coughing, deep breathing exercises q2h *to prevent atelectasis*. · Use incentive spirometer qid. · Use oropharyngeal or tracheal suction prn. · See Mobility, impaired physical, p. 35.	Complications of immobility will be absent or reduced.
Anxiety/fear *Related to:* Insertion of/presence of balloon catheter Dependence on proper functioning of balloon pump Continuous noise of pumping Alteration in body image Inability to control environment Disruption of family life	**ONGOING ASSESSMENT** · Assess level of anxiety/fear and normal coping patterns of patient and significant others. **THERAPEUTIC INTERVENTIONS** · Initiate treatment for Anxiety, p. 4 and Fear, p. 18. · Stay with patient as much as possible. · Explain purpose/functioning of balloon and pump as appropriate. Include significant others *to decrease their feelings of helplessness*. · Prepare patient at times balloon is turned down: when listening to heart, recording baseline pressure, etc. · Provide continuity of care by assigning staff members experienced in balloon functioning of pump *so patient and family feel confident about care rendered*. · Avoid unnecessary conversations about pump function near patient *to increase patient's sense of security*.	Anxiety/fear will be reduced for patient and family.

Intra-aortic balloon pump—cont'd

NURSING DIAGNOSES / DEFINING CHARACTERISTICS	NURSING INTERVENTIONS / *RATIONALES*	EXPECTED OUTCOMES
Gravity of illness; fear of pain/death Financial burden **DEFINING CHARACTERISTICS** Restlessness Vigilant watch over equipment Afraid to sleep Complaining/ uncooperative behavior Withdrawal	• Allow patient as much control of environment as possible (e.g., bathing preference, mealtimes). • Minimize noise in room. • Offer television or music as appropriate *for diversion.* • Keep family informed of patient's condition. • Refer to crisis intervention if necessary.	
Sleep pattern disturbance *Related to:* Increased nursing and medical care Noise from balloon, unfamiliar environment Sleep deprivation Psychological stress caused by illness **DEFINING CHARACTERISTICS** Subjective complaints Restlessness Lethargy Dozing Interrupted sleep Altered mental status, disorientation Irritability	**ONGOING ASSESSMENT** • Assess sleep pattern over past few days. **THERAPEUTIC INTERVENTIONS** • Initiate treatment for Sleep pattern disturbance, p. 50.	Adequate sleep/rest will be achieved.

Knowledge deficit
Related to:
New procedure/ equipment
 	
DEFINING CHARACTERISTICS
Questioning
Verbalized misconceptions
Lack of questions
	ONGOING ASSESSMENT
	• Assess level of understanding of balloon pump by patient/significant others.
	• Assess physical/emotional readiness for learning by patient/significant others.
	
	THERAPEUTIC INTERVENTIONS
	• Take time to provide environment conducive to learning. Advise distracting personnel to leave the room. *These measures facilitate patient's ability to absorb new information.*
	• Provide information about:
	    Rationale for balloon use
	    Insertion procedure
	    Ongoing care related to balloon
	• Include significant others in teaching *to decrease feeling of helplessness and assist them in supporting patient.*
	• Refer more specific questions to cardiac nurse specialist or cardiac surgeon.
		Patient/significant others will verbalize an understanding of the rationale behind insertion of balloon and use of pump.

Originated by: Salvacion P. Sulit, RN, BSN, CCRN
             Christine Hunt, RN

Percutaneous balloon valvuloplasty

(BALLOON DILATION)

Percutaneous balloon valvuloplasty is a procedure that involves the transluminal dilation of stenotic valvular (mitral valve, aortic valve) lesions by using balloon catheters. A percutaneous approach via the femoral artery is used. The procedure is performed under fluoroscopy in the cardiac catheterization laboratory.

NURSING DIAGNOSES / DEFINING CHARACTERISTICS	NURSING INTERVENTIONS / *RATIONALES*	EXPECTED OUTCOMES
Knowledge deficit: prevalvuloplasty *Related to:* New procedure Limited written patient education literature **DEFINING CHARACTERISTICS** Expressed need for more information Multiple questions or lack of questions Anxiousness Restlessness Verbalized misconceptions	**ONGOING ASSESSMENT** • Assess readiness of patient/significant others for teaching/learning. • Note baseline level of knowledge especially of heart anatomy, disease, valvuloplasty procedure, and possible risks/complications. **THERAPEUTIC INTERVENTIONS** • Establish an environment conducive to teaching and learning. • Use available and appropriate teaching materials (e.g., heart model, booklets); *visual aids are effective teaching tools.* • Provide information about: Heart anatomy and physiology Patient's heart problem (mitral or aortic valvular dysfunction) Valvuloplasty: Prevalvuloplasty preparations Procedure Postvalvuloplasty care Expectations/concerns Postvalvuloplasty activity level Discharge instructions: May resume normal activities in 1 wk Notify physician of weight gain, dyspnea, edema *With such knowledge, patient's anxiety level is reduced.* • Include family/significant others in plan of care and teaching *to reduce their feelings of helplessness and increase their ability to support the patient.* • Use appropriate resource persons (e.g., physician, clinical specialists, catheterization lab nurses). • Document teachings as appropriate.	The patient/significant others will verbalize basic understanding of valvuloplasty and the care associated with it.
Anxiety/fear *Related to:* Unfamiliarity with procedure Threat of risks/ complications Patient's personality and coping mechanism **DEFINING CHARACTERISTICS** Restlessness/inability to relax Repeated seeking of assurance Sad expression Irritability Expressed concern Insomnia Overexcitement Constant demands or complaints Denial Uncooperative behavior Increased questioning	**ONGOING ASSESSMENT** • Assess patient's level of anxiety. Note signs and symptoms of anxiety/fear (e.g., tachycardia, tachypnea, increased BP, diaphoresis). • Assess patient's normal coping patterns. **THERAPEUTIC INTERVENTIONS** • Establish rapport. • Offer emotional support/assurance as appropriate. • If necessary, stay with patient during invasive preliminary procedures (Swan-Ganz insertion, etc.). • Provide tactile stimulations, such as holding hands, as necessary. • Remind patient that a nurse will be constantly present in the catheterization lab for physical needs and emotional support. Encourage patient to ask questions. • Clarify in simple terms purpose and procedures for prevalvuloplasty workup (lab tests, Swan-Ganz, etc.) as well as actual procedure. • Be in room when physicians discuss risk/complications of procedure *so that patient's subsequent questions can be answered accurately.* • Establish and maintain an environment that will be conducive to coping: Provide adequate rest periods between care. Provide flexible visiting hours. Maintain continuity of pre- and postvalvuloplasty nursing care *to increase patient's confidence.* Involve the family/significant others with care as appropriate. • Initiate treatment for Anxiety, p. 4 and Fear p. 18	Anxiety/fear will be reduced.

NURSING DIAGNOSES / DEFINING CHARACTERISTICS	NURSING INTERVENTIONS / *RATIONALES*	EXPECTED OUTCOMES
Decreased cardiac output, postvalvuloplasty *Related to:* Possible hemodynamic compromise secondary to severe pulmonary hypertension Fluid volume deficit related to radiographic dye and restricted oral intake before procedure (NPO) Valve tear or rupture, leading to valvular insufficiency **Defining Characteristics** Decrease in BP (as low as 60 mm Hg systolic) Decrease or increase in heart rate Arrhythmias Decrease or increase in RR and change in character (e.g., dyspneic, tachypneic) Increase in PWP, PAP Presence of rales, jugular vein distension Low urine output (<20 cc/hr) Change in mental status/level of consciousness (LOC) Chest pain/palpitations Diaphoresis Clammy skin	**Ongoing Assessment** • Assess patient's hemodynamic status closely: obtain vital signs q15min×4, then q30min×2, then q1h×4 until stable, then q4h. *The first few hours are crucial to recovery. Note and report changes.* • Assess the following parameters as available: pulmonary artery pressure (PAP), pulmonary wedge pressure (PWP), central venous pressure (CVP), cardiac output (CO), venous oxygen saturation (SVO$_2$). • Assess 12-lead ECG on arrival in ICU and monitor each morning. *ECG is necessary to assess changes and to monitor potential arrhythmias.* • Assess heart sounds for change in murmur. • Auscultate lungs. Observe for changes in respiratory pattern and report. • Assess fluid balance closely (strict I & O). • Monitor voiding/urine output closely. Report if there is no voiding for 8 hr or if urine output is less than 20 cc/hr. • Assess urine specific gravity q4h. • Assess for increased restlessness, fatigue, confusion, and disorientation. • Monitor ABGs as necessary. **Therapeutic Interventions** • If signs of hemodynamic compromise are observed, institute treatment for Cardiac output, decreased, p. 9. • Administer O$_2$ therapy *to increase oxygen availability to tissues.* • If cardiac output is decreased secondary to pulmonary hypertension, anticipate use of vasodilators (nitrates, hydralizine) *to reduce pulmonary vascular resistance.* • If cardiac output is decreased secondary to fluid volume deficit, anticipate fluid resuscitation and see following Nursing Diagnosis. • If cardiac output is decreased secondary to valve rupture or tear: Administer afterload reducers (nitroprusside). Anticipate emergency open heart surgery for valve replacement.	Optimum cardiac output will be maintained.
Fluid volume deficit (mild/severe) *Related to:* Secondary to radiographic dye or contrast material causing diuresis Restricted oral intake before procedure (NPO) **Defining Characteristics** Poor skin turgor Decreased urine output/concentrated urine	**Ongoing Assessment** • Assess I & O. • Assess urine specific gravity q4h. • Assess skin turgor, mucous membranes. • Assess vital signs. • Assess mental status. • Assess serum electrolytes. *Sodium increases with dehydration. Potassium is excreted with diuresis.* • Assess BUN and creatinine. **Therapeutic Interventions** • Encourage oral (fluid) intake. • Administer parenteral fluids as ordered via infusion device *to prevent volume overload.*	Optimal fluid balance will be maintained.

Continued.

157

NURSING DIAGNOSES / DEFINING CHARACTERISTICS	NURSING INTERVENTIONS / *RATIONALES*	EXPECTED OUTCOMES
Nervousness and apprehension Dry mucous membranes Decrease BP, increased RR and HR, decreased PWP and CVP Pale, cool, clammy skin Increased thirst Hemoconcentration Increased serum sodium Decreased serum potassium Increased BUN/ creatinine		
Altered peripheral tissue perfusion *Related to:* Thrombus formation Embolization Presence of arterial and venous sheaths Arterial spasm Hematoma formation **DEFINING CHARACTERISTICS** Increased apprehension/ restlessness Presence of hematoma at site of catheter cannulation/insertion Increased heart rate (HR) and respiratory rate (RR), decreased BP Decreased or absent peripheral pulse Decreased temperature of affected extremity Presence of mottling, pallor, and cyanosis in affected extremity Presence of pain in affected leg or cannulation site	**ONGOING ASSESSMENT** • Before procedure, assess and document baseline peripheral pulses, color, temperature, sensation, and movement of extremities. Mark pulses with *X*. • Assess for erythema, tenderness, warmth or change in temperature, edema/ swelling, drainage/secretions. • Assess for cyanosis, mottling, coolness, or change in temperature; pallor; decreased pulses of affected extremity q15min×4, q30min×2, q1h until stable. • Assess pulses with Doppler if unable to palpate and note as such. • Assess movement/mobility and sensation of the affected extremity. • If hematoma is present, note size and circle with date and time *to monitor change*. **THERAPEUTIC INTERVENTION** • Maintain bed rest with head of bed elevated no higher than 30 degrees *to prevent catheter displacement*. • Maintain affected extremity in straight alignment; apply soft restraint prn *as a reminder*. • Provide ROM exercises to unaffected extremity *to prevent venous stasis and thrombus formation*. • Continue prescribed dose of heparin infusion. • Check coagulation tests 2-4hr after return to ICU. Maintain PTT values at 1½ times control *to prevent clot formation*. • Report abnormal PTT values and readjust Heparin drip as prescribed.	Tissue perfusion will be maintained.
Potential for injury: bleeding *Related to:* Arterial trauma Anticoagulation from heparin	**ONGOING ASSESSMENT** • Assess dressing/site of cannulation for presence of bleeding q15min×4, q30min×2, q1h until sheaths removed. • Assess exact amount and location of bleeding if noted. • Assess for signs of retroperitoneal bleeding (e.g., back or thigh pain, loss of peripheral pulses of lower extremity.	Active bleeding is promptly controlled.

NURSING DIAGNOSES / DEFINING CHARACTERISTICS	NURSING INTERVENTIONS / *RATIONALES*	EXPECTED OUTCOMES

DEFINING CHARACTERISTICS
Presence of significant bleeding from site of cannulation and/or dressings
Increased apprehension/restlessness
Increased pallor, cold, clammy skin
Increase HR, decreased BP, increased RR
Changes in mental status
	THERAPEUTIC INTERVENTIONS
	• Maintain bed rest with head of bed no more than 30 degrees *to prevent catheter displacement causing arterial trauma.*
	• Maintain affected extremity in straight position, apply soft restraint prn *as reminder.*
	• Titrate heparin drip as ordered to maintain PTT at 1½ times control. Use infusion device *to prevent overanticoagulation.*
	• If significant bleeding occurs:
	  Remove dressing and apply manual pressure *to provide temporary hemostasis.*
	  Administer IV fluid replacement.
	  Check Hb/Hct as necessary. Replace blood if necessary as prescribed.
	  Notify surgical team for possible emergency surgical repair of artery.
	  Offer emotional support with assurance and explanations.
	• After removal of sheaths:
	  Apply pressure dressing.
	  Apply 5- to 10-lb sandbag.
	  Maintain bed rest with head of bed (HOB) no more than 30 degrees for 6 hr *to promote clot formation.*
	• Allow dangling at bedside; may ambulate 6 hr after sheath removal when no evidence of bleeding.	

Pain *Related to:* Incisional or local pain **DEFINING CHARACTERISTICS** Report and verbalization of discomfort Restlessness/apprehension Moaning Crying Facial mask of pain Diaphoresis Changes in vital signs Fear and guarding behavior	**ONGOING ASSESSMENT** • Solicit patient's description of pain. • Assess pain characteristics: quality, severity, duration, onset, exact location • Assess for relieving factors. • Check incision site for presence or formation of hematoma; see previous Nursing Diagnosis. **THERAPEUTIC INTERVENTIONS** • If dressing too tight, loosen as appropriate. • Assist patient in position changes within activity limitations *to promote overall comfort.* • Apply antipressure devices to bed and provide back rubs *to promote overall comfort.* • Medicate with analgesics (e.g, Tylenol) as prescribed. • Offer support and emotional assurance by staying with patient *to reduce anxiety (may increase pain perception).*	Pain/discomfort will be reduced or promptly relieved.

Originated by: Cynthia Antonio, RN, BSN

Percutaneous transluminal coronary angioplasty

(PTCA; ANGIOPLASTY; BALLOON CATHETERIZATION)

Percutaneous transluminal coronary angioplasty (PTCA) is a nonsurgical procedure in which a balloon-tipped catheter is passed to the coronary artery partially obstructed or blocked by atherosclerotic plaques in order to dilate the vessel to improve blood flow.

NURSING DIAGNOSES / DEFINING CHARACTERISTICS	NURSING INTERVENTIONS / *RATIONALES*	EXPECTED OUTCOMES

Knowledge deficit: pre-PTCA *Related to:* Unfamiliarity with PTCA procedure Information misinterpretation Cognitive limitation **DEFINING CHARACTERISTICS** Request for more information Statement of misconception Increase in anxiety level Lack of questions	**ONGOING ASSESSMENT**
	 • Assess patient's emotional and physical readiness to learn.
	 • Assess patient's knowledge of cardiac anatomy and physiology, coronary artery disease, and PTCA procedure.
	
	 THERAPEUTIC INTERVENTIONS
	 • Use appropriate materials (e.g., illustrations, booklets, heart model, videotape, audiotape) for teaching patient.
	 • Include cardiac clinical nurse specialist, cath lab nurse, coronary care nurses as resource persons.
	 • Provide information about:
	    Heart anatomy and physiology
	    Coronary artery disease
	    Indications for PTCA
	    PTCA preparation
	    PTCA procedure:
	      Procedure room/environment
	      Expected length of procedure
	      Expected discomfort
	    Immediate post-PTCA care:
	      Activity restrictions
	      Routine vital signs
	      Pushing of oral fluids
	      Complications
	    Recovery:
	      Advancing level of activity
	      Discharge 2-3 days after procedure
	      Avoidance of lifting heavy objects for 1 wk
	      Possible return to work in 1 wk
	      Times to notify physician (e.g., chest pain)
	 • Stay with patient when physician explains procedure and evaluates patient. Clarify and reinforce physician's explanation of potential need for CABG surgery.
	 • Encourage patient to verbalize questions and concerns *to correct misunderstanding and misconceptions.*
	 • Allow sufficient time for one-to-one interaction if possible.
	 • Include patient's family/significant others in teaching plan as appropriate.
		Patient will demonstrate basic understanding of heart anatomy and physiology, coronary artery disease, and PTCA procedure.

Chest pain *Related to:* Pre-PTCA: Myocardial ischemia caused by coronary artery disease, coronary artery spasm, possible myocardial infarction	**ONGOING ASSESSMENT**
	 • Assess for characteristics of myocardial ischemia.
	    Quality:
	      Choking, squeezing, aching, "viselike"
	      Intense pressure with heaviness
	      Burning
	      Other
	    Severity: scale 1-10 (10 most severe):
	    Onset: sudden/constant
	    Duration
		Chest pain will be relieved or reduced.

NURSING DIAGNOSES / DEFINING CHARACTERISTICS	NURSING INTERVENTIONS / *RATIONALES*	EXPECTED OUTCOMES

Post-PTCA:
Myocardial ischemia caused by reocclusion of affected coronary artery, coronary artery spasm, possible myocardial infarction
Residual pain from dilation of coronary artery
 	
DEFINING CHARACTERISTICS
Patient reports and verbalizations (see Assessment Criteria)
Restlessness, apprehension
Moaning, crying
Facial mask of pain
Diaphoresis
Change in vital signs: BP, heart rate, respiratory rate
Pallor and weakness
Nausea and vomiting
Fear and guarding behavior
	Location:
	    Anterior chest, usually substernal
	    May radiate to shoulder, arms, jaw, neck, epigastrium
	Precipitating factors:
	    Physical or emotional exertion
	    At rest
	Relieving symptoms
	Associated symptoms (e.g., nausea, vomiting, dyspnea, diaphoresis, anxiety, fatigue)
	
	THERAPEUTIC INTERVENTIONS
	Pre-PTCA:
	• If chest pain occurs, see Angina pectoris, unstable, p. 69.
	• Anticipate need for possible emergency PTCA and/or CABG surgery.
	Post-PTCA:
	• Notify physician of chest pain immediately.
	• Obtain 12-lead ECG stat.
	• Administer medications as ordered:
	    Nitroglycerin
	    Sublingual nifedipine *for spasm*
	    Morphine sulfate
	    Tylenol *for residual pain from dilation of coronary artery*
	• Anticipate need for possible emergency cardiac catheterization and repeat PTCA.
	• Prepare patient for possibility of CABG surgery.	

Altered peripheral tissue perfusion in extremity used for cannulation
Related to:
Post-PTCA:
Mechanical obstruction from arterial and venous sheaths
Arterial vasospasm
Thrombus formation
Embolization
Immobility
Swelling of tissues
Bleeding/hematoma
 	
DEFINING CHARACTERISTICS
Decrease or loss of peripheral pulses
Decrease in skin temperature of extremity
Presence of mottling, pallor, cyanosis, rubor in skin of distal extremity
	ONGOING ASSESSMENT
	Pre-PTCA:
	• Assess and document presence or absence and quality of all distal pulses.
	• Obtain Doppler ultrasonic reading for faint, nonpalpable pulses. Indicate if with Doppler. Mark location of faint pulses with *X for easier location during post-PTCA monitoring.*
	• Assess and document skin color and temperature, presence or absence of pain, numbness, tingling, movement, and sensation of all extremities. *Knowledge of baseline circulatory status of extremities will assist in monitoring for post-PTCA changes.*
	Post-PTCA:
	• Assess presence and quality of pulses distal to arterial cannulation site (radial for brachial artery; dorsalis pedis and/or posterior tibialis pulses for femoral artery) q15min×4, q30min×4, q1h×2, then q2h until stable.
	• Check cannulation site for swelling and hematoma *(may hinder peripheral circulation by constricting vessels).*
	
	THERAPEUTIC INTERVENTIONS
	Post-PTCA:
	• Ensure safety measures to prevent displacement of arterial and venous sheaths *(may compromise circulation or traumatize artery):*
	    Maintain complete bed rest in supine position.
	    Keep cannulated extremity straight at all times. Apply knee immobilizer or soft restraint *to remind patient not to bend it.*
	    Do not elevate HOB more than 30 degrees. Assist with meals, use of bedpan, and position changes appropriate to activity limitations.
		Peripheral tissue perfusion will be maintained in affected extremity.

Continued.

Percutaneous transluminal coronary angioplasty—cont'd

NURSING DIAGNOSES / DEFINING CHARACTERISTICS	NURSING INTERVENTIONS / *RATIONALES*	EXPECTED OUTCOMES
Delayed capillary refill in affected extremity Decrease or loss of sensation and motion	• Continue prescribed dose of heparin infusion *to ensure proper anticoagulation*. Check PTT 4h after start of infusion and after change in dose. Keep PTT 1½-2 times control. • Administer aspirin as prescribed *to prevent platelet aggregation and clot formation*. • Do passive ROM exercises to unaffected extremities q2-4h as tolerated *to prevent venous stasis and joint stiffness*. • Reposition q2h within activity limitations when appropriate *to maintain skin integrity*. • Instruct patient to report presence of pain, numbness, tingling, decrease or loss of sensation and movement immediately. *Important for quick assessment, diagnosis, and treatment*. • Immediately report to physician decrease or loss of pulse, change in skin color and temperature, presence of pain, numbness, tingling, delayed capillary refill, decrease or loss of sensation and motion *(may signify ischemia)*. • Anticipate removal of catheter sheath *(may obstruct blood flow)*. • Prepare for possible embolectomy *to remove blood clot obstructing or compromising circulation*.	

Potential for injury: bleeding
Related to:
Presence of catheter sheaths
Overheparinization
Arterial trauma
 	
DEFINING CHARACTERISTICS
Significant bleeding from cannulation site
Abnormal coagulation values
Restlessness and apprehension
Increased heart rate and respiratory rate
Decreased blood pressure
Hematoma at cannulation site
	ONGOING ASSESSMENT
	• Assess cannulation site for evidence of bleeding (e.g., fresh blood on dressing, oozing, pain/tenderness, swelling, hematoma).
	• Assess for signs of retroperitoneal bleeding (e.g., flank or thigh pain, loss of lower extremity pulses).
	• Monitor vital signs q15min×4, q30min×4, q1h×2, then q2h until stable.
	• Monitor CBC, PT, PTT, and platelets.
	• If significant bleeding occurs:
	   Monitor vital signs at least q15min until bleeding controlled.
	   Monitor for arrhythmias.
	   Observe for circulatory compromise in affected extremity.
	• Note amount of drainage if fresh blood noted on dressing. Circle or outline size of hematoma if noted *to help assess further bleeding*.
	
	THERAPEUTIC INTERVENTIONS
	Before removal of catheter sheaths:
	• Maintain bedrest in supine position with affected extremity straight *to minimize risk of bleeding from cannulation site*.
	• Do not elevate head of bed more than 30 degrees. Observe appropriate positioning for meals, bowel and bladder elimination, and position changes.
	• Avoid sudden movement of affected extremity *to prevent displacement of catheter sheaths (may cause bleeding)*.
	• Instruct patient to apply light pressure on dressing when coughing, sneezing, or raising head off pillow.
	• Instruct patient to notify nurse immediately of signs of bleeding from cannulation site (e.g., feeling of wetness, warmth, "pop" at catheter sheath site, and feeling of faintness).
	• Administer heparin drip via infusion pump *to ensure prescribed dose, depending on PTT result*.
	• If significant bleeding occurs:
	   Turn off heparin drip.
	   Notify physician immediately.
	   Remove dressing and apply manual pressure directly to bleeding site, observing aseptic technique.
	   Anticipate fluid challenge to treat hypotension.
	   Administer protamine sulfate as ordered *to reverse effect of heparin*.
	   Anticipate removal of catheter sheaths.
	   Administer O_2 as appropriate.
	After removal of catheter sheaths:
	• Maintain bed rest in supine position with affected extremity straight for 6 hr.
	• Avoid sudden movement of affected extremity *to facilitate clot formation and wound closure at insertion site*.
		Bleeding will be prevented or reduced.

NURSING DIAGNOSES / DEFINING CHARACTERISTICS	NURSING INTERVENTIONS / *RATIONALES*	EXPECTED OUTCOMES
	• Maintain occlusive pressure dressing on cannulation site. • Apply 5-lb sandbag over dressing on cannulation site for 4 hr. • For 6 hours after removal, do not elevate head of bed more than 30 degrees. • May dangle at bedside, then ambulate 6 hr after sheath removal if no evidence of bleeding.	

Fluid volume deficit
Related to:
Dye-induced diuresis
Restricted fluid intake at least 8 hr before procedure
 	
DEFINING CHARACTERISTICS
Potential:
  Increased urine output
  Thirst
Actual:
  Decreased urine output
  Concentrated urine
  Decreased serum potassium level
  Hemoconcentration
  Increased BUN/creatinine
  Fever
  Dry, sticky mucous membranes
  Poor skin turgor
  Increased serum sodium level
  Increased heart rate and respiratory rate
  Decreased blood pressure
  Pale, cool, clammy skin
  Restlessness, agitation, confusion
  Weight loss
	ONGOING ASSESSMENT
	• Monitor intake and output q1h. *I & O balance must be maintained to prevent hypovolemia/hypervolemia and possible renal dysfunction.*
	• Monitor vital signs as ordered.
	• Observe for changes in mental status.
	• Assess skin turgor and condition of mucous membranes.
	• Monitor serum electrolytes, particularly potassium.
	• Monitor BUN and creatinine *to detect presence of decreasing renal function.*
	• Check for orthostasis when activity resumes.
	• Check urine specific gravity q4h. *Dark urine with high specific gravity may indicate hypovolemia. Light urine with low specific gravity may reflect effects of diuretics, hypervolemia, and/or developing renal failure.*
	• Monitor urine electrolytes as ordered. *Urine sodium differentiates oliguria from dehydration and acute tubular necrosis. Oliguria with low urine sodium indicates dehydration.*
	
	THERAPEUTIC INTERVENTIONS
	• Push oral fluids as tolerated.
	• Administer IV fluids as ordered. Use infusion pump *to ensure patient of prescribed fluid volume and prevent accidental fluid overload.*
	• Give potassium supplement as ordered. *Potassium is excreted through the kidneys. It is important for proper function of skeletal and heart muscles. Slight change in serum levels may cause profound and/or life-threatening arrhythmias.*
	• Provide frequent oral hygiene *to decrease dryness of mouth.*
		Dehydration and renal damage will be prevented.

Incisional pain
Related to:
Incision at cannulation site
Trauma during cannulation
Presence of catheter sheaths
Irritation from catheter sheaths
Tight dressing over cannulation site
	ONGOING ASSESSMENT
	• Assess pain characteristics:
	  Quality
	  Severity
	  Location
	  Onset
	  Duration
	  Precipitating/relieving factors
	  Associated symptoms
	• Assess possible cause of pain.
		Pain/discomfort will be reduced.

Continued.

Percutaneous transluminal coronary angioplasty—cont'd

NURSING DIAGNOSES / DEFINING CHARACTERISTICS	NURSING INTERVENTIONS / *RATIONALES*	EXPECTED OUTCOMES
DEFINING CHARACTERISTICS Complaint of pain or discomfort Restlessness and agitation Facial mask of pain Moaning/crying Rigid nonmoving position Request for pain medication	**THERAPEUTIC INTERVENTIONS** • Instruct patient to report pain as soon as it starts *for early assessment and treatment*. • If pressure dressing too tight, loosen slightly as appropriate. • Change position q2h when appropriate within activity limitations. • Apply antipressure devices to bed and provide back rubs *to promote overall comfort*. • Administer analgesics as ordered and note response. Instruct patient to notify if pain medication is ineffective *so stronger medication can be given as appropriate*. • Provide rest periods for relaxation and sleep. • Use distraction devices (e.g., watching TV; listening to radio; reading book, magazines, newspaper; visiting with family and friends) when applicable. • Respond immediately to patient's complaint of pain. Provide reassurance and emotional support *to help allay fear and apprehension (may contribute to discomfort)*.	

Decreased cardiac output
Related to:
Reperfusion arrhythmias
 	
DEFINING CHARACTERISTICS
Variations in hemodynamic parameters (BP, heart rate, CVP, pulmonary artery pressures, cardiac output, neck veins)
Arrhythmias, ECG changes
Rales, tachypnea, dyspnea, orthopnea, cough, abnormal ABGs, frothy sputum
Decreased urine output
Anxiety, restlessness, syncope, dizziness, weakness, fatigue
Decreased peripheral pulses; cold, clammy skin
Change in mental status
	ONGOING ASSESSMENT
	• Assess and report significant changes in heart rate and rhythm.
	• Assess and report significant changes in:
	    Hemodynamic parameters
	    Breath sounds, respiratory rate
	• Monitor ABGs.
	• Monitor I & O.
	• Assess mental status.
	• Assess peripheral pulses, skin temperature.
	
	THERAPEUTIC INTERVENTIONS
	• See Cardiac output, decreased, p. 9; Cardiac dysrhythmias, p. 74.
		Adequate cardiac output will be maintained.

Anxiety/fear *Related to:* Potentially unsuccessful PTCA requiring immediate or future CABG surgery Potential complications from PTCA	**ONGOING ASSESSMENT** • Assess patient's level of anxiety and normal coping mechanisms. • Assess cause/causes of anxiety. **THERAPEUTIC INTERVENTIONS** • Initiate treatment for Anxiety, p. 4 or Fear, p. 18. • Explain reasons for monitoring in cardiac ICU after procedure. • Inform patient of frequency in checking vital signs, dressing, and presence of pulses. *Preparing patient for what to expect and why may help decrease anxiety level.*	Anxiety will be reduced or relieved.

Percutaneous transluminal coronary angioplasty—cont'd

NURSING DIAGNOSES / DEFINING CHARACTERISTICS	NURSING INTERVENTIONS / *RATIONALES*	EXPECTED OUTCOMES
Admission to cardiac ICU after procedure Frequent assessment and monitoring by nurse **DEFINING CHARACTERISTICS** Patient's verbalization of fear, apprehension, and helplessness Restlessness and agitation Sleeplessness Facial tension Increased heart rate and blood pressure Complaining/ uncooperative behavior Withdrawal	• Assure patient that with his/her cooperation, potential complications will be prevented or immediately handled. • Assist patient to cope effectively with fear and anxiety.	

Originated by: Maureen Kangleon, RN

Swan-Ganz catheterization

(PULMONARY ARTERY PRESSURES; WEDGE PRESSURES; THERMODILUTION; OXYGEN SATURATION)

A multilumen, balloon-tipped, flow-guided catheter inserted into the pulmonary artery for monitoring of pulmonary artery pressure (PAP) and pulmonary capillary wedge pressure (PCWP). It also has the capability of monitoring right atrial pressure (RAP), measuring cardiac output by thermodilution techniques, and monitoring mixed venous saturation via oximetry. The proximal lumen of this catheter can be used solely for intravenous infusion.

NURSING DIAGNOSES / DEFINING CHARACTERISTICS	NURSING INTERVENTIONS / *RATIONALES*	EXPECTED OUTCOMES

Knowledge deficit of patient/significant others
Related to:
Newness, complexity, and urgency of procedure
 	
DEFINING CHARACTERISTICS
Extensive questioning
Excessive anxiety
Inability to talk about procedure
Lack of questioning
	ONGOING ASSESSMENT
	• Assess current level of knowledge.
	• Assess learning capabilities of patient/significant other.
	
	THERAPEUTIC INTERVENTIONS
	• Provide patient/significant others with information about Swan-Ganz catheter:
	    Purpose
	    Insertion procedure
	    Complications
	    Ongoing care
	    Activity restrictions
	• Reinforce previous learning. *The critical care environment can cause sensory overload, sleep deprivation, and anxiety; all affect retention of information.*
		Patient/significant other will verbalize understanding of rationale for use, procedures involved, follow-up care.

Continued.

NURSING DIAGNOSES / DEFINING CHARACTERISTICS	NURSING INTERVENTIONS / *RATIONALES*	EXPECTED OUTCOMES
Potential for cardiac arrhythmias (PVCs) *Related to:* Irritation of ventricular endocardium by catheter during insertion/repositioning Migration of catheter from pulmonary artery to right ventricle Excessive looping of catheter in right ventricle **DEFINING CHARACTERISTICS** Palpitation Dizziness and fainting Shortness of breath Arrhythmia	**ONGOING ASSESSMENT** • Document precatheterization baseline arrhythmias, noting frequency and type. • Observe cardiac monitor continuously for arrhythmias during and after catheter positioning. Transient ventricular arrhythmias are commonly observed while catheter is passed through the right ventricle. • Monitor catheter position on chest x-ray daily and when arrhythmias occur. • Assess insertion site; note length of inserted catheter (check markings). *Change in markings alerts staff of catheter movement.* • Monitor pulmonary artery waveform closely. *Change in waveform to right ventricle tracing signals malpositioned catheter.* • Assess and document amount of air needed to wedge catheter. *Amount increases as catheter migrates to right ventricle, or catheter does not wedge.* • If arrhythmias occur: Assess patient for complaints of dizziness, palpitations, lightheadedness, shortness of breath. Document rhythm strip and notify physician. Observe contributing factors that may have potentiated arrhythmias (e.g., patient/catheter position; other medical problems). **THERAPEUTIC INTERVENTIONS** • Have lidocaine bolus and crash cart available. • Maintain appropriate positioning of extremity if femoral or brachial site is used *to prevent malposition of catheter.* • If catheter slips back to right ventricle, anticipate repositioning (if sterile sleeve in place) or removal and reinsertion of catheter. • Treat arrhythmias as indicated. • See Cardiac dysrhythmias, p. 74.	Occurrence of ventricular arrhythmias will be reduced.
Potential for injury: pulmonary artery infarction or hemorrhage *Related to:* Continuous or prolonged wedging of catheter Overinflation of balloon Migration of catheter to pulmonary capillary seen on x-ray film **DEFINING CHARACTERISTICS** Patient complaint of shortness of breath Hemoptysis	**ONGOING ASSESSMENT** • Monitor pulmonary arterial pressure waveform continuously. *PCWP is only measured intermittently.* • Monitor pulmonary artery position of catheter on x-ray *to verify correct placement.* • Monitor pulmonary artery diastolic pressure instead of wedge pressure when both values are correlated. *This reduces risk of permanent "wedging" of catheter.* **THERAPEUTIC INTERVENTIONS** • Inject only enough air to obtain pulmonary capillary artery wedge pressure. *Waveform will change from PAP to PCWP tracing.* • Do not inflate balloon past recommended volume *to prevent rupture.* Document amount used. • Leave balloon deflated when not directly measuring. • Never forcefully flush catheter. • Do not infuse anything through distal port except standardized continuous flush solution. • If catheter appears permanently wedged: Verify that cause is not false wedge pressure waveform, as with dampening or other technical problems. Have patient take deep breaths, raise arm, turn on left side, cough *to attempt to unwedge.* Notify physician immediately *to pull back catheter to pulmonary artery.* Determine catheter/balloon position on chest x-ray.	Risk of injury is reduced.

NURSING DIAGNOSES / DEFINING CHARACTERISTICS	NURSING INTERVENTIONS / *RATIONALES*	EXPECTED OUTCOMES
Potential for injury: electrical shock *Related to:* Direct low-resistance pathway of current through catheter to heart Current leakage Improperly grounded electrical equipment Frayed cords, exposed wires Wet skin or bed area Invasive catheters **DEFINING CHARACTERISTICS** PVCs, ventricular tachycardia, ventricular fibrillation produced by microshock	**ONGOING ASSESSMENT** • Assess environment for electrical safety. **THERAPEUTIC INTERVENTIONS** Maintain electrical safety standards when rendering care to high-risk patients. • Use as few electrical devices as needed. • Substitute battery-operated machines when possible. • Keep bed linen dry. • Ground electrical equipment *to reduce risk of microshock.*	Risk of electrical shock will be reduced.
Potential for injury: pneumothorax *Related to:* Use of subclavian insertion site Patient movement during insertion **DEFINING CHARACTERISTICS** Shortness of breath Decreased breath sounds on affected side Unequal thoracic wall movement Shift of trachea toward unaffected side	**ONGOING ASSESSMENT** • Assess breath sounds, respiratory pattern, and chest movement before and immediately after insertion. • When checking for catheter placement on x-ray, note lung expansion. **THERAPEUTIC INTERVENTIONS** • Keep patient still during procedure. *Sudden movements increase risks of pneumothorax.* Provide sedatives, local anesthesia, and reassurance as needed. • Provide optimal positioning of insertion area (back/shoulder/subclavian region). • If symptoms of pneumothorax are noted, refer to physician and anticipate chest tube insertion.	Occurrence of pneumothorax will be reduced.
Potential for infection *Related to:* Invasive monitoring Indwelling catheter Manipulation of catheter or connecting tubing Prolonged use of catheter **DEFINING CHARACTERISTICS** Redness at site Swelling Change in local temperature Foul drainage Fever	**ONGOING ASSESSMENT** • Check insertion site for signs of infection. *Foreign body in vascular system increases risk of sepsis.* • Assess vital signs, especially temperature. **THERAPEUTIC INTERVENTIONS** • Change IV tubing per unit policy. • Change IV dressing using sterile technique. • Apply antiseptic ointment to site. • Use caps on all ports of stopcocks. • Encourage removal of catheter or change of insertion site every 3 days. *Prolonged use increases risk.* • If infection occurs, notify physician for removal of catheter and culturing treatment.	Risk of infection will be reduced.

Continued.

NURSING DIAGNOSES / DEFINING CHARACTERISTICS	NURSING INTERVENTIONS / *RATIONALES*	EXPECTED OUTCOMES
Potential pain/ discomfort *Related to:* Thrombophlebitis Venous stasis Dependent edema Catheter irritation Difficult/traumatic insertion **DEFINING CHARACTERISTICS** Report of discomfort Restlessness Irritability Limited movement of extremity Tenderness, swelling at insertion site Edema of extremity	**ONGOING ASSESSMENT** • Check insertion site/extremity for signs of inflammation or discomfort. • Check extremity for swelling or dependent edema. Compare with unaffected extremity. **THERAPEUTIC INTERVENTIONS** • Assist during insertion *so catheter is positioned smoothly and rapidly.* • Maintain optimal position of extremity. Elevate distal portion of extremity *to minimize edema.* • Avoid tight bandaging of affected extremity. Use occlusive but nonconstricting dressing. • *Promote circulation to affected extremity* by performing active/passive ROM, noting limitations of catheter. • Encourage removal of catheter or change of insertion site every 3 days whenever possible. • If pain, phlebitis, or inflammation occurs: Facilitate removal of catheter. Apply warm compresses. Elevate extremity. Give pain medication prn.	Comfort will be maximized.

Originated by: Patricia Hasbrouck-Aschliman, RN, CCRN

Thrombolytic therapy in myocardial infarction

(t-PA; STREPTOKINASE; UROKINASE)

Thrombolytic agents are drugs that activate the fibrinolytic system to dissolve fibrin clots. Thrombolytic therapy is used in the management of acute myocardial infarction secondary to coronary artery thrombus formation.

NURSING DIAGNOSES / DEFINING CHARACTERISTICS	NURSING INTERVENTIONS / *RATIONALES*	EXPECTED OUTCOMES
Chest pain *Related to:* Myocardial infarction **DEFINING CHARACTERISTICS** Patient reports or manifests pain (see Assessment Criteria) Restlessness, apprehension Moaning, crying Facial mask of pain Diaphoresis Change in vital signs: BP, heart rate, respiratory rate Pallor, weakness Nausea and vomiting Fear and guarding behavior	**ONGOING ASSESSMENT** • Assess for characteristics of myocardial pain: Choking, squeezing, aching, "viselike" Intense pressure with heaviness Burning Other • Severity: scale 1-10 (10 most severe) • Onset: Sudden/constant • Duration: At least 30 min; usually 1-2 hr Residual soreness 1-3 days Pain may be intermittent • Location: Anterior chest, usually substernal May radiate to shoulder, arms, jaw, neck, and epigastrium • Precipitating factors: Physical or emotional exertion May occur at rest • Other characteristics: Not relieved by rest or nitrates Not affected by position change or breathing • Assess for indications for the use of thrombolytic agents:	Chest pain will be relieved and salvage of viable myocardium will occur.

NURSING DIAGNOSES / DEFINING CHARACTERISTICS	NURSING INTERVENTIONS / *RATIONALES*	EXPECTED OUTCOMES
	Chest pain less than 6 hr in duration. *Necrosis begins in the endocardium after 20 min of ischemia; transmural necrosis is complete between 4 to 6 hr; thus early intervention may limit infarct size, preserve left ventricular function, and ultimately prolong life.*	
	ECG changes consistent with acute myocardial infarction: ST-segment elevations in at least two contiguous ECG leads.	
	• Assess for contraindications to thrombolytic agents. *Thrombolytic agents will not distinguish a pathologic occlusive coronary thrombus from a protective hemostatic clot.*	
	Assess for increased risk of intracranial bleeding:	
	History of cerebrovascular accident (CVA)	
	Advanced age	
	Severe uncontrolled hypertension	
	Recent intracranial or intraspinal surgery or trauma	
	Intracranial neoplasm, AV malformation, or aneurysm	
	Assess for increased risk of internal bleeding:	
	Active internal bleeding	
	Known bleeding diathesis	
	Recent major surgery or trauma	
	• For streptokinase only:	
	Assess for previous strep infection or previous administration of strep tokinase. *Streptokinase is derived from β-hemolytic streptococci; previous exposure will have activated the patient's immune system; thus streptokinase administration may trigger allergic reaction.*	
	Assess for allergic reaction:	
	Itching	
	Fever, flushing	
	Hives	
	Monitor BP closely during infusion. *Hypotension is a side effect of streptokinase.*	
	• Assess for evidence of reperfusion:	
	Relief of chest pain	
	Normalization of ST segments	
	Reperfusion arrhythmias	
	Late sign: early and high creatinine phosphokinase (CPK) peak (washout)	
	THERAPEUTIC INTERVENTIONS	
	• See Acute myocardial infarction: acute phase (1-3 days), p. 103. Institute measures to relieve pain.	
	• Administer test dose of sublingual nitroglycerin (NTG) tablet *to rule out angina.*	
	• Before streptokinase administration, give hydrocortisone, 100 mg IVP, and Bendadryl, 50 mg IVP, as ordered *as prophylaxis for allergic reaction.*	
	• Administer thrombolytic agent (t-PA, streptokinase, or urokinase) as ordered.	
	• Administer medication via infusion device *to ensure accurate dosage.*	
	• Ensure complete dosage administration by adding 10-20 cc of 0.9 NS to empty IV bag or bottle and infuse at current rate to "flush" tubing.	
	• If signs of reperfusion are not evident and the patient continues to infarct, prepare for possible cardiac catheterization, PTCA, or coronary artery bypass grafting.	
Potential for injury: bleeding *Related to:* Dissolution of protective hemostatic clots Heparin therapy	**ONGOING ASSESSMENT** • Assess all puncture sites for bleeding. • Assess for gingival bleeding. • Assess for bleeding from cuts and abrasions. • Assess for internal bleeding: Monitor vital signs. Observe for presence of occult or frank blood in urine, stool, emesis, and sputum.	Risk for bleeding is reduced.

Continued.

Thrombolytic therapy in myocardial infarction—cont'd

NURSING DIAGNOSES / DEFINING CHARACTERISTICS	NURSING INTERVENTIONS / *RATIONALES*	EXPECTED OUTCOMES

DEFINING CHARACTERISTICS
Surface bleeding
Restlessness
Pallor
Change in vital signs (VS): decreased BP, tachycardia, tachypnea
Decreased urine output
Decreased Hb/Hct, decreased fibrinogen
Increased PTT
Tarry stools
Coffee ground emesis
Hematuria
Hemoptysis
Low back pain, numbness of lower extremities, diminishing pedal pulses (retroperitoneal bleeding)
Confusion
Disorientation
Speech/visual disturbances
Headache

- Assess patient postcardiac catheterization for retroperitoneal bleeding:
    Check pedal pulses.
    Assess for back pain.
    Assess for leg numbness/weakness.
- Assess for intracranial bleeding by frequent monitoring of neurologic status.
- Assess Hb/Hct, fibrinogen, and PTT levels.

THERAPEUTIC INTERVENTIONS
- *To prevent bleeding*:
    Establish all IVs before therapy.
    Insert a heparin lock device with a stopcock *to obtain venous blood samples.*
    Avoid unnecessary arterial or venous punctures or IM injections.
    Avoid noncompressible IV access sites (subclavian, internal jugular). *Any interruption of vascular integrity may cause bleeding secondary to patient's temporary inability to form a hemostatic clot.*
    Avoid discontinuing any arterial/venous lines during thrombolytic infusion and 24 hr after therapy. *The catheters will occlude the puncture sites until coagulation proteins are restores.*
    If arterial/venous puncture is unavoidable, use small-gauge (i.e., 25-gauge) needle and apply direct pressure to all arterial/venous puncture sites for 30 min.
    Apply pressure dressing to all arterial/venous puncture sites.
    Administer prophylactic antiulcer therapy (Mylanta, Tagamet, Zantac, Sucralfate) as ordered *to reduce risk of bleeding from gastritis or stress ulcer (may develop in response to acute MI event).*
    Report abnormal results of Hb/Hct and coagulation studies.
    Obtain type and cross match before therapy as ordered.
    Encourage patient to notify staff of any bleeding.
- Management of minor bleeding (superficial):
    Apply direct pressure *to control bleeding.*
    Gingival bleeding: assist patient with rinsing mouth using ice water *to provide comfort and cause vasoconstriction.*
    Continue medication, infusions; monitor patient.
- Management of major bleeding (frank, GI, intracranial, retroperitoneal):
    Discontinue thrombolytic agent infusion.
    Discontinue heparin infusion. Administer protamine sulfate *to reverse anticoagulant effect of heparin.*
    Notify physician.
    Administer IV fluids as ordered.
    Anticipate blood product replacement.

Potential decreased cardiac output
Related to:
Reperfusion arrhythmias:
    Accelerated idioventricular rhythm (most common)
    Ventricular tachycardia
    Premature ventricular contractions
    Sinus bradycardia
    AV block

DEFINING CHARACTERISTICS
Rapid/slow pulse
Decreased blood pressure

ONGOING ASSESSMENT
- Monitor ECG for heart rate and rhythm. Note any changes.
- Assess for signs of reduced cardiac that may accompany arrhythmia (see Defining Characteristics).

THERAPEUTIC INTERVENTIONS
- Administer prophylactic lidocaine before initiation of thrombolytic therapy *to prevent ventricular ectopy*:
    Lidocaine bolus, 1 mg/kg, as ordered; may repeat
    Lidocaine continuous infusion, 2-4 mg/min, as ordered
- Keep atropine sulfate at bedside *for treatment of bradyarrhythmias commonly associated with reperfusion of right coronary artery (inferior wall MI).*
- Have emergency resusitative equipment and medications readily available. *Any arrhythmia can decompensate into an unstable rhythm such as ventricular tachycardia or ventricular fibrillation with an accompanying compromise in cardiac output.*
- Notify physician of significant arrhythmias.
- Initiate treatment for Cardiac output, decreased, p. 9; Cardiac dysrhythmias, p. 74.

Adequate cardiac output will be maintained.

NURSING DIAGNOSES / DEFINING CHARACTERISTICS	NURSING INTERVENTIONS / *RATIONALES*	EXPECTED OUTCOMES
Dizziness, lightheadedness, syncope Changes in mental state Cool, clammy skin Shortness of breath, cough, rales, chest pain Pallor Fatigue, weakness Increased jugular venous distention (JVD)		
Chest pain *Related to:* Reocculsion of coronary artery (rethrombosis of infarct-related artery) after successful thrombolysis **DEFINING CHARACTERISTICS** Patient report and verbalizations Restlessness, apprehension Moaning, crying Facial mask of pain Diaphoresis Change in vital signs: BP, heart rate, respiratory rate Pallor, weakness Nausea and vomiting Fear and guarding behavior	**ONGOING ASSESSMENT** · Assess for characteristics of myocardial pain. · Assess ECG for ST-segment elevation. · Assess PT/PTT every day and 3-4 hr after any change in heparin dose. **THERAPEUTIC INTERVENTIONS** · Prevention: Maintain infusion of thrombolytic agent at appropriate dose and rate. Administer heparin therapy as ordered. *Concomitant use of heparin reduces risk of reocclusion and thrombosis of infarct-related artery (may develop in response to re-exposure of vessel injury after thrombolysis).* Titrate heparin to maintain PTT at 1.5-2 times control value. Administer antiplatelet agents (aspirin, Persantine) as ordered *to prevent platelet aggregation and subsequent clot formation.* · Recurrence of ischemia: Notify physician of return of any signs and symptoms of myocardial ischemia, Obtain 12-lead ECG. Administer appropriate pharmacologic therapy for treatment of pain (nitrates, morphine sulfate, etc). See Acute myocardial infarction (1-3 days), p. 103. Prepare patient for possible emergency procedures: Repeat administration of thrombolytic agent: *to lyse newly formed occlusive thrombus.* Cardiac catheterization: *to evaluate and diagnose underlying pathology responsible for recurrent myocardial ischemia:* PTCA: *to reduce residual stenosis and improve blood flow* CABG: *to bypass occluded artery*	Chest pain associated with reocclusion will be prevented or treated promptly.
Knowledge deficit *Related to:* New treatment of acute MI Unfamiliarity with disease process, treatment, recovery **DEFINING CHARACTERISTICS** Multiple questions or lack of questions Confusion about events Expressed need for more information	**ONGOING ASSESSMENT** · Assess readiness of patient/significant others for teaching. · Assess baseline knowledge. **THERAPEUTIC INTERVENTIONS** · See Myocardial infarction: acute phase (1-3 days), p. 103. *The patient has experienced an MI and will have the same educational needs as those experiencing an MI managed without thrombolytic therapy.* · Explain to patient/significant others indications for and benefits and risks of thrombolytic therapy. · Inform patient/significant others of possible surface bleeding and bruising as minor side effects. · Instruct patient to report recurrence of chest pain. · Inform patient/significant others of need for frequent inspection for bleeding, VS, and cardiac monitoring.	Patient/significant others will verbalize understanding of patient's condition, healing process of MI, need for observation in CCU, diagnosis of MI, and treatment with thrombolytic agents.

Originated by: Anne Paglinawan, RN, BSN

Transvenous pacemaker, permanent

(CARDIAC PACEMAKER)

A permanent pacemaker is an implanted electronic device that delivers an artificial electrical stimulus to the heart muscle, when needed, for the control of the heart. The stimuli from the pacemaker battery travel through a flexible catheter electrode to the catheter tip, which is usually positioned in the right ventricle (or right atrium). Indications for permanent cardiac pacing include symptomatic chronic heart block, bradyarrhythmias, and refractory tachyarrhythmias.

NURSING DIAGNOSES / DEFINING CHARACTERISTICS	NURSING INTERVENTIONS / *RATIONALES*	EXPECTED OUTCOMES
Potential decreased cardiac output *Related to:* Ventricular arrhythmias caused by ventricular irritation from pacing electrode (lead) Cardiac tamponade resulting from myocardial perforation Permanent pacemaker malfunction caused by: 　Lead displacement 　Battery fault or depletion 　Lead fracture 　Changing myocardial threshold 　Competitive rhythms 　Malfunctioning generator circuitry 　Faulty connection between lead and pulse generator 　Improperly set pacemaker parameters **DEFINING CHARACTERISTICS** Signs of hemodynamic compromise (hypotension, decrease in measured cardiac output, decrease in urine output, confusion, restlessness, dizziness, chest pain, cool skin) and/or congestive heart failure Palpitations Significant decrease (5-10%) in heart rate from preset parameter	**ONGOING ASSESSMENT** If *ECG monitored*: ▪ Assess for proper pacemaker function: 　Capture 　Sensing 　Firing 　Amplitude of pacemaker artifact 　Configuration of paced QRS ▪ Assess for pacemaker-induced arrhythmias. If *unmonitored*: ▪ Assess apical and radial pulses. ▪ Assess patient's hemodynamic status. For *newly implanted pacemaker*: ▪ Check operative note for: 　Type of pacemaker (programmable, ventricular demand, AV sequential, etc.) and prescribed parameters. *Different types may function differently, making evaluation of proper function difficult.* ▪ Monitor chest x-ray and ECG studies after patient returns from OR and as ordered *to verify correct placement and function.* If *pacemaker malfunction* is noted: ▪ Evaluate adequacy of patient's own rhythm. ▪ If patient is not monitored, call for 12-lead ECG. ▪ Monitor for signs of hemodynamic compromise and/or congestive heart failure. If *failure to sense* is noted: ▪ Monitor chest x-ray study *to check position of pacemaker electrode.* ▪ Observe for diaphragmatic contraction (hiccups) and intercostal or abdominal muscle twitching *caused by stimulation of chest wall and diaphragm by dislodged pacemaker or lead.* ▪ Observe for rapid ventricular arrhythmias secondary to pacemaker competition. If *loss of capture* is noted: ▪ Monitor chest x-ray study *to check position of pacemaker electrode.* ▪ Observe for diaphragmatic contraction (hiccups) and intercostal or abdominal muscle twitching *caused by stimulation of chest wall and diaphragm by dislodged pacemaker or lead.* ▪ Observe for rapid ventricular arrhythmias secondary to pacemaker competition. ▪ Assess for factors that increase myocardial threshold (myocardial ischemia, fibrosis at tip of the electrode, electrolyte imbalance, acidosis, some antiarrhythmic drugs). *Threshold represents amount of electrical stimulation needed to initiate paced rhythm.* If *myocardial perforation* is suspected: ▪ Monitor chest x-ray film *for electrode placement.* ▪ Monitor closely for signs of cardiac tamponade. **THERAPEUTIC INTERVENTIONS** If *ECG monitored.* ▪ Keep alarms on at all times. ▪ Record rhythm strips: 　Routine	Optimal cardiac output will be maintained.

NURSING DIAGNOSES / DEFINING CHARACTERISTICS	NURSING INTERVENTIONS / *RATIONALES*	EXPECTED OUTCOMES
Stokes-Adams disease "Runaway" pacemaker (pacer tachycardia) Ventricular arrhythmias Loss of sensing Loss of capture Failure to fire Decrease in amplitude of pacemaker artifact Change in configuration of paced QRS Signs of cardiac tamponade (jugular vein distention, elevated central venous pressure, pulsus paradoxus, quiet heart sounds, signs of decreased cardiac output)	If any malfunction is noted After changes in pacemaker parameters If *pacemaker malfunction* is noted: • Notify physician • If secondary to failure to sense, turn patient on left side *to facilitate stimulation of ventricular muscle wall.* • Initiate basic life support measures as needed. • Prepare IV isoproterenol for standby. *This is a cardiac stimulant to increase heart rate.* • Prepare for temporary pacemaker insertion and other advanced life support measures as needed. • If pacemaker is programmable, call programmer to bedside. *This allows noninvasive adjustment of pacemaker settings.* • Anticipate possible return to OR. • If hemodynamic compromise is noted, see Cardiac output, decreased, p. 9.	
Impaired physical mobility *Related to:* Imposed restriction of activity Reluctance to attempt movement because of pain or fear of injury **Defining Characteristics** Verbalization of inability to perform Limited ROM Complaints of shoulder joint stiffness and pain Muscle weakness, especially of upper extremity on operative side	**Ongoing Assessment** While patient is on bedrest (usually 24-48 hr after insertion): • Auscultate breath sounds and assess respiratory rate, rhythm. • Assess skin integrity; check for signs of redness or tissue ischemia. • Assess for developing thrombophlebitis (increased temperature, redness, swelling, calf pain). • Assess for pulmonary embolism (chest pain, shortness of breath, tachycardia, increased BP). • Observe for signs of discomfort. • Assess for conditional deterrents to mobility. **Therapeutic Interventions** While patient is on bedrest: • Explain necessity for imposed activity restriction *to prevent electrode displacement.* • Encourage patient to turn every 1-2 hr but *not* to right side. • Assist with active ROM exercises to nonaffected extremities tid. • Provide passive ROM to shoulder on *operative* side tid *to prevent "frozen" shoulder.* • Assist patient in using affected extremity to perform ADL; however, caution patient against raising arm over head until instructed to do so *(may cause electrode displacement).* • Encourage patient to cough and deep breathe every hour while awake; incentive spirometry may be used when appropriate *to prevent atelectasis.* • Administer pain medication as ordered and institute other measures *for promotion of pain relief.* • Allow patient to verbalize feelings of fear or pain. Render emotional support, and teach as needed to *decrease reluctance to move extremity on operative side.* • If bed rest will be prolonged, institute prophylactic use of antipressure devices.	Complications of immobility will be absent or reduced.

Continued.

NURSING DIAGNOSES / DEFINING CHARACTERISTICS	NURSING INTERVENTIONS / *RATIONALES*	EXPECTED OUTCOMES

Pain
Related to:
"Frozen" shoulder
Insertion of permanent pacemaker
Self-imposed restriction of movement of extremity on operative side
Lead displacement
 	
Defining Characteristics
Patient/significant other reports discomfort
Request for pain medication
Restlessness, irritability
Guarded or withdrawn behavior
Pallor, increased BP, or diaphoresis
Crying
Grimacing
Reluctance to move
Wound splinted with hands
Limited ROM of shoulder on operative side
Hiccuping (diaphragmatic contraction); intercostal or abdominal muscle twitching
	Ongoing Assessment
	• Observe for objective signs of discomfort (e.g., crying, grimacing).
	• Assess characteristics of source of discomfort, including quality, quantity, location, onset, associated manifestations, precipitating and relieving factors.
	• Assess for hiccups or muscle twitching.
	• Solicit information about effectiveness of pain-relief measures patient has used in the past.
	
	Therapeutic Interventions
	• Anticipate need for pain relief and administer analgesics as ordered.
	• Provide comfort measures:
	  Back rubs
	  Gentle massage to shoulder on operative side
	  Heating pad to shoulder as ordered
	  Relaxation techniques *to decrease muscle tension*
	• Instruct patient to report discomfort.
	• Instruct patient to report effectiveness of interventions.
	• Discuss reasons for self-imposed restriction of movement of extremities on affected side, and teach as needed.
	• If hiccup or muscle twitching is noted:
	  Notify physician
	  Explain that this may be caused by lead displacement
	  Arrange for chest x-ray examination *to check for lead placement* and anticipate repositioning.
	• See Pain, p. 39.
		Discomfort will be relieved or reduced.

Knowledge deficit
Related to:
New procedure/equipment
 	
Defining Characteristics
Questioning
Verbalized misconceptions
Lack of questions
Inappropriate behavior
	Ongoing Assessment
	• Assess patient's level of understanding of pacemaker.
	• Assess patient's readiness for learning.
	
	Therapeutic Interventions
	• Provide environment conducive to learning.
	• Utilize appropriate teaching materials:
	  Pacemaker equipment
	  Manufacturer's pamphlet
	  Enjoy a Fuller Life with Your Pacemaker, an in-hospital television program
	• Include significant others in teaching.
	• Document teaching
	• Refer patient to clinical nurse specialist or physician for further information as needed
	• Provide the following teaching as needed:
	Preoperatively:
	Basic anatomy and physiology of normal conduction system
	Function and use of pacemaker
	Insertion procedure
	Postoperatively:
	Activity limitations:
	  Bed rest as ordered
		Patient will verbalize understanding of need for pacemaker insertion and acceptance of activity limitations.

NURSING DIAGNOSES / DEFINING CHARACTERISTICS	NURSING INTERVENTIONS / *RATIONALES*	EXPECTED OUTCOMES

	Avoidance of over-the-head motion of arms for prescribed time (at least 3 days)
	Avoidance of turning to right side for prescribed time (at least 3 days)
	Notify nurse of any wetness, discoloration, loose dressing
	Notify nurse of any dizziness, headache, confusion, shortness of breath, chest pain, muscle twitching, or hiccups *(may suggest pacemaker malfunction)*
	Need for chest x-ray examination and 12-lead ECG
	Prior to discharge:
	Procedure to take and record pulse daily
	Need for regular follow-up care
	Type of pacemaker inserted (programmable, chamber[s] paced, synchronous or asynchronous)
	Brand name of pacemaker
	Model number
	Pacing rate
	Normal pulse range *(any slowing of rate by more than 5 beats/min may indicate pacemaker battery depletion)*
	Expected pacemaker battery life. Replacement of battery requires approximately 3 days' hospitalization
	Signs and symptoms of pacemaker malfunction
	Signs and symptoms of infection at insertion site
	Notify physician of any signs and symptoms of pacemaker malfunction
	Wound care for insertion sites
	Always carry an ID card with type and model of pacemaker
	Alert any dentist or physician to presence of pacemaker
	Personnel at airport screening area should be made aware that patient has a pacemaker that may trigger the alarm
	Most household appliances and office and shop equipment that are in good repair can be used safely, including:
	  Televisions or radios
	  Toasters, electric can openers, or blenders
	  Washers, dryers, or electric stoves
	  Hair dryers or shavers
	  Heating pads and electric blankets
	  Gardening equipment
	  Electric brooms or vacuum cleaners
	  Microwave ovens (by patients with newer model pacemakers): check with physician or manufacturer's owner manual
	  Copy machines or electric typewriters
	  Light metalworking and woodworking tools
	Avoid equipment that contains powerful magnets or emits high-frequency electrical signals. *They interfere with pacemaker function:*
	  Diathermy or electrocautery equipment
	  High-current industrial machinery
	  Radio and television station transmitting equipment
	If interference with pacemaker function is suspected:
	  Turn off or move away from equipment
	  Pacemaker will resume normal function without permanent effects
	Instruct patient that pacemaker company representatives can make home visits to determine possible sources of electrical interference
	Most activities can be resumed:
	  Traveling or driving a car
	  Having sex
	  Swimming, bowling, fishing, hunting, or golfing
	  Working
	Avoid contact sports (e.g., football, basketball)	

Continued.

Cardiovascular Care Plans

NURSING DIAGNOSES / DEFINING CHARACTERISTICS	NURSING INTERVENTIONS / *RATIONALES*	EXPECTED OUTCOMES
Anxiety *Related to:* Insertion/presence of permanent pacemaker Alteration in body image caused by loss of normal cardiac function or cosmetic appearance of generator and incision line **DEFINING CHARACTERISTICS** Excessive concern about function of pacemaker Increased questioning Restlessness Withdrawal or indifference Increase or self-imposed decrease in activity Fear of sleeping at night Verbal expression of feelings of loss, fear/anxiety, or negative feelings about body Refusal to look at or touch incision or pulse generator site Overexposure or hiding of incision or pulse generator site Refusal to learn about pacemaker, participate in care of incision, or follow instructions about wound care or activity limitations	**ONGOING ASSESSMENT** • Assess level of anxiety. • Assess normal coping patterns. **THERAPEUTIC INTERVENTIONS** • Explain all procedures before they are performed. • Allow patient to verbalize concerns. • Correct knowledge deficits. • Institute measures to promote adequate sleep. • Preoperatively involve patient in decision making for optimal generator placement. *Options for insertion site may be available.* • Request consultation from clergy, social service, or liaison nurse when appropriate. • Initiate treatment for Anxiety, p. 4.	Anxiety level will be decreased.

Potential for infection
Related to:
Alteration in skin integrity caused by permanent pacemaker insertion
 	
DEFINING CHARACTERISTICS
Fever
Redness, drainage, edema, induration, or excessive tenderness at incision line
Elevated WBC with left shift
	ONGOING ASSESSMENT
	• Assess insertion site for signs of infection.
	• Monitor WBC.
	• Monitor temperature.
	• Assess amount and characteristics of Hemovac drainage if present.
	
	THERAPEUTIC INTERVENTIONS
	• Keep dressing dry and intact.
	• Change dressing using sterile technique as per infection control policy until skin closure complete.
	• If Hemovac is in place, record output q8h and as necessary, report excessive drainage.
	• Encourage a high-protein, high-calorie diet unless contraindicated *to facilitate wound healing.*
	• Administer antibiotics as ordered.
	• Before discharge, teach patient:
	    Signs/symptoms of infection
	    Wound care
		Risk of infection will be reduced.

Originated by: Terry Takemoto, RN, MSN, CCRN

Transvenous pacemaker, temporary

Insertion of a specialized electrical device into the right ventricle with the purpose of stimulating cardiac muscle activity.

NURSING DIAGNOSES / DEFINING CHARACTERISTICS	NURSING INTERVENTIONS / *RATIONALES*	EXPECTED OUTCOMES
Potential decreased cardiac output *Related to:* Temporary pacemaker malfunction secondary to: Improperly set pacemaker param- eters Displaced pace- maker lead (cathe- ter) Broken wire Poor electrical con- nections Battery exhaustion Malfunctioning gen- erator circuitry Unsafe environment Change in myocar- dial threshold Competitive rhythms **DEFINING CHARACTERISTICS** Loss of pacemaker capture Loss of pacemaker sensing Loss of pacemaker firing Significant decrease in heart rate Signs of hemody- namic compromise (i.e., hypotension, decreases in cardiac output, restlessness, cool skin, decrease in urine output)	**ONGOING ASSESSMENT** • Assess that prescribed pacemaker parameters are maintained (rate, million-pere (mA), mode, sensitivity). • Monitor ECG continuously for appropriate pacemaker function: Sensing Capturing Firing • If pacemaker is on standby, ensure that pacemaker capture is checked daily and as needed by physician by overriding of spontaneous rhythm. • Assess for pacemaker-induced arrhythmias. • Assess that patient is in an electrically safe environment since the pacemaker lead is in direct contact with the myocardium: All electrical equipment is properly grounded Environment is dry "Exposed" electrode terminals are insulated in rubber glove Patient is in nonelectric bed • If signs of pacemaker malfunction occur, assess patient's hemodynamic status q15-30min until stable. **THERAPEUTIC INTERVENTION** • Keep alarms turned on at all times. • Document spontaneous and paced rhythms during physician rounds: Daily or prn When changes in pacer parameters are instituted • If failure to sense is noted, *pacer is not sensing patient's rhythm and may lead to pacemaker-induced arrhythmias*: Check that power switch is on. Check that dial is *not* on "asynchronous" (pacemaker firing a fixed rate). Check for loose connections. Reposition limb of body. Notify physician of need to adjust sensitivity dial. Check position of lead by chest x-ray examination. • If problem is not corrected and patient's rate is adequate, evaluate whether pacemaker should be turned off (standby) • If loss of capture is noted, pacer is failing to stimulate an electrical response in patient's myocardium: Check all possible connections. Turn patient on left side *to facilitate optimal lead placement*. Increase mA and evaluate effectiveness for capture. • If loss of firing is noted, pacer is not generating an electrical stimulus: Check that power switch is turned on Check "pace" needle on pacemaker box to see that it is fluctuating back and forth If needle is not "pacing", replace batteries in generator. Check all possible connections. Check for electrical interference. Replace generator as needed. • Prepare IV isoproterenol for standby.	Optimal cardiac output will be maintained.

Continued.

Transvenous pacemaker, temporary—cont'd

NURSING DIAGNOSES / DEFINING CHARACTERISTICS	NURSING INTERVENTIONS / *RATIONALES*	EXPECTED OUTCOMES
Impaired physical mobility *Related to:* Imposed restriction secondary to pacemaker insertion and need to guard against any tension on pacing wire **DEFINING CHARACTERISTICS** Reluctance to attempt movement Limited ROM Verbalization of inability to perform activities	**ONGOING ASSESSMENT** · Auscultate breath sounds and assess respiratory rate, rhythm. · Assess skin integrity. Check for signs of redness or tissue ischemia. · Assess for developing thrombophlebitis (e.g., increased temperature, redness, swelling, calf pain). · Assess for pulmonary/embolism (e.g., chest pain, shortness of breath, tachycardia, increased BP). **THERAPEUTIC INTERVENTIONS** · Turn and position q2h, but instruct patient not to turn on right side *to prevent dislodgement of pacer wire*. · Assist with active ROM exercises to nonaffected extremities tid *to reduce risks of immobility*. · Assist patient with modified ROM to extremity with lead insertion tid *to reduce risks of immobility*. · Instruct patient not to raise arm over head if pacemaker lead is in antecubital fossa *to prevent lead displacement*. · Institute prophylactic use of antipressure devices. · Encourage cough and deep breathing q1h while patient is awake *to prevent pulmonary stasis*. · Assist patient to dangle after 24 hr if pacemaker lead is in antecubital fossa *to reduce risks of immobility*. · Ensure that patient maintains strict bed rest with head of bed elevated less than 30 degrees if pacemaker lead is inserted through femoral vein *to prevent lead displacement*.	Complications of immobility will be absent or reduced.

Knowledge deficit
Related to:
New procedure/equipment
 	
DEFINING CHARACTERISTICS
Questioning
Verbalized misconceptions
Lack of questions
Inappropriate behavior
	ONGOING ASSESSMENT
	· Assess patient's level of understanding of pacemaker.
	· Assess patient's readiness for learning.
	
	THERAPEUTIC INTERVENTIONS
	· Provide environment conducive to learning *to facilitate patient's ability to absorb new information*.
	· Use appropriate teaching materials:
	   Temporary pacemaker flip chart
	   Pacemaker equipment
	· Give patient explanation of:
	   Function and use a pacemaker
	   Insertion procedure
	   Activity restrictions
	   Ongoing care related to pacemaker
	· Include significant others in teaching as appropriate *to decrease their feelings of helplessness and increase patient's sense of security and support*.
	· Document teaching.
	· Refer more specific questions to cardiac clinical specialist and physician.
		Patient will verbalize understanding of rationale for use of temporary pacemaker, insertion procedure, and follow-up nursing care.

Anxiety *Related to:* Insertion/presence of temporary pacemaker Dependence on proper functioning of pacemaker Threat to self-concept, especially if patient is pacemaker-dependent and will need a permanent pacemaker	**ONGOING ASSESSMENT** · Assess level of anxiety. · Assess patient's normal coping patterns. **THERAPEUTIC INTERVENTIONS** · Institute treatment for Anxiety, p. 4 · Establish rapport with patient through continuity of care. · Encourage ventilation of feelings/concerns. · Orient to environment, pacemaker equipment *to reduce fear of unknown equipment and alleviate anxiety*. · Adapt care to patient's needs. · Stay with patient as much as possible. · Provide accurate information about purpose/function of pacemaker. · Reassure patient when weaning off pacemaker and especially when terminating.	Anxiety will be reduced.

NURSING DIAGNOSES / DEFINING CHARACTERISTICS	NURSING INTERVENTIONS / *RATIONALES*	EXPECTED OUTCOMES
DEFINING CHARACTERISTICS Patient concern about equipment Increased questioning Restlessness Withdrawal, indifference, uncooperativeness Fear of sleeping at night		
Pain *Related to:* Insertion of temporary pacemaker Subcutaneous irritation by catheter Subsequent restriction in movement of extremity Lead displacement **DEFINING CHARACTERISTICS** Patient/significant other reports discomfort Restlessness, irritability Guarded behavior Pallor, increased BP, diaphoresis Hiccuping (diaphragmatic contraction); intercostal or abdominal muscle twitching	**ONGOING ASSESSMENT** • Assess discomfort characteristics, such as quality, severity, location, onset, associated manifestations, precipitating and relieving factors. • Assess for hiccups or muscle twitching that may occur with lead displacement or excessively high mA. **THERAPEUTIC INTERVENTIONS** • Anticipate need for comfort measures. • Provide comfort measures: position change, back rubs, analgesics as ordered *to increase comfort.* • Turn and position; support dependent parts with pillows. • During dressing change, pad underside of the generator box with 4 by 4 bandages and wrap securely without constricting circulation. • Instruct patient to report pain. • Instruct patient to report effectiveness of intervention. • Explain cause of pain/discomfort. • Initiate treatment for Pain, p. 39. • If hiccups or muscle twitching are noted, call physician to evaluate lead placement *(incorrectly positioned leads may stimulate diaphragm).* Anticipate need to reposition lead.	Optimal comfort will be maintained.
Potential for infection *Related to:* Invasive procedure with possible introduction of bacteria **DEFINING CHARACTERISTICS** Fever Redness, drainage, swelling, tenderness at catheter site Elevated WBC	**ONGOING ASSESSMENT** • Assess catheter site for any pain, redness, moisture, drainage, or bleeding. • Monitor WBC. • Monitor temperature q4h and as needed. • Monitor length of time pacemaker is in place and report to physician after 72 hr. **THERAPEUTIC INTERVENTIONS** • Keeping dressing dry and intact *to prevent contamination with bacteria.* • Change dressing q48h or as needed per infection control policy.	Occurrence of infection will be reduced.

Originated by: Marisa C. Trybula, RN, BSN
              Pat Anderson, RN

Ventricular assist device

(LVAD; RVAD)

Ventricular assist devices (VADs) are flow assistance devices that provide temporary circulatory support for the failing ventricle. The VAD can be inserted in either the right ventricle (RVAD) or left ventricle (LVAD), depending on the site of ventricular failure. Ventricular failure after cardiopulmonary bypass is manifested by poor contractility with resultant low cardiac output, MAP less than 60 mm Hg, cardiac index less than 1.8/min, and elevated filling pressures (increased left atrial pressure [LAP], increased central venous pressure [CVP], or increased RA) depending on the site of injury. Patients who cannot be weaned from cardiopulmonary bypass with an intra-aortic balloon pump, and maximum pharmacologic therapy may require a VAD. With the ventricular assist device in place, blood is diverted away from the atrium, bypassing the ventricle and returning to the patient through the pump. The VAD provides hemodynamic stability until the ventricle can heal and regain its effectiveness as a pump. Optimal postoperative nursing management involves awareness of patient's preoperative history, operative course, and potential problems related to both surgical recovery and insertion of the VAD.

NURSING DIAGNOSES / DEFINING CHARACTERISTICS	NURSING INTERVENTIONS / *RATIONALES*	EXPECTED OUTCOMES
Decreased cardiac output *Related to:* Myocardial dysfunction Postcardiopulmonary bypass resulting in right and/or left ventricular failure	**ONGOING ASSESSMENT** • Monitor hemodynamics: HR, mean arterial pressure (MAP), systolic and diastolic pressure, LAP, PAD, pulmonary capillary wedge pressure (PCWP), right atrial pressure/central venous pressure (RAP, CVP). • Document rhythm strip once per shift. • Monitor assist device flows and cardiac output. • Monitor skin color, temperature, and quality and presence of peripheral pulses. • Monitor strict I & O, daily weights. • Monitor drug infusions as ordered. • Monitor LVAD tubing for kinks and tension *so perfusion is not compromised.*	Optimal cardiac output is maintained.
DEFINING CHARACTERISTICS Left ventricular failure Increased LAP Increased PAD Increased PCWP Tachycardia Decreased BP Decreased CO Sluggish capillary refill Diminished peripheral pulses Changes in chest x-ray Enlarged heart Pulmonary edema Rales Decreased arterial and venous oxygenation Acidosis Decreased urine output Right ventricular failure: Increased RAP Increased CVP	**THERAPEUTIC INTERVENTIONS** • Maintain hemodynamic parameters as ordered: HR _____ to_____ MAP _____ to _____ CVP/RAP _____ to _____ LAP _____ to_____ *Hemodynamic parameters may be maintained by titration of vasoactive drugs and administration of volume such as crystalloids and/or colloids.* • Administer vasopressors as ordered: Use infusion pump *to ensure accuracy.* Administer through central line. Keep drug cards at bedside with patient's name, weight, amount of drug, and rate of infusion. Drugs: *Dopamine:* increased contractility; increased renal blood flow in low doses *Dubutrex:* increased contractility; may slightly vasodilate *Inocor:* increased contractility and vasodilation *Isuprel:* increased HR, contractility; decreased pulmonary resistance for RV failure *Epinephrine:* Strengthens myocardial contractility. Monitor glucose every q4h while on epinephrine. Epinephrine raises blood glucose by promoting conversion of glycogen reserves in liver to glucose and inhibiting insulin release in pancreas. *Nitroglycerin:* dilates coronary vasculature, dilates venous system, prevents coronary spasm.	

NURSING DIAGNOSES / DEFINING CHARACTERISTICS	NURSING INTERVENTIONS / *RATIONALES*	EXPECTED OUTCOMES
Jugular vein distention Decreased BP Decreased CO	*Nipride:* lowers BP, lowers systemic vascular resistance (SVR). *Elevated pressure on new grafts may cause bleeding* *Neosynephrine:* vasoconstricts and increases SVR • Maintain assist device flows as prescribed. If left atrial pressure (LAP) is elevated (for example, >20mm), may need to increase flow of LVAD *to assist failing left ventricle and maintain LAP within prescribed range.* If RVAD is present, may need to increase flow of RVAD *to maintain RA at prescribed range.* • Keep LVAD tubing in full view. Avoid kinking and pulling tubing. Keep patient's hands in safety restraints or mittened as needed *to prevent disconnection of tubing.* • Keep temporary pacemaker at bedside at all times. Attach temporary epicardial wires to pacemaker, which is kept on standby. *Ectopy usually results from irritability caused by ischemia, electrolytic imbalance, or mechanical irritation.* • If cardiac arrest occurs, anticipate/prepare to open chest for cardiac massage. *Cardiac compressions are always contraindicated since dislodgment of cannula results in rapid exsanguination.*	

Potential decreased gas exchange
Related to:
Continuous mechanical ventilation until VAD is removed in OR
Retraction and compression of lungs during surgery
Secretions
Pulmonary vascular congestion
 	
DEFINING CHARACTERISTICS
Abnormal breath sounds
Hypoxemia on ABGs
Increased secretions from endotracheal (ET) tube
Abnormal CXR noting pulmonary infiltrates, effusions, or pulmonary edema
	ONGOING ASSESSMENT
	• Auscultate lung fields.
	• Monitor serial ABGs.
	• Check temperature every hour.
	• Evaluate color, consistency, and amount of sputum.
	• Culture discolored or foul-smelling secretions.
	
	THERAPEUTIC INTERVENTIONS
	• Maintain ventilator settings as ordered:
	    TV 10-15 cc/kg
	    Rate 10-14
	    FIo_2 to maintain Po_2 >80 mm
	    PEEP + 5 cm
	• Adjust ventilator settings as ordered *to maintain ABGs within accepted limits.* PEEP may be increased in increments of 2.5 to maintain adequate oxygenation on FIo_2 of 50%. Patients can usually tolerate up to 20 cm H_2O of PEEP if not hypovolemic or hypotensive.
	• Suction prn.
	• Hyperventilate and hyperoxygenate patients *to prevent desaturation.*
	• Administer sedation as ordered:
	    Morphine sulfate
	    Versed: short-acting central nervous system depressant
	    Pavulon: skeletal muscle relaxant
	    Sedation helps to decrease anxiety (in turn helping decrease myocardial O_2 consumption)
		Optimal gas exchange will be obtained.

Potential fluid volume deficit *Related to:* Total fluid volume may be normal or increased, but because of ECC changes in membrane integrity, fluid leaks into extravascular spaces, causing deficit	**ONGOING ASSESSMENT** • Assess hemodynamics. • Monitor I & O and daily weights. • Check urine specific gravity. • Assess chest tube drainage and report excess. • Check CBC, PT, PTT, as ordered, and active clotting time q2h. • Repeat CBC or spin Hct if bleeding persists. • Assess amount of obvious blood loss from sternum, vein, graft sites, and line sites. • Monitor LVAD and/or RVAD flows. • Monitor electrolytes, BUN, Creatinine, Mg, Ca q6h.	Circulating blood volume will be sufficient to meet metabolic demands.

Continued.

NURSING DIAGNOSES / DEFINING CHARACTERISTICS	NURSING INTERVENTIONS / *RATIONALES*	EXPECTED OUTCOMES
Bleeding caused by coagulopathies from prolonged time on ECC Need for anticoagulation **DEFINING CHARACTERISTICS** Decreased filling pressures, decreased LAP, decreased CVP, decreased RA, decreased PAD, decreased PCWP Decreased BP Tachycardia Decreased urine output with increased specific gravity Increased chest tube drainage Oozing of blood from sternum, vein graft sites, central line sites Bleeding from oral cavity, nasogastric bleeding, or hematuria PT > 15 sec PTT > 90 sec Platelets < 50,000 Increased active clotting time (ACT) Decreased Hbg, decreased Hct	**THERAPEUTIC INTERVENTIONS** • Maintain hemodynamics within parameters set by surgeon. • Milk chest tubes *to maintain patency. Clotted tubes may precipitate cardiac tamponade.* • Maintain patient at prescribed anticoagulation parameter. Notify physician of deviations. • Administer coagulation factors/drugs (FFP, platelets, vitamin K, cryoprecipitate, vasopressin) as ordered *to correct deficiencies.* • Use autotransfusion when possible *to minimize use of bank blood.*	
Potential for infection *Related to:* Invasive lines, catheters, ventricular assist device cannulas Open chest (because of presence of ventricular assist device cannulas, sternum is not closed; sterile barrier to chest must be maintained) **DEFINING CHARACTERISTICS** Fever Increased WBC Redness, swelling, and purulent drainage from incisions, IV sites, central line sites Cloudy, foul-smelling urine	**ONGOING ASSESSMENT** • Assess incisional, chest, and vein graft sites. • Assess central and peripheral line sites *for signs and symptoms of infection.* • Assess hemodynamics, including temperature. • Assess CBC daily. **THERAPEUTIC INTERVENTIONS** • Maintain aseptic technique during procedures *to prevent infection.* • Maintain sterile barrier to chest. Change dressing per unit policy. • Maintain occlusive dressings to central and peripheral line sites. Change dressing per unit policy. • Cap open stopcocks; change if contaminated. • Maintain aseptic technique when entering lines for blood draws or administering medications. • Assure that central line sites are changed q72h. Rotate peripheral IVs. • Change IV bags and tubing per unit protocol. • Draw blood cultures postoperative day 2, as ordered, and if temperature >38.5 °C; obtain urine and sputum cultures as indicated.	Potential for postoperative infection will be reduced.

Ventricular assist device—cont'd

NURSING DIAGNOSES / DEFINING CHARACTERISTICS	NURSING INTERVENTIONS / *RATIONALES*	EXPECTED OUTCOMES
Anxiety/fear of patient/family *Related to:* Insertion of VAD Dependence on proper functioning of VAD Inability to control environment Uncertain prognosis Gravity of illness ICU environment **DEFINING CHARACTERISTICS** Many questions from family Vigilant watch over equipment Restlessness Fear of sleep (if not sedated) Tearfulness, restlessness Wide-eyed appearance Tense appearance	**ONGOING ASSESSMENT** • Assess level of anxiety. **THERAPEUTIC INTERVENTIONS** • Explain purpose/functioning of VAD as appropriate. Include significant others *to decrease their feelings of helplessness.* • Display calm, confident manner *to increase feeling of security.* • Provide continuity of care by assigning staff members experienced in function of assist device *so patient/family feel confident of care rendered.* • Prevent unnecessary conversations about assist device near patient/family *to increase patient's sense of security.* • Keep patient sedated as appropriate. • Encourage visiting by family or significant others *so patient doesn't feel alone.* • Keep family honestly informed of patient's condition. • Refer family to crisis intervention if necessary. • See Anxiety, p. 4.	Anxiety/fear will be reduced.
Potential for injury: thrombus formation *Related to:* Use of ventricular assist device Pooling of blood in ventricles Inadequate anticoagulation **DEFINING CHARACTERISTICS** Presence of mottling, pallor, cyanosis, coolness, pain in affected extremity Change in neurologic status	**ONGOING ASSESSMENT** • Monitor ACT q1-2h as ordered. • Monitor flow function of assist device. *Reduced perfusion facilitates clot formation.* • Assess extremities for color, temperature, quality of pulses. • Assess for signs of peripheral, cerebral, or renal embolization. **THERAPEUTIC INTERVENTIONS** • Regulate heparin drip to maintain ACT between 140-180sec. *Patients with LVADs or both RVAD and LVAD require systemic anticoagulation. Heparin is usually started when mediastinal bleeding is slowed.* • Adjust ACT to 150-200sec during weaning from VAD, when flow rates are reduced.	Potential for injury will be reduced.
Impaired physical mobility *Related to:* Bed rest Imposed restrictions caused by VAD (i.e., head of bed less than 30 degrees) Critical physical condition **DEFINING CHARACTERISTICS** Limited ROM Inability to move purposefully within environment	**ONGOING ASSESSMENT** • Assess skin integrity for signs of redness and tissue ischemia. • Assess for pulmonary complications associated with immobility. **THERAPEUTIC INTERVENTIONS** • Maintain limbs in functional alignment. Support feet in dorsiflexed position • Assist with passive ROM. • Institute prophylactic antipressures devices *to help maintain skin integrity.* • Clean, dry, and moisturize skin. • Apply TED hose as ordered.	Complications of immobility will be absent.

Continued.

Ventricular assist device—cont'd

NURSING DIAGNOSES / DEFINING CHARACTERISTICS	NURSING INTERVENTIONS / *RATIONALES*	EXPECTED OUTCOMES
Alteration in level of consciousness *Related to:* Anesthesia effects Postoperative complications **DEFINING CHARACTERISTICS** Unequal pupils Failure to awaken from anesthesia Focal deficit upon awakening Agitation	**ONGOING ASSESSMENT** · Check pupils. · Check ability to follow commands. · Assess hand grasps. · Determine contributing factors to any changes. **THERAPEUTIC INTERVENTIONS** · Reorient to surroundings as needed. · Record serial assessments. · Notify surgeon immediately of any changes seen in neurologic assessment. · See Consciousness, alteration in level of, p. 234.	Optimal state of consciousness will be maintained.

Pain
Related to:
Restricted mobility
Presence of assist device cannulas, tubes, and catheters
Surgical procedure
 	
DEFINING CHARACTERISTICS
Restlessness
Diaphoresis
Change in HR and/or BP
Facial mask of pain
	ONGOING ASSESSMENT
	· Recognize level of discomfort.
	· Monitor effectiveness of pain medication.
	
	THERAPEUTIC INTERVENTIONS
	· Anticipate need for analgesics or additional methods of pain relief. *Patient may be receiving continuous IV infusion of analgesia to control pain and anxiety. Titrate medication as necessary to keep patient sedated.*
	· Use additional comfort measures when appropriate:
	    Relaxation techniques
	    Reassurance and contact
	    Positive suggestion
	    ROM exercises
	· See Pain, p. 39.
		Discomfort will be reduced.

Decreased cardiac output
Related to:
Atrial, junctional, and ventricular arrhythmias:
Etiology:
  Ischemia
  Irritability of cardiac muscle secondary to manipulation during surgery
  Electrolyte imbalance
 	
DEFINING CHARACTERISTICS
Bradycardia (decreased <60)
Tachycardia (increased >100)
Ectopy (extra beats)
Hypotension
Dizziness
Cool skin
Mental changes
	ONGOING ASSESSMENT
	· Continuously monitor cardiac rhythm.
	· Monitor 12-lead ECG as ordered.
	· Assess electrolytes, especially potassium, magnesium, and calcium.
	
	THERAPEUTIC INTERVENTIONS
	· Keep epicardial pacing wires connected to pulse generator.
	· Administer potassium as ordered *to keep serum level at 4-5 mEq.*
	· Administer magnesium as ordered to keep level >2 mg.
	· Administer calcium as ordered to keep level at 8-10 mg.
	· Reassess electrolyte levels if brisk diuresis occurs.
	· Keep emergency medications readily available (lidocaine, atropine, Isuprel, epinephrine, calcium, verapamil).
	· If cardiac arrest occurs, prepare for open chest procedure. *Cardiac compressions are contraindicated since dislodgment of cannula results in exsanguination. However, defibrillation may be performed safely.*
		Optimal cardiac rhythm and output will be maintained.

Originated by: Linda Kamenjarin, RN, BSN, CCRN
             Meg Gulanick, RN, PhD

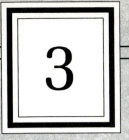

Pulmonary Care Plans

DISORDERS
Adult respiratory distress syndrome
Bronchial asthma
Chronic obstructive pulmonary disease
Pneumonia

Pulmonary thromboembolism
Respiratory failure, acute: secondary to
   chronic obstructive pulmonary disease
Tuberculosis, active

THERAPEUTIC INTERVENTIONS
High-frequency jet ventilation
Mechanical ventilation
Pneumonectomy
Thoracotomy
Tracheostomy

Adult respiratory distress syndrome

(ARDS; SHOCK LUNG; NONCARDIOGENIC PULMONARY EDEMA; ADULT HYALINE MEMBRANE DISEASE; OXYGEN PNEUMONITIS; POST-TRAUMATIC PULMONARY INSUFFICIENCY)

ARDS is a form of respiratory failure that was not recognized as a syndrome until the 1960s, when advances in medical care allowed for prolonged survival of trauma victims who previously would have died. Many causal factors have been related to ARDS (aspiration, trauma, O_2 toxicity, shock, sepsis, disseminated intravascular coagulation (DIC), pancreatitis, etc.), but the exact causative event is unknown. Nursing care must focus upon maintenance of pulmonary function as well as treatment of the causal factor, and even then mortality remains at 50 to 60%.

NURSING DIAGNOSES / DEFINING CHARACTERISTICS	NURSING INTERVENTIONS / *RATIONALES*	EXPECTED OUTCOMES
Ineffective breathing pattern *Related to:* Decreased lung compliance: Low amounts of surfactant Fluid transudation Fatigue and decreased energy: Increased work of breathing Primary medical problem **Defining Characteristics** Dyspnea Shortness of breath Tachypnea Abnormal ABGs Cyanosis Cough Use of accessory muscles	**Ongoing Assessment** · Assess respiratory rate and depth every hour. · Assess for dyspnea, shortness of breath, cough, and use of accessory muscles. *Initially, respiratory rate increases with the decreasing lung compliance. Work of breathing increases greatly as compliance decreases.* · Assess for cyanosis and monitor ABGs. *As the patient becomes fatigued from the increased work of breathing, he/she may no longer be capable of adequately maintaining his/her own ventilation: CO_2 begins to elevate on ABGs.* **Therapeutic Interventions** · Maintain the O_2 delivery system applied to the patient *so that the patient does not desaturate.* · Provide reassurance and allay anxiety: Have an agreed-upon method for calling for assistance, (e.g., call light or bell). Stay with the patient during episodes of respiratory distress. · Keep physician informed of respiratory status. · Anticipate the need for intubation and mechanical ventilation. *Being prepared for intubation prevents full decompensation of patient to cardiopulmonary arrest. Early intubation and mechanical ventilation are recommended.* · See Mechanical ventilation, p. 213, as appropriate.	Optimal breathing pattern will be maintained.
Impaired gas exchange *Related to:* Diffusion defect: Hyaline membrane formation Increased shunting: Collapsed alveoli Fluid-filled alveoli Increased dead space: Microembolization in the pulmonary vasculature **Defining Characteristics** Confusion Somnolence Restlessness Irritability Inability to move secretions Hypercapnia Hypoxia	**Ongoing Assessment** · Assess respirations every hour, noting quality, rate, pattern, depth, and breathing effort. · Assess breath sounds and note changes. · Monitor chest x-ray reports. *Keep in mind that radiographic studies of lung water lag behind clinical presentation by 24 hrs.* · Assess for changes in orientation and behavior. · Closely monitor ABGs and note changes. · Use pulse oximetry *to monitor O_2 saturation and pulse rate continuously.* Keep alarms on at all times. *Pulse oximetry has been found to be a useful tool in the clinical setting to detect changes in oxygenation.* **Therapeutic Interventions** · Use a team approach in planning care with the physician and respiratory therapist. *Timely and accurate communication of assessments is a must to keep pace with the needed ventilator setting changes: F_IO_2 and CPAP.* · Administer sedation, as ordered, *to decrease patient's energy expenditure during mechanical ventilation and to deliver adequate CPAP.* · Combine nursing actions (i.e., bath, bed, and dressing changes) and intersperse with rest periods *to minimize energy expended by patient and to prevent a decreased O_2 saturation.* Temporarily discontinue activity if saturation drops, *to decrease O_2 consumption,* and make any necessary F_IO_2, CPAP, or sedation changes *to improve saturation.*	Impaired gas exchange will be reduced.

Adult respiratory distress syndrome—cont'd

NURSING DIAGNOSES / DEFINING CHARACTERISTICS	NURSING INTERVENTIONS / *RATIONALES*	EXPECTED OUTCOMES
	• Change patient's position q2h *to facilitate movement and drainage of secretions.* • Suction as needed *to clear secretions.*	
Potential decreased cardiac output *Related to:* Positive pressure ventilation **DEFINING CHARACTERISTICS** Variations in hemodynamic parameters (BP, heart rate, CVP, pulmonary artery pressures, cardiac output) Arrhythmias Weight gain, edema Decreased peripheral pulses; cold clammy skin	**ONGOING ASSESSMENT** • Assess vital signs and hemodynamic pressures (CVP, pulmonary artery pressures) q1h; with changes in positive pressure ventilation; and with changes in inotrope administration. • Obtain cardiac output measurement, as ordered, after positive pressure ventilation changes and with inotrope administration change. • Closely monitor ABGs. • See Impaired gas exchange, p. 21. **THERAPEUTIC INTERVENTIONS** • Notify physician of changes in patient status. • Administer inotropic agents as ordered, noting response and observing for side effects. • Administer IV fluids, as ordered, *to maintain optimal fluid balance.* • Anticipate need to decrease level of CPAP *to range that allows improved cardiac output,* if fluid administration and inotropes are not successful. • See Decreased cardiac output, p. 9, as necessary.	Optimal cardiac output will be maintained.
Potential for injury: barotrauma *Related to:* Positive-pressure ventilation Decreased pulmonary compliance **DEFINING CHARACTERISTICS** Crepitus Subcutaneous emphysema Altered chest excursion: asymmetrical chest Abnormal ABGs Shift in trachea Restlessness Evidence of pneumothorax on chest x-ray	**ONGOING ASSESSMENT** • Assess for signs of barotrauma q1h. *Frequent assessments needed since barotrauma can occur at any time and patient will not show signs of dyspnea, shortness of breath, or tachypnea if heavily sedated to maintain ventilation.* • Monitor chest x-ray reports daily and obtain a stat portable chest ray if barotrauma suspected. **THERAPEUTIC INTERVENTIONS** • Notify physician of signs of barotrauma immediately. • Anticipate need for chest tube placement, and prepare as needed. *If barotrauma is suspected, intervention must follow immediately to prevent tension pneumothorax.*	Potential for injury from barotrauma will be reduced.
Potential altered nutrition: less than body requirements *Related to:* Intubation **DEFINING CHARACTERISTICS** Loss of weight >10-20% below ideal body weight Documented inadequate caloric intake	**ONGOING ASSESSMENT** • Obtain and document patient's weight daily. • Obtain nutritional history. • Assess for bowel sounds. • Check for abdominal distention and tenderness. **THERAPEUTIC INTERVENTIONS** • Give enteral or parenteral feedings as ordered. • Refer to appropriate SCP: Nutrition, altered: less than body requirements, p. 37; Enteral tube feeding, p. 308; Total parenteral nutrition (TPN), p. 324	Risk of nutritional deficit will be minimized or prevented.

Continued.

187

NURSING DIAGNOSES / DEFINING CHARACTERISTICS	NURSING INTERVENTIONS / *RATIONALES*	EXPECTED OUTCOMES
Caloric intake inadequate to keep pace with abnormal disease/metabolic state		

Impaired physical mobility *Related to:* Acute respiratory failure Monitoring devices Mechanical ventilation **DEFINING CHARACTERISTICS** Imposed restrictions of movement Decreased muscle strength Limited range of motion (ROM)	**ONGOING ASSESSMENT**
	 • Assess for imposed restrictions of movement.
	 • Assess muscle strength.
	 • Assess range of motion of extremities.
	
	 THERAPEUTIC INTERVENTIONS
	 • Turn and reposition patient q2h.
	 • Maintain limbs in functional alignment (with pillows):
	     Support feet in dorsiflexed position *to prevent footdrop.*
	     Perform/assist with passive ROM exercises to extremities to *prevent contractures.*
	 • Initiate activity increases (dangling, sitting in chair, ambulation) as condition allows
		Optimal physical mobility will be maintained.

Potential impaired skin integrity *Related to:* Prolonged bed rest Immobility Sensory deficit Altered vasomotor tone Altered nutritional state Prolonged intubation **DEFINING CHARACTERISTICS** Actual skin breakdown: Stage I: redness, skin intact Stage II: blisters Stage III: necrosis Stage IV; necrosis involving bones and joints	**ONGOING ASSESSMENT**
	 • Assess bony prominences for signs of threatened or actual breakdown of skin.
	 • Assess around endotracheal (ET) tube for crusting of secretions, redness, or irritation.
	 • Assess for signs of skin breakdown beneath ET-securing tape.
	
	 THERAPEUTIC INTERVENTIONS
	 • Turn and reposition patient q2h.
	 • Institute prophylactic use of pressure-relieving devices.
	 • Maintain skin integrity:
	     If patient is nasally intubated, notify physician if skin is red or irritated or breakdown is noted.
	     If patient is orally intubated, the tube should be repositioned from side to side q24-48h *(will help prevent pressure necrosis on lower lip).*
	 • Provide mouth care q2h.
	 • Keep ET tube free of crusting of secretions.
	 • See Skin integrity, impaired, p. 48 (as needed)
		Skin integrity will be maintained.

Knowledge deficit *Related to:* New equipment New environment New condition	**ONGOING ASSESSMENT** • Evaluate patient's/significant others' understanding of patient's overall condition. • Assess patient's/significant others' readiness for learning	Patient/significant others will demonstrate understanding of serious nature of disease and treatments.

Adult respiratory distress syndrome—cont'd

NURSING DIAGNOSES / DEFINING CHARACTERISTICS	NURSING INTERVENTIONS / *RATIONALES*	EXPECTED OUTCOMES
DEFINING CHARACTERISTICS Increased frequency of questions posed by patient and significant others Inability to respond correctly to questions	**THERAPEUTIC INTERVENTIONS** • Explain all procedures to patient before performing them. *This will help decrease patient's anxiety. Fear of unknown can make patient extremely anxious, uncooperative.* • Orient patient and significant others to ICU surroundings, routines, equipment alarms, and noises. *The ICU is a busy and noisy environment that can be very upsetting to patient/significant others.* • Keep the patient/significant others informed of current patient status. *ARDS is a very serious syndrome with high mortality rates. Significant others must be informed of changes that occur.*	

Originated by: Susan Galanes, RN, MS, CCRN

Bronchial asthma

(STATUS ASTHMATICUS)

Paroxysmal dyspnea accompanied by adventitious sounds (wheezing) caused by swelling and spasm of bronchial tubes. This reversible condition is commonly precipitated by antigen-antibody reactions, respiratory infection, cold weather, physical exertion, emotions, and some drugs.

NURSING DIAGNOSES / DEFINING CHARACTERISTICS	NURSING INTERVENTIONS / *RATIONALES*	EXPECTED OUTCOMES

Ineffective airway clearance
Related to:
Swelling and spasm of bronchial tubes in response to allergies, drugs, stress, infection, inhaled irritants
 	
DEFINING CHARACTERISTICS
 	
Irritability
Retractions
Grunting
Stridor
Nasal flaring
Wheezing
Cough
Dyspnea
Abnormal breath sounds, rate, and depth
Verbalized chest tightness
	ONGOING ASSESSMENT
	• Assess vital signs.
	• Note color changes (lips, buccal mucosa, nail beds).
	• Look for and document signs of respiratory dysfunction:
	    Irritability
	    Retractions
	    Grunting
	    Stridor
	    Nasal flaring
	    Wheezing
	• Evaluate breath sounds.
	• Monitor laboratory work:
	    Theophylline level
	    ABGs
	    CBC
	    Electrolytes
	
	THERAPEUTIC INTERVENTIONS
	• Keep head of bed elevated *to aid lung expansion.*
	• Keep patient as calm as possible.
	• Ensure that respiratory treatments are given as ordered; notify respiratory therapist if need arises:
	    Encourage patient to cough, especially after treatments.
	    Give humidifed O$_2$ as ordered.
	• Give medications and IV fluids as ordered.
	• Use appropriate clinical resources.
	• See Ineffective airway clearance, p. 3
		Respiratory dysfunction will be reduced.

Continued.

Bronchial asthma—cont'd

NURSING DIAGNOSES / DEFINING CHARACTERISTICS	NURSING INTERVENTIONS / *RATIONALES*	EXPECTED OUTCOMES
Potential fluid volume deficit *Related to:* Decreased fluid intake Increased respiratory distress Diaphoresis **DEFINING CHARACTERISTICS** Complaints of thirst Complaints of dryness of lips, mouth Decreased skin turgor Increased specific gravity Decreased urine output < 30 cc/hr Sunken eyes Sunken fontanel in infant Lack of tears in infant	**ONGOING ASSESSMENT** · Monitor vital signs. · Measure I & O. · Assess specific gravity. · Monitor electrolytes. · Assess skin turgor. · Monitor weight. · Assess sputum for color, tenacity, liquification, amount. **THERAPEUTIC INTERVENTIONS** · Encourage oral fluid intake by providing water and preferred liquids at bedside. · Maintain IV infusion at proper rate. *Adequate intake will enhance liquification of bronchial secretions. Thinner, liquid secretions are more easily expectorated.* · Provide assistance with bedpan/commode at frequent intervals. *Some patients decrease intake to decrease frequent need for urination.*	Hydration will be maximized.

Anxiety
Related to:
Respiratory distress
Change in health status
Change in environment
 	
DEFINING CHARACTERISTICS
Complaints of inability to breathe
Verbalized feelings of impending doom
Restlessness
Apprehensiveness
Insomnia
Increased heart rate
Frequent requests for someone to be in room
Diaphoresis
	ONGOING ASSESSMENT
	· Assess anxiety level q4h including:
	  Vital signs
	  Respiratory status
	  Irritability
	  Apprehension
	  Orientation
	
	THERAPEUTIC INTERVENTIONS
	· Help relieve respiratory distress as soon as possible.
	· Explain all procedures to patient before starting.
	· Make patient as comfortable as possible:
	  Be available.
	  Be reassuring.
	· Provide quiet diversional activities.
	· Explain importance of remaining as calm as possible. *Maintaining calm will decrease O_2 consumption and work of breathing.*
	· Explain that nurses will be available if needed.
		Anxiety will be reduced.

Pain/discomfort *Related to:* Excessive exertion of accessory respiratory musculature as result of acute asthma attack	**ONGOING ASSESSMENT** · Monitor respiratory function. · Assess ability to relax. · Assess complaints of pain (degree, location) and intervention effectiveness. · Assess for changes in physical tolerance. *Fatigue may indicate increasing distress and can lead to status asthmaticus and respiratory failure.*	Discomfort will be relieved.

NURSING DIAGNOSES / DEFINING CHARACTERISTICS	NURSING INTERVENTIONS / *RATIONALES*	EXPECTED OUTCOMES

DEFINING CHARACTERISTICS
 	
Complaints of pain when breathing
Complaints of inability to get comfortable
Restlessness
Position of patient
Insomnia
Increased respiratory distress
	THERAPEUTIC INTERVENTIONS
	• Make patient as comfortable as possible:
	   Raise head of bed.
	   Position with pillows.
	   Hold/rock in upright position.
	▪ Be available to:
	   Answer questions simply.
	   Explain procedures.
	• Provide medications as ordered.
	• Explain need to remain as calm as possible.
	• Explain need to inform nurses of discomfort. *Relief of respiratory distress will relieve source of pain.*	

Knowledge deficit
Related to:
Chronicity of disease
Long-term medical management
 	
DEFINING CHARACTERISTICS
 	
Absence of questions
Anxious
Inability to answer questions properly
Ineffective self-care
	ONGOING ASSESSMENT
	▪ Assess knowledge of disease process.
	▪ Assess knowledge of medications.
	▪ Evaluate self-care activities:
	   Preventive care
	   Home management of acute attack
	▪ Assess ability to learn
	
	THERAPEUTIC INTERVENTIONS
	▪ Explain disease to patient/significant others.
	▪ Reinforce need for taking prescribed medications as ordered *to reduce incidence of full-blown attacks*.
	▪ Teach warning signs and symptoms of asthma attack and importance of early treatment of impending attack.
	▪ Reinforce what to do in an asthma attack:
	   Home management
	   Time to go to emergency room
	   Prevention
	▪ Reinforce need of keeping follow-up appointments.
	▪ Refer to social services, if needed.
	▪ Refer to support groups, if needed.
	▪ Address long-term management issues:
	   Environmental controls
	   Avoidance of precipitators
	   Good health habits
		Patient/significant others will verbalize knowledge of disease and its management.

Originated by: Kathleen Jaffry, RN

Chronic obstructive pulmonary disease (COPD)

(CHRONIC BRONCHITIS; EMPHYSEMA)

Chronic obstructive pulmonary disease (COPD) refers to a group of diseases, including chronic bronchitis, asthma, and emphysema, that cause a reduction in expiratory outflow. It is usually a slow, progressive debilitating disease, affecting those with a history of heavy tobacco abuse and prolonged exposure to respiratory system irritants such as air pollution, noxious gases, and repeated upper respiratory tract infections. It is also regarded as the most common cause of alveolar hypoventilation with associated hypoxemia, chronic hypercapnia, and compensated acidosis.

NURSING DIAGNOSES / DEFINING CHARACTERISTICS	NURSING INTERVENTIONS / *RATIONALES*	EXPECTED OUTCOMES

Ineffective airway clearance
Related to:
Hyperplasia and hypertrophy of mucus-secreting glands
Increased mucus production in bronchial tubes
Decreased ciliary function
Thick secretions
Decreased energy and fatigue
Bronchospasm
 	
DEFINING CHARACTERISTICS
"Smoker's cough"
Coarse rales over larger airways
Persistent cough for months
Copious amount of secretions
Wheezing
Loud, prolonged expiratory phase
Dyspnea (air hunger)
	ONGOING ASSESSMENT
	• Auscultate lungs q4h and as needed *to note and document significant change in breath sounds:*
	    Decreased or absent breath sounds may indicate presence of mucous plug or other major airway obstruction.
	    Presence of fine rales may indicate cardiac involvement.
	    Wheezing may indicate increasing airway resistance.
	    Coarse rales indicate presence of fluid along larger airways.
	• Assess characteristics of secretions:
	    Consistency
	    Quantity
	    Color
	    Odor
	• Assess hydration status:
	    Skin turgor
	    Mucous membranes
	    Tongue
	• Monitor accurate I & O:
	    Include accurate approximation of secretions and insensible loss from increased work of breathing.
	    Obtain daily weights.
	• Assess patient's physical strength:
	    Ability to expectorate sputum
	    Ability to use blow bottles or incentive spirometer
	
	THERAPEUTIC INTERVENTIONS
	• Encourage patient to cough out secretions; suction as needed.
	• Assist with effective coughing techniques:
	    Splint chest for comfort.
	    Have patient use abdominal muscles for more forceful cough.
	• Assist in mobilizing secretions *to facilitate airway clearance by:*
	    Increasing room humidification *to liquify secretions.*
	    Administering mucolytic agents in conjunction with respiratory therapist.
	    Performing chest physiotherapy: postural drainage, percussion, and vibration.
	    Encouraging 2-3 L fluid intake unless contraindicated *to prevent dehydration from increased insensible loss and to keep secretions thin.*
	• Anticipate administration of bronchodilators (IV or inhalation) *to relieve bronchoconstriction.*
	• Anticipate intubation and mechanical ventilation if needed. See Mechanical ventilation, p. 213.
	• Demonstrate effective technique in use of blow bottles or incentive spirometer *to conserve energy with positive result.* Emphasize not to overexert self (15-20 times maximum).
	• Perform nasotracheal suctioning as indicated:
	    Use a well-lubricated soft catheter, preferably rubber, *to minimize irritations.*
		Airway will be free of secretions.

NURSING DIAGNOSES / DEFINING CHARACTERISTICS	NURSING INTERVENTIONS / *RATIONALES*	EXPECTED OUTCOMES

Impaired gas exchange
Related to:
Increase in dead space caused by:
  Loss of lung tissue elasticity
  Atelectasis
  Increased residual volume
Increased upper and lower airway resistance caused by:
  Overproduction of secretions along bronchial tubes
  Bronchoconstriction
 	
DEFINING CHARACTERISTICS
Altered I:E ratio (prolonged expiratory phase)
Active expiratory phase: use of accessory muscles of breathing
Decreased vital capacity (VC)
Increased residual volume (RV)
Hypoxemia/hypercapnia
$Pco_2 > 55$ mm Hg
$Po_2 < 55$ mm Hg
Tachycardia
Restlessness
Diaphoresis
Headache
Lethargy
Confusion
Cyanosis
Increase in rate and depth of respiration
Increase in BP
	ONGOING ASSESSMENT
	• Assess for altered breathing patterns:
	  Increased work of breathing
	  Abnormal rate, rhythm, and depth of respiration
	  Abnormal chest excursions
	• Assess for signs and symptoms of hypoxemia/hypercapnia (see Defining Characteristics).
	• Monitor ABGs.
	
	THERAPEUTIC INTERVENTIONS
	• Promote more effective breathing pattern for better gas exchange by:
	  Positioning properly for optimal breathing. *Upright and high Fowler's position will favor better lung expansion; diaphragm is pushed downward. If patient is bedridden, turning from side to side at least q2h will promote better aeration of all lung lobes, thus minimizing atelectasis.*
	  Teaching patient pursed-lip breathing *for more complete exhalation.*
	  Teaching patient to use abdominal and other accessory muscles to exhale *for more forceful exhalation.*
	  Administering bronchodilators as ordered *to decrease work of breathing:*
	    Monitoring for therapeutic and side effects.
	    Monitoring blood levels.
	• Administer low-flow O_2 therapy as indicated (e.g., 2 L/min nasal cannula). If insufficient, switch to high-flow O_2 apparatus (e.g., Venturi mask) for more accurate O_2 delivery. *Higher F_1O_2 may depress hypoxic drive to breathe.*
	• If Po_2 level significantly lower or if Pco_2 level higher than patient's usual baseline (varies from patient to patient), anticipate:
	  Vigorous pulmonary toilet and suctioning
	  Increase in F_1O_2 with use of controlled high-flow system
	  Use of diuretics
	  Possible need for intubation and mechanical ventilation.
	• Assist in performing related procedures and tests (bronchoscopy, pulmonary function tests).
		Hypoxemia/hypercapnia will be reduced.

Altered nutrition: less than body requirements *Related to:* Increased metabolic need caused by increased work of breathing Poor appetite resulting from fever, dyspnea, and fatigue	**ONGOING ASSESSMENT** • Assess patient's caloric requirements. • Assess patient's caloric intake. • Assess for possible cause of poor appetite (see related factors). **THERAPEUTIC INTERVENTIONS** • Compile diet history, including preferred foods and dietary habits. • Consult and work with the dietitian to estimate caloric requirements. • Offer small feedings of nutritious soft foods/liquids frequently. *They are easier to digest and require less chewing.* • Assist patient with meals. • Record amount of food intake (calorie count).	Optimal nutritional status will be maintained.

Continued.

NURSING DIAGNOSES / DEFINING CHARACTERISTICS	NURSING INTERVENTIONS / *RATIONALES*	EXPECTED OUTCOMES
DEFINING CHARACTERISTICS Body weight 20% or more below ideal for height and frame Indifference to food Alteration in ability to taste Caloric intake inadequate for metabolic demands of disease state Muscle wasting Abnormal lab values (e.g., low serum albumin)	· Give frequent oral care. · Instruct patient to avoid very hot/cold foods, gas-producing foods, carbonated beverages *to prevent possible abdominal distention.* · Plan activities to allow rest before eating. · Substitute nasal prongs for O_2 mask during mealtime *to maintain patient's oxygenation.*	
Potential for infection *Related to:* Retained secretions (good medium for bacterial growth) Poor nutrition Impaired pulmonary defense system secondary to COPD Use of respiratory equipment **DEFINING CHARACTERISTICS** Fever, chills Change in characteristics of sputum (consistency, color, amount, odor) Increase in cough Elevated WBC Abnormal breath sounds Rales, wheezing, shortness of breath Signs of failure of right side of heart Nausea, vomiting, diarrhea Anorexia	**ONGOING ASSESSMENT** · Assess patient for signs and symptoms of infection (see Defining Characteristics). · Assess nutritional status: Caloric requirement Caloric intake · Auscultate lungs *to monitor significant changes in breath sounds:* Bronchial breath sounds and rales may indicate pneumonia **THERAPEUTIC INTERVENTIONS** · Document significant change in sputum that may indicate presence of infection: Sudden increase in production Change in color (rusty, yellow, greenish) Change in consistency (thick) · Encourage increase in fluid intake, unless contraindicated, *to maintain good hydration. Insensible loss is markedly increased during infection because of fever and increase in respiratory rate.* · Ensure that O_2 humidifier is properly maintained. Never add new water to old water; *stagnant old water is medium for bacterial growth.* · Minimize retained secretions by encouraging patient to cough and expectorate secretions frequently. If patient unable to cough and expectorate, perform nasotracheal or oropharyngeal suctioning. *Retained secretions provide bacterial growth medium*	Risk for infection will be reduced.
Activity intolerance *Related to:* Imbalance between O_2 supply and demand (demand higher) **DEFINING CHARACTERISTICS** Verbal report of fatigue or weakness	**ONGOING ASSESSMENT** · Assess patient's level of mobility. · Assess patient's respiratory status. **THERAPEUTIC INTERVENTIONS** · See Activity intolerance, p. 2	Optimal activity tolerance will be maintained.

Chronic obstructive pulmonary disease—cont'd

NURSING DIAGNOSES / DEFINING CHARACTERISTICS	NURSING INTERVENTIONS / *RATIONALES*	EXPECTED OUTCOMES
Abnormal heart rate and BP response to activity Exertional discomfort or dyspnea		
Knowledge deficit *Related to:* Recent diagnosis Denial Ineffective past teaching/learning **DEFINING CHARACTERISTICS** Display of anxiety/fear Noncompliance Inability to verbalize health maintenance regime Repeated acute exacerbations Development of complications Misconceptions about health status Multiple questions or none	**ONGOING ASSESSMENT** • Assess readiness to learn. • Assess environmental, social, cultural, and educational factors that may influence teaching plan. • Assess knowledge base. **THERAPEUTIC INTERVENTIONS** • Establish common goals. • Instruct patient in basic anatomy and physiology of respiratory system, with attention to structure and air flow. • Discuss relation of disease process to signs and symptoms patient experiences; Introduce the following words: *mucus, spasm, narrowing, obstruction, elasticity, trapping, inflammation.* • Discuss purpose and method of administration for each medication. • Discuss appropriate nutritional habits. • Discuss concept of energy conservation. Encourage: 　Resting as needed during activities 　Avoiding overexertion/fatigue 　Sitting as much as possible 　Alternating heavy and light tasks 　Carrying articles close to body 　Organizing all equipment at beginning of activity 　Working slowly • Discuss signs/symptoms of infection. • Discuss common factors that lead to exacerbations of lung problems: 　Smoking 　Environmental temperature and humidity • Discuss importance of specific therapeutic measures as listed: 　Breathing exercises 　　*Exercise 1: Purpose: to strengthen muscles of respiration.* 　　　*Technique:* Lie supine, with one hand on chest and one on abdomen. Inhale slowly through mouth, raising abdomen against hand. Exhale slowly through pursed lips while contracting abdominal muscles and moving abdomen inward. 　　*Exercise 2: Purpose: to develop slowed, controlled breathing* 　　　*Technique:* Walk, stop to take deep breath, exhale slowly while walking. 　　*Exercise 3: Purpose: to decrease air trapping and airway collapse.* 　　　*Technique:* For pursed-lip breathing, inhale slowly through nose. Exhale twice as slowly as usual through pursed lips. 　Cough: Lean forward; take several deep breaths with pursed-lip method. Take last deep breath, cough with open mouth during expiration, and simultaneously contract abdominal muscles. 　Chest physiotherapy/pulmonary postural drainage: *Purpose: to facilitate expectoration of secretions and prevent waste of energy.* Demonstrate correct methods for postural drainage: positioning, percussion, vibration. 　Hydration: Discuss importance of maintaining good fluid *intake to decrease viscosity of secretions.* Recommend 1½-2 L/d. 　Humidity: Discuss various forms of humidification *to prevent drying of secretions.* • Discuss home oxygen therapy: 　Use of equipment:	Patient will verbalize understanding of disease process and treatment.

Continued.

Chronic obstructive pulmonary disease—cont'd

NURSING DIAGNOSES / DEFINING CHARACTERISTICS	NURSING INTERVENTIONS / *RATIONALES*	EXPECTED OUTCOMES
	Demonstrate how to open oxygen cylinder, regulate flowmeter, and use humidifier. *Patient or others who will be primarily responsible for O₂ therapy at home should be able to demonstrate process perfectly at least 3 times before discharge.*	

Demonstrate how to open oxygen cylinder, regulate flowmeter, and use humidifier. *Patient or others who will be primarily responsible for O_2 therapy at home should be able to demonstrate process perfectly at least 3 times before discharge.*

Safety precautions: *Oxygen is not combustible itself, but it will feed a fire if one occurs.*

Do not use around a stove or gas space heater.

Do not smoke or light matches around cylinder when O_2 is in use.

Post "No Smoking" sign and call to visitors attention.

Care of humidifier:

Change water in humidifier once a day *to decrease risk of infection.*

• Discuss available resources:

Arrange for visiting nurse to check patient as appropriate.

Refer to local Lung Association if available for support.

Originated by: Lumie L. Perez, RN, BSN, CCRN
Joanne O'Connor, RN, BSN

Pneumonia

(PNEUMONITIS)

Pneumonia is caused by a bacterial or viral infection that results in an inflammatory process in the lungs. It is an infectious process that is spread by droplets or by contact. Predisposing factors to the development of pneumonia include upper respiratory infection, excessive alcohol ingestion, central nervous system depression, cardiac failure, any debilitating illness, chronic obstructive pulmonary disease; at risk are patients who are bedridden, patients with lowered resistance, and hospitalized patients who may develop a superinfection.

NURSING DIAGNOSES / DEFINING CHARACTERISTICS	NURSING INTERVENTIONS / *RATIONALES*	EXPECTED OUTCOMES

Ineffective airway clearance *Related to:* Increased sputum production in response to respiratory infection Decreased energy and increased fatigue resulting from prolonged immobilization, cardiac failure, postoperative effect of general anesthesia, chronic illness, depression of CNS, excessive intake of alcohol Aspiration	**ONGOING ASSESSMENT**
	• Assess breath sounds.
	• Assess respiratory movements and use of accessory muscles.
	• Monitor chest x-ray reports.
	• Monitor sputum Gram's stain and culture and sensitivity reports.
	
	THERAPEUTIC INTERVENTIONS
	• Assist patient with coughing and deep breathing, splinting, as necessary *to improve coughing.*
	• Encourage patient to cough unless cough is frequent and nonproductive. *Frequent nonproductive coughing can result in hypoxemia.*
	• Use positioning *to facilitate clearing secretions.*
	• Use respiratory therapy department for chest physiotherapy and nebulizer treatments, as appropriate.
	• Use humidity *to loosen secretions (humidified O_2 or humidifier at bedside).*
	• Maintain adequate hydration *(fluids are lost by diaphoresis, fever, and tachypnea):*
	    Encourage oral fluids.
	    Administer IV fluids as ordered.
	• Administer medication (e.g., antibiotics, expectorants) as ordered, noting effectiveness.
		Airway will be free of secretions.

NURSING DIAGNOSES / DEFINING CHARACTERISTICS	NURSING INTERVENTIONS / *RATIONALES*	EXPECTED OUTCOMES
DEFINING CHARACTERISTICS Abnormal breath sounds (e.g., rhonchi, bronchial breath sounds) Decreased breath sounds over affected areas Cough Dyspnea Change in respiratory status Infiltrates on chest x-ray film	• Institute suctioning of airway as needed *to remove sputum and mucous plugs.* • Use nasopharyngeal/oropharyngeal airway as needed. • Anticipate possible need for intubation *if condition deteriorates.*	

Impaired gas exchange
Related to:
Collection of mucus in airways
 	
DEFINING CHARACTERISTICS
Dyspnea
Decreased Pao_2
Increased $Paco_2$
Cyanosis
Tachypnea
Air hunger
Tachycardia
Pallor
Decreased activity tolerance
Restlessness
Disorientation/confusion
	ONGOING ASSESSMENT
	• Assess respiratory status:
	  Rate
	  Depth
	  Breath sounds
	  Pattern of respiration
	• Assess skin color and capillary refill.
	• Assess for changes in orientation and note increasing restlessness. *These can be early signs of hypoxia and/or hypercarbia.*
	• Assess for activity changes.
	• Monitor vital sign changes.
	• Monitor ABGs; note differences.
	
	THERAPEUTIC INTERVENTIONS
	• Notify physician if condition worsens.
	• Pace activities to patient's tolerance. *Activities will increase O_2 consumption and should be planned so patient does not become hypoxic.*
	• Maintain O_2 administration device as ordered. *Avoid high concentrations of O_2 in patients with COPD. Hypoxia stimulates drive to breathe.*
	• Anticipate need for intubation, and, possibly, mechanical ventilation if condition worsens.
	• See Mechanical ventilation, p. 213 (as needed).
		Gas exchange will be enhanced.

Infection
Related to:
Invading bacterial/viral organisms
 	
DEFINING CHARACTERISTICS
Elevated temperature
Elevated WBC
Tachycardia
Chills
Positive sputum culture report
Changing character of sputum
	ONGOING ASSESSMENT
	• Elicit patient's description of illness, including:
	  Onset
	  Chills
	  Chest pain
	  Medications *(Patients receiving high dosages of corticosteroids have reduced resistance to infections.)*
	  Recent exposure to illness
	  Alcohol, tobacco, or drug abuse
	  Chronic illness
	• Assess vital signs.
	• Monitor Gram's stain, sputum, culture, and sensitivity reports.
	• Monitor WBC.
	• Monitor temperature. *Continued fever may be caused by:*
	  Drug allergy
	  Drug-resistant bacteria
	  Superinfection
	  Inadequate lung drainage
		Infection will be reduced.

Continued.

Pneumonia—cont'd

NURSING DIAGNOSES / DEFINING CHARACTERISTICS	NURSING INTERVENTIONS / *RATIONALES*	EXPECTED OUTCOMES

	THERAPEUTIC INTERVENTIONS
	· Use appropriate therapy for elevated temperature: antipyretics, cold therapy.
	· Obtain fresh sputum for Gram's stain/culture and sensitivity, as ordered:
	    Instruct patient to expectorate into sterile container. Be sure specimen is coughed up and is not saliva.
	    If patient is unable to cough up specimen effectively, use sterile nasotracheal suctioning with Lukens' tube.
	· Administer prescribed antimicrobial agent(s) on schedule *so blood level is maintained*.
	· Isolate patient as necessary after review of culture and sensitivity results.	

Pain/discomfort
Related to:
Respiratory distress
Coughing
 	
DEFINING CHARACTERISTICS
Complaints of discomfort
Guarding
Withdrawal
Moaning
Facial grimace
Irritability
Anxiety
Tachycardia
Increased BP
Increased temperature
	ONGOING ASSESSMENT
	· Assess complaints of discomfort.
	· Determine quality, severity, location, onset, duration, and precipitating factors for patient's discomfort.
	
	THERAPEUTIC INTERVENTIONS
	· Teach patient to verbalize complaints of discomfort.
	· Examine patient for objective signs of discomfort.
	· Administer appropriate medications to treat cough:
	    Do not suppress productive cough; use moderate amounts of analgesics to relieve pleuritic pain.
	    Use cough suppressants and humidity for dry, hacking cough. *An unproductive hacking cough irritates airways and should be suppressed.*
	· Administer analgesics as ordered and as needed. Encourage patient to take analgesics before discomfort becomes severe *to prevent peak periods of pain*.
	· Evaluate medication effectiveness. Use additional measures to relieve discomfort, including positioning and relaxation.
	· See Pain, p. 39.
		Discomfort will be relieved.

Potential altered levels of consciousness *Related to:* Cerebral hypoxia Meningitis **DEFINING CHARACTERISTICS** Decreasing Pao_2 Change in alertness, orientation, verbal response Agitation Restlessness Irritability	**ONGOING ASSESSMENT** · Assess for presence of defining characteristics; if present, notify physician **THERAPEUTIC INTERVENTIONS** · For decrease in Pao_2, see Impaired gas exchange, p. 21. · See Altered level of consciousness, p. 234. · If appropriate, see Meningitis, p. 250.	Alteration in level of consciousness will be reduced.
Potential anxiety/fear *Related to:* Debilitated condition Air hunger Isolation (if needed) **DEFINING CHARACTERISTICS** Restlessness Constant demands	**ONGOING ASSESSMENT** · Assess for signs of anxiety and fear (see Defining Characteristics). **THERAPEUTIC INTERVENTIONS** · See Anxiety, p. 4 and Fear, p. 18.	Anxiety/fear will be reduced.

NURSING DIAGNOSES / DEFINING CHARACTERISTICS	NURSING INTERVENTIONS / *RATIONALES*	EXPECTED OUTCOMES
Uncooperative behavior Withdrawal Indifference Fear of sleeping		

Potential altered nutrition: less than body requirements
Related to:
Pneumonia, resulting in:
  Increased metabolic needs
  Lack of appetite
  Decreased intake
 	
DEFINING CHARACTERISTICS
Anorexia
Loss of weight
Decreased caloric intake
	ONGOING ASSESSMENT
	• Document patient's actual weight.
	• Obtain nutritional history.
	• Obtain baseline laboratory values:
	  Serum total protein
	  Serum albumin
	  Serum osmolarity
	  Vitamin assays (as appropriate)
	  Mineral and trace element levels (as appropriate)
	
	THERAPEUTIC INTERVENTIONS
	• Maintain bed rest *to decrease metabolic needs.*
	• Increase activity gradually as patient tolerates.
	• Provide high-protein/high-carbohydrate diet.
	• Provide small, frequent feedings.
	• Maintain O_2 delivery system (e.g., nasal cannula if appropriate) while patient eats. *This will help prevent desaturation and shortness of breath, with resultant loss of appetite.*
	• Administer vitamin supplements, as ordered.
	• Administer enteral supplements and parenteral nutrition, as ordered.
	• See Nutrition, altered: less than body requirements, p. 37
		Optimal nutritional status will be maintained.

Diversional activity deficit
Related to:
Isolation
Bed rest
 	
DEFINING CHARACTERISTICS
Patient complaints of:
  Boredom
  Isolation
  Irritability
	ONGOING ASSESSMENT
	• Assess for signs of diversional activity deficit (See Defining Characteristics).
	
	THERAPEUTIC INTERVENTIONS
	• See Diversional activity deficit, p. 17.
		Diversional activities will be available.

Knowledge deficit
Related to:
New condition and procedures
Unfamiliarity with disease process and transmission of disease
 	
DEFINING CHARACTERISTICS
Questions
Confusion about treatment
	ONGOING ASSESSMENT
	• Determine patient's/significant others' understanding of disease process, complications, and treatment.
	• Observe for compliance with treatment regimen.
	
	THERAPEUTIC INTERVENTIONS
	• Provide information to patient/significant others in teaching sessions about need to:
	  Maintain natural resistance to infection through adequate nutrition, rest, and exercise.
	  Avoid contact with people with upper respiratory infections.
	  Obtain immunizations against influenza for the elderly and chronically ill.
		Patient and significant others will demonstrate understanding of disease process and compliance with treatment regimen and isolation procedures.

Continued.

NURSING DIAGNOSES / DEFINING CHARACTERISTICS	NURSING INTERVENTIONS / *RATIONALES*	EXPECTED OUTCOMES

Inability to comply with treatment regimen, including appropriate isolation procedures
 	
Lack of questions
	Use pneumococcal vaccine for those at greatest risk:
	   Elderly patients with chronic systemic disease
	   Patients with COPD
	   Patients with sickle cell anemia
	   Patients who have had splenectomy
	   Patients who have had pneumonectomy and are immunosuppressed
	• Encourage patient/significant others to ask questions.
	• Evaluate understanding of information after teaching sessions *to determine patient's knowledge level.* Repeat teaching as needed *to reinforce information* and provide handouts *for reference.*
	• Instruct patient/significant other on isolation procedure used, *so they understand importance of following procedures for time patient will be in isolation.*	

Originated by: Martha Dickerson, RN, MS, CCRN
           Susan Galanes, RN, MS, CCRN

Pulmonary thromboembolism

(PULMONARY EMBOLUS [PE])

Pulmonary thromboembolism occurs when there is an obstruction in the pulmonary vascular bed (pulmonary artery or one of the branches) caused by blood clots (thrombi). It is one of the most common causes of death in hospitalized patients, resulting from a variety of factors that predispose to intravascular clotting. These include postoperative states, trauma to vessel walls, obesity, diabetes mellitus, infection, venous stasis caused by immobility; postpartum state; and other circulatory disorders. The clinical picture varies according to size and location of the embolus. The primary objective when pulmonary embolism occurs is to prevent recurrence.

NURSING DIAGNOSES / DEFINING CHARACTERISTICS	NURSING INTERVENTIONS / *RATIONALES*	EXPECTED OUTCOMES

Impaired gas exchange
Related to:
Decreased perfusion to lung tissues caused by obstruction in pulmonary vascular bed by embolus
 	
DEFINING CHARACTERISTICS
Increased alveolar dead space
Hypoxemia
Increased alveolar-arterial (A-a) gradient
Increased physiologic shunting
	ONGOING ASSESSMENT
	• Identify and document pertinent data *that aid in early diagnosis:*
	   Risk factors: immobility, postoperative state, cardiomegaly with irregular heartbeat (atrial fibrillation)
	   Most typical physical finding: pleural friction rub
	   Common clinical findings: rales, tachypnea, and tachycardia caused by hypoxemia
	• Assess for alteration in lung function:
	   Hypoxemia:
	     Tachycardia
	     Restlessness
	     Diaphoresis
	     Headache
	     Lethargy/confusion
	     Skin color changes
	   Atelectasis:
	     Diminished chest expansion
	     Limited diaphragm excursion
	     Bronchial/tubular breath sounds
	     Rales
	     Tracheal shift to affected side
		Optimal gas exchange will be maintained.

NURSING DIAGNOSES / DEFINING CHARACTERISTICS	NURSING INTERVENTIONS / *RATIONALES*	EXPECTED OUTCOMES
Dyspnea/tachypnea (respiratory rate ≥ 30/min) Use of accessory muscles Hypocapnia (Pco_2 level < 35 mm Hg) Chest x-ray reflecting atelectasis Rales Decreased breath sounds over involved lung areas Bronchial or tubular breath sounds Pleural friction rub Chest pain (pleuritic) Elevated temperature Hemoptysis	Abnormal lung sounds: Pleural friction rub Rales Work of breathing: Increased respiration rate and depth Increased use of accessory breathing muscles Decreased number of words patient can say between each breath · Assess characteristics of pain: quantity, quality, location, precipitating factors, relieving factors. · Assess for fever. · Monitor ABGs routinely. · Obtain specimens for culture if temperature is $> 102°F$ (rectal) *to identify and treat cause of infection.* **THERAPEUTIC INTERVENTIONS** · Administer O_2 as needed *to prevent severe hypoxemia.* · Position patient properly *to promote optimal lung perfusion. When patient is positioned on side, affected area should not be dependent. Upright and sitting positions optimize diaphragmatic excursions.* · Pace and schedule activities *to conserve energy.* · Use nursing measures to maintain normal body temperature. *Fever causes tachycardia, which increases O_2 demand.*	
Potential decreased cardiac output *Related to:* Failure of right side of heart resulting from pulmonary hypertension Failure of left side of heart secondary to failure of right side **DEFINING CHARACTERISTICS** Failure of right side of heart: Accentuated pulmonic component of second heart sound (S_2) Splitting of S_2 Engorged neck veins, positive hepatojugular reflex Increased CVP readings Palpable liver and spleen Altered coagulation values ECG change associated with right atrial hypertrophy Atrial arrhythmias Pedal edema Weight gain	**ONGOING ASSESSMENT** · Observe and document clinical findings that indicate impending or present failure of right side (see Defining Characteristics). Note: *Embolus causes decreased cross-sectional area of pulmonary vascular bed that results in increased pulmonary resistance. This increases the workload of the right side of the heart.* · Auscultate lung and heart sounds q2-4h *to identify abnormalities indicating impending or present failure of left side of heart (see Defining Characteristics).* Note: *Decreased right ventricular contractility decreases left side blood volume. This decreases left ventricular pumping power if not treated promptly.* · If ECG is monitored, observe for atrial arrhythmias caused by right side strain and for ventricular arrhythmias caused by hypoxemia. · Monitor weight daily. *Gain of 2-3 lb/day is significant for heart failure.* **THERAPEUTIC INTERVENTIONS** · Position patient properly *to promote easier breathing. Sitting and upright position promote better diaphragmatic excursions.* · For massive pulmonary thromboembolism, anticipate the following: Mechanical ventilation (see Mechanical ventilation, p. 213) Insertion of arterial line Insertion of Swan-Ganz catheter (see Swan-Ganz catheter, p. 165) Anticoagulant therapy Thrombolytic therapy Vena caval interruption Pulmonary embolectomy (rarely done) · If cardiac output a problem, see treatment for Cardiac output, decreased, p. 9. · If peripheral edema is present, refer to Skin integrity, impaired, p. 48.	Optimal cardiac output will be maintained.

Continued.

Pulmonary thromboembolism—cont'd

NURSING DIAGNOSES / DEFINING CHARACTERISTICS	NURSING INTERVENTIONS / *RATIONALES*	EXPECTED OUTCOMES
Failure of left side of heart: Fine rales (bases of the lungs) Increased pulmonary artery wedge pressure Presence of S₃; gallop rhythms Frothy secretions Dyspnea Tachycardia Cough Wheezing Orthopnea Hypoxemia Respiratory acidosis ECG changes associated with left atrial hypertrophy		

Potential for bleeding
Related to:
Bleeding secondary to anticoagulant/ thrombolytic therapy
 	
DEFINING CHARACTERISTICS
Petechiae, purpura, hematoma
Bleeding from catheter insertion sites
GI, GU bleeding
Bleeding from respiratory tract
Bleeding from mucous membranes
Decreasing Hb and Hct
	ONGOING ASSESSMENT
	• Assess for signs and symptoms of bleeding (see Defining Characteristics).
	• Assess patient for high-risk bleeding condition:
	    Liver disease
	    Kidney disease
	    Severe hypertension
	    Cavitary tuberculosis
	    Bacterial endocarditis
	• Monitor partial thromboplastin time (PTT) level. *Goal is PTT level at least twice control level.*
	• Monitor IV dosage and delivery system (tubing/pump) to minimize risk of overcoagulation/undercoagulation.
	• Observe patient at all times for signs of bleeding:
	    Keep dressings of IV and arterial sites visible.
	    Use adhesive tape that is not waterproof.
	    Check IV infusion site
	• Estimate and record blood loss.
	
	THERAPEUTIC INTERVENTIONS
	• Administer anticoagulant therapy as ordered (continuous IV heparin infusion).
	• If bleeding occurs, anticipate the following:
	    Stop the infusion.
	    Recheck PTT level stat.
	    Administer protamine sulfate *(heparin antagonist)* as ordered.
	    Take vital signs frequently *to assess status.*
	    Reevaluate dose of heparin on basis of PTT result.
	    Notify blood bank to ensure blood availability if needed.
	• Discontinue anticoagulant infusion cautiously:
	    Taper dose on basis of PTT result, as ordered.
	    Administer oral anticoagulant, usually warfarin (Coumadin), while heparin dose is tapered.
	    Monitor both prothrombin time (PT) and PTT levels.
	    Continue to observe closely for signs of bleeding.
	    Instruct conscious and reliable patients to report signs of bleeding immediately (see Defining Characteristics).
	• Minimize complications of thrombolytic therapy. Be aware of contraindications for thrombolytic therapy:
		Risk for bleeding will be reduced.

NURSING DIAGNOSES / DEFINING CHARACTERISTICS	NURSING INTERVENTIONS / *RATIONALES*	EXPECTED OUTCOMES
	Recent surgery Recent organ biopsy Paracentesis/thoracentesis Pregnancy Recent stroke Recent or active internal bleeding ▪ Institute precautionary measures: 　Use only compressible vessels for IV sites. 　Compress IV sites for at least 10 min and arterial sites for 30 min. 　Discontinue anticoagulants and antiplatelet aggregates before thrombolytic therapy. 　Limit physical manipulation of patients *to prevent disruption of formed blood clots.* 　Pad side rails *to prevent further bleeding injury.* 　Provide gentle oral care. 　Avoid IM injections: *any needle stick is potential bleeding site.* 　Draw all laboratory specimens through existing line. 　Send specimen for type and crossmatch as ordered. ▪ Discuss and provide patient with a list of what to avoid when taking anticoagulants: 　Do not use blade razor (electric razors preferred). 　Do not take new medications without consulting physician, pharmacist, or nurses. 　Do not eat foods high in vitamin K (e.g., dark green vegetables, cauliflower, cabbage, bananas, tomatoes). 　Do not ingest aspirin or other salicylates. ▪ Discuss and give patient list of measures *to minimize recurrence of emboli:* 　Taking medicines as prescribed 　Keeping medical checkup and blood test appointments 　Performing leg exercises as advised, especially during long automobile and airplane trips *to prevent venous stasis* 　Not crossing legs *(pressure alters circulation and may lead to clotting)* 　Use of TED stockings if ordered *to prevent venous stasis* 　Maintenance of adequate hydration *to prevent increased blood viscosity*	
Anxiety *Related to:* Threat of death Change in health status Overall feeling of intense sickness Multiple laboratory tests Increased attention of medical personnel Increasing respiratory difficulty **DEFINING CHARACTERISTICS** Verbalization of anxiety Restlessness, inability to relax Multiple questions Tremors, shakiness Increase in heart rate, BP, and respiratory rate	**ONGOING ASSESSMENT** ▪ Assess level of anxiety. ▪ Assess patient's normal coping mechanisms. **THERAPEUTIC INTERVENTIONS** ▪ Convey sense of empathic understanding through appropriate use of silence and touch. ▪ Encourage patient to ventilate feelings of anxiety. *Understanding patient's feelings of anxiety will guide staff in planning and implementing care plan to allay individualized anxiety.* ▪ Support previously effective coping mechanisms. ▪ Provide adequate rest: 　Organize activities (e.g., morning care, meals, hospital staff rounds, treatments). 　Decrease sensory stimulations: 　　Dim lights when appropriate. 　　Remove unnecessary equipment from room *to maintain more relaxed environment.* 　　Limit visitors and phone calls *(to prevent tiring). Patients feel obligated to entertain (may be physically and emotionally taxing).* ▪ Administer pain medicines or sedatives as indicated *to assist in allaying anxiety.* ▪ Explain reasons for multiple laboratory tests and increased medical personnel attention. ▪ See Anxiety, p. 4, as needed.	Anxiety will be decreased.

Continued.

NURSING DIAGNOSES / DEFINING CHARACTERISTICS	NURSING INTERVENTIONS / *RATIONALES*	EXPECTED OUTCOMES
Tense/anxious appearance Crying Withdrawal Denial		

Knowledge deficit
Related to:
New medical condition
 	
DEFINING CHARACTERISTICS
Expresses inaccurate perception of health status
Verbalizes deficiency in knowledge
Multiple questions or none
	ONGOING ASSESSMENT
	· Assess learning ability.
	· Assess present knowledge of illness:
	    Severity
	    Prognosis
	    Risk factors
	    Therapy
	· Assess patient's readiness for learning:
	    Past acute stage of illness
	    Expression of desire to learn
	
	THERAPEUTIC INTERVENTIONS
	· Facilitate the learning process. Inform patient/significant others of the following:
	    Etiology of the problem
	    Effects of pulmonary embolus on body functioning
	    Common risk factors:
	        Immobilization
	        Trauma: hip fracture, major burns
	        Certain heart conditions
	        Oral contraceptives
	· Instruct patient/significant others about medications, their actions, dosages, and side effects.
	· Discuss and give patient list of signs and symptoms of excessive anticoagulation:
	    Easy bruising
	    Severe nosebleed
	    Black stools
	    Blood in urine or stools
	    Joint swelling and pain
	    Coughing up of blood
	    Severe headache
		Patient will understand importance of medications, signs of excessive anticoagulation, and means to reduce risk of bleeding and recurrence of emboli.

Originated by: Lumie L. Perez, RN, BSN, CCRN

Respiratory failure, acute: secondary to chronic obstructive pulmonary disease

Acute respiratory failure is a life-threatening inability to maintain adequate pulmonary gas exchange. The chronic obstructive pulmonary disease patient has a significant decrease in pulmonary reserves, and any physiologic stress may result in acute respiratory failure.

NURSING DIAGNOSES / DEFINING CHARACTERISTICS	NURSING INTERVENTIONS / *RATIONALES*	EXPECTED OUTCOMES
Ineffective breathing pattern *Related to:* Hypoxia Acidosis Obstructed airway secondary to retention of secretions Pulmonary infection Congestive heart failure resulting from pulmonary hypertension **DEFINING CHARACTERISTICS** Shortness of breath Retention of CO_2 O_2 below 50 mm Hg Increased restlessness and irritability Tachycardia Dyspnea Tachypnea Cyanosis Respiratory depth changes Frequent wheezing and increased severity of coughing Decrease in level of consciousness (LOC) may occur as respiratory insufficiency increases in severity	**ONGOING ASSESSMENT** • Review respiratory health history. • Monitor and record vital signs every hour and notify physician of abnormalities. Note any irregularity of pulse. • Observe for changes in patient's respiratory status, including rate, depth, changes heard during auscultation, and in respiratory effort. • Assess for productive cough, including amount expectorated, frequency, color. • Observe for signs of hypoxia (e.g., dyspnea, increased pulse, changes in LOC, restlessness, and cyanosis). • Observe for signs of increased P_{CO_2} (e.g., asterixis or tremors). • Monitor ABGs carefully and notify physician of abnormalities. • Observe for intercostal retractions and marked use of accessory muscles. • Auscultate lungs and assess breath sounds for wheezing, rales, or rhonchi. **THERAPEUTIC INTERVENTIONS** • Administer O_2 as needed. For patients with severe COPD, give O_2 cautiously, preferably with a Venturi device *(a high-flow O_2 delivery system with a stable F_1O_2 unaffected by patient's respiratory rate or tidal volume). COPD patients who chronically retain CO_2 depend upon "hypoxic drive" as their stimulus to breathe. When applying O_2, close monitoring is imperative to prevent unsafe increases in patient's Pa_{O_2}, which would result in apnea.* • Position patient with proper body alignment *for optimal chest excursion and breathing pattern.* • Maintain adequate airway; position patient *to prevent mechanical obstruction from tongue.* • Pace activities *to prevent fatigue.* • Maintain planned rest periods.	Adverse changes in breathing pattern will be reduced.
Potential ineffective airway clearance *Related to:* Respiratory failure requiring intubation **DEFINING CHARACTERISTICS** Rales Rhonchi Wheezes Cough	**ONGOING ASSESSMENT** • Assess for significant alterations in breath sounds (e.g., rhonchi, wheezes). After intubation, auscultate lungs for bilateral breath sounds *to assure that ET tube not in right main stem bronchus or in esophagus.* • Assess for changes in ventilation rate or depth. Obtain chest x-ray study after intubation *to determine ET tube placement.* **THERAPEUTIC INTERVENTIONS** • Instruct and/or change patient's position q2h *to mobilize secretions.* • Provide humidity (when appropriate) via bedside humidifier/humidified O_2 therapy *(will prevent drying of secretions).* • Instruct patient to deep breathe adequately and to cough effectively.	Airway will be free of secretions.

Continued.

NURSING DIAGNOSES / DEFINING CHARACTERISTICS	NURSING INTERVENTIONS / *RATIONALES*	EXPECTED OUTCOMES

Dyspnea
Change in rate or depth of ventilation
	• Use nasotracheal suction for patients who cannot clear secretions.
	• When necessary, prepare for intubation:
	  Position patient appropriately and have necessary equipment readily available.
	  Instruct patient who is awake and alert, *since explanation is essential for total cooperation.*
	  Stay with patient *to allay anxiety.*
	  Institute suctioning via ET tube as necessary.
	  See Mechanical ventilation, p. 213, as appropriate.	

Potential for infection *Related to:* Suctioning of airway Endotracheal intubation **DEFINING CHARACTERISTICS** Increased WBC Increased temperature Change in bronchial secretions: amount, thickness, color	**ONGOING ASSESSMENT** • Monitor and document temperature q4h and notify physician of temperature > 38.5°C. *Note: If patient is receiving steroid therapy, detecting infections may be more difficult.* • Monitor WBC level and notify physician of abnormalities. • Observe patient's secretions for color, thickness, and amount. Notify physician of any abnormalities. • Monitor sputum cultures and sensitivities. **THERAPEUTIC INTERVENTIONS** • Use conscientious bronchial hygiene, good handwashing techniques, and sterile suctioning. *Many infections are transmitted by hospital personnel.* • Administer mouth care (e.g., Cepacol, mouth swabs, Chloraseptic mouth spray). q2h and as needed. *This will help limit oral bacterial growth and promote patient comfort.* • Institute airway suctioning as needed. *Accumulation of secretions can lead to invasive process.* • Maintain patient's personal hygiene, nutrition, and rest *to increase natural defenses.*	Risk of infection will be reduced.

Potential altered levels of consciousness
Related to:
Increased Paco$_2$ and/or decreased Pao$_2$
 	
DEFINING CHARACTERISTICS
Restlessness
Anxiety
Confusion
Somnolence
	ONGOING ASSESSMENT
	• Observe and document:
	  Increased restlessness
	  Increased anxiety
	  Confusion
	  Somnolence
	• Check pupils for size, shape, and reaction to light.
	• Obtain initial BP, and monitor serial BP. *Hypoxia/hypercarbia may cause initial hypertension with restlessness and progress to hypotension and somnolence.*
	
	THERAPEUTIC INTERVENTIONS
	• See Consciousness, altered level of, p. 234
		Optimal level of consciousness will be maintained.

Anxiety
Related to:
Threat of death
Change in health status
Change in environment
Change in interaction patterns
Unmet needs
 	
DEFINING CHARACTERISTICS
Restlessness
Diaphoresis
Pointing to throat (possibly unable to speak)
	ONGOING ASSESSMENT
	• Assess patient for signs indicating increased anxiety.
	
	THERAPEUTIC INTERVENTIONS
	• If patient unable to speak because of respiratory status:
	  Provide pencil and pad.
	  Establish some form of nonverbal communication if patient too sick to write. *Maintaining an avenue of communication is important to alleviate anxiety.*
	• Assist patient by:
	  Explaining mechanical ventilation
	  Explaining alarm systems on monitors and ventilators
	  Reassuring patient of your presence
	• Display a confident, calm manner and tolerant, understanding attitude.
	• Allow family/significant others to visit; involve them in care.
	• Use other supportive measures (e.g., medications, psychiatric liaison, clergy, social services) as indicated.
		Absence or decrease in anxiety will be evidenced.

NURSING DIAGNOSES / DEFINING CHARACTERISTICS	NURSING INTERVENTIONS / *RATIONALES*	EXPECTED OUTCOMES
Uncooperative behavior Withdrawal Vigilant watch on equipment		
Knowledge deficit *Related to:* Unfamiliarity with disease process and treatment **DEFINING CHARACTERISTICS** Multiple questions Lack of concern Anxiety Noncompliant of medication/health care orders, e.g., smoking	**ONGOING ASSESSMENT** • Evaluate patient's perception and understanding of disease process. • Assess patient's knowledge of O_2 therapy, deep breathing, and coughing. **THERAPEUTIC INTERVENTIONS** • Encourage patient to verbalize feelings and questions. • Explain disease process to patient and correct misconceptions. • Discuss need for monitoring equipment and frequent assessments. *Patient must be aware that this is an acute episode of respiratory failure*. • Explain all tests and procedures before they occur. • Explain necessity of O_2 therapy, including its limitations. • Instruct patient to deep breathe and cough effectively. • See Chronic obstructive pulmonary disease, p. 192, *for long-term teaching needs, as appropriate*.	Patient will verbalize understanding of disease process, procedures, and treatment.

Originated by: Linda Marie St. Julien, RN, MS
                 Susan Galanes, RN, MS, CCRN

Tuberculosis, active

(TB)

A disease of the lung caused by tubercle bacillus, which is infectious, contagious, and curable.

NURSING DIAGNOSES / DEFINING CHARACTERISTICS	NURSING INTERVENTIONS / *RATIONALES*	EXPECTED OUTCOMES
Ineffective breathing pattern *Related to:* Decreased lung volumes Increased metabolism as result of high fever Frequent productive cough and hemoptysis Nervousness, fear of suffocation **DEFINING CHARACTERISTICS** Increased work of breathing: tachypnea, use of accessory muscles, retractions, diaphoresis, tachycardia	**ONGOING ASSESSMENT** • Assess respiratory status. Note depth, rate and character of breathing q4h. • Check for increased work of breathing. • Assess cough (productive, weak, or hard). • Assess nature of secretions; color, amount, consistency. • Auscultate lungs for presence of normal and abnormal breath sounds q4h. • Monitor vital signs q4h. Note time of temperature spikes. • Monitor ABGs **THERAPEUTIC INTERVENTIONS** • Administer O_2 as ordered (*decreases work of breathing*). • Push fluids and promote hydration *to liquify secretions for easy expectoration*. • Induce sputum with heated aerosol if needed *to expedite diagnosis and start early treatment*. • Maintain semi-Fowler's position *to facilitate easy breathing*.	An effective breathing pattern will be maintained.

Continued.

Tuberculosis, active— cont'd

NURSING DIAGNOSES / DEFINING CHARACTERISTICS	NURSING INTERVENTIONS / *RATIONALES*	EXPECTED OUTCOMES
Purulent or bloody expectoration Increased anxiety, nervousness, fear, or anger secondary to dyspnea		

Actual infection
Related to:
Active pulmonary TB
 	
DEFINING CHARACTERISTICS
Purulent or bloody expectoration
Temperature spikes
Positive culture report
	ONGOING ASSESSMENT
	· Check amount, color, and consistency of sputum.
	· Monitor temperature q4h.
	· Monitor sputum cultures.
	
	THERAPEUTIC INTERVENTIONS
	· Observe respiratory isolation:
	  Keep sputum cups at bedside.
	  Dispose of secretions properly.
	  Keep tissues at bedside.
	  Have patient cover mouth when coughing *to decrease airborne contaminants*.
	  Use masks:
	    Anyone entering patient's room should wear a mask.
	    If patient is transported out of room, for any reason, should wear mask.
	  Keep door to room closed at all times and post isolation sign where visible.
	  Place respiratory isolation sticker on chart.
	  Assist visitors to follow appropriate isolation techniques *to prevent spread of infection*.
	· Administer medications as ordered.
		Infection will be treated and risk of spread reduced.

Diversional activity deficit *Related to:* Isolation **DEFINING CHARACTERISTICS** Verbal expression of boredom Preoccupation with illness Frequent use of call light Excessive complaints	**ONGOING ASSESSMENT** · Assess for presence of defining characteristics. · Assess understanding of need for isolation. **THERAPEUTIC INTERVENTIONS** · Encourage questions, conversation, and ventilation of feelings. · Address fears about communicability of disease and need for isolation *so patient will understand need for isolation and know it is temporary*. · Encourage visitors to involve patient in activities (e.g., conversation, card games, board games). · Arrange for television in room, when possible. · Arrange occupational therapy in room. · See Diversional activity deficit, p. 17.	Boredom will be reduced.

Altered nutrition: less than body requirements
Related to:
Chronically poor appetite caused by:
  Fever
  Coughing
  Shortness of breath
	ONGOING ASSESSMENT
	· Assess nutritional status on admission through diet history and physical exam.
	· Assess for possible causes of malnutrition.
	· Assess laboratory values:
	  Serum albumin
	  Serum protein
	  Leukocyte count
	  Urine protein
	  Urine glucose
	· Obtain admission weight and daily weight for 1 wk, then weekly weights.
		Optimal nutritional status will be maintained.

Tuberculosis, active— cont'd

NURSING DIAGNOSES / DEFINING CHARACTERISTICS	NURSING INTERVENTIONS / *RATIONALES*	EXPECTED OUTCOMES
DEFINING CHARACTERISTICS Wasted appearance Unintentional weight loss	**THERAPEUTIC INTERVENTIONS** • Provide high-protein, high-calorie diet and nutritional supplements *for muscle building and tissue healing*. • Explain importance of good nutrition while taking TB medications. • See Nutrition, altered: less than body requirements, p. 37.	

Noncompliance to therapeutic regimen
Related to:
Patient value system: Health and spiritual beliefs, cultural beliefs, and cultural influences
Prolonged therapy
Inadequate follow-up
Patient and provider relationship
 	
DEFINING CHARACTERISTICS
TB reactivation shown on chest x-ray and sputum examination
Poor nutritional status: signs of malnutrition; not feeling well
Drug-resistant organism seen in culture and sensitivity
Verbal cue by patient/ significant others of noncompliance
	ONGOING ASSESSMENT
	• Assess patient for evidence of noncompliance:
	  Weight loss
	  Increased coughing
	  Thick, green-gray purulent sputum
	  Drug-resistant organism on culture and sensitivity
	• Identify causes of noncompliance.
	• Obtain sputum for culture and sensitivity studies *to determine proper combination of drugs to be reinstituted*.
	
	THERAPEUTIC INTERVENTIONS
	• Adapt respiratory isolation techniques to home environment.
	• Arrange for social service involvement for patient and family.
	• Discuss with patient/significant others importance of following therapeutic regimen.
		Optimal compliance with treatment will be achieved.

Knowledge deficit
Related to:
Unfamiliarity with disease process and new treatment methods
 	
DEFINING CHARACTERISTICS
Verbalization of incorrect information
Statement of lack of understanding/asking questions
Evidence of noncompliance with therapeutic regimen related to lack of information
	ONGOING ASSESSMENT
	• Assess knowledge of TB.
	• Assess readiness and interest to learn about topics related to TB.
	
	THERAPEUTIC INTERVENTIONS
	• Teach patient the following: *A patient with knowledge of disease will be more likely to be compliant with the treatment regimen.*
	  Detection
	  Transmission
	  Signs/symptoms
	  Treatment and length of therapy
	  Prevention
	  Importance of compliance with therapy
	  Health regimen to follow after discharge
	    Clinic appointments
	    Sources of free medication
	    ADL
	    Resource telephone numbers
	• Reinforce respiratory isolation technique. (Refer to interventions and rationale of Nursing Diagnosis: *Actual infection*, p. 208).
		Patient will verbalize basic knowledge of TB.

Originated by: Annie F. Jenkins, RN
Remedios S. Garces, RN, BSN

High-frequency jet ventilation

(HFJV)

HFJV is a type of mechanical ventilation that uses high-frequency rates (40 to 150 cycles/min are approved by FDA for adults, as nonexperimental) with very low tidal volumes (3-5 ml/kg) to achieve ventilation (30-35 L/min ventilation). It is useful for patients with bronchopleural fistulas, and large pulmonary air leaks and is indicated for patients who have failed on conventional ventilation.

NURSING DIAGNOSES / DEFINING CHARACTERISTICS	NURSING INTERVENTIONS / *RATIONALES*	EXPECTED OUTCOMES

Impaired gas exchange (requiring HFJV) *Related to:* Adult respiratory distress syndrome Barotrauma Aspiration pneumonitis Bronchopleural fistula **Defining Characteristics** Hypercapnia Hypoxia Abnormal ABGs Presence of increased intrathoracic pressures (measured by esophageal balloon and manometer) Low pulmonary compliance exhibited by high peak pressures (≥ 55 cm H_2O)	**Ongoing Assessment**
	 • Assess respiratory rate, rhythm, and character q1h.
	 • Auscultate lungs q1h to check for aeration before and after jet ventilation.
	 • Observe for abnormal breathing patterns (Cheyne-Stokes, Kussmaul, sternal retractions).
	 • Assess level of consciousness and level of anxiety.
	 • Assess skin color (presence/absence of cyanosis), temperature, capillary refill, and peripheral perfusion.
	 • Monitor vital signs q1h, watching for increased central venous pressure, increased pulmonary capillary wedge pressure (PCWP), decreased BP, and decreased cardiac output. Notify physician if these occur.
	 • Monitor for complaints of pain, which may increase respirations, making patient ventilation more difficult. Assess location and duration.
	 • Monitor ABGs frequently or as indicated (i.e., after changes in F_1O_2, rate, drive pressure, or continuous positive airway pressure).
	 • Monitor cardiac output as indicated or ordered, especially after ventilator changes or changes in patient's condition.
	
	 Therapeutic Interventions
	 • Administer O_2 as ordered and indicated.
	 • Obtain informed consent for jet therapy if possible.
	 • Prepare patient for intubation with Hi-Lo Jet Tracheal Tube (National Catheter Co.). *This endotracheal tube has two additional ports: for jet driveline and for continuous intratracheal pressure monitoring. Note: Hi-Lo Jet Tracheal Tube outer diameter is half-size larger than conventional ET tubes (e.g., 7.5 Hi-Lo single-lumen cuffed ET tube = 7.0 Hi-Lo Jet Tracheal Tube).*
	     Administer sedation and neuromuscular blocking agent (e.g., diazepam [Valium], pancuronium [Pavulon], or succinylcholine) as ordered.
	     Provide comfort measures/reassurance (verbal and nonverbal contact).
	     Obtain baseline status before instituting therapy (PCWP, cardiac output, and ABGs) as ordered.
	 • Maintain adequate blood volume, treating any sources of hemorrhage or changes in vascular compartments with appropriate fluids (i.e., blood, crystalloid, colloid) as ordered.
	 • Combine nursing actions (i.e., bath, bed, and dressing changes) *to minimize patient energy expenditive and allow frequent rest periods.*
	 • Provide frequent attendance *(few alarms on present jet system to detect patient disconnect or low volumes). Be prepared to use Ambu bag in case of emergency failure of machinery or acute change in condition. Ambu bag ventilation may be difficult because of decreased compliance and elasticity.*
	 • Administer antibiotics and medications as ordered.
	 • Administer pain relievers as ordered, and provide other comfort measures as needed.
	 • Be aware that sedation to maintain ventilation control will decrease with jet ventilation. *Most patients on HFJV have cessation of ventilatory effort at supraphysiologic ventilatory rates.* However, when weaning back to conventional ventilation, need for sedation may recur.
		Optimal gas exchange will be maintained.

NURSING DIAGNOSES / DEFINING CHARACTERISTICS	NURSING INTERVENTIONS / *RATIONALES*	EXPECTED OUTCOMES
Ineffective airway clearance *Related to:* Presence/irritation by ET tube Secretions Drying of mucosa Decreased energy and fatigue **DEFINING CHARACTERISTICS** Abnormal breath sounds Change in rate, depth, and character of respirations Tachypnea Cough Cyanosis Dyspnea or shortness of breath	**ONGOING ASSESSMENT** ▪ Assess for alteration in airway clearance. ▪ Assess ET tube placement and adequacy of cuff to prevent air leakage. *Underinflation may cause aspiration of oral secretions. Overinflation of cuff may obliterate perfusion to left or right bronchus causing ABG deterioration.* Notify respiratory therapist to check cuff pressure. Notify physician of problems with ET tube maintenance (e.g., placement, suctioning, cuff). **THERAPEUTIC INTERVENTIONS** ▪ Institute aseptic suctioning of airway as needed *to prevent airway obstruction. Potential for mucous plug is present because of drying of mucosa from high-frequency ventilation* (respiratory therapist will maintain humidification). ▪ Turn off jet ventilator or disconnect during suctioning; *otherwise increased airway resistance may increase potential for pneumothorax.* ▪ Be aware that respiratory therapist will use Ambu bag or "sigh" q1h, with jet off, *to prevent atelectasis or atrophy of respiratory muscles as result of low tidal volume.*	Airway will be free of secretions.
Potential for injury: barotrauma *Related to:* Pressure-cycled ventilation High-peak airway pressures **DEFINING CHARACTERISTICS** Crepitus Subcutaneous emphysema Altered chest excursion: asymmetrical chest Abnormal ABGs Shift in trachea Restlessness Chest x-ray report shows evidence of pneumothorax	**ONGOING ASSESSMENT** ▪ Assess for signs of barotrauma q1h. *Frequent assessments are needed (barotrauma can occur at any time; patient may not show signs of dyspnea, shortness of breath, or tachypnea while on HFJV).* ▪ Monitor chest x-ray reports daily; obtain stat portable chest x-ray if barotrauma suspected. **THERAPEUTIC INTERVENTIONS** ▪ Notify physician of barotrauma signs immediately. ▪ Anticipate need for chest tube placement; prepare as needed. If *barotrauma is suspected, intervention must follow immediately to prevent tension pneumothorax.*	Potential for injury from barotrauma will be reduced.
Potential impaired skin integrity *Related to:* Prolonged bed rest Immobility Sensory deficit Altered vasomotor tone and/or altered nutritional state Prolonged intubation	**ONGOING ASSESSMENT** ▪ Assess bony prominences for signs of threatened or actual skin breakdown. ▪ Assess around ET tube for crusting of secretions, redness, or irritation. ▪ Assess for signs of skin breakdown beneath ET-securing tape. **THERAPEUTIC INTERVENTIONS** ▪ Institute changes in position carefully *because of limitations in length of ventilator tubing (designed to minimize compressible volume, increasing efficiency). Changes in position may change ability to ventilate patient but should be made q2h.* ▪ Institute prophylactic use of pressure-relieving devices. ▪ See Skin integrity, impaired, p. 48 (as needed).	Skin integrity will be maintained.

Continued.

Pulmonary Care Plans

NURSING DIAGNOSES / DEFINING CHARACTERISTICS	NURSING INTERVENTIONS / *RATIONALES*	EXPECTED OUTCOMES
DEFINING CHARACTERISTICS Actual skin breakdown: Stage I: redness, skin intact Stage II: blisters Stage III: necrosis Stage IV: necrosis involving bones and joints	• Change ET tube securing tape when loosened or soiled. If patient is nasally intubated, notify physician of red or irritated skin or of breakdown. If patient is orally intubated, tube should be repositioned from side to side q24-48h (*will help prevent pressure necrosis on lower lip*). • Provide mouth care q2h. • Keep ET tube free of crusting of secretions.	
Potential altered nutrition: less than body requirements *Related to:* Intubation	**ONGOING ASSESSMENT** • Obtain and document patient's weight daily. • Obtain nutritional history. • Assess for bowel sounds. • Check for abdominal distention and tenderness.	Nutritional deficit will be reduced or prevented.
DEFINING CHARACTERISTICS Loss of weight ≥ 10-20% below ideal body weight Documented inadequate caloric intake Caloric intake inadequate to keep pace with abnormal disease/metabolic state	**THERAPEUTIC INTERVENTIONS** • Give enteral or parenteral feedings as ordered. Refer to Nutrition, altered: less than body requirements, p. 37; Enteral tube feeding, p. 308; Total parenteral nutrition (TPN), p. 324.	
Knowledge deficit *Related to:* New equipment New environment	**ONGOING ASSESSMENT** • Evaluate patient's/significant others understanding of patient's overall condition and need for jet ventilation. • Evaluate readiness for learning of patient/significant others.	Patient/significant others will demonstrate understanding of rationale for jet ventilation.
DEFINING CHARACTERISTICS Increased frequency of questions of patient and significant others Inability to respond correctly to medical personnel's questions	**THERAPEUTIC INTERVENTIONS** • Explain all procedures to patient before performing them, especially during period of intubation and start of jet ventilation. *This will help to decrease patient's anxiety. Fear of unknown could otherwise result in extreme patient anxiety with uncooperativeness.* • Provide reassurance of safety of jet ventilatory system. • Orient and reorient patient to ICU surroundings, routines, equipment alarms, and noises. *The ICU is a busy and noisy environment that can be very upsetting to patient who doesn't know what noises and alarms mean.* • Include significant others in explanations of jet therapy. • Allow patient to ventilate feelings through alternative methods of communication (sign language, written messages, alphabet board). • Explain methods/procedures of "weaning off" HFJV. Be aware that sedation, which may have been used before jet therapy, may have to be reinstituted during weaning process. Reassure that sedation is not meant as punishment but may provide easier transition to conventional ventilation and eventual extubation.	

Originated by: Carol Ann Rooks, RN, BSN
            Susan Galanes, RN, MS, CCRN

Mechanical ventilation

The patient requiring mechanical ventilation must have an artificial airway (endotracheal [ET] tube or tracheostomy). A mechanical ventilator will facilitate movement of gases into and out of the pulmonary system (ventilation), but it cannot ensure gas exchange at the pulmonary and tissue levels (respiration). It provides either partial or total ventilatory support for patients with respiratory failure.

NURSING DIAGNOSES / DEFINING CHARACTERISTICS	NURSING INTERVENTIONS / *RATIONALES*	EXPECTED OUTCOMES
Altered gas exchange/breathing pattern requiring mechanical ventilation *Related to:* Acute respiratory failure: Pneumonia Chronic obstructive pulmonary disease (COPD) Acute respiratory distress syndrome (ARDS) Tuberculosis Pulmonary embolus Pulmonary edema Airway obstruction Copious amounts of secretions Drug overdosage Diabetic coma Uremia Various CNS disorders Smoke inhalation Aspiration Chest trauma Status asthmaticus Guillian-Barré Myasthenia gravis **DEFINING CHARACTERISTICS** pH < 7.35 Po_2 < 50-60 $Pco_2 \geq$ 50-60 Decreased available Hb resulting in decreased O_2 content Changes in mental status Increased or decreased respiratory rate Apnea Inability to maintain airway (i.e., depressed gag, depressed cough, emesis)	**ONGOING ASSESSMENT** • Assess vital signs q1h and prn. *Hypotension, tachycardia, and tachypnea may result from hypoxia and/or hypocarbia.* • Assess lung sounds q1-2h *(allows early detection of deterioration or improvement)*. Listen closely for rhonchi, rales, wheezing, and diminished breath sounds in each lobe, assessing right to left, *to compare lung sounds*. Reassess lung sounds after coughing/suctioning *to determine improvement or clearance*. • Assess breathing rate, pattern, depth; note position assumed for breathing. • Observe ABGs for abrupt changes or deteriorations. Normal ranges: pH 7.35-7.45 Po_2 80-90 torr Pco_2 35-45 torr O_2 saturation 85-98% O_2 content 16-23 vol% HCO_3 23-29 mEq/L Base excess 0 $\pm$ 2 mEq/L • Assess for changes in mental status and LOC. *Signs of hypoxia include anxiety, restlessness, disorientation, somnolence, lethargy, and/or coma.* • Assess skin color, checking nail beds and lips for cyanosis. • Use pulse oximetry, as available, *to monitor O_2 saturation continuously*. • Observe laboratory data, especially noting changes in Hb, electrolytes, and blood glucose. • If patient has hemodynamic monitoring, assess pressures q1h; notify physician if outside prescribed ranges. • After intubation, assess for ET tube position: Inflate cuff until no audible leaks are heard. *Cuff pressure should not exceed 30 mm Hg. Cuff overinflation increases incidence of tracheal erosions.* Auscultate for bilateral breath sounds while patient is being manually ventilated by Ambu bag *to assure good ET tube position. If diminished breath sounds are present over left lung field, ET tube is most likely below carina, in right main stem bronchus, and must be pulled back.* Observe for abdominal distention *(may indicate gastric intubation; can follow CPR when air is inadvertently blown/bagged into esophagus as well as trachea)*. Ensure that chest x-ray is obtained *to determine ET tube placement.* **THERAPEUTIC INTERVENTIONS** Before intubation: • Maintain patient's airway: Encourage patient to cough and deep breathe. If coughing and deep breathing not effective, use nasotracheal suction as needed *to clear airway.* Use oral or nasal airway as needed *to prevent tongue from occluding oropharynx.* See Airway clearance, ineffective, p. 3. Provide O_2 therapy as ordered and indicated. *Increasing O_2 tension in alveoli may result in more O_2 diffusion into capillaries.* Coordinate respiratory therapy treatments. • Place patient in high Fowler's position, if tolerated, to *promote lung expansion.* • Notify physician: If vital signs are out of prescribed range or trending from baseline Immediately for signs of impending respiratory failure	Alteration in gas exchange will be reduced.

Continued.

NURSING DIAGNOSES / DEFINING CHARACTERISTICS	NURSING INTERVENTIONS / *RATIONALES*	EXPECTED OUTCOMES
Forced vital capacity <10 cc/kg) Rales, rhonchi, wheezing Diminished breath sounds	• Prepare for endotracheal intubation: Notify respiratory therapist to bring mechanical ventilator. If possible, before intubation, explain to patient: Need for intubation Steps involved Temporary inability to speak Prepare equipment: ET tubes of various sizes; note size used Benzoin and waterproof tape or other methods *for securing ET tube* 20-cc syringe *for inflating balloon after ET tube positioned* Local anesthetic agent (e.g., Cetacaine spray, cocaine, lidocaine [Xylocaine] spray or jelly, and cotton tip applicators) *for comfort and suppression of gag reflex* Sedation as prescribed by physician *to decrease combative resistance to intubation* Stylet *to make ET tube firmer and give additional support to direction* Magill forceps Laryngoscope and blades Ambu bag and mask connected to oxygen *to provide assisted ventilation with 100% O$_2$* Suction equipment *to maintain clear airway* Oral airway if patient is being orally intubated *to prevent occlusion or biting of ET tube* Bilateral soft wrist restraints *to prevent self-extubation of ET tube* Assist with intubation: • Place patient in supine position, hyperextending neck (if not contraindicated) and aligning patient's oropharynx, posterior nasopharynx, and trachea. • Oxygenate and ventilate patient as needed before and after each intubation attempt. If intubation is difficult, physician will stop periodically so oxygenation will be maintained. After intubation: • Continue with manual ventilation until ET tube is stabilized. • *To prevent patient from biting down on ET tube,* insert oral airway for orally intubated patient. • Assist in securing ET tube (if in proper placement per examination). • Institute aseptic suctioning of airway. • Place patient on mechanical ventilator with setting as ordered by physician. • Apply bilateral soft wrist restraints as needed, explaining reason for use. *Although all patients do not require restraints to prevent extubation, many do.* • Anticipate need for nasogastric (NG) suction if abdominal distention present.	
Potential for injury *Related to:* Improper ventilator settings Improper alarm settings Disconnection of ventilator **DEFINING CHARACTERISTICS** Reduction of Po$_2$ Increase in Pco$_2$ Acidosis Tachypnea Apnea	**ONGOING ASSESSMENT** • Check ventilator settings q1h *to see that patient is receiving correct:* Mode: Synchronized intermittent mandatory ventilation (SIMV) Controlled mandatory ventilation (CMV) Assist control (AC) Rate of mechanical breaths Tidal volume F$_I$O$_2$ Continuous positive airway pressure Pressure support **THERAPEUTIC INTERVENTIONS** • Notify respiratory therapist of discrepancy in ventilator settings immediately. • Listen for alarms, know range in which ventilator will alarm, and respond to alarms.	Injury will be prevented.

NURSING DIAGNOSES / DEFINING CHARACTERISTICS	NURSING INTERVENTIONS / *RATIONALES*	EXPECTED OUTCOMES
Changes in mental state Tachycardia	High peak pressure alarm: 　If patient is agitated, give sedation as ordered. Auscultate breath sounds; institute suctioning as needed. Notify respiratory therapist and physician if high pressure alarm persists. *(may indicate decrease in lung compliance or partial airway obstruction).* Low pressure alarm *indicates possible disconnection or mechanical ventilatory malfunction.* 　If disconnected, reconnect patient to mechanical ventilator. 　If malfunctioning, remove patient from mechanical ventilator and use Ambu bag. Notify respiratory therapist to correct malfunction. Low exhale volume *indicates patient is not returning delivered tidal volume (i.e., leak or disconnection).* 　Reconnect patient to ventilator if disconnected, or reconnect exhale tubing to the ventilator. If problem is not resolved, notify physician and respiratory therapist. 　Check cuff volume by assessing whether patient can talk or make sounds around tube or whether exhaled volumes are significantly less than volumes delivered. To correct, slowly reinflate cuff with air until no leak is detected. Notify respiratory therapist to check cuff pressure: *Cuff pressure should be maintained at <30 mm* Hg. *Maintenance of low-pressure cuffs prevents many tracheal complications formerly associated with ET tubes.* Notify physician if leak persists. *ET tube cuff may be defective, requiring physician to change tube.* Apnea alarm *is indicative of disconnection or absence of spontaneous respirations.* 　If disconnected, reconnect patient to ventilator. 　If apnea persists, use Ambu ventilation; notify physician.	
Ineffective airway clearance *Related to:* Endotracheal intubation **Defining Characteristics** Copious secretions Abnormal breath sounds Dyspnea	**Ongoing Assessment** • Assess breath sounds q1h and as needed. • Note quantity, color, consistency, and odor of sputum. **Therapeutic Interventions** • Institute suctioning of airway as needed. • Turn patient q2h *to mobilize secretions.* • Use sterile saline instillations during suctioning as needed *to help facilitate removal of tenacious sputum.*	Airway will remain patent.
Impaired verbal communication *Related to:* Endotracheal intubation **Defining Characteristics** Patient inability to communicate verbally because of intubation Difficulty in being understood with nonverbal methods Increasing frustration and/or anxiety	**Ongoing Assessment** • Assess patient's ability to use nonverbal communication. **Therapeutic Interventions** • Provide nonverbal means of communication: 　Writing equipment 　Communication board 　Artificial larynx 　Generalized list of questions/answers • Reassure patient that inability to speak *is temporary effect of ET tube's passing vocal cords.* • See Communication, impaired, p. 11.	Nonverbal means to express needs and concerns will be attained.

Continued.

NURSING DIAGNOSES / DEFINING CHARACTERISTICS	NURSING INTERVENTIONS / *RATIONALES*	EXPECTED OUTCOMES
Potential anxiety/fear *Related to:* Inability to breathe adequately without support Inability to maintain adequate gas exchange Fear of unknown outcome **DEFINING CHARACTERISTICS** Restlessness Fear of sleeping at night Uncooperative behavior Withdrawal Indifference Vigilant watch on equipment	**ONGOING ASSESSMENT** · Assess for signs of fear/anxiety. **THERAPEUTIC INTERVENTIONS** · Display confident, calm manner and understanding attitude. · Inform patient of alarms in ventilatory system and reassure patient of close proximity of health care personnel *to respond to alarms.* · Reduce distracting stimuli *to provide quiet environment.* · Encourage visiting by family/friends. · See Anxiety, p. 4 and Fear, p. 18 as appropriate.	Fear/anxiety will be reduced.
Potential decreased cardiac output *Related to:* Mechanical ventilation Positive-pressure ventilation **DEFINING CHARACTERISTICS** Hypotension Tachycardia Arrhythmias, ECG changes Anxiety, restlessness Decreased peripheral pulses Weight gain, edema	**ONGOING ASSESSMENT** · Assess vital signs and hemodynamic parameters (CVP, pulmonary artery pressures, cardiac output). *Mechanical ventilation can cause decreased venous return to heart, resulting in decreased cardiac output (may occur abruptly with ventilator changes: rate, tidal volume, or positive-pressure ventilation). Close monitoring during ventilator changes is imperative.* · Assess skin color, temperature; note quality of peripheral pulses. · Assess fluid balance through: 　Daily weights 　I & O: *After initial decrease in venous return to heart, volume receptors in right atrium signal decrease in volume, which triggers increase in antidiuretic hormone release from posterior pituitary and kidney retention of H_2O* · Assess mentation. **THERAPEUTIC INTERVENTIONS** · Maintain optimal fluid balance. *Fluid challenges may initially be used to add volume. However, if pulmonary artery pressures rise and cardiac output remains low, fluid restriction may be necessary.* · Notify physician immediately of signs of decrease in cardiac output and anticipate possible ventilator setting changes. · Administer medications (diuretics, inotropic agents, bronchodilators) as ordered. · See Cardiac output, decreased, p. 9.	Cardiac output will be maintained.
Potential impaired skin integrity *Related factors to:* Prolonged intubation **DEFINING CHARACTERISTICS** "Crusting" of secretions around ET tube	**ONGOING ASSESSMENT** · Observe skin for buildup of secretions, redness, or breakdown. **THERAPEUTIC INTERVENTIONS** · If patient is nasally intubated, notify physician of red or irritated skin or breakdown. · If patient orally intubated, tube should be repositioned from side to side q24-48h. · Support ventilator tubing *to prevent pressure on nose or lips.* · Change tape when loosened or soiled.	Skin integrity will be maintained.

NURSING DIAGNOSES / DEFINING CHARACTERISTICS	NURSING INTERVENTIONS / *RATIONALES*	EXPECTED OUTCOMES
Redness or irritation around ET tube and/or beneath securing tape Skin breakdown under or around ET tube and/or tape	• Provide mouth care q2h (e.g., may use 1:1 H_2O_2 and H_2O, and mouthwash afterward). *This will help decrease oral bacteria and prevent crusting of secretions.*	
Altered nutrition: less than body requirements *Related to:* Endotracheal intubation **DEFINING CHARACTERISTICS** Loss of weight with or without caloric intake ≥10-20% below ideal body weight Documented inadequate caloric intake Caloric intake inadequate to keep pace with abnormal disease/metabolic state	**ONGOING ASSESSMENT** • Document weight on admission and every day. • Obtain nutritional history. • Assess for bowel sounds. • Check for abdominal distention and tenderness; if present, notify physician *(may indicate paralytic ileus, bowel obstruction, or acute abdomen).* **THERAPEUTIC INTERVENTIONS** • Give enteral or parenteral feedings as ordered. *Be aware that patients with elevated CO_2 need low-carbohydrate diet to reduce CO_2 production. Use specially formulated enteral feeding formula, which provides low carbohydrate, high polyunsaturated fats, moderate protein, and high calories.* • Refer to Nutrition, altered: less than body requirements, p. 37; Enteral tube feeding, p. 308; Total parenteral nutrition, p. 324.	Nutritional deficit will be reduced or prevented.
Potential for infection *Related to:* ET intubation Suctioning of airway **DEFINING CHARACTERISTICS** Increased temperature Increased WBC Changes in tracheal secretions, color, consistency, and amount Tachycardia Infiltrates on chest x-ray.	**ONGOING ASSESSMENT** • Monitor temperature q4h; notify physician of temperature >38.5° C. • Monitor WBC and notify physician of elevation. • Monitor sputum culture and sensitivity reports. **THERAPEUTIC INTERVENTIONS** • Maintain aseptic suctioning techniques *to lessen probability of infection acquisition.* • Administer antibiotics as ordered.	Risk of infection will be reduced.
Knowledge deficit *Related to:* New treatment New environment **DEFINING CHARACTERISTICS** Multiple questions Lack of concern Anxiety	**ONGOING ASSESSMENT** • Assess patient's/significant others' perception and understanding of mechanical ventilation. **THERAPEUTIC INTERVENTIONS** • Allow patient/significant other to express feelings and ask questions. • Explain that patient will not be able to eat or drink while intubated but assure him/her that alternative measures (i.e., gastric feedings or hyperalimentation) will be taken to provide nourishment. *Risk of aspiration is high if patient eats or drinks while intubated.*	Patient/significant others will state basic understanding of mechanical ventilation and care involved.

Continued.

Pulmonary Care Plans

NURSING DIAGNOSES / DEFINING CHARACTERISTICS	NURSING INTERVENTIONS / *RATIONALES*	EXPECTED OUTCOMES
	· Explain to patient/significant others necessity for procedures (e.g., obtaining ABGs.) · Explain to patient inability to talk while intubated: *ET tube passes through vocal cords and attempts to talk can cause more trauma to cords.* · Explain that alarms may periodically sound off, which may be normal, and staff will be in close proximity. · Explain need for frequent assessments (i.e., vital signs, auscultation of breath sounds.) · Explain probable need for restraints *to gain cooperation to prevent accidental extubation.* · Explain need for suctioning as appropriate.	

Originated by: Michelle McGhee, RN, BSN
　　　　　　　　Susan Galanes, RN, MS, CCRN

Pneumonectomy

(LOBECTOMY)

Surgical removal of a lung performed for lung cancer. Five-year survival rate is 20%. Pneumonectomy may be combined with radiation and/or chemotherapy.

NURSING DIAGNOSES / DEFINING CHARACTERISTICS	NURSING INTERVENTIONS / *RATIONALES*	EXPECTED OUTCOMES
Ineffective breathing pattern *Related to:* Thoracotomy incision Pain Void in thoracic cavity Fatigue **Defining Characteristics** Asymmetrical chest excursion Dyspnea Use of accessory muscles for breathing Shallow respirations Splinting Complaints of pain	**Ongoing Assessment** · Monitor rate and depth of respirations. · Note asymmetry of chest wall movement during respirations. · Assess degree to which altered breathing pattern is compromising ventilation: 　　Note cyanosis. 　　Check ABGs. **Therapeutic Interventions** · Position patient *so that remaining lung expansion is facilitated* (i.e., position patient on operated side). · Assist patient in performing deep-breathing and coughing exercises: 　　Head of bed (HOB) elevated 　　Use of pillow or hands to splint incision 　　Use of incentive spirometry or stair-step inspirations · Administer pain medication as indicated. · See Breathing pattern, ineffective, p. 8.	Effective breathing pattern will be achieved.
Potential impaired gas exchange *Related to:* Loss of lung Altered breathing pattern Retained secretions	**Ongoing Assessment** · Monitor breath sounds. · Note changes in level of consciousness or behavior consistent with hypoxia. · Monitor ABGs. **Therapeutic Interventions** · Administer oxygen as ordered.	Optimal gas exchange will be maintained.

NURSING DIAGNOSES / DEFINING CHARACTERISTICS	NURSING INTERVENTIONS / *RATIONALES*	EXPECTED OUTCOMES
DEFINING CHARACTERISTICS Restlessness Hypoxia Abnormal breath sounds Change in LOC	- Encourage coughing *to remove retained secretions.* - Suction if necessary. - See Gas exchange, impaired, p. 21.	

Pain
Related to:
Incision
 	
DEFINING CHARACTERISTICS
Complaints of pain
Grimacing
Self-imposed limitation on activity
Restlessness
Withdrawal
	ONGOING ASSESSMENT
	- Assess pain:
	    Quality
	    Severity
	    Location
	    Onset
	    Duration
	    Precipitating/relieving factors
	- Solicit techniques patient considers useful in pain prevention/relief.
	- Assess degree to which pain interferes with treatment plan.
	
	THERAPEUTIC INTERVENTIONS
	- Anticipate need for pain medications *to prevent peak episodes of pain and coincide with/facilitate ambulation and breathing exercises.*
	- Use nonpharmacologic methods of pain management (e.g., positioning, distraction, touch).
	- Reinforce techniques to support incision during movement and breathing/coughing.
	- See Pain, p. 39.
		Pain will be reduced.

Anxiety *Related to:* Unknown results of surgical pathology Possible need for further cancer therapy Cancer diagnosis **DEFINING CHARACTERISTICS** Multiple questions Lack of questions Sleep disturbance Facial tension Restlessness Trembling	**ONGOING ASSESSMENT** - Assess patient's anxiety. - Explore previously successful methods of managing anxiety. - Assess presence and helpfulness of social support system in managing anxiety. **THERAPEUTIC INTERVENTIONS** - Encourage ventilation of concerns. - Give accurate concise information as available. - Answer questions simply and honestly. - Repeat information as often as necessary. *Anxious individuals frequently fail to comprehend or remember what they are told or may be "shopping" for more information.* - See Anxiety, p. 4.	Anxiety will be reduced.
Potential for injury: mediastinal shift *Related to:* Void created by removal of diseased lung Shifting of thoracic contents Accumulation of drainage **DEFINING CHARACTERISTICS** Hypoxia Low cardiac output	**ONGOING ASSESSMENT** - Assess for midline position of trachea. - Check vital signs. - Monitor I & O. - Monitor ABGs. **THERAPEUTIC INTERVENTIONS** - Position patient on operated side. *Pooling and consolidation on the operated side are desired outcomes; dependent position facilitates process while enhancing remaining lung function.* - Be prepared to administer resuscitative efforts in event of mediastinal shift. - See Decreased cardiac output, p. 9; Cardiac dysrhythmias, p. 74.	Potential for mediastinal shift is reduced

Continued.

Pneumonectomy—cont'd

NURSING DIAGNOSES / DEFINING CHARACTERISTICS	NURSING INTERVENTIONS / *RATIONALES*	EXPECTED OUTCOMES
Tachycardia Arrhythmias Hypotension Trachea not at midline		

NURSING DIAGNOSES / DEFINING CHARACTERISTICS	NURSING INTERVENTIONS / *RATIONALES*	EXPECTED OUTCOMES
Potential for infection *Related to:* Surgical incision History of radiation and/or chemotherapy Cancer **DEFINING CHARACTERISTICS** Elevated temperature Redness, pain, purulent discharge associated with incision Elevated WBC	**ONGOING ASSESSMENT** · Assess wound condition, noting redness, pain, swelling, or discharge. · Monitor WBC. · Monitor vital signs. · Culture drainage from wound or other invasive sites as ordered. **THERAPEUTIC INTERVENTIONS** · Perform all dressing changes using sterile technique. · Administer antibiotics and antipyretics as ordered. · Encourage high-calorie, high-protein intake. *Development of local and systemic infections is prevalent in malnourished patients and fever increases basal metabolic rate, thereby increasing caloric need.*	Risk of infection will be reduced.

Knowledge deficit
Related to:
No previous similar experience
 	
DEFINING CHARACTERISTICS
Multiple questions
Lack of questions
Verbalized misconception(s)
Behavior(s) indicative of knowledge deficit (e.g., continued smoking)
	ONGOING ASSESSMENT
	· Assess patient's learning readiness.
	· Determine patient's knowledge of etiology of disease and need for behavior modification *to protect remaining lung*.
	
	THERAPEUTIC INTERVENTIONS
	· Instruct patient/significant other about known causes of lung cancer:
	    Cigarette smoking
	    Air pollution
	    Industrial pollutants
	· Stress importance of avoiding these *to protect remaining lung and improve oxygenation*.
	· Instruct patient/significant other to seek professional advice for:
	    Dyspnea
	    Fever/chills
	    Unusual wound drainage/change in wound appearance
	    Loss of appetite/unintentional weight loss
	· Instruct patient/significant other in administration and potential side effects of medications and/or home oxygen.
	· Reinforce need for/encourage compliance with recommended follow-up therapies.
	· Refer patient to American Cancer Society for informational support.
		Patient/significant other will verbalize understanding of posthospitalization care.

Originated by: Debra Terry, RN

Thoracotomy

(CHEST SURGERY; THORACIC SURGERY)

A surgical opening into the thorax for biopsy, excision, drainage, and/or correction of defects.

NURSING DIAGNOSES / DEFINING CHARACTERISTICS	NURSING INTERVENTIONS / *RATIONALES*	EXPECTED OUTCOMES

Potential ineffective breathing pattern *Related to:* Malfunctioning chest tube drainage system Positive pressure in pleural space secondary to surgical incision Collapse of lung on affected side (partial or complete) **Defining Characteristics** Dyspnea Shortness of breath Tachypnea Altered chest excursion	**Ongoing Assessment**
	• Perform complete respiratory assessment and repeat frequently.
	• Obtain vital signs, noting early signs of respiratory insufficiency; document and report abnormal parameters to physician.
	• Perform complete assessment of closed chest drainage system; repeat frequently:
	  Check the H_2O seal for:
	    Correct fluid level
	    Presence/absence of fluctuation. *Absence of fluctuation indicates obstruction or lung reexpansion and must always be investigated.*
	    Presence of air leaks; document and report to physician. *Bubbling in H_2O seal chamber indicates air leak, which may be present because the lung has not yet expanded or because of a persistent air leak. There may be leak in system before H_2O seal drainage (e.g., loose tubing connection or air leak around entrance site of tube).*
	  Check suction control chamber for correct fluid level as specified. *Amount of suction (negative pressure) being applied to pleural space is regulated by amount of fluid in suction control chamber, not amount dialed on Emerson/wall suction.*
	  Measure the output in closed chest drainage system.
	  Accurately report drainage of bright red blood of 100 ml/hr for 2 hr consecutive.
	  Document color, amount, and characteristics of output.
	
	Therapeutic Interventions
	• Position chest drainage system below patient's chest level. *Gravity will aid in drainage and prevent backflow into chest.*
	• Make sure tubing is free of kinks and clots. Milk tubing from insertion site downward.
	• Set Emerson suction machine correctly (if the system is connected to vacuum suction); 30 mm Hg = 20 L/air is recommended. *If system disconnected from vacuum suction, it merely functions as large drain with H_2O seal preventing air from entering pleural space.*
	• Do not clamp chest tubes unless:
	  Physician has ordered clamping
	  Closed chest drainage system is being changed to new system
	  System becomes disconnected or H_2O seal is disrupted. *Clamping chest tubes is dangerous because tension pneumothorax may occur*
		Optimal breathing pattern will be maintained.

Ineffective airway clearance *Related to:* Incisional pain **Defining Characteristics** Complaint of pain Refusal to cough Diminished breath sounds Splinting of respirations	**Ongoing Assessment**
	• Assess patient for subjective complaints of discomfort or pain.
	• Perform respiratory assessment, noting signs of hypoventilation.
	
	Therapeutic Interventions
	• Instruct patient in.
	  Use of pillow or hand splints when coughing
	  Use of "huff" or stair step ventilations and/or spirometry
	  Importance of early ambulation and/or frequent position changes. *These methods will help patient maintain adequate lung expansion, thus preventing buildup of secretions and atelectasis.*
	• Administer medication as ordered, offering pain medication before patient asks for it *to prevent peak periods of pain.*
	• Assist patient with ambulation/position changes. *Note:* Patient with pneumonectomy should never be positioned with remaining lung in dependent position *(would compromise respiratory excursion of remaining lung).*
	• Assist patient in performing coughing and breathing maneuvers q1h.
		Airway will be free of secretions.

Continued.

221

NURSING DIAGNOSES / DEFINING CHARACTERISTICS	NURSING INTERVENTIONS / *RATIONALES*	EXPECTED OUTCOMES
Impaired physical mobility: arm on affected side *Related to:* Incisional pain and/or edema Decreased strength **DEFINING CHARACTERISTICS** Limited ROM Reluctance to attempt movement	**ONGOING ASSESSMENT** · Ask patient to raise arm on affected side laterally, documenting degree of ROM present. **THERAPEUTIC INTERVENTIONS** · Instruct patient to perform arm circles, with arm moving in a 360° arc *(will help maintain mobility and strength to arm on affected side)*. · Document progress.	Full ROM of affected extremity will be attained.
Pain *Related to:* Incisional pain **DEFINING CHARACTERISTICS** Patient report of pain Guarding behavior Relief/distraction behavior (moaning, crying, restlessness, irritability, alteration in sleep pattern) Facial mask of pain Alteration in muscle tone (listless/flaccid; rigid/tense) Autonomic responses not seen in chronic stable pain (e.g., diaphoresis, change in BP, pulse rate, pupillary dilation, increased/decreased respiratory rate, pallor)	**ONGOING ASSESSMENT** · Assess for presence of defining characteristics. · Assess pain characteristics: Quality Severity Location Onset Duration Precipitating/relieving factors **THERAPEUTIC INTERVENTIONS** · Anticipate need for analgesics *to prevent peak periods of pain:* At periodic intervals and before activities (e.g., repositioning, ambulation, coughing, and deep breathing) · Respond immediately to complaints of pain by administering analgesics as ordered, and evaluating effectiveness. · Provide scheduled rest periods *to promote comfort, sleep, and relaxation.*	Discomfort will be relieved.
Knowledge deficit *Related to:* Unfamiliarity with discharge activity **DEFINING CHARACTERISTICS** Patient/significant others unable to restate appropriate discharge activity Patient/significant others verbalize questions/concerns regarding discharge activities	**ONGOING ASSESSMENT** · Assess knowledge base and readiness for learning. **THERAPEUTIC INTERVENTIONS** · Instruct patient/significant others to: Have patient resume normal activities gradually (e.g., begin with short walks rather than stair climbing) as approved by physician. Avoid inhaling noxious or harmful respiratory irritants, especially cigarette smoke. *Respiratory irritants can cause bronchoconstriction with resultant irritating cough and rapid shallow respiratory rate.* Keep follow-up appointments with physician. Report complaint of shortness of breath or dyspnea at once. · Ask the patient/significant others verbally to reiterate activity plan. · Give written discharge information.	Patient will be able to resume activities based on limits of existent pulmonary disease, prevent further damage from respiratory irritants, and recognize signs and symptoms of respiratory distress.

Originated by: Dorothy Lewis, RN,C, BSN

Tracheostomy

A surgical opening into the trachea that is used to prevent or relieve airway obstruction and/or to serve as an access for suctioning and for mechanical ventilation.

NURSING DIAGNOSES / DEFINING CHARACTERISTICS	NURSING INTERVENTIONS / *RATIONALES*	EXPECTED OUTCOMES

Ineffective airway clearance *Related to:* Thick secretions Fatigue; weakness Patient uncooperativeness Patient confusion Tracheostomy **DEFINING CHARACTERISTICS** Increasing restlessness and irritability Change in mental status Pallor, cyanosis Diaphoresis Tachypnea Increased work of breathing: use of accessory muscles, intercostal retractions, nasal flaring	**ONGOING ASSESSMENT**
	 • Assess for evidence of respiratory distress (tachypnea, nasal flaring, and increased use of accessory muscles of respiration).
	 • Assess vital signs q4h and prn. Notify physician if outside prescribed range.
	 • Auscultate chest *for normal and adventitious sounds.*
	 • Assess for changes in mental status (increasing lethargy, confusion, restlessness, and irritability).
	 • Record amount, color, and consistency of secretions.
	
	 THERAPEUTIC INTERVENTIONS
	 • Keep suction equipment and Ambu at bedside.
	 • Provide humidified air *to prevent drying and crusting of secretions:*
	 • Administer O$_2$ as needed.
	 • Encourage patient to cough out secretions.
	 • Institute suctioning of airway as needed *to clear secretions.*
	   Instill 2-5 cc of sterile saline if secretions are thick *(helps loosen secretions and induce coughing).*
	   Administer O$_2$ between suctioning *to prevent hypoxemia.*
	 • Administer stoma care:
	   Clean inner cannula with hydrogen peroxide and saline.
	   Keep stoma clean and dry using sterile dressings.
	   Secure outer cannula with twill tie, using square knot on side of neck.
	 • Keep spare tracheostomy tube of same size and brand at bedside.
	 • Keep tracheal obturator taped at HOB *for emergency use.*
	 • Maintain inflated tracheostomy cuff:
	   Immediately after operation
	   If patient on mechanical ventilation
	   If patient prone to regurgitate and aspirate; cuff should be deflated at other times *to prevent tracheal erosion*
		Patent airway will be maintained.

Potential impaired gas exchange *Related to:* Pneumothorax (during insertion; apices of lungs are at risk for damage) Superimposed infection Copious tracheal secretions Tracheostomy leak **DEFINING CHARACTERISTICS** Shortness of breath Tachypnea Increased work of breathing Anxiety Diaphoresis, pallor Hyperventilation Decreased breath sounds	**ONGOING ASSESSMENT** • Monitor respirations, pulse, and temperature q4h and assess changes. • Assess changes in orientation and behavior pattern. • Auscultate breath sounds q4h. • Monitor ABGs and note changes. • Check tracheostomy cuff for inflation; if leak present, notify physician. **THERAPEUTIC INTERVENTIONS** • Stay with patient; notify physician of signs of respiratory distress. • Maintain adequate airway. • Place patient in semi- to high Fowler's position *to promote full lung expansion.* • Administer humidified O$_2$ as needed *to maintain oxygenation and prevent drying of mucosal membranes.* • If abnormal breath sounds present, use tracheal suction as needed *to clear secretions.* • Assist in proper positioning when portable chest x-ray film is needed *so that entire lung field will be x-rayed and optimal lung expansion will occur.* • Set up chest tube placement as needed *to evacuate air from the pleural cavity and re-expand collapsed lung.*	Adequate gas exchange will be maintained.

Continued.

NURSING DIAGNOSES / DEFINING CHARACTERISTICS	NURSING INTERVENTIONS / *RATIONALES*	EXPECTED OUTCOMES
Adventitious breath sounds Intercostal retractions Fever Tachycardia Audible tracheostomy cuff leak Behavior changes		
Potential altered nutrition: less than body requirements *Related to:* Possible dysphagia secondary to tracheostomy Depression Anorexia Fatigue **DEFINING CHARACTERISTICS** Loss of weight with or without adequate caloric intake > 10-20% under ideal body weight Caloric intake inadequate to keep pace with abnormal disease/metabolic state	**ONGOING ASSESSMENT** · Compare admission weight to present weight. · Obtain nutritional history. · Assess patient's present nutritional intake: oral feeding, enteral, parenteral. **THERAPEUTIC INTERVENTIONS** · If signs of altered nutrition present, see Altered nutrition: less than body requirements, p. 37. · Refer to Enteral feedings, p. 308; Total parenteral nutrition, p. 324, as appropriate.	Optimal nutrition will be maintained
Potential for infection *Related to:* Surgical incision of tracheostomy **DEFINING CHARACTERISTICS** Wound inability to heal Abnormal appearance of wound drainage Purulent wound drainage Fever and chills Elevated WBC count Stoma red, warm, and tender to touch	**ONGOING ASSESSMENT** · Observe stoma for erythema, exudates, odor, and crusting lesions. If present, culture stoma and notify physician. · Assess vital signs q4h; notify physician of abnormalities. · Assess laboratory values of WBC and differential. · Assess for fever and chills; monitor blood cultures. **THERAPEUTIC INTERVENTIONS** · Provide routine tracheostomy care q8h and prn *to prevent airway obstruction and infection.* · Do not allow secretion pooling around stoma. Suction area or wipe with aseptic technique *to keep stoma clean and dry.* · Keep skin under tracheostomy ties clean and dry *to prevent skin irritation.* · Apply hydrocolloid dressing beneath tracheostomy ties *to prevent excoriation.* · If signs of infection present, apply topical antifungal or antibacterial agent as ordered.	Potential for infection will be reduced.

Tracheostomy—cont'd

NURSING DIAGNOSES / DEFINING CHARACTERISTICS	NURSING INTERVENTIONS / *RATIONALES*	EXPECTED OUTCOMES
Impaired verbal communication *Related to:* Tracheostomy **Defining Characteristics** Difficulty in making self understood Withdrawal Restlessness Frustration	**Ongoing Assessment** ▪ Assess patient's ability to understand spoken word. ▪ Assess patient's ability to express ideas. **Therapeutic Interventions** ▪ Provide call light within easy reach at all times. ▪ Obtain room close to nurse's station *to ensure easy staff observation of patient.* ▪ Provide patient with pad and pencil. Use picture or alphabet board for patient unable to write. ▪ Provide patient with reassurance and patience *to allay frustration.* ▪ Consult speech therapist for possible artificial larynx. ▪ See Communication, impaired, p. 11.	Alternative methods of communication will be facilitated.
Knowledge deficit *Related to:* New procedure/ intervention in hospital **Defining Characteristics** Anxiety Lack of questioning Increased questioning Expressed need for more information	**Ongoing Assessment** ▪ Assess patient's/significant others' knowledge of tracheostomy. ▪ Assess patient's/significant others' ability to provide adequate home health care. ▪ Assess interest and readiness to learn. **Therapeutic Interventions** ▪ Discuss patient's need of tracheostomy and its particular purpose. ▪ Begin teaching skills one at a time and reinforce daily. *Patient/significant others can begin to acquire skills at pace that is not overwhelming.* ▪ Provide instruction on sterile tracheostomy care and suctioning; include step-by-step care guidelines.	Patient/significant others will demonstrate skills appropriate for tracheostomy.

Originated by: Pam Harston, RN
Remedios S. Garces, RN, BSN

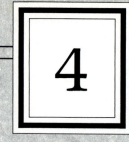

Neurologic Care Plans

DISORDERS
Amyotrophic lateral sclerosis (ALS)
Cerebral artery aneurysm:
   preoperative/unclipped
Consciousness, altered level of
Dementia

Dysphagia
Guillain-Barré syndrome
Intracranial infection
Low back pain
Meningitis
Multiple sclerosis (MS)

Myasthenia gravis: acute crisis phase
Normal pressure hydrocephalus
Parkinsonism
Seizure activity

THERAPEUTIC INTERVENTIONS
Craniotomy

Amyotrophic lateral sclerosis (ALS)

(LOU GEHRIG'S DISEASE; MOTOR NEURON DISEASE; PROGRESSIVE BULBAR PALSY; PROGRESSIVE MUSCULAR ATROPHY)

Amyotrophic lateral sclerosis (ALS), commonly called Lou Gehrig's disease, is a progressive disease that attacks specialized nerve cells called motor neurons, which control the movement of muscles via the anterior horns of the spinal cord and the motor nuclei of the lower brain stem. There is usually progressive paralysis, with death occurring within 3-5 years.

NURSING DIAGNOSES / DEFINING CHARACTERISTICS	NURSING INTERVENTIONS / *RATIONALES*	EXPECTED OUTCOMES

Anxiety
Related to:
Irreversible and terminal disease process
Threat to self-concept
Threat to or change in health status, socioeconomic status, role
 	
DEFINING CHARACTERISTICS
Restlessness
Increased awareness
Increased questioning
Insomnia
Increased glancing about
Increased tension
Scared, wide-eyed appearance
Shakiness
Regretfulness
Focus on self
Poor eye contact
Overexcitement/ jitteriness
Rattled behavior
Distressed behavior
Increased perspiration
Apprehension
Uncertainty
Feelings of inadequacy
Expressed concern about changes in life events
Trembling
Constant demands
	ONGOING ASSESSMENT
	• Assess patient's level of anxiety (mild, severe). Note signs and symptoms, including nonverbal communication.
	• Assess patient's normal coping patterns (by interview with patient/ significant others).
	
	THERAPEUTIC INTERVENTIONS
	• Display confident, calm manner and tolerant, understanding attitude.
	• Establish rapport with patient, especially through continuity of care.
	• Encourage ventilation of feelings, concerns about dependency.
	   Listen carefully; sit down if possible.
	   Give unhurried attentive appearance; be aware of defense mechanisms used (denial, regression, etc.)
	• Review coping skills used in past. *The nurse should be aware of own feelings of anxiety. Acknowledge fear; do not deny or reassure patient that everything will be all right.*
	• Use supportive measures (e.g., medications, clergy, social service).
	• Allow expressions of fear/anxiety without internalizing *(may increase feelings of depression, anxiety, regression, etc.)*
	• Encourage patient to talk; ask open-ended questions *to allow expansion, clarification of feelings.*
	• Provide accurate information about disease, medications, test/procedures, and self-care.
	• Give patient and family compassionate and caring support.
	• Allow expressions of frustrations about loss and eventual outcome. *Depression is normal and expected in this setting.*
	• Understand that patient may have inappropriate behaviors (e.g., outbursts of laughing/crying.)
		Anxiety will be reduced to manageable level.

Ineffective airway clearance *Related to:* Dysarthria Aspiration Progressive bulbar palsy Respiratory muscle atrophy	**ONGOING ASSESSMENT** • Assess breath sounds and respiratory movement q2h or more often as indicated. • Observe for signs of respiratory distress (e.g., increased respiratory rate; restlessness). • Observe for signs/symptoms of infection (change in sputum color, amount, character; increased WBC). • Observe for shallow or absent respirations requiring artificial ventilation (see Ineffective airway clearance, p. 3).	Effective airway clearance is maintained.

Continued.

NURSING DIAGNOSES / DEFINING CHARACTERISTICS	NURSING INTERVENTIONS / *RATIONALES*	EXPECTED OUTCOMES
DEFINING CHARACTERISTICS Patient report of breathing difficulty Abnormal breath sounds: rales (crackles), rhonchi, wheezes Periods of apnea	**THERAPEUTIC INTERVENTIONS** • Elevate head of bed (HOB); change position q2h and prn. • Increase fluid intake to 2000 ml daily within level of cardiac reserve *to keep secretions thin and promote lung expansion.* • Encourage warm liquids *(loosen secretions).* • Discourage use of oil-based products around nose *to prevent aspiration into lungs.* • Suction as needed.	
Impaired gas exchange, *Related to:* Aspiration Dysarthria **DEFINING CHARACTERISTICS** Sense of impending doom Headache Dyspnea Restlessness Irritability Hypoxia Hypercarbia	**ONGOING ASSESSMENT** • Note respiratory rate, depth, use of accessory muscles, pursed-lip breathing. • Auscultate breath sounds; note areas of decreased as well as adventitious breath sounds. • Assess level of consciousness (LOC), mentation changes. • Monitor vital signs q4h. • Monitor ABGs. • See Impaired gas exchange, p. 21. **THERAPEUTIC INTERVENTIONS** • *Promote optimal chest expansion and drainage of secretions* by frequent position changes and encouragement of deep breathing/coughing exercises, HOB elevated. • Maintain I & O *for mobilization of secretions but avoid fluid overload.* • Provide/monitor oxygen therapy as ordered. • If patient mechanically ventilated, see Mechanical ventilation, p. 213.	Gas exchange will be maximized.
Impaired physical mobility *Related to:* Increasing motor weakness caused by paralysis Spasticity of extremities Limited ROM Fatigue Neuromuscular impairment Imposed restrictions of movement **DEFINING CHARACTERISTICS** Intolerance to activity, decreased strength and endurance Inability to move purposefully within the physical environment (including bed mobility, transfer, and ambulation) Impaired coordination, limited ROM, decreased muscle strength control, and/or muscle mass	**ONGOING ASSESSMENT** • Assess ROM, muscle strength, previous activity level, gait, coordination, and movement. • Assess patient's current level of dependence. • Assess patient's requirements for assistive devices, amount of help in transfer from bed or chair to bathroom. • Evaluate patient's ability to perform ADL. • Assess patient's endurance in performing ADL. **THERAPEUTIC INTERVENTIONS** • Position patient for optimum comfort and *to facilitate ventilation and prevent skin breakdown.* Reposition regularly. • Maintain adequate exercise program: active/passive ROM *to prevent venous stasis, maintain joint mobility and good body alignment, and prevent foot-drop and contractures.* • Provide skin care every day and prn. Wash and dry skin well; use gentle massage and lotion *to stimulate circulation.* • Encourage patient's and significant other(s)' involvement in care: help them learn ways to manage problems of immobility. • Refer to physical therapy as indicated. • Alternate periods of activity with adequate rest periods *to prevent fatigue.* • Encourage participation in activities, occupational/recreational therapy. • Provide safety measures as indicated by individual situation. • See Impaired physical mobility, p. 35.	Optimal physical mobility will be maintained.

NURSING DIAGNOSES / DEFINING CHARACTERISTICS	NURSING INTERVENTIONS / RATIONALES	EXPECTED OUTCOMES

Urinary retention, incontinence
Related to:
Neuromuscular impairment
Urinary tract infection
 	
DEFINING CHARACTERISTICS
Incontinence
Frequency
Retention
Dysuria
Nocturia
Urgency
	ONGOING ASSESSMENT
	· Assess patient's ability to sense need to void.
	· Monitor amount and frequency of output.
	· Monitor for signs of urinary tract infection: burning, frequent voiding of ≤100 cc of foul-smelling cloudy urine.
	· Assess need for assistive devices:
	  Diapers
	  External catheter (males)
	· Check frequently for bladder distention; observe for overflow/dribbling *to prevent complications of infection and/or autonomic hyperflexia.*
	
	THERAPEUTIC INTERVENTIONS
	· Institute appropriate bladder training program, depending on patient's amount of control.
	· *Prevent bladder overdistention* by use of indwelling or intermittent catheter.
	· Investigate alternatives (e.g., intermittent catheterization, drugs, voiding maneuvers, use of diapers, external catheters) when possible.
	· Maintain acidic environment by use of vitamin C, cranberry juice *to discourage bacterial growth.*
	· Instruct patient in perineal exercises *to help strengthen sphincter control.*
	· Encourage significant other(s) to participate in routine care.
	  Encourage patient to limit fluids after 6 p.m. *(decreases need to void at night).*
	  Instruct/assist to void at precise timed intervals *to prevent overdistention and strengthen perineal muscles.*
	  Monitor I & O for at least 24 hr when indwelling catheter removed.
	  Wake to void at night.
	  Respond to call light quickly if patient unable to delay voiding.
	  Offer/assist with urinal/bedpan/commode.
	· Instruct in complications necessitating interventions.
		Adequate bladder emptying is achieved.

Constipation, incontinence *Related to:* Impaired neuromuscular control Physical immobility Inadequate fluid intake **DEFINING CHARACTERISTICS** Abdominal pain Urgency Frequency Inability to retain feces Lack of awareness of need to defecate Passage of watery stools	**ONGOING ASSESSMENT** · Auscultate abdomen for presence, location, and characteristics of bowel sounds every shift. · Assess diet and nutritional status. · Check for fecal impaction. · Identify pathophysiologic factors present. **THERAPEUTIC INTERVENTIONS** · Decrease stress/anxiety. · Provide for changes in dietary intake that may precipitate diarrhea. · Administer drugs as indicated *to decrease gastrointestinal motility and minimize fluid loss.* · Encourage oral intake of fluids (e.g., juices or commercial preparations [Gatorade] and bouillion.) · Maintain perianal skin integrity. · Do pericare with each bowel movement. · Apply lotion/ointment/skin barrier as needed. · Expose area to air. · Encourage increased intake in bulk/fiber. · Give stool softeners as indicated/needed. · Promote exercise program as individually able *to increase muscle tone/strength.* · Establish bowel program: regular time for defecation (usually 30 min after eating), glycerine suppositories, and/or digital stimulation.	Normal bowel pattern/function is re-established-maintained.

Continued.

Amyotrophic lateral sclerosis—cont'd

NURSING DIAGNOSES / DEFINING CHARACTERISTICS	NURSING INTERVENTIONS / RATIONALES	EXPECTED OUTCOMES
Altered nutrition: less than body requirements *Related to:* Progressive bulbar palsy Tongue atrophy/ weakness Dysphagia Decreased salivation **DEFINING CHARACTERISTICS** Dysphagia (difficulty in swallowing) Loss of appetite Loss of weight Choking during meals	**ONGOING ASSESSMENT** • Assess swallowing, presence/absence of gag reflex daily. • Assess nutritional status. • Inquire about food and fluid preferences. • Assess weight loss; inquire about weight gain/loss over past few weeks/ months. • Assess tissue turgor, mucous membranes, muscular weakness, and tremors. • Evaluate serum electrolyte reports, total protein albumin levels for imbalance. • See Nutrition, altered: less than body requirements, p. 37. **THERAPEUTIC INTERVENTIONS** • Encourage intake of food patient can swallow; provide frequent small meals and supplements. • Instruct patient not to talk while eating. • Encourage patient to chew thoroughly and eat slowly. • Maintain patient in high Fowler's position during and after meals *to minimize risk of aspiration.* • Provide sufficient fluids with meals. *Decreased salivation makes swallowing of certain foods difficult.* • Prepare environment *so that it will be well ventilated, uncluttered, cheerful, distraction-free.*	Adequate nutritional intake is maintained.

Impaired verbal communication
Related to:
Dysarthria
Tongue weakness
Nasal tone to speech
 	
DEFINING CHARACTERISTICS
Difficulty in articulating words
Inability to express self clearly
	ONGOING ASSESSMENT
	• Determine the degree of speech difficulty by assessing:
	   Ability to speak spontaneously
	   Endurance of ability to speak
	• Assess patient's ability to use alternative methods of communication (i.e., spelling board, finger writing, eye blinks, signal system, word cards).
	• See Impaired communication, p. 11.
	
	THERAPEUTIC INTERVENTIONS
	• Use close-ended questions requiring only yes/no response *to minimize effort, conserve energy, and decrease anxiety.*
	• Allow patient time to respond.
	• Anticipate needs *to decrease feelings of helplessness.*
	• Consult speech therapist for additional help.
	• Praise accomplishments.
	• Offer family opportunity to ask questions about communication problem.
	• Inform patient/family about dysarthria and its effects on speech and language ability.
		Alternate methods of communication are facilitated.

Impaired skin integrity *Related to:* Immobility Increasing motor weakness Progressive muscular paralysis Urinary/fecal incontinence External, mechanical factors (e.g., shearing) Altered circulation Altered metabolic state	**ONGOING ASSESSMENT** • Assess skin color, temperature, texture, turgor, moisture daily. • Assess for presence/absence of skin breakdown. • Assess current skin care rendered. • See Skin integrity, p. 48 impairment of actual/potential. **THERAPEUTIC INTERVENTIONS** • Document signs of tissue ischemia (redness and changes in skin color); treat immediately. • Maintain skin hygiene, using mild soap, drying gently and thoroughly, and lubricating with lotion or emollient as indicated. • Massage around bony prominences gently. • Administer adequate nutrition and hydration. • Use skin barriers (e.g., Duoderm) on skin exposed to irritating secretions, excretions *for protection.* • Provide prophylactic pads, pillows, waterbeds *to increase circulation to skin and alter/eliminate pressure.*	Optimal skin integrity will be maintained.

NURSING DIAGNOSES / DEFINING CHARACTERISTICS	NURSING INTERVENTIONS / RATIONALES	EXPECTED OUTCOMES
DEFINING CHARACTERISTICS Disruption of skin surface Destruction of skin layers Altered sensation Altered skin turgor (change in elasticity)	• Turn and reposition q1-2h. • Provide passive ROM exercises, especially when patient immobile. • Keep bedclothes dry; use nonirritating materials; keep bed free of wrinkles, crumbs, etc. • Assist patient/significant other(s) to learn importance of effective skin care in preventing problems.	
Knowledge deficit *Related to:* Unfamiliarity with disease process and management **DEFINING CHARACTERISTICS** Lack of questions Multiple questions Misconceptions	**ONGOING ASSESSMENT** • Assess patient's/significant others' knowledge of disease process, diagnostic tests, treatment, outcome. • Evaluate knowledge/awareness of community support groups **THERAPEUTIC INTERVENTIONS** • Provide information about: Disease process: *Progressive degenerative motor disease of unknown cause that interferes with motor activities (may include lower cranial nerves: swallowing, speech, and respiration).* Diagnostic testing: EMG, muscle biopsy, pulmonary function, etc. Home care planning Nutrition Communication aids ALS support groups: ALS Society of America 15300 Ventura Blvd., Ste. 315 Sherman Oaks, CA 91403 National ALS Foundation, Inc. 185 Madison Ave. New York, NY 10016 Muscular Dystrophy Assoc., Inc. 810 Seventh Ave. New York, NY 10019	Patient/family demonstrate knowledge of ALS, progressive course, nutritional and respiratory needs, and available community resources.

Originated by: Lela Starnes, RN

Cerebral artery aneurysm: preoperative/unclipped

(SUBARACHNOID HEMORRHAGE [SAH]; INTRAPARENCHYMAL HEMORRHAGE; INTRACRANIAL ANEURYSM)

Thin-walled blisters, 2 mm to 3 cm in size, protruding from the arteries of the circle of Willis or its major branches, located predominantly at bifurcation of vessels. It is presumed to be the result of developmental defects in the media and elastica. The intima bulges outward, covered only by adventitia, and eventually rupture may occur.

NURSING DIAGNOSES / DEFINING CHARACTERISTICS	NURSING INTERVENTIONS / *RATIONALES*	EXPECTED OUTCOMES

Altered cerebral tissue perfusion *Related to:* Subarachnoid hemorrhage Ruptured aneurysm Vasospasm Cerebral edema
 	
 DEFINING CHARACTERISTICS
 Severe headache (unlike any experienced before) Unconsciousness: transitory or lasting Nuchal rigidity Mental confusion, drowsiness Seizures Transitory or fixed neurologic signs (numbness, speech disturbance, paresis) Hypertension, *which may accentuate or aggravate any vascular weakness, although not necessarily a causative factor in aneurysm development or rupture*
	ONGOING ASSESSMENT
	 • Complete an initial assessment of patient's symptoms. *Time of onset is important in assessing time of initial bleed and subsequent hemorrhages, and it may influence timing of surgery.*
	 • Complete baseline assessment of neurologic status and deficits.
	 • Assess for seizure activity, noting:
	     Time of onset
	     Localization of seizure
	     Postictal state
	 • Assess for meningeal signs:
	     Nuchal rigidity
	     Photophobia
	
	 THERAPEUTIC INTERVENTIONS
	 • Administer anticonvulsants as ordered:
	     Dilantin: PO/IV. Give slow IV push *(not faster than 50 mg/min). Cannot be given in D_5W (precipitation occurs). Must be given slowly to prevent cardiac arrhythmias/arrest.*
	     Valium: Give slow IV infusion, *no faster than 10 mg/min, to prevent respiratory arrest.* Also monitor heart rate and BP.
	     Phenobarbital: PO/IV/IM 100-200 mg/day in divided doses. *May cause drowsiness.*
	 • Place patient on bed rest in private room if possible *to allow quiet environment, minimize startling noises that may increase BP.*
	 • Keep lighting subdued *because of photophobia associated with subarachnoid hemorrhage.*
	 • Limit visitors.
	 • Administer stool softeners *to prevent straining, which may increase intracranial pressure (ICP).*
	 • Administer antihypertensive agents as ordered.
	 • Encourage liquid intake if cardiovascular status and electrolytes within normal limits. *Dehydration seems to have an adverse effect on cerebral vasospasm.*
		Maximal cerebral perfusion will be achieved.

Altered levels of consciousness *Related to:* Vascular spasm/ ischemia Hemorrhage or re-bleed Cerebral edema Hydrocephalus	**ONGOING ASSESSMENT** • Assess for signs of altered levels of consciousness. • Record serial assessments. *LOC is most sensitive and reliable index of change in patient with neurologic disease or injury.* **THERAPEUTIC INTERVENTIONS** • Maintain airway patency. *Hypoxia and/or hypercapnea can cause increased cerebral blood flow and intracranial pressure.* • See Consciousness, altered level of, p. 234.	Optimal state of consciousness will be maintained.

NURSING DIAGNOSES / DEFINING CHARACTERISTICS	NURSING INTERVENTIONS / *RATIONALES*	EXPECTED OUTCOMES
DEFINING CHARACTERISTICS Change in alertness, orientation, verbal response, eye opening, motor response, memory impairment, judgment impairment, agitation, inappropriate affect, impaired thought processes, Glasgow Coma Scale Score < 11		
Potential for injury *Related to:* Alterations in autoregulation Elevated BP **DEFINING CHARACTERISTICS** Systolic BP < 100 or > 150 mm Hg Diastolic BP < 60 or > 90 mm Hg Mean BP < 90 or > 100 mm Hg	**ONGOING ASSESSMENT** · Closely monitor BP and other hemodynamics, including central venous pressure (CVP), PCWP, cardiac output. **THERAPEUTIC INTERVENTIONS** · Provide bed rest and quiet environment by closing doors, keeping lights low and noise level minimum, and limiting visitors. Provide private room if possible. · Administer antihypertensives as ordered; keep BP in prescribed range. *Sodium nitroprusside may be used initially. Changing to oral antihypertensives requires caution (possibility of sudden hypotension with methyldopa or clonidine therapy).*	Risk for rebleed will be reduced.
Knowledge deficit *Related to:* Unfamiliarity with pathology, treatment, prevention of rebleed **DEFINING CHARACTERISTICS** Multiple questions Lack of questions Misconceptions	**ONGOING ASSESSMENT** · Assess level of understanding. · Assess readiness for learning. **THERAPEUTIC INTERVENTIONS** · Explain possible causes of hypertension to patient/significant others. · Explain to patient/significant others rationale for limitation of length and frequency of visits *to provide most quiet and restful environment possible to prevent excitement/stimulation associated with changes in BP and ICP.* · Explain to patient/significant others need to avoid nicotine. *Nicotine has vasospastic effect on blood vessels; thus increases risk of hemorrhage or vasospasm.* · Explain necessity to avoid Valsalva's maneuver. Stress importance of exhaling when pulled up in bed and avoiding coughing and straining at stool. Provide stool softener if necessary. · Teach patient/family about diet and stress management: Diet: low-salt, low-fat Stress: understanding cause of stress and ways to prevent/cope · Discuss studies (e.g., computerized axial tomography [CAT], cerebral angiography, cerebral blood flow) ordered and explain each to patient/family	Patient will understand diagnostic process, treatment, and prevention of rebleed.
Potential for injury *Related to:* Complications of antifibrinolytic therapy **DEFINING CHARACTERISTICS** Deep vein thrombosis	**ONGOING ASSESSMENT** · Monitor patient for side effects of drug. Monitor coagulation studies. · Monitor for signs/symptoms of: Deep vein thrombosis: pain in lower extremities, positive Homan's sign, increased extremity circumference, increased temperature Dehydration: decreased CVP (< 5 cm H_2O), poor skin turgor, dry mucous membranes Pulmonary emboli: dyspnea, tachycardia, wheezing, chest pain, hemoptysis, right axis deviation on ECG. If pulmonary infarct occurs, pleural effusion, friction rub, and fever may be noted	Risk of complications of antifibrinolytic therapy will be reduced.

Continued.

Cerebral artery aneurysm: preoperative/unclipped—cont'd

NURSING DIAGNOSES / DEFINING CHARACTERISTICS	NURSING INTERVENTIONS / RATIONALES	EXPECTED OUTCOMES
Dehydration as result of volume contraction Pulmonary emboli Side effects of aminocaproic acid (Amicar) therapy: headache, dizziness, nausea, tinnitus, cramps, skin rash, diarrhea, malaise	**THERAPEUTIC INTERVENTIONS** • Administer antifibrinolytic agents as ordered *(inhibit fibronolysis; prevent clot degradation and potential rebleed:* Aminocaproic acid: initial dose 5 g orally or by *slow* IV infusion followed by 1-2 g/h. Total daily dose 36-48 g/24 hr. • Replace fluid, as ordered, *to prevent dehydration.* • Explain purpose of drug therapy to patient/significant others. • Explain possible side effects of drug to patient/significant others: nausea, cramps, diarrhea, dizziness, headache, rash, deep vein thrombosis, pulmonary emboli.	
Impaired physical mobility *Related to:* Prolonged bed rest **DEFINING CHARACTERISTICS** Inability to move purposefully within physical environment Decreased muscle strength Imposed restriction of movement (e.g., medical protocol)	**ONGOING ASSESSMENT** • Assess muscle strength and coordination. • See Impaired physical mobility, p. 35. **THERAPEUTIC INTERVENTIONS** • Encourage deep breathing exercises 10 times/hr while awake. • Encourage foot plantar flexion and dorsiflexion exercises 10 times/hr when awake. *These exercises stimulate antagonistic muscle groups, promote venous flow, and help decrease bone demineralization.* • Instruct patient and family to avoid Valsalva maneuver. As patient is turned or pulled up in bed, instruct to exhale *to prevent straining and increased ICP, increased BP.* • Instruct to avoid isometric and vigorous active ROM exercises in preoperative period *to minimize possibility of increasing BP.* • Instruct patient and family in activity restrictions.	Optimal physical mobility will be maintained with reduced risk of hypertension and rebleed.

Originated by: Carol Ann Rooks, RN, BSN

Consciousness, altered level of

(COMA; IMPAIRED MENTAL STATUS; UNRESPONSIVENESS)

Normal consciousness can be defined as the condition of the normal person when awake. In this state, the patient is fully responsive to stimuli and indicates by behavior and speech that he/she has an accurate awareness of himself/herself and the environment. There are two components of consciousness: (1) arousal or wakefulness, which reflects the integrity of the reticular activating system (RAS) located in the upper brain stem and diencephalon; and (2) cognition or awareness, which reflects the integrity of the cortical cerebral hemisphere.

NURSING DIAGNOSES / DEFINING CHARACTERISTICS	NURSING INTERVENTIONS / RATIONALES	EXPECTED OUTCOMES
Altered level of consciousness *Related to:* *Structural:* Stroke Head trauma Tumor Cerebral edema Increased ICP	**ONGOING ASSESSMENT** • Assess level of consciousness/responsiveness as indicated. • Determine contributing factors to any change (e.g., anesthesia, medications, awakening from sound sleep, not understanding questions). • Assess patient's/significant others' understanding of events surrounding change in LOC. • Assess potential for physical injury. • Assess vital signs, especially respiratory status.	Optimal state of consciousness will be maintained.

NURSING DIAGNOSES / DEFINING CHARACTERISTICS	NURSING INTERVENTIONS / *RATIONALES*	EXPECTED OUTCOMES
Metabolic: Anoxia Profound hypogly- cemia Hypercalcemia **DEFINING CHARACTERISTICS** Change in alertness, orientation, verbal response, eye open-ing in response to command, motor response Memory judgment Impaired judgment Agitation Inappropriate affect Impaired thought pro-cesses Glasgow Coma Scale Score < 11	**THERAPEUTIC INTERVENTIONS** · Record serial assessments. Report/record change or deterioration. · Keep side rails up at all times, bed in low position, and functioning call light within reach. · If restraints are needed, patient must be positioned on side, never on back. *Restraints should be used judiciously (may increase agitation/anxiety and contribute to increased ICP).* · Reorient to environment as needed *to decrease apprehension and anxiety. Short-term memory may be affected by pathologic etiology.* · Explain all nursing activities before initiating. · Protect patient from possible injury (seizure activity, decreased corneal re-flex, decreased blink, decreased gag reflex, airway obstruction/aspiration). · Avoid contributing to confusion/disorientation by agreeing with misinter-pretations. *Reality orientation decreases false sensory perception and en-hances patient's sense of personal dignity and self-esteem.* · Use calendars, television, radio, clocks, lights *to help with reorientation.* · Call neurologic resource personnel if instructions needed. · Involve patient/significant others in goal setting and care planning. · Encourage significant others to provide familiar things (e.g., pictures, paja-mas). · Consult rehabilitation medicine and social service departments as needed. · Encourage and support verbalization by patient and significant others.	

Originated by: Marilyn Magafas, RN,C, BSN, MBA
Karen Moyer, RN, MS, CCRN, CNA
Kathryn S. Bronstein, RN, PhD, CS
Linda Arsenault, RN, MSN, CNRN

Dementia

(ALZHEIMER'S DISEASE; MULTI-INFARCT DEMENTIA [MID])

Dementia: Evidence of intellectual dysfunction related to a variety of factors, including some pathophysiologic factors. Approximately 5% of persons > 65 years of age suffer from dementia. Alzheimer's disease: An irreversible disease of the central nervous system that manifests as a cognitive dis-order. The etiology of Alzheimer's disease is unknown. This care plan addresses needs for patients with a wide variety of dementia, of which Alzheimer's is a type.

NURSING DIAGNOSES / DEFINING CHARACTERISTICS	NURSING INTERVENTIONS / RATIONALES	EXPECTED OUTCOMES

Potential for vio-lence: self-directed or directed at oth-ers
Related to:
Impaired perception of reality
Impaired frustration tolerance
Decreased self-esteem
Perceived threat to self
	ONGOING ASSESSMENT
	· Assess *cognitive* factors that may contribute to development of violent be-haviors, including:
	    Decreased ability to solve problems
	    Alteration in sensory/perceptual capacities
	    Impairment in judgment
	    Psychotic or delusional thought patterns
	    Impaired concentration or decreased response to redirection
	· Assess *physical* factors:
	    Physical discomfort
	    Sensory overload (overstimulation)
	    Changes in body posture (increased muscle tension, making fists, guard-ing self)
		Potential for violence will be reduced.

Continued.

Dementia—cont'd

NURSING DIAGNOSES / DEFINING CHARACTERISTICS	NURSING INTERVENTIONS / *RATIONALES*	EXPECTED OUTCOMES

Alteration in sleep/rest pattern
Impaired self-expression, verbal and nonverbal
Anxiety
Impaired coping skills
Decreased sense of personal boundaries
Drug intoxication or idiosyncratic reaction
hysical discomfort
Overstimulation
 	
DEFINING CHARACTERISTICS
Nonaggressive behaviors:
  Wandering/pacing
  Restlessness/ increased motor activity
  Climbing out of bed
  Changing clothes/ disrobing
  Pulling at dressing/ tubes
  Handwringing/ handwashing
Verbally aggressive behaviors, including:
  Cursing
  Yelling
  Screaming
  Unintelligible/ repetitious speech
  Threatening/ accusing
Physically aggressive behaviors, including:
  Hitting
  Kicking
  Spitting/biting
  Throwing objects
  Pushing/pulling others
  Fighting
	Motor activity/restlessness/repetitive behaviors
	Changes in tone of voice
	• Assess *emotional* factors:
	  Inability to cope with frustrating situations
	  Expressions of low self-esteem
	  Noncompliance with treatment plan
	  History of aggressive behaviors as means of coping with stress
	
	THERAPEUTIC INTERVENTIONS
	• Involve patient on a cognitive level as much as possible. Begin with least restrictive measures and progress to most restrictive measures
	  Level I: Nonaggressive behaviors
	    Give verbal feedback and institute interpersonal approaches.
	    Consider environmental measures to be taken *to reduce sensory stimulation.*
	    Evaluate impact of medication regimen on behaviors in terms of contribution to agitation. *Neuroleptics may cause extrapryamidal side effects (EPS), manifested as restlessness.* Consider use of medications prescribed for agitation.
	    Speak in slow, clear, soothing tones. Make comments brief and to the point.
	    Consider distracting the patient.
	  Level II: Verbally aggressive behaviors:
	    Consider use of verbal control; may be feedback about behavior (for less cognitively impaired), distraction (for cognitively impaired), or limit setting (although this may increase agitation at times).
	    Consider allowing patient more personal space. If memory span is short, leaving room briefly may decrease agitation.
	    Acknowledge fear of loss of control; evaluate use of touch and hand holding.
	    If wandering/pacing behaviors present, evaluate need to provide visual supervision, especially if patient expresses need to leave unit.
	    Provide diversional activity (e.g., folding towels, handling worry beads, walking with the patient).
	  Level III: Physically aggressive behaviors:
	    Permit verbalization of feelings associated with agitation.
	    Offer acceptable alternatives to behaviors such as undressing by suggesting that patient dress.
	    If patient poses potential threat of injury to self or others, consider use of physical restraints.
	    Use soft restraints such as cloth wrist, hand, leg, belt, or vest types (restraints always used in conjunction with full side rails secured in the up position). Refer to policy and procedure manual for application of restraints.
	    Use leather restraints only if agitation has reached point that soft restraints inadequate to protect patient from injury.	

Bathing/grooming, feeding self-care deficit:
Related to:
Alteration in cognition, including:
  Impaired memory
  Disorientation
  Memory deficits
  Impaired judgment
  Impaired sense of social self
	ONGOING ASSESSMENT
	• Assess cognitive deficits/behaviors that would create difficulty in:
	  Bathing self
	  Performing oral hygiene
	  Selecting and putting on appropriate clothing
	  Choosing food menu items and feeding self
	• Assess level of independence in completing self-care.
	• Assess need for supervision/redirection during self-care.
	
	THERAPEUTIC INTERVENTIONS
	• Stay with patient during self-care activities if judgment is impaired *to promote safety and provide necessary redirection.*
		Self-care abilities are maximized.

NURSING DIAGNOSES / DEFINING CHARACTERISTICS	NURSING INTERVENTIONS / *RATIONALES*	EXPECTED OUTCOMES

DEFINING CHARACTERISTICS
Requires assistance with at least one of the following:
  Bathing
  Oral hygiene
  Dressing/grooming
  Feeding
Denies need for personal hygiene measures
Refuses to change clothes or wears more than one set
Unable to assist in personal care because of motor deficits/confusion
	• Provide simple, easy-to-read list of self-care activities to complete each day (brush teeth, comb hair, etc.).
	• Assist, as needed, with perineal care each morning and evening (or after each episode of incontinence).
	• Assist, as needed, in selecting clothing. Allow patient to choose if at all possible.
	• Encourage to dress as independently as possible. Provide easy-to-wear clothes (elastic waistbands, snaps, large buttons, Velcro closures) *to facilitate*.
	• Assist in selection of nutritious, high-bulk foods. Allow patient to choose food he/she prefers if possible *to promote adequate intake*.
	• Assist in setup of meal as needed (opening containers, cutting food).
	• If judgment is impaired, cool hot liquids to palatable temperatures before serving.
	• Limit number of choices of food on plate or tray *to reduce number of necessary decisions*.
	• Provide easy-to-eat finger foods if motor coordination impaired.
	• Provide nutritious between-meal snacks if nutritional intake inadequate.
	• Follow established routines for self-care if possible.
	• If patient refuses a task, use distraction techniques; break the task into smaller steps; use calm, unhurried voice to offer praise and encouragement. Humor also works sometimes.	

Impaired social interaction
Related to:
Alteration in cognition, including:
  Impaired sense of social self
  Memory deficits
  Impaired judgment
  Disorientation
  Social isolation
 	
DEFINING CHARACTERISTICS
Change in patterns of social interaction, including:
  Language/behaviors inappropriate to social situations
  No relationships with others
	ONGOING ASSESSMENT
	• Assess cognitive deficits/behaviors that interfere with forming relationships with others.
	• Assess previously adaptive patterns of interaction.
	• Assess potential to interact in community day care situation after discharge.
	
	THERAPEUTIC INTERVENTIONS
	• Within context of nurse-patient relationship, provide regular opportunity for frequent brief contacts.
	• Discuss subjects in which patient is interested, but which do not require extensive recall.
	• When discussing past experiences, assist patient in connecting them with here-and-now.
	• Support participation in social activities appropriate to patient's level of cognitive functioning.
	• Redirect patient when behaviors become socially embarrassing.
	• If patient expresses delusional ideas, focus on reality-based interactions. Do not correct patient's ideas or confront them as delusional.
	• Consider impact of milieu on social interaction. Avoid milieu that is overstimulating (noise, lights, activity, etc.).
	• Involve patient in developing a daily schedule that includes time for social activity and quiet time. Consider patient's talents, interests, and abilities when developing daily program.
	• Provide information on community day-care programs *that will help patient maintain social interaction*.
		Social interaction is enhanced.

Impaired home maintenance/ management
Related to:
Alteration in cognition:
  Impaired memory
  Disorientation
  Memory deficits
	ONGOING ASSESSMENT
	• Assess cognitive deficits/behaviors making it difficult to:
	  Prepare meals
	  Feed self
	  Use utensils
	  Cut food
	  Drink from cup
	  Recognize signs of hunger
	  Maintain attention while eating
		Aspects of home maintenance/ management will be adequately addressed.

Continued.

Dementia—cont'd

NURSING DIAGNOSES / DEFINING CHARACTERISTICS	NURSING INTERVENTIONS / *RATIONALES*	EXPECTED OUTCOMES
DEFINING CHARACTERISTICS Requires assistance with at least one of the following: 　Food/fluid intake 　Personal hygiene/ dressing 　Toileting Disorientation in familiar surroundings Need for supervision in potentially hazardous situations Family caregiver concerns about caring for patient at home	• Assess level of independence in completing: 　Bathing/oral hygiene 　Dressing/grooming 　Toileting • Assess frequency of: 　Disorientation 　Wandering 　Becoming lost in familiar surroundings • Assess motor, sensory, and cognitive deficits to determine safety needs. • Assess family/caregiver's: 　Understanding of patient's needs/deficits 　Resources to provide adequate supervision and behavior management 　Ability to cope 　Internal/external support systems **THERAPEUTIC INTERVENTIONS** • Involve patient/family/caregiver in all home planning. • Identify alternate methods of meal preparation to facilitate independent feeding (e.g., finger foods, group dining if available, precooked meals, home-delivered meals). • Discuss potential need for supervision of ADLs, including feeding. • Discuss ways to minimize environmental hazards in home. • Discuss need to wear identification bracelet at all times. • Assist in developing daily schedule that allows rest and activity periods. • Suggest daily supervised exercise/walking program *to decrease wandering behavior*. • Teach about home security devices *to decrease chances of patient's wandering from home*. • Recommend procedure for getting help should patient become lost. • Identify and encourage correction of obstacles/hazards in home. • Help family identify and mobilize available support networks *to facilitate home patient care*. • Provide information about support groups available to family members. • Provide literature/references related to caring for cognitively impaired persons in home. • Discuss available home health and community services. • See Home maintenance/management, impaired, p. 27.	
Altered patterns of urinary elimination: potential incontinence *Related to:* Alteration in cognition Neurogenic bladder Lack of sensation or urge to void **DEFINING CHARACTERISTICS** Inability to control urination Palpable bladder Residual urine of more than 50 cc Dribbling	**ONGOING ASSESSMENT** • Assess *physiologic* factors that may contribute to incontinence pattern, including: 　Urinary frequency/urgency 　Urinary retention 　Distended bladder 　Symptoms of urinary tract infection (UTI) 　Amount voided, color and odor of urine • Assess *behavioral* factors that may contribute to incontinence pattern, including: 　Impaired judgment 　Disorientation 　Agitation 　Depression 　Decreased attention span • Assess for perineal skin integrity. • Obtain specimens and residual urine as indicated. **THERAPEUTIC INTERVENTIONS** • Maintain record of intake and output, including pattern of voiding. • Report symptoms of UTI or urinary retention to physician. • Push fluids (depending on medical status). • Medicate as prescribed and assess response to medication.	Reasonable pattern/ method of urinary elimination is achieved.

NURSING DIAGNOSES / DEFINING CHARACTERISTICS	NURSING INTERVENTIONS / *RATIONALES*	EXPECTED OUTCOMES
	• Maintain patency of external or indwelling catheters if in place. • Administer diuretic medication in morning if ordered; *be aware that administration of diuretics and psychotropic medications may alter urinary elimination.* • Establish bladder program acceptable to patient/caretaker. • Direct patient to toilet q2-3h during day. • Use urinal/bedside commode at night. • Reduce fluid intake after 8 p.m. • *Maintain skin integrity* by assisting the patient as needed in perineal care after each voiding. • Request and use protective skin creams as needed. • Use protective clothing and incontinent pads as necessary during day. *Incontinence pads are available in several forms and sizes from simple sanitary napkin size to adult diaper size.* • Avoid using incontinent pads (obstruct air flow to perineal area at night). • See Urinary tract infections, p. 361; Urinary retention, p. 61.	

Potential bowel incontinence
Related to:
Alteration in cognition
Spontaneous bowel evacuation
Low-bulk diet
Chronic constipation
Immobility
 	
DEFINING CHARACTERISTICS
Uncontrolled bowel elimination
Lack of sensation or urge to eliminate
Abdomen firm or distended
Bowel evacuation in socially unacceptable places
	ONGOING ASSESSMENT
	• Assess *physiologic* factors that may contribute to incontinence, including:
	  Constipation
	  Diarrhea
	  Frequent expulsion of small amounts of formed stool
	  Alteration in baseline bowel sounds
	  Alteration in frequency of bowel elimination patterns
	• Assess *behavioral* factors that may contribute to incontinence, including:
	  Impaired judgment
	  Disorientation
	  Agitation
	  Depression
	  Decreased attention span
	• Assess skin integrity in perineal and buttock areas.
	
	THERAPEUTIC INTERVENTIONS
	• Maintain daily record of bowel elimination. Note amount, consistency, and frequency:
	  Consider patient's food preferences when planning diet high in bulk and fiber.
	  Provide fluid intake (depending on medical status).
	  Involve patient in daily exercise program.
	  Establish bowel program that may include bulk laxatives, stool softeners, suppositories, or enemas if necessary.
	  Locate patient near a bathroom and clearly mark the door "Bathroom".
	• Take patient to toilet after breakfast *to take advantage of increased bowel motility at this time.*
	• Provide privacy.
	• Be aware of nonverbal cues that may indicate patient need to evacuate the bowel (e.g., restlessness, pulling clothes, holding hand over the rectal area, and using fingers to disimpact stool from the rectum).
	• Use incontinence pads and protective clothing as necessary during daytime.
	• Avoid using incontinence pads (*obstruct air flow to buttock area*) at night.
	• Be aware that *many psychotropic medications used to control agitated behaviors may contribute to constipation.*
		Establishment of regular bowel evacuation pattern will be achieved.

Originated by: Kim Mackey, RN, BS
Sylvia Kupferer, RN, MS

Dysphagia

(IMPAIRED SWALLOWING; POTENTIAL FOR ASPIRATION)

The state in which an individual has decreased ability to pass fluids and/or solids from the mouth to the stomach voluntarily.

NURSING DIAGNOSES / DEFINING CHARACTERISTICS	NURSING INTERVENTIONS / *RATIONALES*	EXPECTED OUTCOMES
Altered nutrition: less than body requirements *Related to:* *Neuromuscular:* Decreased or absent gag reflex Decreased strength or excursion of muscles involved in mastication Perceptual impairment Facial paralysis *Mechanical:* Edema Tracheostomy tube Tumor Fatigue Limited awareness Reddened irritated oropharyngeal cavity (stomatitis) **DEFINING CHARACTERISTICS** Documented inadequate caloric intake Weight loss Loss of appetite Regurgitation of food	**ONGOING ASSESSMENT** Swallowing: • Assess presence/absence of gag and cough reflexes. • Assess strength of facial muscles. • Assess for residual food in mouth after eating. • Assess regurgitation of food/fluid through nares. • Assess choking during eating/drinking. Nutritional status: • Inquire about food and fluid preferences. • Observe for drooling or complaint about appetite. Weight loss: • Assess patient's admission weight and compare to normal range for age and height. • Inquire about weight gain/loss over past few weeks/months. • Document amount of weight loss since diagnosed. • Evaluate and document 24-hr oral I & O. • Compare normal caloric requirements and body weight to present. Dehydration: • Assess tissue turgor, mucous membranes, muscular weakness, and tremors. • Evaluate serum electrolyte reports, total protein, and albumin levels and imbalances. **THERAPEUTIC INTERVENTIONS** • Before mealtime, provide adequate rest periods. *Fatigue can further contribute to swallowing impairment.* • Remove or reduce environmental stimuli (television, radio) *so patient can concentrate on swallowing.* • Provide analgesics, if appropriate, before feeding *so patient is relaxed and can concentrate.* • Provide oral care before feeding. Clean and insert dentures before each meal. • Place suction equipment at bedside *(aspiration is potential complication).* • If decreased salivation is contributing factor: Before feeding, swab oral cavity with lemon-glycerin or encourage patient to suck tart-flavored hard candy. *Tart flavors stimulate salivation.* Use artificial saliva. *During feeding:* • Encourage intake of food patient can swallow; provide frequent small meals and supplements. *Foods with consistency of pudding, hot cereal, and semisolid food are most easily swallowed because of consistency and weight. Thin foods are most difficult; gravy or sauce added to dry foods facilitates swallowing.* • Instruct patient not to talk while eating. • Encourage patient to chew thoroughly and eat slowly. Provide patient with direction/reinforcement until he/she has swallowed each mouthful *to keep focus on task.* • Maintain patient in high Fowler's position with head flexed slightly forward during meals. *Upright position facilitates gravity flow of food/fluid through alimentary tract. Aspiration less likely to occur with head tilted slightly forward (position narrows airway).* • Encourage high-calorie diet that includes all food groups, as appropriate. Avoid milk, milk products, and chocolate *(can lead to thickened secretions.)*	Adequate nutritional intake will be achieved.

NURSING DIAGNOSES / DEFINING CHARACTERISTICS	NURSING INTERVENTIONS / *RATIONALES*	EXPECTED OUTCOMES

	• Identify food given to patient before each spoonful.
	• Proceed slowly, giving small amounts; whenever possible, alternate servings of liquids and solids *to help prevent foods from being left in the mouth*.
	• If food is pouched, encourage patient to turn head to unaffected side and manipulate tongue to paralyzed side *to clean out residual food*.
	• If patient has had a cerebrovascular accident (CVA):
	    Place food in back of mouth, on unaffected side.
	    Gently massage unaffected side of throat.
	• Place whole or crushed pills in custard, gelatin, etc. (First ask pharmacist which pills should not be crushed).
	• Encourage patient to feed self as soon as possible.
	• If oral intake not possible or inadequate, initiate alternative feedings (e.g., nasogastric feedings, gastrostomy feedings, hyperalimentation).
	Follow-up:
	• Initiate dietary consultation for 72-hr calorie count, food preferences.
	• Initiate speech pathology consultation for swallowing impairment evaluation and patient assistance.	

Potential ineffective breathing pattern *Related to:* Pulmonary aspiration **DEFINING CHARACTERISTICS** Dyspnea Shortness of breath Tachypnea Fremitus Cyanosis Cough Nasal flaring Respiratory depth changes Altered chest excursion Use of accessory muscles Pursed-lip breathing/ prolonged expiratory phase Increased anteroposterior diameter	**ONGOING ASSESSMENT** • Assess gag reflex before each feeding. • Assess patient's ability to swallow small amount of water *(if aspirated, little or no harm to patient occurs)*. • Assess breath sounds and respiratory status q4h *for clinical evidence of aspiration*. **THERAPEUTIC INTERVENTIONS** • Maintain patent airway. • Stay with patient during feeding as appropriate. • Assist and teach patient to maintain position best suited to optimal lung expansion. • Encourage slow deep breathing exercises 10 times/hr while awake *to promote full lung expansion and prevent atelectasis*. • Suction prn. *With impaired swallowing reflexes, secretions can rapidly acumulate in posterior pharynx and upper trachea and increase risk of aspiration*. • See Ineffective breathing pattern, p. 8.	Risk of aspiration is reduced.

Knowledge deficit
Related to:
New problem (dysphagia)
New nutritional needs
 	
DEFINING CHARACTERISTICS
Inability to practice good nutritional habits
Multiple questions
Lack of questions
	ONGOING ASSESSMENT
	• Assess the following:
	    Swallowing difficulty and cause
	    Patient's ability to feed self
	    Family knowledge
	    Nutrition knowledge
	
	THERAPEUTIC INTERVENTIONS
	• Inform patient/significant others of problem and its effect on swallowing.
	• Discuss with and demonstrate to patient/significant others the following:
	    Avoidance of certain foods or fluids
	    Upright position during eating
	    Allowance of time to eat slowly and chew thoroughly
	    Provision of high-calorie meals
		Patient and significant other will verbalize/ demonstrate understanding of adequate nutritional intake.

Continued.

NURSING DIAGNOSES / DEFINING CHARACTERISTICS	NURSING INTERVENTIONS / *RATIONALES*	EXPECTED OUTCOMES
	Use of fluids to help facilitate passage of solid foods	
	Monitoring of patient for weight loss or dehydration. *Fluid intake should equal 2-3 L/day; weight loss of 5 lb/wk over 2 wk should be reported to physician*	
	• Facilitate dietary counseling from hospital dietitian.	
	• Help patient/significant other set realistic goals *to prevent feelings of frustration and disappointment.*	
	• Provide name and telephone number of primary nurse and physician and information on when to call.	
	• Instruct significant others in emergency techniques for choking *so they can intervene should aspiration occur.*	
	• Discuss feelings about body image and life-style changes.	

Originated by: Patsy McDonald, RN

Guillain-Barré syndrome

Guillain-Barré syndrome is a rapidly evolving, reversible, paralytic illness of unknown origin. The disease is thought to be autoimmune and has been reported to be related to the occurrence of varicella, Epstein Barr virus, and swine flu vaccines and to follow respiratory or gastrointestinal illnesses, mumps, and mycoplasma pneumonia. The disease occurs as a result of destruction of peripheral nerve myelin sheaths. The onset of neurologic symptoms is abrupt, with a tendency for the paralysis to ascend the body symmetrically. Paralysis may last 4 weeks or longer. Recovery tends to be slow.

NURSING DIAGNOSES / DEFINING CHARACTERISTICS	NURSING INTERVENTIONS / *RATIONALES*	EXPECTED OUTCOMES
Ineffective breathing pattern *Related to:* Increasing weakness of respiratory muscles Progression to total motor paralysis resulting in respiratory failure	**ONGOING ASSESSMENT** • Assess respiratory rate, pattern, and depth. • Monitor tidal volume and vital capacity daily and prn. *A significant amount of respiratory muscle insufficiency may exist without being apparent clinically.* • Monitor ABGs and watch closely for development of hypercapnia and hypoxia. • Observe for mental status changes *(may indicate change in adequacy of ventilation).*	Optimal breathing pattern will be maintained.
DEFINING CHARACTERISTICS Shortness of breath Decreasing tidal volume Decreasing vital capacity Dyspnea Tachypnea Hypercapnia Hypoxia Change in mental status	**THERAPEUTIC INTERVENTIONS** • Elevate head of bed (HOB) *for optimal ventilatory excursion.* • Anticipate need for intubation and mechanical ventilation if respirations become shallow with decreasing tidal volume and vital capacity. *Intercostal and diaphragmatic paralysis produces progressive alveolar hypoventilation, which can occur within 36 hr. Patient may not be disturbed by weakness because of gradual onset and slow progression.* • See Mechanical ventilation, p. 213, as appropriate.	

Guillain-Barré syndrome—cont'd

NURSING DIAGNOSES / DEFINING CHARACTERISTICS	NURSING INTERVENTIONS / *RATIONALES*	EXPECTED OUTCOMES
Potential for aspiration: *Related to:* Ascending muscle paralysis **DEFINING CHARACTERISTICS** Depressed gag and cough reflexes Dysphagia	**ONGOING ASSESSMENT** • Assess for presence of gag and cough reflexes every shift. • Assess for difficulty in swallowing every shift and before oral intake. *Paralysis of the ninth and tenth cranial nerves may occur.* **THERAPEUTIC INTERVENTIONS** • Notify physician immediately of noted decreases in cough and gag reflexes or difficulty in swallowing. *Early intervention protects airway and prevents aspiration.* • Assist patient with oral intake *to detect abnormalities early.*	Aspiration will be prevented.
Ineffective airway clearance *Related to:* Increasing muscle weakness Loss of gag or cough reflex **DEFINING CHARACTERISTICS** Abnormal breath sounds (rales, rhonchi, wheezes) Changes in respiratory rate or depth Cough Cyanosis Dyspnea	**ONGOING ASSESSMENT** • Auscultate lungs for breath sounds every shift. • Assess respiratory rate and depth. • Assess effectiveness and productivity of cough. **THERAPEUTIC INTERVENTIONS** • Elevate HOB *to promote effective coughing.* • If cough ineffective, use oropharyngeal or tracheal suction as needed *to clear secretions.* • Anticipate need for intubation and mechanical ventilation *to maintain airway.* • See Mechanical ventilation, p. 213.	Airway clearance will be maintained.
Potential decrease in cardiac output *Related to:* Vasomotor instability Autonomic dysfunction that reflects involvement of myelinated preganglionic fibers and ganglia. **DEFINING CHARACTERISTICS** Instability of BP (increased or decreased) Dysrhythmias Decreased peripheral pulses Confusion, agitation, restlessness Anxiety Fatigue, lethargy	**ONGOING ASSESSMENT** • Monitor BP and heart rate continuously. • Continuously monitor ECG rhythm for dysrhythmia development. • Assess peripheral pulses. • Observe for profuse diaphoresis or loss of sweating. • Observe for mental status changes and signs of fatigue/lethargy. • Monitor pulmonary artery wedge pressure and cardiac output, as available. **THERAPEUTIC INTERVENTIONS** • Administer inotropic medications as ordered *to maintain hemodynamic parameters* (heart rate, BP, cardiac output, CVP, pulmonary artery pressures). *Patients are prone to labile heart rate and BP as a result of autonomic dysfunction.* • Place patient on sequential or Venodyne pump to legs *to increase venous return, decrease peripheral pooling of blood, and decrease risk of thrombosis.* • Maintain adequate ventilation; provide O_2 as needed.	Cardiac output will be maximized.

Impaired physical mobility
Related to:
Muscle weakness or total paralysis as a result of disease process
	ONGOING ASSESSMENT
	• Assess motor strength and reflexes, checking for:
	  Level of progression
	  Symmetry
	  Ascending paralysis
	  Paresthesia
	• Assess baseline ROM; note deterioration or improvement.
		Optimal physical mobility will be maintained.

Continued.

■ **Guillain-Barré syndrome—cont'd**

NURSING DIAGNOSES / DEFINING CHARACTERISTICS	NURSING INTERVENTIONS / *RATIONALES*	EXPECTED OUTCOMES
DEFINING CHARACTERISTICS Symmetrical weakness Hyporeflexia Ascending paralysis Verbalized generalized weakness	**THERAPEUTIC INTERVENTIONS** • Turn and reposition patient q2h. • Maintain limbs in functional alignment and begin passive ROM *to prevent contractures.* • Use physical therapy *to help maintain muscle tone.*	
Potential impairment of skin integrity *Related to:* Complete bed rest Impaired physical mobility Paresthesia **DEFINING CHARACTERISTICS** Stage I: redness, skin intact Stage II: blisters Stage III: necrosis Stage IV: necrosis involving joints, bones, and body cavities	**ONGOING ASSESSMENT** • Assess skin integrity every shift, noting color, moisture, texture, and temperature. **THERAPEUTIC INTERVENTIONS** • Maintain good skin care, keeping skin clean and moist. • Turn q2h according to established schedule. • Provide prophylactic use of pressure-relieving devices *to help prevent skin breakdown.*	Skin integrity will be maintained.
Altered nutrition: less than body requirements *Related to:* Dysphagia Paralysis **DEFINING CHARACTERISTICS** Loss of weight with or without adequate caloric intake Documented inadequate caloric intake Caloric intake inadequate to keep pace with abnormal diseases/metabolic rate	**ONGOING ASSESSMENT** • Obtain nutritional history. • Obtain daily weights. • Assess nutritional needs, consulting dietitian when appropriate. **THERAPEUTIC INTERVENTIONS** • See Enteral tube feeding, p. 282; Total parenteral nutrition, p. 297, as appropriate.	Optimal caloric intake will be maintained.
Constipation *Related to:* Increasing muscle weakness/paralysis **DEFINING CHARACTERISTICS** Decrease in soft formed stools Abdominal pain Fecal impaction Abdominal distention Nausea/vomiting	**ONGOING ASSESSMENT** • Assess bowel sounds every shift. • Assess frequency of bowel movements, checking color, consistency, and amount. • Observe for nausea/vomiting, abdominal pain, or distention. • Assess for presence of fecal impaction, as needed. **THERAPEUTIC INTERVENTIONS** • Provide adequate fluid intake as ordered *to prevent dehydration.* • Administer prescribed medications, as needed. • See Constipation, p. 12.	Constipation will be prevented.

Guillain-Barré syndrome—cont'd

NURSING DIAGNOSES / DEFINING CHARACTERISTICS	NURSING INTERVENTIONS / *RATIONALES*	EXPECTED OUTCOMES
Anxiety/fear *Related to:* Change in health status Fear of unknown **DEFINING CHARACTERISTICS** Restlessness Fear Crying Trembling Withdrawal Facial tension	**ONGOING ASSESSMENT** - Assess level of fear/anxiety. - Assess normal coping patterns (by interview with patient/significant other). **THERAPEUTIC INTERVENTIONS** - Display a confident, calm manner *to reassure patient.* - Allow patient to verbalize feelings through talking, writing, or using alphabet board. - Keep patient informed of condition and treatment regimen *to help decrease anxiety.* - Reduce distracting stimuli *to provide quiet environment.* - Provide diversional activities (e.g., television, books, radio, magazines) as appropriate.	Anxiety/fear will be reduced.
Knowledge deficit *Related to:* New disease **DEFINING CHARACTERISTICS** Request for information Multiple questions Lack of questions	**ONGOING ASSESSMENT** - Assess readiness to learn. - Assess current knowledge of illness. - Assess level of understanding of therapeutic regimen. **THERAPEUTIC INTERVENTIONS** - Ensure physical comfort and maintain quiet atmosphere *to provide environment conducive to learning.* - Establish rapport with patient and significant other. - Explain disease process as simply as possible. - Inform patient/significant other of treatment regimen. *Patient/significant other must be aware that prognosis for recovery is good, but recovery tends to be slow.*	Patient/significant other will state a basic understanding of disease and its treatment.

Originated by: Pamela Paramore, RN, BSN
              Susan Galanes, RN, MS, CCRN

Intracranial infection

(ENCEPHALITIS; BRAIN ABSCESS; CENTRAL NERVOUS SYSTEM INFECTION)

Intracranial infection may be the result of encephalitis (inflammation of the brain/meninges) or abscess (a localized collection of pus in the brain or its membranes).

NURSING DIAGNOSES / DEFINING CHARACTERISTICS	NURSING INTERVENTIONS / *RATIONALES*	EXPECTED OUTCOMES
Hyperthermia *Related to:* Brain infection Encephalitis Brain abscess **DEFINING CHARACTERISTICS** Fever 39° C or > 102° F Increased WBC Nuchal rigidity Altered level of consciousness (LOC)	**ONGOING ASSESSMENT** - Monitor temperature q4h. - Monitor WBC daily or as ordered. - Evaluate LOC. - Evaluate motor-sensory status. - Monitor peak/trough levels of antibiotics as ordered. - Monitor I & O. - Monitor serum Na and osmolality (*index of hydration/dehydration*) as ordered. - Check and record urine specific gravity. *Patient may become dehydrated because of fever and conservative fluid administration with concern for cerebral edema.* - Monitor IV insertion site closely for signs of infiltration, thrombosis, phlebitis.	Normothermia will be maintained.

Continued.

Intracranial infection—cont'd

NURSING DIAGNOSES / DEFINING CHARACTERISTICS	NURSING INTERVENTIONS / *RATIONALES*	EXPECTED OUTCOMES
Irritability Motor-sensory abnormalities Chills Malaise Headache Localized redness/swelling (e.g., along a suture line or area of injury)	**THERAPEUTIC INTERVENTIONS** · Administer tepid sponge baths prn for temperature $> 39°$ C. · Apply cooling blanket for temperature $> 39.5°$ C. · Administer antipyretics as ordered; document patient response. *Fever increases cerebral metabolic demand.* · Provide mouth care and lubrication q1h. · Administer antibiotics on strict administration schedule *to maintain therapeutic blood levels, reduce virulence, eradicate pathogen, and prevent swings in antibiotic blood levels.* · Change IV site per hospital policy.	
Potential for seizures *Related to:* Cerebral irritation Focal edema Cerebritis Ventriculitis **DEFINING CHARACTERISTICS** Involuntary repetitive motor/sensory movement/spasticity Repetitive psychomotor activity Change in alertness, orientation, verbal response, eye opening, motor response. Aspiration of oral secretions/gastric fluid, food.	**ONGOING ASSESSMENT** · Monitor for seizure activity. · Monitor anticonvulsant levels. · Evaluate patency of airway, monitor rate, and rhythm of respirations. **THERAPEUTIC INTERVENTIONS** · Document seizure pattern and frequency of occurrence. Notify physician as appropriate (i.e., *first seizure, repetitive seizures; seizure pattern that varies may indicate need for anticonvulsant medications re-evaluation and/or further neurologic evaluation*). · After motor activity has ceased, roll patient to side/semiprone position *to promote gravity drainage of secretions.* · Suction prn *to prevent aspiration.* · Administer anticonvulsants as ordered. · See Seizure activity, p. 263.	Potential for physical injury will be reduced.

Altered cerebral tissue perfusion
Related to:
Cerebral edema
Increased intracranial pressure
 	
DEFINING CHARACTERISTICS
Headache
Vomiting
Change in LOC (confusion, disorientation, somnolence, lethargy, coma)
Pupillary changes
Impaired memory, judgment, thought processes
Glasgow Coma Scale score < 11
Seizures
Motor sensory deficits
	ONGOING ASSESSMENT
	· Evaluate neurologic parameters as follows:
	    Assess LOC, Glasgow Coma Scale.
	    Determine factors contributing to LOC change (i.e., *awakening from sleep, sedation, seizure*).
	    Monitor pupillary size, reaction to light.
	· Monitor motor strength and coordination.
	· Assess ability to follow simple/complex commands.
	· Evaluate presence/absence of protective reflexes: swallow, gag, blink, cough, etc.
	
	THERAPEUTIC INTERVENTIONS
	· Ask patient to tell you his/her name, location, month/year.
	· Record Glasgow Coma Scale score serially.
	· Report persistent deterioration in LOC. *If LOC decreases, treatment may need to be changed, new treatment instituted, or additional tests obtained.*
	· Reorient to environment prn.
	· Position with HOB elevated 30-45° with head in neutral alignment. *If actual/potential increased ICP, positioning with elevated HOB will promote venous outflow from brain and help decrease ICP.*
	· See Altered level of consciousness, p. 234.
		Optimal cerebral tissue perfusion will be maintained.

NURSING DIAGNOSES / DEFINING CHARACTERISTICS	NURSING INTERVENTIONS / *RATIONALES*	EXPECTED OUTCOMES
Altered nutrition: less than body requirements *Related to:* Altered level of consciousness Infection with increased metabolic activity	**ONGOING ASSESSMENT** • Monitor caloric intake and food; record every meal. *Provides objective data on types, amounts consumed.* • Monitor appropriate laboratory parameters (i.e., serum albumin, iron, total protein, and electrolytes) 2-3 times/wk. • Monitor I & O every shift.	Optimal caloric intake will be maintained.
DEFINING CHARACTERISTICS Weight loss (10-20% of ideal body weight) Decreased serum albumin Decreased serum transferrin or total iron binding capacity Decreased total protein Electrolyte imbalance Poor appetite/intake	**THERAPEUTIC INTERVENTIONS** • Weigh patient on admission and qod. • Assist with meals prn. • Elevate HOB for meals and for 1 hr after meals. *Helps prevent epigastric discomfort/feeling of fullness and minimize potential for aspiration.* • Provide adaptive/assistive devices (plate guard, special padded utensils, splints). • Encourage family/friends to visit. *Being with others may promote PO intake; others may be able to encourage/assist.* • Consult dietitian as appropriate. • See Altered nutrition: less than body requirements, p. 37.	
Knowledge deficit *Related to:* New treatment Possible surgical drainage	**ONGOING ASSESSMENT** • Assess patient's/significant others' knowledge base and readiness for teaching/learning. • Assess patient's mental status (orientation, thought processes, memory, insight, judgment). • See Knowledge deficit, p. 33.	Patient/significant others will verbalize a basic understanding of medical diagnosis, treatment, and safety measures.
DEFINING CHARACTERISTICS Patient/significant others verbalize questions/concerns Incorrect/inaccurate information conveyed	**THERAPEUTIC INTERVENTIONS** • Provide explanations at patient's/significant others' level of understanding. • Encourage patient's/significant others' questions. • Instruct patient/significant others in principles of antibiotic therapy, effects and possible side effects, maintenance of therapeutic levels, and duration of treatment. *This involves patient/significant others, making them educated consumers, and helps decrease anxiety/fear.*	

Originated by: Linda Arsenault, RN, MSN, CNRN

Low back pain

(DISK HERNIATION; SPINAL STENOSIS; BACK TRAUMA)

A syndrome characterized by pain and tenderness in the muscles or their attachments in the lower lumbar, lumbosacral, or sacroiliac regions. Pain may be referred to one or both legs if nerve root compression occurs. This phenomenon is called radiculopathy. The most common cause is intervertebral disk herniation. Other causes of low back pain include uterine or prostatic disorders, infection, arthritis, and metastatic cancer.

NURSING DIAGNOSES / DEFINING CHARACTERISTICS	NURSING INTERVENTIONS / *RATIONALES*	EXPECTED OUTCOMES
Altered neurologic status *Related to:* Disk herniation (herniated nucleus pulposus) Spinal stenosis Osteoarthritis Mechanical instability Back trauma Infection Metastatic cancer	**ONGOING ASSESSMENT** • Evaluate history/onset: Injury/spontaneous Work-related Unknown • Assess neurologic and vascular status of lower extremities: Pulses Temperature Movement and strength Sensation Equality of foot strength Pratt's symptom, Homan's sign Reflexes (knee, ankle, Babinski)	Optimal neurologic functioning will be achieved.
DEFINING CHARACTERISTICS Low back pain Radiating pain into lower extremities Paresthesia Weakness in lower extremity Bladder/bowel incontinence Decreased/absent deep tendon reflex Limited straight leg raising Urinary retention	• Assess bladder/bowel functioning: I & O Dribbling Incontinence Rectal sphincter tone Retention • Inquire about previous episodes, hospitalization, and treatment: Bed rest Pelvic traction Transcutaneous nerve stimulation Heat/massage Exercise program Medications • Inquire about previous tests, dates, and results, if known: Myelogram CT scan Electromyogram Lumbosacral x-ray studies Sedimentation rate Magnetic resonance imaging (MRI) scan • Inquire about previous surgery for low back pain: Chemonucleolysis Lumbar laminectomy Fusion • Inquire about location of pain/radiation: Location Aggravating factors Alleviating factors **THERAPEUTIC INTERVENTIONS** • Reinforce need for bed rest as indicated. • Provide bedside commode or assist patient to bathroom as needed. • Apply pelvic traction: 15-20 lb 4 times/day as ordered. • Elevate knees about 10-20 degrees *to relieve sciatic stretch and promote comfort.* • Assist patient with application of lumbosacral corset, if appropriate, *to promote proper body alignment.*	

NURSING DIAGNOSES / DEFINING CHARACTERISTICS	NURSING INTERVENTIONS / *RATIONALES*	EXPECTED OUTCOMES

	• Evaluate motor strength, reflexes, sensory status q4-6h *for improvement or deterioration of neurologic status.*
	• Teach and encourage the following exercises q1h:
	   Quad sets (isometric contraction of anterior thigh muscles with knee in extension)
	   Ankle ROM
	   Toe movement
	• Send patient to physical therapy via stretcher if indicated.	

Pain *Related to:* Low back pain Disk herniation Muscle spasm, strain **Defining Characteristics** Complaints of discomfort Decreased physical activity Slow, guarded movement Irritability, restlessness, altered sleep pattern Palpable muscle spasm	**Ongoing Assessment** • Evaluate for signs of discomfort. • Inquire about previous episodes, hospitalization, and treatment. **Therapeutic Interventions** • Anticipate need for pain medication/muscle relaxant as ordered; document effects. *Attention to pain relief promotes trust, increases confidence, and facilitates patient independence.* • Apply heating pad with setting on low heat as ordered. • If characteristics are present, see Pain, p. 39.	Pain will be relieved or discomfort reduced.
Impaired physical mobility *Related to:* Pain Muscle weakness Imposed bed rest **Defining Characteristics** Difficulty with movement and position changes; inability to move Reluctance to attempt movement Limited ROM Decreased muscle strength	**Ongoing Assessment** • Evaluate for signs of alteration in mobility. • Assess for potential complications of immobility (e.g., phlebitis, pulmonary embolism, altered skin integrity). **Therapeutic Interventions** • If signs of altered mobility are present, see Impaired physical mobility, p. 35.	Complications associated with immobility will be reduced.

Knowledge deficit
Related to:
Unfamiliarity of causes of low back pain and rehabilitation of back
 	
Defining Characteristics
Multiple questions
Misconceptions
	Ongoing Assessment
	• Evaluate patient's knowledge of:
	   Body mechanics (bending from waist, lifting objects, rotating spine)
	   Cause of low back pain (if known)
	   ADL
	   Discharge instructions
	
	Therapeutic Interventions
	• Discuss causes of low back pain (e.g., *repeated stress on lower back, poor body mechanics.*)
	• Define disk herniation.
	• Discuss symptoms of disk herniation (e.g., *lower back pain, radiation of pain, weakness, changes in sensation.*)
		Patient/significant others will be able to verbalize/demonstrate understanding of low back pain, potential causes, and recommended ADL modifications.

Continued.

■ **Low back pain—cont'd**

NURSING DIAGNOSES / DEFINING CHARACTERISTICS	NURSING INTERVENTIONS / *RATIONALES*	EXPECTED OUTCOMES
	• Discuss recommended alterations in life-style:	
	When to return to work; when to resume driving	
	Date and time of follow-up appointment	
	Name and telephone number of physician	
	Recreational restrictions	
	• Discuss exercises for muscle strengthening. *Strong muscles help support back; proper muscle tone can improve posture and reduce chances of recurring muscle strain:*	
	Isometric abdominal and gluteal muscle exercises begin 7-10 days after surgery	
	Flexion-extension exercises initiated per physician's instructions	
	• Discuss ADL guidelines with patient:	
	Sleeping: *Recommend a firm mattress. Sleeping on the side with knees and hips flexed is preferable to sleeping on the back or abdomen.*	
	Bathing: Showers are preferable to tub baths. *If tub baths important to patient, instruct in avoiding flexing lower back when getting into and out of tub.*	
	Bending: Instruct patient to squat rather than bend at waist.	
	Lifting: When physician allows resumption of lifting (recommend not more than 20 lb) instruct patient to squat, hold object close to body, straighten knees, and *never* lift anything heavy above waist.	
	Reaching: Instruct patient not to reach or strain to pick up object; to rise to level required; to avoid movements such as bending backward, twisting to reach telephone, or crouching over desk.	
	Sexual activities: Recommend abstinence for about 3 wks. Then for about 8-12 wk, the patient should assume underlying position with pillow under buttocks. Alternative: woman lies on side with knees bent, man lying behind and facing back.	
	If lower back pain occurs, instruct patient to go to bed and rest back.	

Originated by: Vicki Chester, RN, BSN, MBA
              Linda Arsenault, RN, MSN, CNRN

Meningitis

(MENINGOENCEPHALITIS; MENINGOCEREBRITIS)

Inflammation/infection of the membranes of the brain or spinal cord caused by bacteria, viruses, or other organisms. Encephalitis is an inflammation or infection of the brain and meninges.

NURSING DIAGNOSES / DEFINING CHARACTERISTICS	NURSING INTERVENTIONS / *RATIONALES*	EXPECTED OUTCOMES
Altered cerebral tissue perfusion *Related to:* CNS infection Cerebral edema Hydrocephalus Increased intracranial pressure (ICP)	ONGOING ASSESSMENT • Assess for signs of infection: Fever Increased WBC Chills Emesis • Assess for meningeal signs: Nuchal rigidity Headache Pain with flexion or neck	Optimal cerebral perfusion will be maintained.

NURSING DIAGNOSES / DEFINING CHARACTERISTICS	NURSING INTERVENTIONS / *RATIONALES*	EXPECTED OUTCOMES

DEFINING CHARACTERISTICS
Fever
Elevated WBC
Rash
Chills
Emesis
Seizures
Nuchal rigidity
Headache
Photophobia
Impaired mentation
	Kernig's sign
	Brudzinski's sign
	Photophobia
	Hyperirritability
	• Assess for neurologic deficits:
	    Change in LOC using Glasgow Coma Scale
	    Cranial nerve paresis
	    Seizure activity
	
	THERAPEUTIC INTERVENTIONS
	• Report temperature > 39° C.
	• Maintain normothermia with tepid sponge bath and antipyretics or hypothermia blanket as ordered.
	• Document baseline and serial neurologic assessment q1-4h. Report alteration in mentation, seizures, bradycardia, increasing BP *(one or more of these events may indicate increasing intracranial pressure with decrease in cerebral perfusion pressure)*.
	• Administer antibiotics and antiemetics as ordered.
	• Isolate patient if appropriate (e.g., *bacterial meningitis for 24-48 hr after start of antibiotic therapy)*.	

Pain
Related to:
Meningeal irritation
Increased ICP
 	
DEFINING CHARACTERISTICS
Headache
Photophobia
Nuchal rigidity
Irritability
	ONGOING ASSESSMENT
	• Assess for:
	    Headache
	    Photophobia
	    Restlessness
	    Irritability
	• Evaluate response to analgesics.
	
	THERAPEUTIC INTERVENTIONS
	• Restrict visitors as appropriate.
	• Reduce noise in environment.
	• Keep patient's room darkened and ask family to bring in sunglasses *to minimize effects of photophobia*.
	• Administer analgesics as ordered.
	• Discourage Valsalva maneuver (e.g., *instruct patient to exhale when moving up in bed; provide stool softeners to prevent increased cerebral blood flow and increased ICP)*.
	• See Pain, p. 39.
		Comfort will be maintained.

Potential fluid volume deficit *Related to:* Reduced LOC Lack of oral intake Fever **DEFINING CHARACTERISTICS** Poor skin turgor Increased urine specific gravity Decreased urine output Change in mental status Tachycardia Hypotension Increased BUN Hypernatremia	**ONGOING ASSESSMENT** • Assess skin turgor. *Loss of interstitial fluid causes loss of skin elasticity.* • Monitor intake and output. • Monitor weight. *Changes may reflect fluid volume changes.* • Monitor serum electrolytes, urine specific gravity, and blood urea nitrogen (BUN). **THERAPEUTIC INTERVENTIONS** • Encourage fluid intake as appropriate. Patient may require intravenous or nasogastric feedings. *To ensure hydration, average daily fluid loss is 1500 cc urine, 200 cc stool, and 700 cc perspiration/respiration/insensible water loss.* • Provide oral care, lubrication to lips. • Document and report changes in BP, heart rate. *Reduction in circulating blood volume can cause changes in vital signs.*	Optimal fluid volume will be maintained.

Continued.

NURSING DIAGNOSES / DEFINING CHARACTERISTICS	NURSING INTERVENTIONS / *RATIONALES*	EXPECTED OUTCOMES
Increased serum osmolality Increased urine specific gravity		
Potential altered nutrition: less than body requirements *Related to:* Reduced oral intake Vomiting Loss of appetite **DEFINING CHARACTERISTICS** Weight loss Documented reduction in intake	**ONGOING ASSESSMENT** - Assess patient's ability to swallow. - Inquire about food and fluid preferences. - Assess patient's admission weight and compare to normal range for age and height. - Monitor I & O. - Compare normal caloric requirements for body weight to present weight. - Weigh every other day. **THERAPEUTIC INTERVENTIONS** - Encourage food intake. Provide frequent small meals and supplements as tolerated. *Patient may experience sense of fullness related to decreased digestive secretions or altered glucose metabolism. Smaller meals may facilitate gastric emptying and improve appetite.* - Administer IV fluids as ordered. - Assist patient with eating as appropriate. - Provide adaptive or assistive devices as needed. - Consult dietitian when appropriate. - See Altered nutrition: less than body requirements, p. 37.	Weight loss will be reduced and nutritional requirements maintained.
Knowledge deficit *Related to:* Lack of prior similar experience **DEFINING CHARACTERISTICS** Probing questions Request for information	**ONGOING ASSESSMENT** - Assess patient's/significant other's current knowledge - Assess readiness for learning. **THERAPEUTIC INTERVENTIONS** - Discuss need for calm, quiet environment and restriction of visitors *to conserve energy and minimize discomfort.* - Discuss course/prognosis as appropriate. - Identify exposed contacts; refer for prophylactic treatment if appropriate. - See Knowledge deficit, p. 33.	Patient will understand disease process.

Originated by: Kathryn S. Bronstein, RN, PhD, CS
Linda Arsenault, RN, MSN, CNRN

Multiple sclerosis (MS)

(DISSEMINATED SCLEROSIS; DEMYELINATING DISEASE)

A chronic progressive nervous system disease characterized by scattered patches of demyelination and glial tissue overgrowth in the white matter of the brain and spinal cord. Among the clinical symptoms associated with multiple sclerosis are extremity weakness, visual disturbances, ataxia, tremor, uncoordination, sphincter impairment, and impaired position sense. Remissions and exacerbations are also associated with the disease.

NURSING DIAGNOSES / DEFINING CHARACTERISTICS	NURSING INTERVENTIONS / *RATIONALES*	EXPECTED OUTCOMES
Impaired physical mobility *Related to:* Decreased motor strength Tremors Spasticity secondary to multiple sclerosis **DEFINING CHARACTERISTICS** Unsteady gait Dizziness Spasticity Weakness of extremities Incoordination Intention tremor Paraparesis	**ONGOING ASSESSMENT** • Assess patient's girth, muscle strength, weakness, coordination, and balance. • Inquire about falls, use of assistive devices, and decrease in muscle strength. **THERAPEUTIC INTERVENTIONS** • Encourage ambulation with assistance/supervision. • Schedule rest periods *to decrease fatigue.* • Consult physical therapist and occupational therapist *for use of assistive/ambulatory devices and ADL evaluation.* • Encourage self-care as tolerated; assist when necessary. • Avoid rushing patient. • Place belongings within reach. • Use adaptive techniques and equipment from occupational therapy department. These may include: Wrist weight Use of proximal rather than upper extremities Adaptive equipment such as stabilized plates and nonspilling cups Stabilization of extremity and training patient to use trunk and head to compensate for impaired function • Encourage stretching exercises daily. • Administer antispasmodics as ordered.	Optimal mobility will result.
Sensory perceptual alterations: visual *Related to:* Multiple sclerosis **DEFINING CHARACTERISTICS** Diplopia Blurred vision Nystagmus Visual loss Scotomas (blind spots)	**ONGOING ASSESSMENT** • Assess for visual impairment and effect on ADL. **THERAPEUTIC INTERVENTIONS** • Orient patient to environment. • Place objects within reach. • Provide eyepatch for diplopia; encourage alternating patch from eye to eye *to eliminate diplopia temporarily.* • Instruct patient to rest eyes when fatigued. • Advise of availability of large-type reading materials and talking books. • Place call light within reach with side rails up and bed in low position. • Place sign over the bed; indicate visual impairment in chart and kardex. • See Visual impairment, p. 492.	Optimal visual ability with decreased risk of injury will be attained.
Urinary retention *Related to:* Neuromuscular impairment secondary to multiple sclerosis **DEFINING CHARACTERISTICS** Frequency Urgency Hesitancy Abdominal distention Pain	**ONGOING ASSESSMENT** • Inquire about symptoms of frequency, urgency, abdominal distention, pain, and recurrent urinary tract infections. **THERAPEUTIC INTERVENTIONS** • Measure urine output; catheterize for residual urine as indicated. *Note: Residual urine > 100 ml predisposes patient to urinary tract infections.* • Initiate individualized bladder training program; instruct patient about Credé method, intermittent catheterization, signs and symptoms of urinary tract infection, time of voiding. • Recommend vitamin C and liberal intake of cranberry juice *to acidify urine and reduce bacterial growth.* • See Urinary retention, p. 61.	Reduced risk of developing urinary tract infections will be achieved.

Continued.

Multiple sclerosis—cont'd

NURSING DIAGNOSES / DEFINING CHARACTERISTICS	NURSING INTERVENTIONS / *RATIONALES*	EXPECTED OUTCOMES
Constipation *Related to:* Spinal cord involvement **DEFINING CHARACTERISTICS** Straining at stools Frequent but nonproductive desire to defecate Abdominal distention Hemorrhoids Small, hard stool	**ONGOING ASSESSMENT** • Evaluate bowel habits. **THERAPEUTIC INTERVENTIONS** • Initiate bowel training program as needed with uniform daily time. *Regularity is necessary to establish reflex assistance.* • Encourage high fluid intake ($\geq$ 2000 ml/day) and bulk diet. • See Constipation, p. 12.	Regular bowel elimination will be achieved.
Potential impaired skin integrity *Related to:* Sensory changes **DEFINING CHARACTERISTICS** Hypoalgesia Paresthesia Loss of position sense	**ONGOING ASSESSMENT** • Assess skin integrity. • Inquire about areas of body with decreased sensation. **THERAPEUTIC INTERVENTIONS** • Avoid heat, cold, and pressure. • Instruct patient to test bath water with unaffected extremity. • Instruct patient to notice foot placement when ambulating *to compensate for decreased position sense.* • See Potential impaired skin integrity, p. 48.	Absence of skin breakdown, burns, or decubitus formation will be achieved.
Body image disturbance/loss of self-esteem *Related to:* Physical and psychosocial changes **DEFINING CHARACTERISTICS** Anxiety Depression Noncompliance Poor eye contact Refusal to participate in care/treatment Fears regarding level of independence	**ONGOING ASSESSMENT** • Assess quality and quantity of verbalizations about self-image. • Observe for changes in behavior and/or level of functioning. • Note patient's/significant others' report of change in self-concept. **THERAPEUTIC INTERVENTIONS** • Make frequent, unhurried patient contact. • Provide patient opportunity to ask questions and talk about feelings. • Include patient in care planning. • Support patient's efforts to maintain independence. • Use referral sources (e.g., liaison psychiatry service) when appropriate *to facilitate patient's attempts at coping.*	External source of discomfort and anxiety will be reduced.
Knowledge deficit *Related to:* Unfamiliarity with the disease process and management **DEFINING CHARACTERISTICS** Verbalization of misconceptions Questioning Noncompliance	**ONGOING ASSESSMENT** • Assess patient's/significant others' knowledge of disease, exacerbations, remissions, and medical regimen. **THERAPEUTIC INTERVENTIONS** • Reassure patient/significant others that most MS patients do not become severely disabled. • Instruct patient/significant others when to contact health team (e.g., urinary symptoms; exacerbations; motor, sensory, visual disturbances). • Offer referral for counseling services when indicated. • Instruct patient/significant others about: Purpose of steroid therapy (*decreases edema and acute inflammatory response within evolving plaque*)	Patient/significant others will verbalize understanding of disease process, medications used, and adverse effects.

NURSING DIAGNOSES / DEFINING CHARACTERISTICS	NURSING INTERVENTIONS / *RATIONALES*	EXPECTED OUTCOMES
	Side effects (e.g., sodium retention, fluid retention, pedal edema, hypertension, gastric irritation) Measures to control side effects (e.g., low-sodium diet, daily weighing, leg elevation, support hose, blood pressure monitoring, antacids, adequate rest, and avoidance of contact with persons with infectious disease) Importance of maintaining most normal activity level possible. Avoidance of hot baths *(increases metabolic demands and may increase weakness)* Sleeping in a prone position *to decrease flexion spasms* Need to inspect areas of impaired sensation for serious injuries	

Originated by: Corea Hodge, RN

Myasthenia gravis: acute crisis phase

(MYASTHENIC CRISIS; CHOLINERGIC CRISIS)

Myasthenia gravis is a chronic disorder of neuromuscular transmission of the voluntary muscles. The exact etiology is unknown, but it is theorized to be an autoimmune disorder affecting postsynaptic receptor sites. It occurs at all ages, with females affected twice as often as males, and the highest incidence in the third decade of life. It is characterized by muscular weakness and easy fatigability, most frequently affecting the facial, oculomotor, laryngeal, pharyngeal, and respiratory muscles. An acute crisis can be precipitated by failure to take anticholinesterase medication (myasthenic crisis), overdosage of anticholinesterase drugs (cholinergic crisis), emotional stress, surgery, fatigue, some drugs, and influenza.

NURSING DIAGNOSES / DEFINING CHARACTERISTICS	NURSING INTERVENTIONS / *RATIONALES*	EXPECTED OUTCOMES

Potential for injury: muscle weakness
Related to:
Myasthenic/cholinergic crisis secondary to alteration in transmission of acetylcholine across neuromuscular synapse preventing transmission of nerve impulse
 	
DEFINING CHARACTERISTICS
Myasthenic crisis:
  Dysphagia with potential for aspiration
  Diplopia and ptosis
  Generalized weakness and rapid fatigability
	ONGOING ASSESSMENT
	• Assess patient's ability to speak and swallow; presence of ptosis and diplopia; degree of proximal muscle strength; presence of cough and gag reflexes; respiratory status (rate, depth, excursion, presence of shortness of breath/dyspnea).
	• Check for dysphagia before any oral medications or meals. *To prevent aspiration,* hold medications and meals with any questionable dysphagia or lack of gag/cough reflex; and notify physician.
	• Check for presence of diplopia and ptosis at least each shift and as needed.
	• Check hand grasp and degree patient is able to raise arms/legs, at least q6h and whenever changing anticholinesterase dosage (usually ½ - 1 hr after administration) *to monitor effectiveness and prevent cholinergic crisis.* Record length of time patient is able to hold position. Notify physician of decrease in strength, especially after dosage change.
	• Have patient count from one upward; record point at which speech becomes unintelligible.
	
	THERAPEUTIC INTERVENTIONS
	• *Maintain levels of anticholinesterase* by giving medications exactly on time. Observe for signs and symptoms of overdosage (see Defining Characteristics), *since medication needs may fluctuate day to day.*
	• Assist patient with ADL as needed; plan activities around period of optimal strength (usually 1-2 hr after anticholinesterase dose).
		Complications of muscle weakness will be reduced.

Continued.

Myasthenia gravis: acute crisis phase—cont'd

NURSING DIAGNOSES / DEFINING CHARACTERISTICS	NURSING INTERVENTIONS / *RATIONALES*	EXPECTED OUTCOMES
Dyspnea Difficulty speaking, often with nasal quality Restlessness Difficulty chewing Cholinergic crisis: Same as above, with: Muscular fasciculations Increased bronchial secretions Nausea/vomiting Abdominal cramping with diarrhea Increase in tearing and perspiration	· Place patient in room near nursing station *for easy access.* · Prevent precipitating factors in crisis (e.g., infection, overdosage, emotional crisis); plan frequent rest periods. · Use resources as appropriate (e.g., physical therapy, splints/Stryker boots as needed). Turn q2h if patient lacks strength. · Instruct patient to inform nursing staff/physician of change in muscle strength or respiratory difficulty after anticholinesterase medication. · If signs of crisis occur, determine time of onset in relation to last anticholinesterase medication *to help determine which reaction (crisis) is occurring.*	
Ineffective airway clearance *Related to:* Inability to clear secretions because of weakness of respiratory muscles resulting from myasthenic or cholinergic crisis and/or intubation **DEFINING CHARACTERISTICS** Abnormal breath sounds Inadequate ABGs as evidenced by change in patient's baseline values Weak, nonproductive cough Increased airway pressures Shallow respirations Tachypnea/bradypnea Cyanosis Complaints of shortness of breath and/or dyspnea	**ONGOING ASSESSMENT** · Establish patient's baseline: Respiratory rate Depth of respirations Use of respiratory muscles and/or accessory muscles · Monitor forced vital capacity (FVC) and tidal volume as ordered; notify physician of significant change (e.g., FVC < 1.0). · Auscultate lungs q4h and as needed for presence of, change in breath sounds. *Early detection of changes is important to prevent accumulation of secretions and/or atelectasis.* · Assess for neurologic change (e.g., increase in drowsiness, confusion, agitation, or anxiety), *which may indicate respiratory acidosis or hypoxemia.* **THERAPEUTIC INTERVENTIONS** · Perform nasotracheal suctioning, or suction via endotracheal tube (if present), using sterile technique *to clear airway of secretions.* · Draw ABGs as ordered or with significant change in respiratory status. Notify physician. · Reposition patient q2h *to mobilize secretions.* · Avoid any unnecessary activities that increase fatigue (especially during crisis). · Coordinate activities and respiratory treatments to correspond with peak action of medication, such as neostigmine (Prostigmine) and pyridostigmine (Mestinon) *(anticholinesterase drugs that improve neuromuscular transmission and muscle strength).* · Have suction equipment and emergency intubation equipment readily available. · Instruct patient in need to breathe deeply and cough during periods of optimal strength *to prevent complications of respiratory infections.* · Explain all procedures and alarms (especially ventilator alarms).	Airway clearance will be maintained.
Anxiety *Related to:* Fear of unknown and inability to express fears and needs Impaired verbal communication	**ONGOING ASSESSMENT** · Assess patient's level of anxiety and understanding of illness. · Assess patient's normal coping patterns by interviewing patient/significant others. **THERAPEUTIC INTERVENTIONS** · Have some form of communication system for patients with severe dysarthria and/or tracheal tubes (e.g., paper, pencil; letter, number, picture board; blinking of eyes to indicate yes/no). *This will help alleviate anxiety related to inability to communicate verbally.*	Anxiety will be reduced.

NURSING DIAGNOSES / DEFINING CHARACTERISTICS	NURSING INTERVENTIONS / *RATIONALES*	EXPECTED OUTCOMES
DEFINING CHARACTERISTICS Restlessness Tachypnea, tachycardia Alteration in BP Dilated pupils Withdrawal Fear of sleep	· Encourage patient who is able to speak to ventilate his/her feelings. · Have call light readily available at all times. · Explain all procedures to patient beforehand. · Explain reason for ventilator alarms (*one of patients' major fears is malfunctioning ventilator*). · Reassure patient with endotracheal intubation that he/she will be able to speak after extubation. *Patient needs to know inability to communicate verbally is temporary, caused by endotracheal tube's passing through vocal cords.* · See Communication, p. 11.	
Potential altered nutrition: less than body requirements *Related to:* Inability to swallow or chew because of weakness of bulbar muscles Lack of appetite resulting from side effects of anticholinesterase medications (i.e., abdominal cramping, nausea, vomiting, and diarrhea) **DEFINING CHARACTERISTICS** Loss of weight Lack of appetite Choking or gagging when attempting to swallow Absence of gag reflex Complaints of nausea/vomiting Diarrhea	**ONGOING ASSESSMENT** · Assess patient's ability to swallow and chew. · Assess for presence of nausea, vomiting, abdominal cramping, or diarrhea. · Check patient's ability to chew and swallow before meals. **THERAPEUTIC INTERVENTIONS** · Withhold meal if swallowing impaired. Plan meal around peak action of medication (usually 1 hr after dose). *Anticholinesterase medications improve neuromuscular transmission, thereby increasing muscle strength. Chance of aspiration is lessened by giving meals during peak medication action.* · Give patient who has difficulty in chewing soft or liquid diet. · Give atropine or anticholinergic drug (i.e., Donnatal) as ordered *to decrease side effects of anticholinesterase medication (be aware that anticholinergic drugs can mask symptoms of overdosage and therefore precipitate cholinergic crisis).* · Instruct patient in side effects of anticholinesterase and anticholinergic medications. · Encourage patient to eat well-balanced diet when possible and space meals during periods of optimal muscular strength. · Instruct patient to report significant changes in swallowing ability *to enable early detection of difficulties and prevent aspiration.* · If patient is intubated or unable to swallow effectively, prepare to feed patient via nasogastric tube. See SCP in Ch. 1: Altered nutrition: less than body requirements, p. 37; Enteral tube feeding, p. 308.	Optimal nutritional requirements will be maintained.
Knowledge deficit *Related to:* Unfamiliarity with disease process, treatment **DEFINING CHARACTERISTICS** Multiple questions Lack of questions Misconceptions	**ONGOING ASSESSMENT** · Assess patient's/significant others' knowledge base and readiness for learning. **THERAPEUTIC INTERVENTIONS** · Instruct patient in difference between cholinergic and myasthenic crisis (see Defining Characteristics, Potential for injury, p. 255). · Teach patient factors precipitating crisis and ways to avoid them (*knowledgeable patient is more likely to assist in care to prevent crisis*). · Instruct in signs and symptoms of pending or recurring pulmonary problems and ways to avoid precipitating factors (e.g., avoiding those with upper respiratory infection/smokers). · Instruct patient to avoid drugs that could cause problems: quinidine, mycin-antibiotics, procainamide, quinine, phenothiazides, barbiturates, tranquilizers, narcotics, alcohol (*may precipitate crisis*).	Patient will effectively demonstrate knowledge of disease process, cholinergic/myasthenic crisis, precipitating factors, and good pulmonary care.

Originated by: Donna Raymer, RN, BSN, CCRN

Normal pressure hydrocephalus

Nonresorptive or malresorptive hydrocephalus leading to brain compression with normal intracranial pressure. The condition is thought to be caused by a disturbance of cerebrospinal fluid absorption caused by cisternal adhesions possibly after meningitis, subarachnoid hemorrhage, or sinus thrombosis. It causes varying degrees of mental deterioration, gait disturbance, and urinary incontinence. About one-third of patients are thought to benefit from surgical shunting.

NURSING DIAGNOSES / DEFINING CHARACTERISTICS	NURSING INTERVENTIONS / *RATIONALES*	EXPECTED OUTCOMES

Altered thought processes
Related to:
Physiologic changes secondary to:
  Past history of subarachnoid hemorrhage
  Inflammatory process
  Remote head injury
  Decreased brain resiliency
  Meningitis
  Sinus thrombosis
 	
DEFINING CHARACTERISTICS
Dementia
Decreased recent memory
Slowness of speech or paucity of speech
Impaired judgment
	ONGOING ASSESSMENT
	• Evaluate premorbid behavior.
	• Assess long-term memory, attentiveness, attention span, and retention of information.
	• Assess orientation to person, time, place.
	• Assess speech pattern *(often slow speech, use of few words in response to questions, and little spontaneity).*
	• Assess effect and behavior *(often apathetic, flat effect with decreased insight into illness).*
	THERAPEUTIC INTERVENTIONS
	• Reorient to surroundings as necessary.
	• Provide clock/calendar for room.
	• Explain treatments and nursing care slowly and simply, asking patient to repeat explanation *(allows verification of understanding).*
	• Allow patient time to answer questions *(allows time to assimilate information and organize responses).*
	• See Altered thought processes, p. 52.
		Maximal communication and orientation will be achieved.

Potential for injury: trauma
Related factors:
Physiologic changes related to NPH
 	
DEFINING CHARACTERISTICS
Spastic gait
Ataxia
Urinary incontinence
Mental status changes
	ONGOING ASSESSMENT
	• Evaluate gait, ambulation, safety needs.
	• Assess posture, balance, coordination.
	• Evaluate premorbid pattern of elimination.
	• Assess mental status, including memory, judgment, comprehension, insight.
	• Evaluate skin integrity daily with special attention to bony prominences and shins of legs where patient may have bumped into objects.
	THERAPEUTIC INTERVENTIONS
	• Apply soft restraints (e.g., Posey vest) as needed, especially at night.
	• Maintain bed in low position with all side rails up.
	• Assist patient in ambulating from bed to chair or bathroom. Indicate number of people needed to assist patient.
	• Minimize environmental barriers such as chairs, waste cans.
	• Place needed articles within reach (e.g., water, call light, glasses, tissue).
	• Establish a program for urinary elimination:
	  Keep urinal/bedpan within patient's reach.
	  Offer urinal/bedpan to patient q2-4h.
	  Encourage ample fluids: 2-3 L every day.
	  Limit fluid intake after 8 p.m. *to reduce need to get up and use washroom.*
	• Consult physical therapist, dietitian as ordered/needed.
		Risk of falls and injury will be reduced.

NURSING DIAGNOSES / DEFINING CHARACTERISTICS	NURSING INTERVENTIONS / *RATIONALES*	EXPECTED OUTCOMES

Knowledge deficit
Related to:
Uncertain course of disease, diagnosis, test, and treatment
 	
DEFINING CHARACTERISTICS
Questioning
Verbalization of misconceptions
	ONGOING ASSESSMENT
	• Evaluate understanding by patient/significant other of disease process, diagnostic tests, treatments, and outcome.
	
	THERAPEUTIC INTERVENTIONS
	• Explain disease process (altered brain fluid absorption with consequent changes in ability to walk, behavior, memory, speech, and control of urination).
	• Instruct family about communication with patient, safety needs, and need for frequent offering of urinal/bedpan.
	• Explain diagnostic tests to patients and family and repeat explanations as necessary:
	  CT scan
	  Lumbar puncture
	  Skull films
	• Give patient/significant others booklet of shunting procedure.
	• Discuss signs and symptoms of shunt malfunction
	  Increased mental deterioration
	  Increased gait disturbance
	  Urinary incontinence
		Patient/significant others will be able to verbalize or demonstrate understanding of disease process.

Originated by: Corea Hodge, RN

Parkinsonism

(PARALYSIS AGITANS)

A chronic neurologic disorder affecting the extrapyramidal system of the brain responsible for control of regulation of movement. The clinical manifestations are tremor, rigidity, slowness of movement, bent posture, shuffling gait, masklike facial expressions, and muscle weakness affecting writing, speaking, eating, chewing, and swallowing.

NURSING DIAGNOSES / DEFINING CHARACTERISTICS	NURSING INTERVENTIONS / *RATIONALES*	EXPECTED OUTCOMES
Impaired physical mobility *Related to:* Neuromuscular impairment Decreased strength and endurance **DEFINING CHARACTERISTICS** Tremors Muscle rigidity Decreased ability to initiate movements (akinesis) Impaired coordination of movement Limited ROM Impaired ability to carry out ADL Postural disturbances	**ONGOING ASSESSMENT** • Evaluate baseline activity level. • Assess ability to carry out ADL. • Assess posture, coordination, resting tremors, and movements. **THERAPEUTIC INTERVENTIONS** • Maintain side rails in up position. • Allow sufficient time for ADL. • Encourage and allow sufficient time for hygiene and self-care; assist as needed. • Supervise and assist with ambulation at least three times per day. • Encourage patient to lift feet and take large steps while walking *to improve balance and minimize shuffling*. • Remove environmental barriers while patient is ambulating. • Encourage ROM to all joints twice daily. • Consult physical and occupational therapists about aids *to facilitate ADL and safe ambulation*.	Optimal level of functioning and minimal complications of immobility will be achieved.

Continued.

NURSING DIAGNOSES / DEFINING CHARACTERISTICS	NURSING INTERVENTIONS / *RATIONALES*	EXPECTED OUTCOMES
Impaired verbal communication *Related to:* Dysarthria **Defining Characteristics** Difficulty in articulating words Monotonous voice tones Slow, slurred speech Stammered speech	**Ongoing Assessment** · Evaluate ability to communicate and understand spoken words. · Assess ability to write/understand written words/pictures. **Therapeutic Interventions** · Allow patient time to articulate. · Encourage patient to read aloud. · Encourage face and tongue exercises. · Consult speech therapist if indicated. · Place call light and other articles (tissues, water, glasses) within reach. · Avoid speaking loudly unless patient is deaf. · Maintain eye contact when speaking (*promotes focus and attention and encourages patient*). · See Impaired verbal communication, p. 11.	Alternative methods of communication will be facilitated and maximal communication skills will be realized.
Altered nutrition: less than body requirements *Related to:* Difficulty swallowing Choking spells Drooling Regurgitation of food/ fluids through nares **Defining Characteristics** Documented intake below required caloric level Weight loss	**Ongoing Assessment** · Assess degree of swallowing difficulty: Fluids Solids · Assess nutritional status: Height Weight · Weigh patient three times per week. · Record I & O. **Therapeutic Interventions** · Place patient in a high Fowler's position for eating and drinking. · Supervise patient during meals. · Allow time for meals; avoid rushing patient. Offer high-calorie, low-volume supplements between meals *to provide additional caloric intake.* · Encourage fluids: 2000 ml/day. · Place suction machine at bedside *for emergency use.* · Assist with oral hygiene after meals. · Consult dietitian for needed changes in food consistency and for caloric counts. · Consult the speech therapist to evaluate swallowing. · See Altered nutrition: less than body requirements, p. 37.	Adequate caloric and fluid intake will be achieved.
Ineffective breathing pattern *Related to:* Decreased muscle strength Decreased chest area **Defining Characteristics** Dyspnea Shortness of breath Tachypnea Cough Cyanosis Altered chest excursion	**Ongoing Assessment** · Evaluate respiratory rate, depth, pattern. · Assess for dyspnea. · Assess for changes in orientation and restlessness. · Assess for skin color, temperature, and capillary refill. · Assess breath sounds. **Therapeutic Interventions** · Position patient upright if tolerated *to promote increased ventilation of lower lobes.* · Encourage sustained deep breaths by *emphasizing slow inhalation, holding of end-inspiration for a few seconds, and passive exhalation.* · See Ineffective breathing pattern, p. 8.	Respiratory status within limitations of disease is maintained.
Constipation/ diarrhea *Related to:* Drug therapy Inactivity	**Ongoing Assessment** · Assess home pattern of elimination and compare to present pattern. · Evaluate usual dietary habits, eating schedule, intake of liquid and food. · Assess activity level (*prolonged bed rest, lack of exercise contribute to constipation*).	Constipation/diarrhea will be relieved.

NURSING DIAGNOSES / DEFINING CHARACTERISTICS	NURSING INTERVENTIONS / *RATIONALES*	EXPECTED OUTCOMES
DEFINING CHARACTERISTICS Straining at stools Passage of liquid fecal steepage Abdominal distention Fecal incontinence	· Evaluate bowel sounds every shift. · Evaluate current medications that may contribute to constipation/diarrhea. **THERAPEUTIC INTERVENTIONS** · Encourage bulk in diet: raw fruits, vegetables, salads, grains, fiber. · Encourage fluid intake 2-3 L/day if not medically contraindicated. · See Constipation, p. 12; Diarrhea, p. 16.	
Potential urinary retention *Related to:* Drug therapy **DEFINING CHARACTERISTICS** Decreased (< 30 ml/ hr) or absent urinary output for consecutive 2 hr Frequency, hesitancy, urgency, and incontinence Lower abdominal distention Urinary tract infections	**ONGOING ASSESSMENT** · Evaluate previous pattern of voiding. · Inspect lower abdomen for distention. · Evaluate intervals between voiding. · Assess amount, frequency, character, color, odor, specific gravity. · Evaluate current medications that may contribute to urinary problems. · Evaluate I & O. **THERAPEUTIC INTERVENTIONS** · Place bedpan/urinal/bedside commode within reach. · Have patient listen to running water, place hands in warm water, or pour warm water over perineum *to stimulate urination.* · Institute intermittent catheterization or Foley catheter as indicated. · See Urinary retention, p. 61.	Optimal pattern of urine elimination is maintained.
Self concept disturbance *Related to:* Changes in body image Dependence **DEFINING CHARACTERISTICS** Minimal eye contact Self-deprecating statements Anger Expression of guilt	**ONGOING ASSESSMENT** · Assess perception of self. · Assess level of anxiety. · Assess normal coping pattern. · Evaluate support system. **THERAPEUTIC INTERVENTIONS** · Encourage patient to verbalize fears and concerns. Listen attentively *to facilitate development of trust.* · Consider effect of loss of significant persons and include in discussion. · Explore strengths and resources with patient. · Avoid overprotection of individual; promote social interaction as appropriate. · Clarify patient's misconceptions and provide accurate information. · Provide privacy as needed. · See Self concept disturbance, p. 46.	Patient will recognize self-maligning statements and begin to verbalize positive expression of self-worth.
Knowledge deficit *Related to:* Uncertain cause of disease and treatment **DEFINING CHARACTERISTICS** Multiple questions Lack of questions Apparent confusion over condition	**ONGOING ASSESSMENT** · Evaluate patient's/significant others' understanding of disease process, diagnostic tests, treatments, and outcomes. · Assess patient's/significant others' anxiety level. **THERAPEUTIC INTERVENTIONS** · Encourage communication with family/significant others. · Involve family/significant others in care and instructions. · Reinforce physician's explanation of disease, causes, symptoms, and treatments. · Discuss feelings about symptoms: tremors, drooling of saliva, slurred speech. · Encourage independence and avoid overprotection by permitting patient to do things for self: self-care, feeding, dressing, ambulation. · Discuss with patient, family/significant others:	Patient/significant others will demonstrate understanding of patient's disability and special needs with regard to disease process, activity, exercises, ambulation, medication, diet, and elimination.

Continued.

NURSING DIAGNOSES / DEFINING CHARACTERISTICS	NURSING INTERVENTIONS / *RATIONALES*	EXPECTED OUTCOMES
	Medication:	

Medication:
  Dosage, frequency, administration, action, and toxic effects: orthostatic hypotension, nausea and vomiting, abnormal involuntary movements, changes in mental status, and shortness of breath.
  Those to be taken with meals.
  Limitation of high-protein foods such as milk, meat, fish, cheese, eggs, peanuts, grains, and soybeans for patients taking Levodopa.
Diet:
  Provide high-caloric, soft diet.
  Cut food for patient.
  Place utensils within easy reach.
  Use blender for thick foods.
  Use brace for severe tremors occurring during meals.
  Maintain 2000-ml/day liquid intake.
  Offer frequent small feedings.
  Use straws and bibs for excessive drooling.
  Instruct patient to swallow slowly and take small bites of food.
Activity:
  Plan rest periods.
  Encourage passive and active ROM exercises to all extremities.
  Encourage family/significant others to participate in physical therapy exercises of stretching and massaging muscles.
  Encourage daily ambulation outdoors but avoidance of extreme hot and cold weather.
  Encourage patient to practice lifting feet while walking, using heel-toe gait, and swing deliberately while walking.
  Avoid sitting for long periods of time.
  Encourage patient to dress daily, avoid clothing with buttons (use zippers instead) and shoes with laces or snaps or velcro.
  Offer diversional activities depending on extent of tremors and disability: read, watch television, hobbies.
  Prevent falls by clearing walkways of furniture and throw rugs and provide side rails on stairs.
Speech therapy:
  Instruct patient to speak slowly and practice reading aloud in an exaggerated manner.
Oral hygiene: Perform q2-4h and prn *(especially if drooling)* and have tissues accessible to patient.
Elimination:
  Institute voiding measures as needed.
  Institute bladder control program as needed.
  Raise toilet seats with side rails at home *to facilitate sitting or standing.*
  Avoid constipation; encourage fluids, use of natural laxatives (prune juices and roughage) and stool softeners as needed

Originated by: Marian D. Cachero-Salavrakos, RN, BSN

Seizure activity

(CONVULSIONS; EPILEPSY)

A seizure is an occasional, excessive disorderly discharge of neuronal activity. Recurrent seizures (epilepsy) may be classified as (1) partial, (2) generalized, or (3) unclassified.

NURSING DIAGNOSES / DEFINING CHARACTERISTICS	NURSING INTERVENTIONS / *RATIONALES*	EXPECTED OUTCOMES
Potential for injury *Related to:* Seizure activity Postictal state Altered LOC Impaired judgment **DEFINING CHARACTERISTICS** Increased rhythmic motor activity, jerking of arms and legs Repetitive psychomotor activity Tonic-clonic movements Change in alertness, orientation, verbal response, eye opening, motor response Aspiration of oral secretions	**ONGOING ASSESSMENT** • Assess frequency, duration, and type of seizure activity. • Note the following: 　Change in LOC 　Patient's preceding seizure activity 　Place where seizure started 　Epileptic cry 　Automatism 　Length of seizure 　Head and eye turning 　Pupillary reaction 　Associated falls 　Foam from mouth 　Urinary or fecal incontinence 　Cyanosis 　Postictal state 　Any postseizure focal abnormality (e.g., Todd's paralysis) **THERAPEUTIC INTERVENTIONS** • Document observations and frequency of seizures; notify physician as indicated. • Roll patient to side after cessation of muscle twitching *to prevent aspiration.* • If patient is in bed: 　Pad side rails. 　Remove sharp objects from bed. 　Keep bed in low position. • If patient is on floor, remove furniture or other potentially harmful objects from area. • Do not restrain patient. *Physical restraint applied during seizure activity can cause pathogenic trauma.*	Potential for physical injury will be reduced.
Altered health maintenance *Related to:* Perceptual and/or cognitive impairment Lack of fine motor ability Lack of material resources Physiologic derangement **DEFINING CHARACTERISTICS** Inadequate serum anticonvulsant levels (below therapeutic range) Intake altered to the degree of affecting medication intake Vomiting Demonstrated inability to take or obtain medications	**ONGOING ASSESSMENT** • Assess perceptual and cognitive abilities. • Note alterations in fine motor ability. • Inquire as to material resources that would influence ability to obtain medications (money or transportation). • Assess for presence/history of prolonged vomiting. • Monitor blood levels of anticonvulsant. **THERAPEUTIC INTERVENTIONS** • Administer anticonvulsant as ordered during hospitalization. • Suggest alternate routes to physician if patient is vomiting. • Involve significant others/friends/social support in solving home care needs, where appropriate. • Consult social service as appropriate. *May be helpful in securing transportation or applying for financial assistance necessary for compliance.*	Therapeutic level of anticonvulsant will be maintained.

Continued.

Seizure activity—cont'd

NURSING DIAGNOSES / DEFINING CHARACTERISTICS	NURSING INTERVENTIONS / *RATIONALES*	EXPECTED OUTCOMES
Potential disturbed self-esteem *Related factors:* Seizure activity Dependence on medications **DEFINING CHARACTERISTICS** Nonparticipation in therapy Lack of responsibility for self-care Self-destructive behavior Lack of eye contact	**ONGOING ASSESSMENT** · Assess feelings about self and disease. · Assess perceived implications of disease and need for long-term therapy. **THERAPEUTIC INTERVENTIONS** · Encourage ventilation of feelings. · Incorporate family and significant others in care plan. *May be helpful in assisting/giving support.* · Assist patient and others in understanding nature of disorder. · Dispel common myths and fears about convulsive disorders.	Effect of convulsant disorder on self-esteem will be reduced.

Knowledge deficit
Related to:
Lack of exposure
Information misinterpretation
Unfamiliarity with information resources
 	
DEFINING CHARACTERISTICS
Verbalization of problem
Inappropriate or exaggerated behavior
Request for information
Statement of misconception
	ONGOING ASSESSMENT
	· Assess patient's/significant others' knowledge of disease and treatment.
	· Assess readiness for learning *so that information is presented when comprehension will be optimal.*
	
	THERAPEUTIC INTERVENTIONS
	· Discuss disease process.
	· Review with patient need for medication and schedule:
	    Right medication at right time and dosage
	    Drug levels
	    Danger of seizure activity with abrupt withdrawal
	    Possible side effects and interactions of medication
	· Educate patient in safety measures:
	    Diving
	    Swimming
	    Medic-Alert tag
	    Home safety
	· Refer to Epilepsy Foundation.
	· See Knowledge deficit, p. 33.
		Patient will understand and be able to verbalize disease process, treatment, and safety measures.

Originated by: Kathryn S. Bronstein, RN, PhD, CS

Craniotomy

(CRANIECTOMY; BURR HOLE; THEPHENATION)

Surgical opening of a part of the cranium to gain access to disease or injury affecting the brain, ventricles, or intracranial blood vessels.

NURSING DIAGNOSES / DEFINING CHARACTERISTICS	NURSING INTERVENTIONS / *RATIONALES*	EXPECTED OUTCOMES
Altered cerebral tissue perfusion *Related to:* Cerebral edema Intracranial bleeding	**ONGOING ASSESSMENT** · Assess and document baseline level of consciousness: pupillary size, position, reaction to light; motor movement and strength of limbs; and vital signs. *Early detection of changes is necessary to prevent permanent neurologic dysfunction.* · Compare current assessment to previous assessment. Report any deviations.	Optimal cerebral perfusion will be maintained.

NURSING DIAGNOSES / DEFINING CHARACTERISTICS	NURSING INTERVENTIONS / *RATIONALES*	EXPECTED OUTCOMES

Cerebral ischemia/ infarction
Increased ICP
Metabolic abnormalities
Hydrocephalus
 	
DEFINING CHARACTERISTICS
Changed LOC
Changed pupillary size, reaction to light, deviation
Focal or generalized motor weakness
Presence of pathologic reflexes (Babinski)
Seizures
Increased BP and bradycardia
Changed respiratory pattern
	• Evaluate contributing factors to change in responsiveness; re-evaluate in 5-10 min *to see whether change persists as a result of such factors as anesthesia, medications, awakening from sound sleep, not understanding question.*
	• Check head dressing for presence of drains. *Intraventricular drains, self-contained bulb suction and drainage system (e.g., Jackson-Pratt) are most commonly used. All drains and catheters should be secured to patient/bed to prevent falls to floor, negative gravity suctioning, and increased risk of bleeding or dislodging of drain.*
	• Evaluate function of catheter monitoring ICP.
	• Evaluate for lash reflex.
	• Assess current medications and compare to preoperative medications, with specific attention to thyroid replacement, anticonvulsants, and steroids.
	• Monitor CBC, electrolytes, and ABGs. Report ABGs:
	   $Po_2 < 80$ mm Hg
	   $Pco_2 > 45$ mm Hg
	   CBC: Hct < 30
	   Electrolytes: Na <130, >150
	   Glucose <80 or >200
	
	THERAPEUTIC INTERVENTIONS
	• Report temperature >39° C. Maintain normothermia with tepid sponge bath/antipyretics or hypothermia blanket as ordered. Turn blanket off at temperature of 100° F rectally (38° C).
	• Maintain HOB at 30 degrees.
	• Turn and reposition patient on side, with head supported in neutral alignment, q2h. Avoid neck flexion/rotation *to prevent venous outflow obstruction and increased ICP.*
	• Reorient patient to environment as needed.
	• If soft restraints needed, position patient on side, never on back.
	• Avoid nursing activities that may trigger increased ICP (straining, strenuous coughing, positioning with neck in flexion, head flat).
	• If patient has difficulty closing eye (cranial nerve VII palsy), administer artificial tears (methyl-cellulose drops) q2h. Glad Plastic wrap or Saran or facsimile can be applied over eye *to protect exposed cornea and prevent dryness.*
	• See Altered level of consciousness, p. 234.	

Potential fluid volume deficit *Related to:* Diabetes insipidus **DEFINING CHARACTERISTICS** Urine output >200 ml for consecutive 2 hr Urine specific gravity <1.005 Thirst Increased serum Na >145 mEq/L Increased serum osmolarity >300	**ONGOING ASSESSMENT** • Monitor I & O q1h with specific attention to fluid volume infused over output. Report urine output >200 ml/hr for consecutive 2 hr. • Check urine specific gravity q2-4h. *Specific gravity is decreased to <1.005 with diabetes insipidus.* • Monitor serum and urine electrolytes and osmolarity. **THERAPEUTIC INTERVENTIONS** • Replace fluid output as directed. • Administer vasopressin (Pitressin) *(exogenous synthetic antidiuretic hormone that causes decreased urinary output)* as ordered. • See Fluid volume deficit, p. 20. • See Diabetes insipidus, p. 374.	Optimal fluid volume will be maintained.

Continued.

Craniotomy—cont'd

NURSING DIAGNOSES / DEFINING CHARACTERISTICS	NURSING INTERVENTIONS / *RATIONALES*	EXPECTED OUTCOMES
Fluid volume excess *Related to:* Syndrome of inappropriate antidiuretic hormone secretion Free-H$_2$O excess **DEFINING CHARACTERISTICS** Changed sensorium Decreased serum Na <130 Decreased serum osmolarity <285 Increased urine Na Seizures	**ONGOING ASSESSMENT** ▪ Assess patient for fluid volume excess *(usually determined by hyponatremia/hyposmolarity). Edema is usually not present in syndrome of inappropriate antidiuretic hormone (SIADH).* ▪ Monitor serum and urine electrolytes and osmolarity daily. ▪ Monitor I & O **THERAPEUTIC INTERVENTIONS** ▪ Restrict PO/IV fluids as ordered. *Fluid restriction of 1-1.5 L/day usually corrects hyponatremia associated with SIADH. Intravenous D$_5$ W is inappropriate because of excess free water.* ▪ Weigh patient QOD. ▪ See SIADH, p. 392; Seizure activity, p. 263.	Optimal fluid balance will be maintained.
Potential impaired physical mobility *Related to:* Decreased LOC Weakness/paralysis of extremities Imposed restrictions **DEFINING CHARACTERISTICS** Inability to move purposefully within physical environment Decreased muscle strength Impaired coordination; verbalization of inability to perform Limited ROM	**ONGOING ASSESSMENT** ▪ Assess for alteration in mobility. **THERAPEUTIC INTERVENTIONS** ▪ Do not position patient in prone or semiprone position *(increases intrathoracic pressure; may increase ICP).* ▪ Encourage active ROM of affected joints *to maintain muscle strength and prevent contractures.* ▪ Establish turning schedule *to prevent skin breakdown, respiratory complications, bone demineralization, and muscle wasting.* ▪ See Mobility, impaired physical, p. 35.	Mobility will be maximized.
Ineffective airway clearance *Related to:* Decreased LOC **DEFINING CHARACTERISTICS** Abnormal breath sounds Change in rate, depth of respirations; tachypnea Cough, cyanosis, dyspnea Change in respiratory rhythm	**ONGOING ASSESSMENT** ▪ Assess for signs of ineffective airway clearance. **THERAPEUTIC INTERVENTIONS** ▪ Suction prn. However, *nasotracheal suctioning is contraindicated for patient having surgery proximal to frontal sinuses (i.e., pituitary tumor, basal frontal meningioma, basal skull fracture). This can result in introduction of catheter tip into brain or allow bacterial communication.* ▪ See Airway clearance, ineffective, p. 3. ▪ See Breathing pattern, ineffective, p. 8.	Airway will be free of secretions.

NURSING DIAGNOSES / DEFINING CHARACTERISTICS	NURSING INTERVENTIONS / *RATIONALES*	EXPECTED OUTCOMES

Potential for injury: seizures *Related to:* Intracranial bleeding Infarction Tumor Trauma
 	
 DEFINING CHARACTERISTICS Focal and/or generalized seizures with/without loss of consciousness
	ONGOING ASSESSMENT
	 • Observe for seizure activity. Record and report observations:
	   Note time and signs of seizures.
	   Observe parts involved: order of involvement and character of movement.
	   Check deviation of eyes; note change in pupillary size.
	   Assess airway and respiratory pattern.
	   Note tonic-clonic stages.
	   Assess postictal state (e.g., loss of consciousness, loss of airway)
	 THERAPEUTIC INTERVENTIONS
	 • Pad side rails. Protect head from injury *to ensure safety.*
	 • Maintain airway during postictal state. Turn patient on side; suction as needed.
	 • Maintain minimal environmental stimuli:
	   Noise reduction
	   Curtains closed
	   Private room (when available/advisable)
	   Dim lights
	 • Administer anticonvulsants as indicated. *Dilantin can only be administered PO/IV. When given IV it should be administered in NS. It will precipitate in any dextrose solution. Infuse no faster than 50 mg/min to prevent hypotension. IV valium is often used to control recurrent seizures and should not be administered any faster than 10 mg/min to prevent respiratory compromise.*
		Risk of seizures will be reduced.

Knowledge deficit *Related to:* New procedures and treatments **DEFINING CHARACTERISTICS** Patient/significant others verbalize questions and concerns	**ONGOING ASSESSMENT** • Assess patient's/significant others' knowledge and readiness for learning. **THERAPEUTIC INTERVENTIONS** • Discuss change in body image related to head dressing and loss of hair, potential for and duration of facial edema. • Discuss need for monitoring equipment and frequent assessments. • Explain unit visiting hours and reasons for restrictions. • Instruct in deep breathing and leg exercises. • Explain use of medications such as dexamethasone (Decadron), anticonvulsants, antibiotics. • Discuss need for frequent assessment, reorientation, etc. • Encourage significant others to participate in reorientation, rehabilitation. • Reinforce discussion of neurologic definitions/progress given by physician to significant others.	Patient/significant others will verbalize understanding of postoperative expectations and experiences.

Originated by: Robert Rowlands, RN

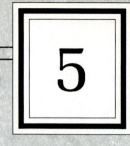

Gastrointestinal and Digestive Care Plans

DISORDERS
Acute abdomen
Appendicitis/appendectomy
Cirrhosis
Diverticular disease
Enterocutaneous fistula
Gastrointestinal bleeding
Hemorrhoids/herniorraphy
Hiatal hernia

Inflammatory bowel disease
Obesity, simple
Pancreatitis: acute
Peptic ulcer

THERAPEUTIC INTERVENTIONS
Cholecystectomy
Colon resection

Enteral tube feeding
Fecal ostomy
Gastrectomy
Gastric restrictive procedure for morbid
    obesity
Pancreaticoduodenectomy
Surgical tubes/drains
Total parenteral nutrition

Acute abdomen

A condition characterized by abdominal pain, vomiting, anorexia, constipation or diarrhea, changes in bowel sounds, and fever. Accurate diagnosis depends on thorough physical assessment, appropriate testing, and observation. Treatment depends on etiology.

NURSING DIAGNOSES / DEFINING CHARACTERISTICS	NURSING INTERVENTIONS / *RATIONALES*	EXPECTED OUTCOMES

Pain
Related to:
Pancreatitis
Thrombosis
Strangulating/infarcted bowel
Renal/biliary colic
Ruptured aneurysm
Appendicitis
Peritonitis
Diverticulitis
Obstruction
Gastroenteritis
 	
DEFINING CHARACTERISTICS
Complaints of abdominal pain
Restlessness
Insomnia
Guarding behavior
Self-focusing
Moaning
Crying
Autonomic responses not seen in chronic stable pain (e.g., diaphoresis, changes in vital signs, pupillary dilation)
	ONGOING ASSESSMENT
	· Assess pain: degree, location, sudden or gradual onset.
	· Assess for precipitating and relieving factors.
	· Monitor for changes in type, degree, location of pain.
	· Evaluate effectiveness of interventions.
	
	THERAPEUTIC INTERVENTIONS
	· Make patient as comfortable as possible:
	    Respond immediately to complaints of pain.
	    Place in semi-Fowler's position.
	    Support with pillows.
	    Provide analgesics as ordered.
	    Explain need to remain as calm as possible.
	    Use techniques patient identifies as helpful.
	· Be available to answer questions, explain procedures, and prepare for tests.
	· Explain need to inform nurse of any change in discomfort. *Changes may indicate complications (e.g., ruptured appendix).*
	· Notify physician if interventions ineffective.
		Pain will be reduced.

Anxiety
Related to:
Change in health status
Change in environment
Suddenness of illness
 	
DEFINING CHARACTERISTICS
Restlessness
Apprehensiveness
Facial tension
Increased questioning/awareness
Difficulty in sleeping
Fear of unknown
Change in vital signs
	ONGOING ASSESSMENT
	· Monitor anxiety level:
	    Assess vital signs.
	    Assess behavior for Defining Characteristics.
	· Document signs and symptoms, including nonverbal communication.
	· Assess usual coping patterns and support system.
	
	THERAPEUTIC INTERVENTIONS
	· Establish rapport through continuity of care.
	· Encourage ventilation of feelings, concerns. Acknowledge anxiety of this and other feelings.
	· Explain importance of remaining as calm as possible. *Relaxation of abdominal muscles may help decrease pain severity.*
	· Explain that nurse always available if needed.
	· Explain all procedures before starting.
	· Provide comfort measures (e.g., reassurance, quiet environment, and medications).
		Anxiety will be reduced.

Continued.

Acute abdomen— cont'd

NURSING DIAGNOSES / DEFINING CHARACTERISTICS	NURSING INTERVENTIONS / *RATIONALES*	EXPECTED OUTCOMES
Potential fluid volume deficit *Related to:* NPO status Diaphoresis Vomiting Diarrhea Increased metabolic need **DEFINING CHARACTERISTICS** Decreased urine output Increased urine specific gravity Thirst Tachycardia Weakness Dry mucous membranes Poor skin turgor, tenting Hemoconcentration	**ONGOING ASSESSMENT** • Monitor vital signs, skin turgor, mucous membranes. • Assess I & O, urine specific gravity. • Monitor weight; record daily. • Monitor lab values. • Observe for complications and notify physician. **THERAPEUTIC INTERVENTIONS** • Maintain IV fluid infusion *to prevent dehydration.* • Insert NG tube and attach to *low suction to ease persistent vomiting.* • Measure gastric output and provide cc for cc IV replacement fluid, usually 0.45 NS or 0.9 NS.	Risk of dehydration will be reduced.

Altered gastrointestinal function/ elimination *Related to:* Acute abdominal condition
 	
 DEFINING CHARACTERISTICS Vomiting Pain Diarrhea/constipation Abdominal distention Change in bowel sounds
	ONGOING ASSESSMENT
	 • Assess vital signs, abdominal circumference, and bowel sounds at least q4h.
	 • Maintain accurate I & O, including emesis, gastric output.
	 • Assess emesis for color, frequency, odor, consistency, blood.
	 • Assess stools for color, frequency, amount, consistency, blood.
	 • Monitor lab work:
	     CBC
	     Electrolytes
	     Amylase
	     BUN/creatinine
	     Sedimentation rate
	 • Assess for changes in pain characteristics.
	
	 THERAPEUTIC INTERVENTIONS
	 • Maintain IV fluids.
	 • Insert and monitor NG tube if ordered.
	 • Maintain NPO unless otherwise stated.
	 • Explain all procedures.
	 • Prepare for and assist with diagnostic tests: x-rays, peritoneal tap.
	 • Provide comfort measures.
	 • Notify physician immediately of changes in condition; *may indicate emergency requiring surgical intervention.*
		Gastrointestinal function/elimination will be maximized.

Potential ineffective airway clearance *Related to:* Pain Abdominal distention **DEFINING CHARACTERISTICS** Guarded breathing because of pain Dyspnea Tachypnea	**ONGOING ASSESSMENT** • Assess vital signs. • Assess respiratory function: rate, quality, pattern, depth, use of accessory muscles. • Ausculate lung fields at least q4h to assess airway clearance. • Assess for abdominal distention. **THERAPEUTIC INTERVENTIONS** • Position to *facilitate lung expansion.* • Encourage patient to change position *to facilitate drainage and air exchange.* • Encourage coughing and deep breathing or use of incentive spirometer *to enhance airway clearance and pulmonary toilet.* • Notify physician of abdominal distention and respiratory difficulty.	Risk of complications because of ineffective airway clearance will be reduced.

NURSING DIAGNOSES / DEFINING CHARACTERISTICS	NURSING INTERVENTIONS / *RATIONALES*	EXPECTED OUTCOMES

Knowledge deficit
Related to:
Acuity of illness
New diagnosis
 	
DEFINING CHARACTERISTICS
Anxiety
Questioning
Anger/hostility
Withdrawal/depression
Noncompliance
	ONGOING ASSESSMENT
	• Assess knowledge of:
	   Illness
	   Medications
	   Management of disorder
	• Assess previous experience and health teaching.
	• Assess ability to learn. Explore attitude and feelings about change.
	• Assess ability to perform tasks.
	
	THERAPEUTIC INTERVENTIONS
	• Provide physical comfort and quiet environment to *enhance ability to concentrate on teaching*.
	• Establish mutual objectives/goals.
	• Allow time for integration of material.
	• Provide home care information:
	   Home management
	   Prevention
	   Follow-up
	   Signs/symptoms necessitating ER visit
	• Provide consultation referrals as needed, including appropriate support/self-help groups.
		Patient will understand current illness, treatment, and home care management.

Originated by: Kathleen Jaffry, RN

Appendicitis/ appendectomy

An infection of the appendix that causes inflammation and pain, appendicitis is a surgical problem. If left untreated, it can lead to rupture of infected appendix and peritonitis.

NURSING DIAGNOSES / DEFINING CHARACTERISTICS	NURSING INTERVENTIONS / *RATIONALES*	EXPECTED OUTCOMES

Preoperative pain
Related to:
Inflamed appendix
 	
DEFINING CHARACTERISTICS
Progressive increase in abdominal pain
Periumbilical pain that radiates to right lower quadrant (RLQ)
Rebound tenderness
	ONGOING ASSESSMENT
	• Assess abdomen for:
	   Location of pain
	   Migration of pain and time involved
	• Assess attempts at pain relief and their effects.
	
	THERAPEUTIC INTERVENTIONS
	• Assist to a comfortable position. *Any position that does not put tension on abdomen usually preferred.*
	• Provide ice pack. Do not provide heat *(may cause appendix rupture)*.
	• Provide analgesics when ordered. *Analgesics may not be ordered before definitive diagnosis.*
		Pain will be reduced.

Infection *Related to:* Bacterial invasion and inflammation of appendix	**ONGOING ASSESSMENT** • Assess vital signs, especially temperature. • Assess for GI symptoms. • Assess I & O and recent PO intake. • Evaluate lab results, especially WBCs.	Infection will be reduced.

Continued.

Appendicitis/appendectomy— cont'd

NURSING DIAGNOSES / DEFINING CHARACTERISTICS	NURSING INTERVENTIONS / *RATIONALES*	EXPECTED OUTCOMES
DEFINING CHARACTERISTICS Elevated temperature Anorexia Nausea, vomiting Constipation RLQ pain Elevated white cell count	**THERAPEUTIC INTERVENTIONS** • Provide support in controlling GI symptoms: NPO Deep breathing and relaxation Cool cloth to forehead Ice pack for abdomen. *If patient complains of feeling constipated, never administer cathartics or enemas (may cause appendicial rupture and peritonitis).* • Prepare for surgical intervention per policy. • Administer antibiotics if ordered.	
Potential fluid volume deficit *Related to:* Vomiting NPO in preparation for surgery **DEFINING CHARACTERISTICS** Dry mucous membranes Thirst Decreasing urine output	**ONGOING ASSESSMENT** • Assess for signs of dehydration. • Maintain I & O. **THERAPEUTIC INTERVENTIONS.** • Provide lip moisturizer. • Provide ice chips, if allowed. • Maintain IV fluids *to prevent dehydration caused by emesis and NPO.*	Normal fluid volume will be maintained.
Potential postoperative infection *Related to:* Surgical procedure **DEFINING CHARACTERISTICS** Fever Increased WBC From incision site: Redness Swelling Drainage Tenderness Foul odor	**ONGOING ASSESSMENT** • Assess incision site q8h for: Redness Swelling Drainage (note color and amount) Tenderness Foul odor • Assess vital signs q4h, especially temperature. • Monitor lab values. **THERAPEUTIC INTERVENTIONS** • Notify physician of infection symptoms. • Keep incision clean and dry after initial dressing changes *to prevent introduction of bacteria into incision site.* • Administer antipyretics and antibiotics as ordered.	Risk of infection will be decreased.
Pain *Related to:* Incision **DEFINING CHARACTERISTICS** Verbal complaints of pain and discomfort Tachycardia Tachypnea Elevated BP Facial grimacing Little or no movement Guarding of abdomen Withdrawal	**ONGOING ASSESSMENT** • Solicit patient's description of pain. • Assess pain characteristics: Quality Severity Location Duration • Assess relief obtained from analgesics. • Refer to Pain, p. 39. **THERAPEUTIC INTERVENTIONS** • Anticipate need for analgesics or additional methods of pain relief. • Instruct patient to prevent tension on suture line by: Splinting Bending legs	Pain will be relieved or reduced.

Appendicitis/appendectomy— cont'd

NURSING DIAGNOSES / DEFINING CHARACTERISTICS	NURSING INTERVENTIONS / *RATIONALES*	EXPECTED OUTCOMES

Diaphoresis	• Provide additional methods of pain relief:
	  Maintain quiet, relaxed atmosphere.
	  Alternate rest periods with activity.
	  Reposition.
	  Provide psychosocial support.
	  These provide ways to decrease external stimulation and maximize analgesic effects.	

Potential fluid volume deficit *Related to:* NPO Increased metabolic requirements Bleeding from operative site Intraoperative fluid loss **DEFINING CHARACTERISTICS** Dry mucous membranes Concentrated urine Decreased urine output Increased sodium level Frequent emesis Tachycardia Hypotension Hemoconcentration Thirst Restlessness Excessive bleeding from incision site	**ONGOING ASSESSMENT** • Maintain strict I & O. • Monitor daily weights. • Monitor vital signs. • Assess incision site for bleeding. • Monitor electrolytes. • Refer to Fluid volume deficit, p. 20. **THERAPEUTIC INTERVENTIONS** • Maintain adequate hydration through parenteral and oral routes. *Oral intake may not be well tolerated until bowel sounds present.* • Report urine output <30 ml/hr for 2 consecutive hr. • Report significant bleeding to physician.	Adequate fluid and electrolyte balance will be maintained.

Potential ineffective airway clearance
Related to:
Anesthesia
Pain
 	
DEFINING CHARACTERISTICS
Abnormal breath sounds
Frequent congested cough
Tachypnea
Dyspnea
	ONGOING ASSESSMENT
	• Assess respirations for:
	  Rate
	  Quality
	  Depth
	  Pattern
	  Use of accessory muscles
	• Assess cough for:
	  Frequency
	  Type
	• Assess sputum for:
	  Color
	  Consistency
	  Amount
	• Auscultate lungs q4h to assess air exchange.
	• See Airway clearance, ineffective, p. 3; Gas exchange, impaired, p. 21.
	
	THERAPEUTIC INTERVENTIONS
	• Encourage patient to change position in bed frequently.
	• Elevate HOB 30-45 degrees.
	• Encourage patient to deep breathe and cough and use the incentive spirometer at least q2h *to promote adequate lung expansion.*
		Airway will be free of secretions.

Continued.

NURSING DIAGNOSES / DEFINING CHARACTERISTICS	NURSING INTERVENTIONS / *RATIONALES*	EXPECTED OUTCOMES
	- Instruct patient on how to splint abdominal incision. *Patient may be apprehensive about breathing and coughing exercises because of tension on suture line and fear of pain.* - Provide humidity if needed *to aid in liquification of secretions.*	
Anxiety *Related to:* Emergency surgery Hospitalization **DEFINING CHARACTERISTICS** Frequent questions Calls nurse often Withdrawal Anger/hostility Restlessness Tension Tachypnea Elevated BP Tachycardia	**ONGOING ASSESSMENT** - Assess patient's level of anxiety. - Assess patient's pattern of coping. - Assess involvement of family or significant other. - See Anxiety, p. 4. **THERAPEUTIC INTERVENTIONS** - Establish rapport with patient and family/significant other *to enhance trust and confidence.* - Encourage ventilation of feelings and concerns. - Approach patient in calm, relaxed manner. - Reassure patient that nurses always present if needed. - Medicate for pain as needed *(pain may contribute to anxiety).*	Patient will exhibit decreased level of anxiety.

Knowledge deficit
 Related to:
 Lack of previous similar experiences
 	
 DEFINING CHARACTERISTICS
 Lack of questions
 Too many questions
 Inability of patient/ significant other to verbalize home care steps
	ONGOING ASSESSMENT
	 - Assess patient's level of understanding.
	 - Assess patient's ability to learn.
	 - Assess patient's physical ability to care for self.
	
	 THERAPEUTIC INTERVENTIONS
	 - Encourage patient to ask questions.
	 - Provide information about surgery, postoperative care, and convalescence *to decrease anxiety and promote trust.*
	 - Evaluate understanding of information after teaching sessions *to assess knowledge retained.*
	 - Instruct patient in the following before discharge:
	     Incision care
	     Bathing
	     Exercising
	     Proper diet
	     Time to notify physician
		Patient and family will understand importance of adhering to medical regimen to prevent postoperative complications.

Originated by: Ruth E. Novitt-Schumacher, RN,C, MSN

Cirrhosis

(LAËNNEC'S CIRRHOSIS; HEPATIC ENCEPHALOPATHY; ASCITES)

A chronic disease characterized by scarring of the liver. Cirrhosis of the liver is the eighth leading cause of death among men age 40-60.

NURSING DIAGNOSES / DEFINING CHARACTERISTICS	NURSING INTERVENTIONS / *RATIONALES*	EXPECTED OUTCOMES
Altered nutrition: less than body requirements *Related to:* Poor eating habits Excess alcohol intake Lack of financial means Altered hepatic metabolic function Inadequate bile production Nausea, vomiting, anorexia **DEFINING CHARACTERISTICS** Documented inadequate dietary intake Weight loss Muscle wasting, especially in extremities Skin changes consistent with vitamin deficiency (flaking, loss of elasticity) Coagulopathies	**ONGOING ASSESSMENT** • Obtain weight history. • Assess for weight distribution. *Actual weight may remain steady while muscle mass deteriorates and ascitic fluid accumulates.* • Document intake. • Monitor serum electrolytes and albumin/protein levels. • Monitor glucose levels. • Monitor coagulation profile. **THERAPEUTIC INTERVENTIONS** • Provide diet high in calories from carbohydrate source. *Aberrant protein metabolism in failing liver can cause hepatic encephalopathy.* • Schedule small frequent meals. • Assist with meals as needed. • Provide dietary/pharmacologic vitamin supplementation. *If bile production is impaired, absorption of fat soluble vitamins A, D, E, and K will be inadequate.* • Provide enteral or parenteral nutritional support as ordered, using carbohydrates as calorie source. • See Nutrition, altered: less than body requirements, p. 37.	Optimal nutritional status will be achieved.

Excess extravascular fluid volume: ascites
 Related to:
 Increased portal venous pressure
 Hypoalbuminemia
 Low serum oncontic pressure
 Aldosterone imbalance
 	
 DEFINING CHARACTERISTICS
 Increasing abdominal girth
 Ballottement (fluid wave) on abdominal assessment
 Taut abdomen, dull to percussion
	ONGOING ASSESSMENT
	 • Assess for presence of ascites:
	     Measure abdominal girth daily, taking care to measure at same point consistently.
	     Check abdomen for dullness on percussion.
	     Check for ballottement.
	 • Monitor serum albumin and globulin levels.
	 • Assess for signs of portal hypertension:
	     History of upper GI bleeding
	     Spider nevi
	 • Record I & O.
	 • Assess for side effects of massive ascites:
	     Limited mobility
	     Decreased appetite
	     Inadequate lung expansion
	     Altered body image
	     Self-care deficit
	
	 THERAPEUTIC INTERVENTIONS
	 • Restrict fluid and sodium intake as ordered.
	 • Administer diuretics cautiously *as excess fluid is extravascular; aggressive diuresis can lead to dehydration and acute tubular necrosis or hepatorenal syndrome.*
		Extravascular fluid volume excess will be relieved.

Continued.

Cirrhosis— cont'd

NURSING DIAGNOSES / DEFINING CHARACTERISTICS	NURSING INTERVENTIONS / *RATIONALES*	EXPECTED OUTCOMES

	• Assist with paracentesis as needed.
	• For peritoneovenous shunt (LaVeen shunt, Denver shunt), facilitate shunt function by:
	    Applying abdominal binder.
	    Encouraging use of blow bottle or incentive spirometer. *Inspiring against resistance and use of abdominal binder increase intraperitoneal pressures, causing valve in shunt to open, allowing ascitic fluid to shunt into vascular space.*
	• Administer spironolactone as ordered.
	• If side effects of massive ascites present, see Mobility, impaired physical, p. 35 and Body image disturbance, p. 6.	

Potential fluid volume deficit Overly aggressive diuresis GI bleeding Poor oral intake Coagulopathies **DEFINING CHARACTERISTICS** Dark, tea-colored urine Concentrated urine Poor skin turgor Hematemesis Melena Hematochezia Stool and/or gastric contents guaiac-positive Falling blood pressure	**ONGOING ASSESSMENT** • Monitor vital signs; check for orthostatic changes. • Monitor I & O; note urine specific gravity. • Test any emesis, gastric aspirate, or stool for blood. • Note any loss of blood from GI tract; document amount. • Monitor coagulation profile. **THERAPEUTIC INTERVENTIONS** • Administer IV fluids and/or blood products as ordered. • Hold diuretics. • See Gastrointestinal bleeding, p. 284.	Fluid volume will remain adequate.

Potential altered thought processes
Related to:
Hepatic encephalopathy
Delirium tremens
Acute intoxication
Hepatic metabolic insufficiency
 	
DEFINING CHARACTERISTICS
Altered attention span
Inability to give accurate history
Inability to follow commands
Disorientation to person, place, and/or time
Delusions
Inappropriate behavior
	ONGOING ASSESSMENT
	• Monitor blood alcohol level on admission.
	• Monitor blood ammonia levels. *Ammonia is a cerebral toxin that contributes to changed LOC.*
	• Note time since last ingestion of alcohol. *Delirium tremens can occur up to 7 days after last alcohol intake.*
	• Assess for signs/symptoms of hepatic encephalopathy; note stage.
	• Document improvement/deterioration in level of encephalopathy.
	• Monitor for evidence of violent, hallucinatory, and/or delusional thought.
	• Monitor lab values.
	• Monitor I & O.
	• Evaluate factors that may increase cerebral sensitivity to ammonia (infections, acid-base imbalances).
	
	THERAPEUTIC INTERVENTIONS
	• Protect patient from physical harm:
	    Pad side rails.
	    Keep bed in low position.
	    Restrain, if necessary.
	    Administer sedatives (*nonhepatic metabolism*) as ordered; document effectiveness; notify physician if dosage needs adjustment.
	    Prevent oversedation *that may precipitate coma.*
		Thought processes will remain normal.

Cirrhosis— cont'd

NURSING DIAGNOSES / DEFINING CHARACTERISTICS	NURSING INTERVENTIONS / *RATIONALES*	EXPECTED OUTCOMES
Self- or other-directed violence Inappropriate affect Evidence of hepatic encephalopathy: *Stage I:* Minor mental aberrations Confusion *Stage II:* Asterixis Apraxia *Stage III:* Lethargy alternating with combativeness Stupor EEG slowing *Stage IV:* Coma Further EEG slowing Fetor hepaticas Altered hepatic enzymes Altered liver function studies	• Orient patient to time, place, and person: 　Place calendar and clock in room. 　Provide environmental stimulation (television, radio, newspaper, visitors). • Provide emotional support by reassuring patient of physiologic cause of confusion. • Decrease intestinal bacteria content: 　Administer nonabsorbable antibiotics (neomycin, kanamycin) as ordered. 　Administer lactulose as ordered *to alter colonic pH and stimulate evacuation.* • Decrease ammonigenic potential: 　Order low-protein diet (20-40 g/day). 　Check drugs for ammonia content. 　Clean intestines of any old blood (lavage, suction, enemas). • See Thought process, altered, p. 52.	
Potential impaired gas exchange *Related to:* Decreased lung excursion related to ascites Aspiration secondary to vomiting, retching Altered LOC **DEFINING CHARACTERISTICS** Restlessness Irritability Altered ABGs Confusion Change in mentation	**ONGOING ASSESSMENT** • Assess respirations; note quality, rate, depth, use of accessory muscles, position assumed for ease of breathing, and apparent impact of ascitic abdomen. • Monitor ABGs. • Assess for changes in orientation and/or behavior. **THERAPEUTIC INTERVENTIONS** • Administer O_2 as ordered. • Assist patient to most effective position for breathing. *Elevating HOB to 30 degrees facilitates diaphragmatic excursion by displacing ascitic fluid from chest.* • Assist patient in eating/drinking *to minimize risk of aspiration.* • Withhold oral food/fluid from patient if LOC altered. • Suction if necessary. • Encourage turning, coughing, and deep breathing. • See Gas exchange, impaired, p. 21.	Optimal gas exchange will be achieved.
Pain, itching *Related to:* Jaundice Elevated bilirubin levels **DEFINING CHARACTERISTICS** Icteric skin, sclerae Itching/scratching Restlessness	**ONGOING ASSESSMENT** • Assess for jaundice. • Monitor liver function tests, especially bilirubin levels. *Unexcreted bilirubin moves by diffusion into subcutaneous and cutaneous structures and irritates the tissue, causing histamine release and itching.* • Assess itchiness and scratching. **THERAPEUTIC INTERVENTIONS** • Keep skin clean and well moisturized. • Discourage scratching *(can introduce pathogens and cause localized infection).* • Place mitts on patient if scratching cannot be discouraged by other means. • Administer antihistamines as ordered.	Itching will be relieved.

Continued.

Cirrhosis— cont'd

NURSING DIAGNOSES / DEFINING CHARACTERISTICS	NURSING INTERVENTIONS/ *RATIONALES*	EXPECTED OUTCOMES
Potential impaired skin integrity *Related to:* Immobility related to altered LOC Anasarca Poor nutritional status Poor personal hygiene Icteric skin Exposure to outside environment **DEFINING CHARACTERISTICS** Taunt, shiny skin Jaundiced skin Evidence of scratching Redness over bony prominences Stage I or greater areas of breakdown Evidence of poor personal hygiene Dirty clothes Dirt on body Dirt on feet Body odor Emaciated appearance	**ONGOING ASSESSMENT** · Assess skin for redness, excoriation, especially over bony prominences. · Assess for peripheral and generalized edema. · Assess patient's ability to provide self-care and initiate movement. · Assess weight and general nutritional status **THERAPEUTIC INTERVENTIONS** · Keep skin clean and well moisturized. · Institute pressure relief device(s) for patients confined to bed for long periods. · Handle edematous extremities gently *to minimize pitting.* · Institute turning schedule if patient immobile/unconscious. · Provide low-protein, high-calorie, high-carbohydrate diet. · Encourage fluid intake within limits of medical treatment plan. · See Skin integrity, impaired, p. 48.	Optimal skin integrity will be maintained.

Knowledge deficit *Related to:* New disease New complications of long-standing disease
 	
DEFINING CHARACTERISTICS Multiple questions Lack of questions Repeated admissions Evidence of inability to care for self
	ONGOING ASSESSMENT
	· Assess readiness to learn.
	· Assess available support systems.
	· Assess resources, ability to provide housing, food, medical care.
	· Assess need for readiness for alcohol rehabilitation.
	
	THERAPEUTIC INTERVENTIONS
	· Teach patient/significant other the following:
	   Effects of alcohol intake/abstinence
	   Need for high-calorie, low-protein diet *to facilitate regeneration of damaged liver cells*
	   Signs and symptoms of complications of cirrhosis:
	     Abdominal pain
	     Vomiting, anorexia
	     Loss of blood from GI tract
	     Generalized bleeding (from gums, skin, GU tract)
	     Changes in level of consciousness
	· Teach patient/significant other dose, administration schedule, expected actions, and possible side effects of prescribed medications.
	· Refer to alcohol rehabilitation program, if appropriate.
		Patient will verbalize understanding of disease and complications.

Originated by: Denise Myles, RN,C
        Urakay Campbell, RN
        Audrey Klopp, RN, PhD, ET

Diverticular disease

(DIVERTICULITIS; DIVERTICULOSIS)

A diverticulum is a saclike weakening in the wall of the bowel. Diverticulitis is the inflammation of diverticula and the condition in which an individual has many diverticula present. Diverticulosis may remain asymptomatic or may present as alternating diarrhea/constipation, peritonitis (if a diverticulum perforates), or a life-threatening GI hemorrhage (10 to 20%). Management is generally medical, although 25% of patients are treated surgically for diverticulitis.

NURSING DIAGNOSES / DEFINING CHARACTERISTICS	NURSING INTERVENTIONS / *RATIONALES*	EXPECTED OUTCOMES

Pain
 Related to:
 Inflamed diverticulum
 Perforated diverticulum
 Peritonitis
 Spastic bowel contractions
 	
 DEFINING CHARACTERISTICS
 Grimacing
 Moaning
 Tenderness in left lower abdominal quadrant
 Suprapubic pain
 Abdominal rigidity
	ONGOING ASSESSMENT
	 • Assess abdominal pain:
	    Location
	    Quality
	    Severity
	    Precipitating factors
	    Progress
	 • Investigate perception of precipitating factors and possible history of diverticulosis. *Long-standing history of constipation and/or diarrhea may indicate undiagnosed diverticulosis.*
	 • Assess recent diet history.
	
	 THERAPEUTIC INTERVENTIONS
	 • Assist patient to position of comfort.
	 • Administer analgesics as ordered.
	 • Use nonpharmacologic methods of pain management.
	 • See Pain, p. 39; and Acute abdomen, p. 269.
		Pain will be relieved.

Anxiety *Related to:* New disease Recurrence of old disease Hospitalization Possible surgery Uncertain outcome **DEFINING CHARACTERISTICS** Restlessness Trembling Worried facial expression Repeated requests for information	**ONGOING ASSESSMENT** • Assess level of anxiety. • Elicit perception of events and likely outcomes. • Explore previous methods of coping with anxiety. • Assess availability of social support system. **THERAPEUTIC INTERVENTIONS** • Provide accurate information so patient understands. • Answer questions honestly. • Help patient mobilize previously successful coping strategies. • Minimize environmental factors (noise, light, odors) *that may worsen anxiety*. • Encourage/support family/significant others in patient support. • See Anxiety, p. 4.	Anxiety will be managed.
Potential for infection *Related to:* Perforated diverticulum Peritonitis **DEFINING CHARACTERISTICS** Extreme abdominal pain	**ONGOING ASSESSMENT** • Assess abdominal pain. • Note rigidity on abdominal examination. • Auscultate for bowel sounds. • Monitor WBC. • Monitor vital signs, especially temperature. **THERAPEUTIC INTERVENTIONS** • Notify physician if defining characteristics present. *Peritonitis usually a surgical emergency*. • Prepare for possible surgery.	Risk of infection will be reduced.

Continued.

NURSING DIAGNOSES / DEFINING CHARACTERISTICS	NURSING INTERVENTIONS / *RATIONALES*	EXPECTED OUTCOMES
Rigid, boardlike abdomen on palpation Fever Elevated WBC Absent bowel sounds	· Administer antibiotics and antipyretics as ordered. · Administer IV fluids as ordered. · Maintain NPO status and functional NG tube. · See Acute abdomen, p. 269.	
Potential fluid volume deficit *Related to:* Hemorrhage from diverticulum **DEFINING CHARACTERISTICS** Decreased blood pressure Increased heart rate Change in LOC Dry mucous membranes Decreased urine output Blood in stool (visible or occult)	**ONGOING ASSESSMENT** · Monitor vital signs. · Monitor LOC, noting changes that may indicate fluid volume deficit. · Maintain careful I & O records. · Assess and document blood loss from GI tract. **THERAPEUTIC INTERVENTIONS** · Administer IV fluids and/or blood products as ordered. · Prepare for surgery or transfer to monitored area. *Hypovolemic patients may be volume resuscitated and prepared for surgery in critical care area unless hemorrhage life-threatening and patient too unstable to be moved or taken directly to surgery.* · See Fluid volume deficit, p. 20; and Gastrointestinal bleeding, p. 284.	Optimal fluid volume will be maintained.

Knowledge deficit
Related to:
New disease
Recurrence of old disease
 	
DEFINING CHARACTERISTICS
Multiple questions
Lack of questions
Verbalized need for more information
Observed selection of inappropriate diet
	ONGOING ASSESSMENT
	· Assess readiness to learn.
	· Assess understanding of causes and management of diverticular disease.
	
	THERAPEUTIC INTERVENTIONS
	· Teach patient/significant other the following:
	  Role of dietary fiber *in producing fecal bulk and facilitating peristaltic movement in bowel*
	  Necessity of reporting abdominal pain and/or GI tract blood loss
	  Use of prescribed pharmacologic fiber sources *(Some individuals with diverticulosis tolerate increased bulk poorly and may need prescribed dosage altered.)*
	· Document teaching and patient's response.
		Patient/significant other will verbalize understanding of long-term management of diverticular disease.

Originated by: Sheila Winfield, RN, BSN

Enterocutaneous fistula

Communication between any portion of the gastrointestinal tract and the skin. Fistulae may occur spontaneously or post-operatively and may be treated medically or surgically.

NURSING DIAGNOSES / DEFINING CHARACTERISTICS	NURSING INTERVENTIONS / *RATIONALES*	EXPECTED OUTCOMES
Actual impaired skin integrity; Potential impaired skin integrity *Related to:* Continuous contact of bowel secretions with skin Altered nutritional/metabolic state **DEFINING CHARACTERISTICS** Patient complains of burning, itching Skin is red, tender Skin is excoriated	**ONGOING ASSESSMENT** • Assess skin condition: Redness Excoriation Tenderness • Assess secretion amount, quality, and pH. **THERAPEUTIC INTERVENTIONS** • See Skin integrity, impaired, p. 48. • Maintain intact perifistulous skin. *Dressing method:* Protect wound edges with Duoderm or Stomahesive barriers. Change dressing as frequently as necessary *to keep wound edges dry.* Use alternate methods (net panties, Montgomery straps) *to hold dressing in place. Adhesives can further compromise skin integrity.* *Pouch method:* Choose appropriate pouch by evaluating: Skin condition Size and shape of abdomen Presence of current or recent sutures Fistula site Characteristics of fistula drainage Clean and prepare perifistulous skin. *Skin preparation most important step in pouching fistula.* Prepare pattern; apply Stomahesive or Duoderm. Fashion pouch; apply over skin barrier. Attach to gravity drainage if indicated. *Skin barrier is protected, pouch will last longer if drainage channeled from skin seal.* Keep pouch emptied routinely if not connected to gravity. Change as necessary when leakage occurs. *Suction method (if neither pouch nor dressings maintain dryness):* Obtain permission from physician to place soft, fenestrated catheter near fistula site. Position and anchor catheter. Connect to low, intermittent suction device.	Potential for altered skin integrity will be reduced.
Potential fluid volume deficit *Related to:* Loss of fluid via fistula NPO status	**ONGOING ASSESSMENT** • Assess hydration status every shift: Skin turgor Mucous membranes I & O Weight Laboratory values Vital signs Subjective indicators • Monitor serum and urine osmolality and specific gravity.	Fluid volume and electrolyte balance will be maintained.

Continued.

281

NURSING DIAGNOSES / DEFINING CHARACTERISTICS	NURSING INTERVENTIONS / *RATIONALES*	EXPECTED OUTCOMES
DEFINING CHARACTERISTICS Decreased urine output Concentrated urine Dry mucous membranes Decreased venous filling Weight loss Increased heart rate Decreased skin turgor Abnormal electrolyte profile Complaints of thirst Complaints of weakness, dizziness Change in mental status	**THERAPEUTIC INTERVENTIONS** · Document and report to physician signs/symptoms of electrolyte imbalance and dehydration. · Administer parenteral fluids as ordered. · Offer ice chips and fluids as ordered/tolerated by patient. · Administer anticholinergeric drugs as ordered *to inhibit intestinal secretion*. · See Fluid volume deficit, p. 20.	
Altered nutrition: less than body requirements *Related to:* Nutritional loss from fistula(s) Decreased or bypassed absorptive surface Prolonged therapeutic withholding of nutrients **DEFINING CHARACTERISTICS** Complaints of weakness Weight loss Negative nitrogen balance Low serum albumin Low total iron-binding capacity (TIBC) Scaling skin	**ONGOING ASSESSMENT** · See Nutrition, altered: less than body requirements, p. 37. · Assess nitrogen balance. · Assess serum TIBC and serum albumin. · If patient has hyperalimentation line, inspect insertion site for redness, swelling, oozing, and tenderness. · Weigh patient daily. · Check electrolytes daily. **THERAPEUTIC INTERVENTIONS** · Administer hyperalimentation per order. · Maintain flow rate. *If administration to be stopped or resumed for any reason, change flow rate to 50% normal rate for at least 1 hr to allow appropriate pancreatic response.* · Change occlusive dressing and tubing q48h or as situation dictates.	Adequate nutritional status will be maintained.
Body image disturbance *Related to:* Continuous fecal drainage Fecal odor Necessity of pouch, dressings, and/or suction catheter	**ONGOING ASSESSMENT** · Note verbal indications of altered self-concept/body image. · Note patient's willingness to socialize with family, friends, staff, other patients. · Note patient's involvement in self-care. · Note defensive behaviors about appearance.	Body image disturbance is reduced.

Enterocutaneous fistula— cont'd

NURSING DIAGNOSES / DEFINING CHARACTERISTICS	NURSING INTERVENTIONS / *RATIONALES*	EXPECTED OUTCOMES
DEFINING CHARACTERISTICS Verbalized concern of altered pattern of excretion Resistance to environmental change Reluctance to look at or touch pouch Altered socialization Nonparticipation in therapy Lack of eye contact	**THERAPEUTIC INTERVENTIONS** · Encourage verbalization. · Talk with patient empathetically. · Provide adequate site care *so odor is minimized or eliminated.*	
Potential anxiety *Related to:* Prolonged hospitalization Appearance of fistula/pouch Painful uncomfortable pouch/dressing changes Prolonged nutritional support Prolonged isolation from family, friends, and work Possible need for surgery **DEFINING CHARACTERISTICS** Increased questioning Facial tension Verbalized anxiety Constant demands Restlessness Lack of participation in self-care Inability to accept care from others Derogatory comments about self Increased heart rate, respiratory rate Insomnia	**ONGOING ASSESSMENT** · See Anxiety, p. 4. · Assess for defining characteristics. **THERAPEUTIC INTERVENTIONS** · Discuss present status/anticipated therapy. · Explain usual therapy course. · Provide simple explanations and reassurance. *Understanding how and why procedures are done may help decrease fear/anxiety.* · Take time to listen to fears, concerns. · Point out progress, however slight (e.g., decrease in drainage). · Assist patient in using usual coping behaviors. · Express normalcy of such feelings about self under circumstances. · Verbalize for nonverbal patient. · Reinforce that once fistula healed, elimination returns to normal. · Institute appropriate odor-control measures. · Initiate consultation with occupational/physical therapist *to provide opportunity for exercise and activity.* · Encourage use of distractions (television, radio, newspapers).	Anxiety/fear will be reduced.

Originated by: Florencia Isidro-Sanchez, RN, BSN

Gastrointestinal bleeding

(LOWER GASTROINTESTINAL BLEED; UPPER GASTROINTESTINAL BLEED; ESOPHAGEAL VARICES; ULCERS)

Loss of blood from the GI tract is most often the result of erosion or ulceration of the mucosa but may be the result of arteriovenous (AV) malformation, malignancies, increased pressure in the portal venous bed, or direct trauma to the gastrointestinal tract. Alcohol abuse is a major etiologic factor in GI bleeding.

NURSING DIAGNOSES / DEFINING CHARACTERISTICS	NURSING INTERVENTIONS / *RATIONALES*	EXPECTED OUTCOMES
Actual fluid volume deficit *Related to:* *Upper GI bleeding* (mouth, esophagus, stomach, duodenum) caused by: Gastric ulcer Duodenal ulcer Gastritis Esophageal varices Mallory-Weiss tear Blunt or penetrating trauma Cancer *Lower GI bleeding* (small or large intestine, rectum, anus) caused by: Tumors Inflammatory bowel disease (diverticular disease, Crohn's disease, ulcerative colitis) A-V malformations Blunt or penetrating trauma Hemorrhoids *Generalized GI bleeding:* Systemic coagulopathies Radiation therapy Chemotherapy Family history of GI bleeding **DEFINING CHARACTERISTICS** Hematemesis, observed or reported Melena Hematochezia (bright red blood per rectum) History of recent violent retching Abdominal pain History of alcohol abuse	**ONGOING ASSESSMENT** • Monitor color, consistency of hematemesis, melena, or rectal bleeding; encourage patient to describe unwitnessed blood loss accurately using common household measures (e.g., a cupful a spoonful, a pint). • Obtain history of use/abuse of substances known to predispose to GI bleeding: 　Aspirin 　Aspirin-containing drugs 　Nonsteroidal anti-inflammatory drugs 　Ibuprofen-containing drugs 　Alcohol 　Steroids • Monitor BP for orthostatic changes (from patient lying prone to high Fowler's). Note orthostatic hypotension significance: 　*>10 mm Hg drop: circulating blood volume decreased by 20%.* 　*>20-30 mm Hg drop: circulating blood volume decreased by 40%.* • Assess for signs/symptoms of fluid volume deficit. • Monitor coagulation profile. • Monitor Hb and Hct. • Monitor liver function studies. • Obtain diet history **THERAPEUTIC INTERVENTIONS** • Start one or more large-bore IVs. *Rapid volume expansion necessary to prevent/treat hypovolemia complications; IV medication and/or blood component administration is likely.* • Insert NG tube *for stomach lavage, to monitor continuing blood loss closely, and for medication administration.* • Lavage stomach until clots no longer present, return is clear, using room temperature saline. *Iced saline may cause undesirable ischemic changes in gastric mucosa.* • Provide volume resuscitation with crystalloids or blood products as ordered; monitor cardiopulmonary response to volume expansion. *Patients with history of alcohol abuse may have alcohol-related cardiomyopathies.* • Assist with/coordinate diagnostic procedures performed *to identify bleeding site:* 　Endoscopy: *provides direct visualization of esophagus, stomach, and duodenum. Procedure must precede x-rays requiring barium ingestion to maximize visualization by endoscopist.* 　Sigmoidoscopy/proctoscopy/colonoscopy; *provides direct visualization of rectum and colon.* 　Barium studies: 　　Barium swallow: *indirect visualization of esophagus, stomach, and small intestine* 　　Barium enema: *indirect visualization of colon* 　　Small bowel follow-through: *indirect visualization of small intestine* 　Angiography *(may be diagnostic or performed for arterial line placement to infuse vasoconstrictive medications locally; will be inconclusive diagnostically unless bleeding >0.5 cc/min).* After angiography, dress site with pressure dressing for at least 8 hr. Connect arterial line left in place to pressure/flush system or to vasopressin drip. See Nursing Diagnosis, Potential for injury p. 286.	Optimal fluid volume will be maintained.

NURSING DIAGNOSES / DEFINING CHARACTERISTICS	NURSING INTERVENTIONS / *RATIONALES*	EXPECTED OUTCOMES
History of aspirin, steroid, nonsteroid, or ibuprofen use/ abuse Orthostatic changes Tachycardia Hypotension Change in LOC Thirst Dry mucous membranes Altered coagulation profile	• Administer vitamin K as ordered *to allow coagulation factor production.* • Administer antacids and H$_2$ receptor antagonists (i.e., Cimetadine, Zantac) *to suppress gastric/duodenal secretions.* • Arrange/assist with transfer of patient to monitored area if hemodynamically unstable. • Guard against inadvertent administration of drugs that may potentiate further bleeding. *If in critical care area:* • Prepare for insertion of Sengstaken-Blakemore tube for the patient bleeding from esophageal/gastric varices. • See Fluid volume deficit, p. 20.	
Anxiety *Related to:* Blood loss Hurried activity/care Uncertain outcome **DEFINING CHARACTERISTICS** Tense facial appearance Multiple questions No questions Restlessness Crying Requests constant attendance by health care personnel	**ONGOING ASSESSMENT** • Assess level of anxiety. • Solicit expression(s) of anxiety cause. • Explore previous methods patient considers successful in managing anxiety (if possible). • Assess presence and helpfulness of social support system in managing anxiety. **THERAPEUTIC INTERVENTIONS** • Encourage verbalization/expressions of anxiety. • Keep patient informed of status and related information. *Patient's view pending transfer from one area to another as a sign of deterioration.* • Answer questions honestly and simply, repeating information when necessary. • See Anxiety, p. 4.	Anxiety/fear will be reduced.
Potential for pain *Related to:* Invasive therapies Diagnostic procedures Vomiting Diarrhea **DEFINING CHARACTERISTICS** Verbalizes pain/ discomfort Facial grimacing Restlessness	**ONGOING ASSESSMENT** • Assess specific sources of discomfort. • Ask patient what measure(s) he/she believes might provide comfort. **THERAPEUTIC INTERVENTIONS** • Tape/stabilize all tubes, drains, and catheters *to minimize movement causing discomfort.* • Provide frequent oral hygiene *to remove blood/emesis and moisten mucous membranes.* • For patient with traction helmet for stabilization of Sengstaken-Blakemore tube, pad parts contacting skin *to minimize occurrence of skin friction and/ or ischemia.* • Provide meticulous perineal care after all bowel movements. • For patient with any indwelling nasogastric tube, moisten external nares with water-soluble lubricant at least once per shift *to reduce adherence of mucus (can dry and cause irritation).* • Change linens as necessary *to minimize discomfort and reduce unpleasant melenic odor.* • Use analgesics with caution *so LOC changes related to fluid volume deficit may be carefully evaluated.* • See Pain, p. 39.	Pain will be relieved.
Potential altered skin integrity *Related to:* Bed rest Frequent stooling	**ONGOING ASSESSMENT** • Assess condition of skin at least q2h. **THERAPEUTIC INTERVENTIONS** • Turn patient side to side as hemodynamic status allows.	Skin will remain intact.

Continued.

Gastrointestinal bleeding— cont'd

NURSING DIAGNOSES / DEFINING CHARACTERISTICS	NURSING INTERVENTIONS / *RATIONALES*	EXPECTED OUTCOMES
Hypovolemia leading to skin ischemia Poor nutritional status **DEFINING CHARACTERISTICS** Red, irritated skin Poor capillary refill Broken epidermis	· Place pressure relief device(s) beneath patient. · Do not allow patient to sit on bedpan for long periods. · Clean perianal skin with soap and water after each bowel movement; dry well. · Apply liquid film barrier to perianal area *so no direct skin contact with stool*. · Minimize use of plastic linen protectors (*harbor moisture and enhance maceration*). · See Skin integrity, impaired, p. 48.	
Potential for injury: complications of vasopressin (Pitressin) therapy *Related to:* Vasoconstriction Antidiuretic effect of vasopressin **DEFINING CHARACTERISTICS** Anginal pain ST-segment changes on ECG Sinus bradycardia Tremors Sweating Vertigo Pounding in head Abdominal cramps Circumoral pallor Nausea/vomiting Flatus Urticaria Fluid retention	**ONGOING ASSESSMENT** · Assess for side effects of vasopressin. · Monitor vital signs. · Assess peripheral pulses (rate, regularity) and capillary refill. · Assess for abdominal distention; record abdominal girth. **THERAPEUTIC INTERVENTIONS** · Administer vasopressin per order. · If side effects occur: 　Stop infusion of vasopressin drip. *IV vasopressin preparation is short-acting; cessation of administration diminishes adverse effects rapidly.* 　Have atropine on hand for decreased heart rate. 　Provide patient comfort and assurance.	Potential risk of injury related to vasopressin therapy is reduced.
Potential altered level of consciousness (LOC) *Related to:* Elevated cerebral toxin levels Altered metabolic liver function Increased cerebral sensitivity **DEFINING CHARACTERISTICS** Lethargy Confusion Somnolence Fever Acid-base imbalance	**ONGOING ASSESSMENT** · Assess for changes in level of consciousness. · Monitor ammonia levels. · Monitor acid-base balance. · Monitor temperature. **THERAPEUTIC INTERVENTIONS** · Reduce toxins available to the cerebral circulation by: 　Lavaging stomach *to remove blood*. 　Giving enemas *to remove blood*. 　Administering nonabsorbable antibiotics as ordered *to reduce intestinal bacteria count (thus reducing ammonia production)*. · Administer antipyretics as ordered. · Correct acid-base balance. · See Consciousness, altered level of, p. 234.	Normal LOC will be maintained.
Knowledge deficit *Related to:* First GI bleed Unfamiliar environment	**ONGOING ASSESSMENT** · Assess patient's/significant other's understanding of GI bleeding cause and treatment. · Assess understanding of need for long-term follow-up and possible lifestyle changes.	Patient/significant other understand cause(s) and management of GI bleeding.

Gastrointestinal bleeding— cont'd

NURSING DIAGNOSES / DEFINING CHARACTERISTICS	NURSING INTERVENTIONS / *RATIONALES*	EXPECTED OUTCOMES
DEFINING CHARACTERISTICS Multiple questions Lack of questions Verbalized misconceptions	**THERAPEUTIC INTERVENTIONS** • Explain procedures necessary for diagnosis and/or treatment before they are performed. *Understanding need for unpleasant procedures may help patient comply/participate and increase yield/effectiveness of treatment or procedure.* • Encourage/stress importance of avoidance of substances containing: 　Aspirin 　Alcohol 　Nonsteroidal anti-inflammatory drugs 　Ibuprofen 　Steroids • Teach patient dose, administration schedule, expected actions, and possible adverse effects of medications that may be prescribed for long periods. *Drugs given to decrease gastric acid production may be prescribed indefinitely; patients must understand that cessation of bleeding or other symptoms does not mean need for medication has ended.* • Refer patient to alcohol rehabilitation if indicated.	

Originated by: Marion C. Wallis, RN, CCRN
　　　　　　　Lou Ann Ary, RN, BSN

Hemorrhoids/ hemorrhoidectomy

(RECTAL POLYPS; PILES)

Hemorrhoids are the vascular tumors formed in the rectal mucosa caused by the presence of dilated blood vessels. Treatment varies with condition, including banding, laser, and surgical ligation.

NURSING DIAGNOSES / DEFINING CHARACTERISTICS	NURSING INTERVENTIONS / *RATIONALES*	EXPECTED OUTCOMES
Excess fluid volume, in superior (internal) and/or inferior (external) hemorrhoidal plexus *Related to:* Increased intravenous pressure in hemorrhoidal plexus **DEFINING CHARACTERISTICS** Large, firm lumps protruding from rectum Presence of large, firm lumps on rectal examination Anal itching Painless, intermittent bleeding Constant discomfort and bleeding	**ONGOING ASSESSMENT** • Solicit patient's history of signs/symptoms of hemorrhoids. *Severe bleeding and/or pain may indicate proctoscopy to diagnose internal hemorrhoids versus rectal polyps.* • Examine rectal area for external hemorrhoids: 　Skin-covered, emerging from external anal tissue. 　Protruding from anal canal, covered by rectal mucosa. **THERAPEUTIC INTERVENTIONS** • Encourage patient to avoid prolonged standing or sitting *(causes blood pooling and thrombosis).* • Treat diarrhea/constipation (see Diarrhea, p. 16 or Constipation, p. 12.) • Discuss patient's life-style and predisposing factors to hemorrhoid development: 　Prolonged occupational standing or sitting 　Straining caused by diarrhea, constipation, vomiting, sneezing, and coughing 　Heart failure 　Hepatic disease (abscess, hepatitis, cirrhosis) 　Loss of muscle tone (old age, rectal surgery, pregnancy, episiotomy, anal intercourse) 　Alcoholism 　Anorectal infections	Complications/ progression will be reduced.

Continued.

287

NURSING DIAGNOSES / DEFINING CHARACTERISTICS	NURSING INTERVENTIONS / *RATIONALES*	EXPECTED OUTCOMES
Rectal discomfort	• Discuss self-care issues: 　Bowel elimination 　Manual reduction of hemorrhoidal prolapse 　Dietary habits (provide dietary consultation if necessary)	
Pain *Related to:* Thrombosis of external hemorrhoids or hemorrhoidal prolapse **DEFINING CHARACTERISTICS** Sudden rectal pain Large, firm lumps protruding from rectum Postoperative pain	**ONGOING ASSESSMENT** • Assess onset, duration, type of pain. • Elicit comfort factors used in past. • Examine rectal area. **THERAPEUTIC INTERVENTIONS** • Provide local anesthetic as ordered. • Provide cold compresses. • Encourage warm sitz baths. • Administer analgesics as ordered for intractable pain (see Pain, p. 39). *Pain will be present until thrombosis is resolved.*	Pain/discomfort will be relieved or reduced.
Potential for injury *Related to:* Bleeding hemorrhoids Preoperative or postoperative hemorrhoidal bleeding Postoperative status or surgical procedure **DEFINING CHARACTERISTICS** Sudden, severe rectal bleeding Frequent, recurrent rectal bleeding (preoperative) Postoperative bleeding Pallor Weakness, fatigue	**ONGOING ASSESSMENT** *Preoperative care* • Assess onset and cause of bleeding. • Obtain history of past bleeding, frequency. • Assess vital signs q4h. • Examine rectal area; assess amount of bleeding: 　Small, moderate, or profuse 　Number of pads soaked • Assess Hct, Hb if anemia suspected in patient bleeding for a long time. *Postoperative care* • Examine rectal area for hematoma, swelling, drainage, and excessive bleeding. **THERAPEUTIC INTERVENTIONS** *Preoperative care* • Provide gentle rectal hygiene and minimal manipulation *to prevent tearing thin rectal tissue.* Do *not* take rectal temperature. • Notify physician of large blood loss, vital sign changes. • Anticipate need for type and cross match. • Prepare patient for surgery if indicated. *Postoperative care* • Administer medications as ordered (*Metamucil to increase stool bulk*). • Keep wound site clean by changing pads as needed and providing sitz baths if appropriate.	Rectal bleeding will be avoided or reduced.
Knowledge deficit *Related to:* New condition No previous surgical intervention **DEFINING CHARACTERISTICS** Requests for information Repeated episodes of bleeding or thrombosis	**ONGOING ASSESSMENT** • Assess current level of understanding. • Assess ability to comprehend. **THERAPEUTIC INTERVENTIONS** • Instruct patient on importance of regular bowel habits. • Discuss good anal hygiene: 　Suggest use of plain, nonscented white toilet paper. 　Encourage use of medicated astringent pads for cleansing. 　Discuss avoidance of hand soaps and vigorous washing with hand towels. *Soap can irritate rectal mucosa. Vigorous washing can disrupt thin tissues and cause bleeding.* • Provide dietary information/consultation.	Patient expresses understanding of treatment and prevention.

Hemorrhoids/hemorrhoidectomy— cont'd

NURSING DIAGNOSES / DEFINING CHARACTERISTICS	NURSING INTERVENTIONS / *RATIONALES*	EXPECTED OUTCOMES

	• Discuss other predisposing factors:
	    Occupational
	    Disease-oriented
	    Sexual habits
	• If patient to have surgical or other intervention, provide accurate preoperative instruction; discuss postprocedural expectations.
	• Upon discharge, provide patient with follow-up appointment and important telephone numbers.	

Originated by: Michele Knoll Puzas, RN,C, MHPE

Hernia/herniorrhaphy

A hernia is a protrusion of an organ through a congenital or acquired weakness in the abdominal wall. More frequent in men than women, hernias can be inguinal, labial, scrotal, femoral, umbilical, or incisional in origin. Surgical correction prevents incarceration and strangulation of protruding bowel, which are emergencies.

NURSING DIAGNOSES / DEFINING CHARACTERISTICS	NURSING INTERVENTIONS / *RATIONALES*	EXPECTED OUTCOMES
Preoperative: altered tissue integrity *Related to:* Break in continuity of musculature **DEFINING CHARACTERISTICS** Abnormal abdominal bulge Hernia may or may not be reducible Hernia may or may not be painful	**ONGOING ASSESSMENT** • Assess for presence of abnormal bulges in abdominal wall. • Assess size and reducibility of bulge. *Small hernias may present only with increased abdominal pressure (cough, straining).* • Assess for pain. *Pain with fever, swelling, and vomiting may indicate strangulated bowel.* **THERAPEUTIC INTERVENTIONS** • Notify physician if hernia is new phenomenon *so appropriate treatment will be initiated.* • Notify physician of signs of complications. • Prepare patient for surgical intervention.	Further tissue damage will be prevented.

Postoperative potential for infection
Related to:
Surgical incision
 	
DEFINING CHARACTERISTICS
Elevated temperature, pulse, and respiratory rate
Presence of drainage, odor, redness, and/or swelling of incision
	ONGOING ASSESSMENT
	• Assess incision line and/or dressing for cleanliness, approximation, swelling, hematoma, redness, drainage, and odor.
	• Assess vital signs, especially temperature, q4h.
	• Obtain culture if drainage from incision *to facilitate treatment.*
	
	THERAPEUTIC INTERVENTIONS
	• Keep operative site clean and dry by:
	    Changing dressing when soiled and at least every day.
	    Preventing urine and stool contamination.
	• Avoid pressure on operative site.
	• Administer antipyretics for temperature >38.5° C (rectal) per order.
	• Administer antibiotics as ordered *to prevent infection.*
		Risk of infection will be decreased.

Continued.

289

NURSING DIAGNOSES / DEFINING CHARACTERISTICS	NURSING INTERVENTIONS / *RATIONALES*	EXPECTED OUTCOMES

Ineffective airway clearance *Related to:* Medications, anesthesia, and pain
 	
 DEFINING CHARACTERISTICS Presence of rales, rhonchi, and wheezes Tachypnea Dyspnea and apnea Cyanosis Ineffective cough Inability to cough voluntarily
	ONGOING ASSESSMENT
	 • Assess breath sounds for:
	   Quality
	   Rate
	   Depth
	 • Assess for symptoms of respiratory distress: retractions; rales, rhonchi, and wheezing; cyanosis; decreased/increased respiratory rate.
	 • See Airway clearance, ineffective, p. 3.
	
	 THERAPEUTIC INTERVENTIONS
	 • Provide humidity at bedside by humidifier/humidified O_2 *to liquify secretions.*
	 • Suction nasopharynx as needed.
	 • Reposition frequently.
	 • Encourage coughing, deep breathing, and use of incentive spirometer *to promote lung expansion.*
		Airway will be free of secretions.

Pain *Related to:* Surgery
 	
 DEFINING CHARACTERISTICS Crying Restlessness Listlessness Irritability Poor appetite Altered sleep pattern Verbalized complaint of discomfort
	ONGOING ASSESSMENT
	 • Observe for:
	   Type and level of pain
	   Behavioral changes, irritability, restlessness, fretfulness, inability to soothe
	 • Assess effectiveness of analgesics administered.
	 • See Pain, p. 39.
	
	 THERAPEUTIC INTERVENTIONS
	 • Avoid direct pressure on incision.
	 • Provide comfort measures:
	   Quiet atmosphere
	   Analgesics as ordered
	 • Provide diversional activities if helpful, *to divert focus from pain and its source.*
		Pain will be reduced.

Potential fluid volume deficit *Related to:* Preoperative NPO Postoperative discomfort **DEFINING CHARACTERISTICS** Irritability Skin turgor poor to fair Dry mucous membranes Decreased urine output (<30 cc/hr) Weight loss Poor appetite	**ONGOING ASSESSMENT** • Assess for defining characteristics. • See Fluid volume deficit, p. 20. **THERAPEUTIC INTERVENTIONS** • Administer analgesics before meals. • Provide well-balanced diet and adequate fluids. • Encourage family participation at meals. *Mealtime a social occasion; intake may be better in social atmosphere.*	Potential for dehydration will be reduced.
Potential urinary retention *Related to:* Tissue swelling Anesthesia	**ONGOING ASSESSMENT** • Assess for evidence of urine output q2h. • Assess urine for appearance, color, volume, specific gravity. • See Urinary retention p. 61.	Normal pattern of urine elimination will be maintained.

NURSING DIAGNOSES / DEFINING CHARACTERISTICS	NURSING INTERVENTIONS / *RATIONALES*	EXPECTED OUTCOMES

DEFINING CHARACTERISTICS
Irritability
Pain
Abdominal/bladder distention
Restlessness
Absence of urine
Poor intake
	THERAPEUTIC INTERVENTIONS
	• Initiate measures to facilitate voiding:
	  Encourage fluids as tolerated.
	  Use warmth to relax sphincter (warm compress).
	  Use Crede's method.
	  Administer analgesics as ordered.
	• Notify physician of urine output <30 cc/hr *to facilitate treatment and prevent undue complications.*
	• Anticipate need to perform urinary catheterization.	

Knowledge deficit
Related to:
Hospitalization
Surgery and postoperative care
 	
DEFINING CHARACTERISTICS
Withdrawal
Depression and silence
Helplessness
Crying
Anxiety and tension
Demanding attitude
Frequent/repeated questions
	ONGOING ASSESSMENT
	• Assess for:
	  Previous surgery, hospitalization experience
	  Current understanding of surgery
	• Assess support system:
	  Family members
	  Relatives and friends
	  Clergy
	
	THERAPEUTIC INTERVENTIONS
	• Encourage communication and expression.
	• Encourage family involvement in care.
	• Explain home care of operative site:
	  Wash only with warm water.
	  Prevent contamination.
	  Do not remove Steristrips (will come off by themselves). *Early removal may hinder incision site healing.*
	• Explain possible postoperative complications:
	  Need to check for increased bleeding and drainage from operative site.
	  Need to check for symptoms of infection: elevated temperature, increased drainage, foul odor.
		Patient will verbalize understanding of treatment plan, home care responsibilities, and complications.

Originated by: Andrea So, RN, BSN
Ruth Novitt-Schumacher, RN,C, MSN

Hiatal hernia

(GASTROESOPHAGEL REFLUX [GER]; ESOPHAGITIS; HEARTBURN)

Sliding of a portion of the stomach through the normal opening in the diaphragm into the thoracic cavity, often accompanied by an incompetent gastroesophageal sphincter. Hiatal hernia occurs most frequently in older females.

NURSING DIAGNOSES / DEFINING CHARACTERISTICS	NURSING INTERVENTIONS / *RATIONALES*	EXPECTED OUTCOMES

Pain: heartburn
Related to:
Reflux of gastric contents secondary to:
  Weakening of esophageal muscles
Esophageal cancer
Kyphoscoliosis
Diaphragm malformation
Ascites
	ONGOING ASSESSMENT
	• Assess for complaints of:
	  Heartburn
	  Chest pain
	  Regurgitation
	• Assess pain characteristics:
	  Quality
	  Severity
	  Location
	  Onset
		Discomfort from gastric reflux will be reduced.

Continued.

NURSING DIAGNOSES / DEFINING CHARACTERISTICS	NURSING INTERVENTIONS / *RATIONALES*	EXPECTED OUTCOMES

Pregnancy
Any increase in intra-abdominal pressure (tumors)
 	
DEFINING CHARACTERISTICS
Heartburn, usually worse in recumbent position
Chest pain
Regurgitation
Facial mask of pain
Decreased physical activity
Guarding behavior
Moaning
Alteration in sleep pattern
Irritability
Diaphoresis
Change in pulse rate
Change in blood pressure
	Duration
	Precipitating factors
	Relieving factors
	
	THERAPEUTIC INTERVENTIONS
	• Enhance gravity *to keep stomach and gastric contents out of thoracic cavity:*
	   Elevate HOB at least 15 degrees.
	   Apply shock blocks to HOB.
	   Use pillows behind back for support.
	• Respond quickly to pain/discomfort complaints.
	• Provide quiet and restful environment *to reduce amount of gastric acid secretion.*
	• Structure patient's activities to provide time for rest.
	• Instruct patient to avoid:
	   Straining during bowel movement
	   Wearing restricting clothes
	   Bending forward
	   Coughing
	   Lifting heavy objects
	• Administer laxatives or stool softeners as ordered.
	• Discourage smoking *(stimulates acid production and decreases bicarbonate secretions).*
	• Administer antacids as ordered.	

Potential altered nutrition: less than body requirement
Related to:
Gastric reflux
Pain
 	
DEFINING CHARACTERISTICS
Weight less than ideal body weight
Documented inadequate caloric intake
Recent weight loss
	ONGOING ASSESSMENT
	• Document patient's actual weight on admission and daily.
	• Obtain nutritional history.
	• Assess dental status.
	• Document foods known to cause symptoms.
	• Assess patient's willingness to change diet habits.
	• Assess whether meal partner/food preparer understands nutrition requirements.
	• Monitor blood and urine (electrolytes, BUN, creatinine, CBC, glucose).
	• Maintain strict I & O.
	• Monitor caloric count if initiated by dietitian.
	
	THERAPEUTIC INTERVENTIONS
	• Order bland diet.
	• Instruct patient:
	   To eat frequent, small meals
	   To avoid eating for minimum of 2 hr before lying down
	   To eat slowly *(These measures decrease gastric reflux.)*
	• Instruct patient to avoid spicy foods, fruit juices, alcohol, bedtime snacks, coffee, other foods that produce symptoms.
	• Encourage reducing diet for overweight patient. *(Will decrease abdominal pressure)*
	• Consult dietitian for patient teaching:
	   Foods to avoid
	   Foods high in spices
	   Caloric requirements to reduce weight
	   Food preparation
	• Assist patient with meals when needed.
		Optimal weight will be maintained.

Hiatal hernia— cont'd

NURSING DIAGNOSES / DEFINING CHARACTERISTICS	NURSING INTERVENTIONS / *RATIONALES*	EXPECTED OUTCOMES
Knowledge deficit *Related to:* Unfamiliarity with diagnostic workup, disease process, and treatment **DEFINING CHARACTERISTICS** Lack of questions Multiple questions Verbalization of mis-information	**ONGOING ASSESSMENT** • Evaluate patient's level of understanding of: 　Diagnostic workup 　Disease process 　Treatment 　Long-term follow-up care • Explain to patient/significant others that *increased understanding reduces anxiety and stress-mediated gastric acid secretion.* **THERAPEUTIC INTERVENTIONS** • Explain to patient: 　Pathophysiology of hernia. 　Use of medications, including purpose, proper administration, side effects. 　Diagnostic test, including purpose and special instructions: 　　Chest x-ray film shows air behind heart 　　Barium study detects outpouching, which will contain barium 　　Endoscopy and biopsy reveal perforation 　　Esophageal abnormalities 　　pH studies detect gastric reflux 　　Guaiac test detects blood in stool 　　CBC to determine possible blood loss	Patient will verbalize understanding of diagnostic workup and management.

Originated by: Carolyn Bolton, RN, BS

Inflammatory bowel disease

(CROHN'S DISEASE; ULCERATIVE COLITIS)

The term inflammatory bowel disease (IBD) refers to a cluster of specific bowel pathologies whose symptoms are often so similar as to make diagnosis difficult and treatment empirical. Crohn's disease is associated with involvement of all four layers of the bowel and may occur anywhere in the GI tract, although it most commonly occurs in the small bowel. Ulcerative colitis involves the mucosa and submucosa only and occurs only in the colon. Etiology is unknown for both diseases. Incidence is usually in the 15- to 30-year-old age group. Diverticular disease occurs frequently in persons over age 40; seems to be etiologically related to high-fat, low-fiber diets; and occurs almost exclusively in the colon. IBD is treated medically. If medical management fails or complications occur, surgical resection and possible fecal diversion will be undertaken.

NURSING DIAGNOSES / DEFINING CHARACTERISTICS	NURSING INTERVENTIONS / *RATIONALES*	EXPECTED OUTCOMES
Abdominal pain, joint pain *Related to:* Bowel inflammation and contractions of diseased bowel or colon Systemic manifestations of IBD	**ONGOING ASSESSMENT** • Assess pain: 　Duration 　Location 　Frequency 　Occurrence/onset 　Severity (scale 1-10, 10 most severe) • Solicit patient's perception of measures to control pain. • Auscultate bowel sounds. • Check abdomen for rebound tenderness. • Evaluate patient's perception of dietary impact on abdominal pain. *Many IBD patients cannot tolerate dairy products.*	Pain will be relieved.

NURSING DIAGNOSES / DEFINING CHARACTERISTICS	NURSING INTERVENTIONS / *RATIONALES*	EXPECTED OUTCOMES
DEFINING CHARACTERISTICS Reports of intermittent colicky abdominal pain associated with diarrhea and chronic joint pain Abdominal rebound tenderness Chronic joint pain Hyperactive bowel sounds Pallor Diaphoresis Anxiety Restlessness Fatigue Malaise Abdominal distention Pain and cramps associated with eating	**THERAPEUTIC INTERVENTIONS** · Use techniques patient has found helpful in relieving discomfort. · Provide adequate rest periods *to facilitate sleep, comfort, and relaxation.* · Administer medications as ordered; evaluate and document effectiveness; observe for signs of untoward effects. · Institute use of diversional activities, hobbies, relaxation techniques, and psychosocial support systems *to facilitate comfort and relaxation.* · Make necessary alterations in diet.	
Altered nutrition: less than body requirements *Related to:* Malabsorption Zinc deficiency Increased nitrogen loss with diarrhea Decreased intake Poor appetite **DEFINING CHARACTERISTICS** Nausea Diarrhea >10-20% below ideal body weight Decreased/normal serum calcium, K^+, vitamins K and B_{12}, folic acid, and zinc Muscle wasting Pedal edema Skin lesions Poor wound healing	**ONGOING ASSESSMENT** · Document patient's actual weight on admission (do not estimate). · Obtain nutritional history. · Assess for skin lesions, skin breaks, tears, decreased skin integrity, and edema of extremities. · Assess serum electrolytes, Ca^+, vitamins K and B_{12}, folic acid, and zinc levels *to determine actual or potential deficiencies.* · Assess patterns of elimination: color, amount, consistency, frequency, odor, and presence of steatorrhea. · Monitor I & O **THERAPEUTIC INTERVENTIONS** · Consult dietitian to review nutritional history, monitor calorie count, and assist in menu selection. · Encourage active/passive ROM to patient's tolerance. · Keep room as odor-free as possible. · Administer vitamin/mineral supplements as ordered *to compensate for deficiencies.* · Encourage family members to bring food patient enjoys and *to enhance social nature of mealtime.*	Optimal nutritional state will be maintained.

NURSING DIAGNOSES / DEFINING CHARACTERISTICS	NURSING INTERVENTIONS / *RATIONALES*	EXPECTED OUTCOMES
Potential fluid volume deficit: *Related to:* Presence of excessive diarrhea/nausea/vomiting Blood loss from inflamed bowel mucosa Poor oral intake **DEFINING CHARACTERISTICS** Weight loss Decreased skin turgor Hypotension Concentrated urine Bloody stools	**ONGOING ASSESSMENT** • Assess hydration status: skin turgor, mucous membranes, I & O, weight, and vital signs. • Document hemoccult-positive stools or obvious presence of bloody diarrhea. • Monitor Hb and Hct if patient is bleeding. **THERAPEUTIC INTERVENTIONS** • Administer medications as ordered, noting possible reactions. *Azulfidine affects inflammatory response; corticosteroids may be used for both anti-inflammatory and immunosuppressive benefits.* • Administer IV fluids if patient unable to maintain adequate oral intake. • See Fluid volume deficit, p. 20; and Gastrointestinal bleeding, p. 284.	Normal fluid volume will be maintained.
Potential impaired skin integrity *Related to:* Decreased nutritional status Frequent loose stools **DEFINING CHARACTERISTICS** Reddened or irritated areas over bony prominences Excoriated perianal skin	**ONGOING ASSESSMENT** • Assess skin integrity, noting color, texture, moisture, and temperature. • Assess perianal skin daily. **THERAPEUTIC INTERVENTIONS** • Use prophylactic pressure-relieving devices on bed, chairs. • Encourage sitz baths *(promote perianal hygiene, comfort)*. • Use liquid skin barrier film on perianal region *for protection from diarrheal stool*.	Skin will remain intact.
Potential for infection *Related to:* Poor nutritional status Immunosuppression from steroid therapy **DEFINING CHARACTERISTICS** Decreased total lymphocyte count Poor wound healing Frequent "colds," flu Fever or lack of fever with other signs of infection	**ONGOING ASSESSMENT** • Monitor vital signs. • Monitor WBC. • Assess frequency of infectious episodes. • Assess wounds for signs of healing. **THERAPEUTIC INTERVENTIONS** • Maintain good handwashing and encourage patient to do same *to prevent nosocomial infection*. • Encourage well-balanced diet as tolerated. • Discourage visits from individuals with colds, flu, sore throat, or fever. • See "Granulocytopenia, p. 505; Excessive Glucocorticoids: Cushing's Syndrome, p. 381.	Risk of infection in immunocompromised patient is reduced.

Continued.

Gastrointestinal and Digestive Care Plans

NURSING DIAGNOSES / DEFINING CHARACTERISTICS	NURSING INTERVENTIONS / *RATIONALES*	EXPECTED OUTCOMES

Knowledge deficit
Related to:
Need for continuous and long-term management of chronic disease
Change in health care needs related to remission/ exacerbation of disease
 	
DEFINING CHARACTERISTICS
Multiple questions by patient/significant others related to disease process and management
Noncompliance with earlier therapy
Depression
Anxiety
	ONGOING ASSESSMENT
	• Assess patient's/significant other's understanding of IBD and necessary management.
	
	THERAPEUTIC INTERVENTIONS
	• Allow uninterrupted time with patient *to enhance communication and facilitate learning.*
	• Discuss disease process and management.
	• Encourage patient/significant others to verbalize disease process, management, concern, fears, and feelings. Document patient's understanding.
	• Make appropriate referrals:
	    Dietary
	    Psychiatric counseling
	    Ostomy association
	• Refer to Grief over long-term illness/disability, p. 618.
		Patient/significant other will verbalize understanding of disease and management.

Originated by: Vivian Jones, RN

Obesity, simple
(OVERWEIGHT)

Weight is 20% or more above ideal body weight for height and frame.

NURSING DIAGNOSES / DEFINING CHARACTERISTICS	NURSING INTERVENTIONS / *RATIONALES*	EXPECTED OUTCOMES

Altered nutrition: more than body requirements
Related to:
Food intake exceeds metabolic needs; not caused by hypothalamic disorder
 	
DEFINING CHARACTERISTICS
Body weight 20% or more above ideal for height and frame
Dysfunctional eating pattern
	ONGOING ASSESSMENT
	• Obtain detailed weight history, including:
	    Onset of obesity
	    Family history of obesity
	    Numbers and types of diets tried
	    Patterns of gaining and losing weight
	• Document, record patient's actual height and weight.
	• Determine caloric requirements and include in diet elements of balanced calorie-reduced diet.
	• Reassess calorie requirements whenever patient's weight plateaus *(metabolic rate decreases in response to prolonged decreased caloric intake).*
	• Assess level of nutritional knowledge.
	• Note type and amount of routine exercise.
	• Identify whether patient sees weight as problem.
	• Identify presence of associated diseases (e.g., hypertension, diabetes).
	
	THERAPEUTIC INTERVENTIONS
	• Set realistic weight goals. *Approximately 1-2 lb/wk is reasonable and will produce more permanent weight loss.*
	• Encourage patient to keep a food diary, including time food was eaten, amount eaten, where food was eaten, and associated feelings.
		A desirable weight with corresponding reduction of existing illness factors will be achieved.

Obesity, simple— cont'd

NURSING DIAGNOSES / DEFINING CHARACTERISTICS	NURSING INTERVENTIONS / *RATIONALES*	EXPECTED OUTCOMES
	• Devise aerobic activity program that enhances weight loss and is suitable to patient's needs. • Provide information about healthy diet, metabolic activity, and relationship between obesity and associated illnesses. • Develop list of substitute activities for eating to curtail or diminish overeating. • Stress importance of structured meal plan. • Support patient's efforts; offer frequent encouragement. • Encourage and enlist patient's cooperation in all decision making *to increase likelihood of success.*	
Body image disturbance *Related to:* Distortion between one's mental and physical images Psychosocial factors (e.g., depression, anxiety, stress) **DEFINING CHARACTERISTICS** Low self-esteem Expression of negative feelings about body size and shape	**ONGOING ASSESSMENT** • Explore and assess patient's view of self and body. • Determine patient's motivation for weight loss. • Explore functions of overeating and obesity (e.g., attempt to achieve emotional satiety or defense against intimacy). **THERAPEUTIC INTERVENTIONS** • Encourage verbalizations of feelings and perceptions of self and body. • Convey attitude of understanding and acceptance of patient's feelings about physical self. • Assist patient to acknowledge and identify feelings that lead to overeating and develop substitute activities. *Help patient recognize that overeating can be triggered by unpleasant feeling states.* • Encourage patient to care for self through appropriate grooming and dressing. • Be aware/deal with own negative feelings and reactions toward obesity. • When appropriate, encourage patient to join support groups, such as Overeaters' Anonymous, where ongoing support and social contact can be received.	Acceptance of self and body as is rather than an idealized image will be manifested.

Originated by: Nancy Staples, RN, BSN

Pancreatitis, acute

A nonbacterial inflammatory process of autodigestion of pancreatic tissue by pancreatic enzymes, resulting in edema, necrosis, and hemorrhage. It may be treated medically and/ or surgically.

NURSING DIAGNOSES / DEFINING CHARACTERISTICS	NURSING INTERVENTIONS / *RATIONALES*	EXPECTED OUTCOMES

Pain
Related to:
Inflammation of pancreas and surrounding tissue
Biliary tract disease (spasm of Vater's ampulla)
Common channel involving biliary/ pancreatic duct
Duodenal content reflux
	ONGOING ASSESSMENT
	• Assess, document, and report to physician pain characteristics:
	  Quality
	  Location
	  Onset
	  Duration
	  History of previous attack
	• Assess precipitating and relieving factors.
	• Observe for increased abdominal distention:
	  Auscultate abdomen for bowel sounds q2h.
	  Report decrease or absence of bowel sounds.
	  Extravasation of pancreatic enzymes causes paralytic ileus.
	• Observe sclera and skin for jaundice.
	• Observe stool for fat, absence of bile, odor.
		Pain will be relieved or reduced.

NURSING DIAGNOSES / DEFINING CHARACTERISTICS	NURSING INTERVENTIONS / *RATIONALES*	EXPECTED OUTCOMES

Excessive alcohol intake
Abdominal trauma/ surgery
Infectious process
Drugs
 	
DEFINING CHARACTERISTICS
Epigastric pain or umbilical pain radiating to back/shoulders
Pain not relieved/ worsened by certain narcotics
Increasing pain in supine position
Pain aggravated by food
Abdominal distention with rebound tenderness
Increased heart rate
Splinted respirations
Extreme restlessness
Decreased or absent bowel sounds
	THERAPEUTIC INTERVENTIONS
	• Reduce pancreatic stimulus by maintaining patient NPO or with nasogastric tube to low suction as ordered. *Oral intake causes vagally stimulated pancreatic secretion.*
	• Anticipate need for pain medication.
	• Respond immediately to complaints of pain.
	• Administer medication, such as anticholinergic drugs *(mimic sympathetic stimulation and quiet pancreatic secretion); avoid MSO$_4$ derivatives (may cause spasms of sphincter of Oddi, increasing pain).*
	• Keep environment conducive to rest.
	• Use repositioning and back rubs *to soothe.*
	• Maintain bed rest.
	• Administer oral hygiene.
	• Use other measures for controlling discomfort:
	    Provide reassurance.
	    Explain all procedures.
	    Encourage communication with significant others.
	    Remain with extremely anxious or confused patient.
	• See Pain, p. 39.	

Fluid volume deficit
Related to:
Vomiting
Decreased intake
Shifting of fluids to extravascular space
 	
DEFINING CHARACTERISTICS
Nausea and vomiting
Abdominal distention
Fever
Hypotension
Tachycardia
Ileus
	ONGOING ASSESSMENT
	• Monitor vital signs q2h if stable, more frequently if unstable. *Fluid volume deficit occurs rapidly; subtle vital sign changes may indicate profound fluid volume deficit.*
	• Assess hydration status, including skin turgor, daily weight, hemodynamic parameters.
	• Observe for complications of dehydration.
	• Monitor serum and urine amylase levels as ordered.
	• Monitor serum calcium levels. *Calcium ions may become trapped in fat surrounding inflamed pancreas, reducing amount available to circulation.*
	
	THERAPEUTIC INTERVENTION
	• Maintain circulatory volume; replace fluid and electrolyte losses:
	    Administer IV fluid as ordered.
	    Administer volume expanders or blood transfusion as ordered by physician.
	• Keep body metabolism of patient low:
	    Maintain bed rest.
	    Maintain body temperature in desired range.
	• Institute seizure precautions if Ca^{++} falls below 8.5.
	• See Fluid volume deficit, p. 20.
		Fluid volume and electrolyte balance will be maintained.

Potential ineffective breathing pattern *Related to:* Pain Abdominal distention or ascites Abdominal trauma or surgery Extravasation of pancreatic enzymes	**ONGOING ASSESSMENT** • Assess respiratory rate and breath sounds q2h. • Assess quality of respirations (depth, ease). • Note use of accessory muscles for breathing. • Assess position patient assumes for normal/easy breathing. • Assess for dyspnea. • Note retractions and flaring nostrils. • Assess for changes in orientation level.	An effective breathing pattern will be maintained.

NURSING DIAGNOSES / DEFINING CHARACTERISTICS	NURSING INTERVENTIONS / *RATIONALES*	EXPECTED OUTCOMES
DEFINING CHARACTERISTICS Dyspnea Shortness of breath Splinted respirations Tachypnea Cyanosis	**THERAPEUTIC INTERVENTIONS** • Assist patient to semi-Fowler's or side-lying position. *Pancreatic pain often referred to middle of back; these positions improve breathing patterns by minimizing discomfort.* • See Breathing pattern, ineffective, p. 8.	

Potential alteration in skin integrity
 Related to:
 Dehydration
 Restricted/limited activity
 	
 DEFINING CHARACTERISTICS
 Poor skin turgor
 Evidence of stage I pressure areas
	ONGOING ASSESSMENT
	 • Assess skin integrity:
	    Note color, moisture, and temperature.
	    Ask patient about burning or itching.
	 • Note patient's prescribed activity level:
	    Bed rest
	    Turning from side to side
	 • Assess nutritional status. *Patients with pancreatitis often have history of alcohol abuse (predisposes patient to poor nutritional status).*
	
	 THERAPEUTIC INTERVENTIONS
	 • Institute prophylactic pressure-relief device.
	 • See Skin integrity, impaired, p. 48.
		Skin integrity will be maintained.

Knowledge deficit
 Related to:
 Disease process of acute pancreatitis
 Strange environment
 	
 DEFINING CHARACTERISTICS
 Multiple questions about causes of pain, NPO or special diet, prognosis
 Questioning indicating lack of information about hospital policies and procedures
 Repeat admissions to hospital with recurrent bouts of pancreatitis
	ONGOING ASSESSMENT
	 • Assess patient's/significant others' understanding of disease process, particularly potentially controllable behaviors *that may trigger episodes of pancreatitis.*
	 • Assess patient's/significant others' knowledge of hospital/unit visiting hour policy, source for patient's condition report, and relevant hospital procedures.
	
	 THERAPEUTIC INTERVENTIONS
	 • Explain hospital policies/procedures to patient/significant others:
	    Visiting hours
	    Number of visitors
	    Telephone number for inquiry about patient's condition
	 • Orient patient to bedside environment.
	 • Explain necessary procedures.
	 • Instruct patient/significant others of importance of calm and comfortable environment. *Emotions can cause vagally mediated outpouring of pancreatic enzymes, causing more pain and increasing possibility of complications.*
		Patient and family will verbalize understanding of procedures and environment.

Originated by: Malu N. Viloria, RN, BSN
                Susan Galanes, RN, MS, CCRN

Peptic ulcer

(GASTRIC ULCER)

Erosion of lower esophageal, gastric, or duodenal mucosa by acidic gastric secretions.

NURSING DIAGNOSES / DEFINING CHARACTERISTICS	NURSING INTERVENTIONS / *RATIONALES*	EXPECTED OUTCOMES
Altered tissue integrity *Related to:* Decreased mucosal resistance Defective mucus Inadequate mucosal blood flow Overproduction of gastric secretions Chronic gastritis Gastric irritants: aspirin, alcohol, caffeine, tobacco Dysfunctional pylorus (usually in elderly) **DEFINING CHARACTERISTICS** Pain (midepigastric) Indigestion or heartburn GI bleeding Diagnosis or history of peptic ulcer Family history	**ONGOING ASSESSMENT** · Assess for signs/symptoms of ulcerations (see Defining Characteristics). · Assess for events surrounding exacerbations and remission of symptoms. **THERAPEUTIC INTERVENTIONS** · Assist with diagnostic evaluations as appropriate: Upper GI x-ray examinations Gastric secretory studies Upper GI endoscopy Stools for occult blood Esophagogastroduodenoscopy *Exact location of ulcer predetermines treatment modalities.* · Administer medications as ordered, *to prevent tissue erosion:* Antacids Cimetidine: *decreases gastric secretions* Anticholinergics for duodenal ulcers: *decrease gastric acid production* Sedatives/tranquilizers: *for gastric ulcers only* · Provide quiet, restful environment. *Stress and activity tend to increase gastric secretion.*	Mucosal erosion will be reduced.
Pain *Related to:* Lesion in gastric mucosa exposed to gastric secretions (hydrochloric acids, pepsin) **DEFINING CHARACTERISTICS** Patient reports or verbalizes pain (see Ongoing Assessment)	**ONGOING ASSESSMENT** · Assess for site and type of pain: Heartburn Indigestion Back pain (pancreatic involvement) Burning in throat Localized midepigastric pain · Assess for onset and duration of pain. · Assess for predisposing factors: Large meals Ingestion of aspirin, alcohol, coffee, orange juice Psychogenic factors · Solicit techniques for relief of pain: Eating Antacids Analgesics **THERAPEUTIC INTERVENTIONS** · Provide medications as ordered *to decrease gastric acid secretion:* Antacids Sedatives Analgesics · Maintain quiet, nonstressful environment. · Provide small frequent meals, 4-6/day, *to dilute gastric acid.* · Encourage fluids (nonacidic) between meals. · Encourage patient to lie down after meals. *Activity increases gastric acid secretion.* · See Pain, p. 39.	Discomfort will be relieved or decreased.

NURSING DIAGNOSES / DEFINING CHARACTERISTICS	NURSING INTERVENTIONS / *RATIONALES*	EXPECTED OUTCOMES
Altered nutrition: less than body requirements *Related to:* Decreased intake caused by pain (gastric ulcers) **DEFINING CHARACTERISTICS** Less than body requirements: Loss of weight Inadequate caloric intake Pain upon eating More than body requirements: Weight gain Reported dysfunctional eating pattern Increased intake to relieve discomfort (duodenal ulcers)	**ONGOING ASSESSMENT** • Perform nutritional assessment. • Document admission weight. • Obtain nutritional history **THERAPEUTIC INTERVENTIONS** • Consult dietitian when appropriate. • Document I & O, appetite. *Ulcer patients may under- or overeat to control symptoms.* • Provide small meals, 4-6/day. • See Nutrition, altered: less than/more than body requirements, pp. 37-38.	Good nutritional habits will be realized.
Potential for injury: hemorrhage *Related to:* Perforation of gastric mucosal membrane **DEFINING CHARACTERISTICS** Frank, continual loss of bright red blood in emesis Evidence of blood in stool (black, tarry, bright maroon)	**ONGOING ASSESSMENT** • Assess vital signs q2h. • Assess emesis and stool for presence, amount of blood. • Maintain strict I & O. • Monitor electrolytes, CBC, and bleeding times **THERAPEUTIC INTERVENTIONS** • If bleeding occurs, report immediately (*potentially life-threatening*). • Anticipate need for type and cross, lavage and/or surgical intervention.	Potential effects of gastric perforation and hemorrhage will be reduced.
Knowledge deficit *Related to:* Cause and prevention of peptic ulcers New conditions Unfamiliarity with treatment regimen **DEFINING CHARACTERISTICS** Frequent exacerbations Inability to verbalize causative and preventive factors Maintenance of dysfunctional destructive habits	**ONGOING ASSESSMENTS** • Assess level of understanding and ability to learn. • Assess current habits: dietary, smoking, drinking, medications. **THERAPEUTIC INTERVENTIONS** • Discuss ulceration site and common causative factors. *Exacerbation is common, especially in the noncompliant patient.* • Discuss pain control, eating habits, and use of antacids and analgesics: Discuss avoidance of aspirin and aspirin-containing products. Warn patients of change in bowel habits caused by magnesium (diarrhea) or aluminum (constipation) in antacids. Discuss use and side effects of anticholinergics (if appropriate). Discuss avoidance of caffeine and alcohol, especially during exacerbation. Encourage patients to stop smoking *to prevent increased gastric acid secretion and decreased pancreatic bicarbonate secretion.* • Discuss signs/symptoms of perforation and hemorrhage. • Discuss availability of emergency care. • Discuss follow-up care; provide appropriate names and phone numbers if questions arise.	Patient will verbalize causative and preventive health care factors.

Originated by: Michele Knoll Puzas, RN,C, MHPE

Cholecystectomy

(GALLBLADDER SURGERY)

Surgical removal of the gallbladder, usually performed as the result of acute cholecystitis, which may or may not be accompanied by the presence of gallstones.

NURSING DIAGNOSES / DEFINING CHARACTERISTICS	NURSING INTERVENTIONS / *RATIONALES*	EXPECTED OUTCOMES
Potential intravascular fluid volume deficit *Related to:* Excessive wound drainage Excessive nasogastric (NG) tube output Excessive third-space fluid losses Postoperative hemorrhage Excessive T-tube drainage **DEFINING CHARACTERISTICS** Increased heart rate Hypotension Hemoconcentration Dry mucous membranes Thirst Apprehension Concentrated urine Change in LOC Edema	**ONGOING ASSESSMENT** • Monitor vital signs; note trends denoting dehydration or shocklike states. • Assess LOC. • Monitor I & O. • Assess surgical dressings for amount and character of drainage. • Assess T tube: Stabilization Patency Amount, color, and character of output • Assess NG tube: Patency Amount, color, and character of output • Weigh patient. **THERAPEUTIC INTERVENTIONS** • Maintain patency and function of NG tube. *Accumulation of gastric secretions may trigger increased bile production.* • Administer IV fluids as ordered. • See Fluid volume deficit, p. 20; Surgical tubes/drains, p. 322.	Normal fluid volume will be maintained.
Potential infection *Related to:* Bacterial invasion through incision and/ or T-tube insertion site Bile leak into peritoneum **DEFINING CHARACTERISTICS** Obviously displaced T tube Absence of bile flow Complaints of abdominal pain Elevated WBC Jaundice Fever Redness, pain, swelling, or drainage from incision(s)	**ONGOING ASSESSMENT** • Monitor temperature and WBC. • Assess patency and placement of T tube. • Monitor and record bile drainage. *Note: Bile drainage should be bright yellow to dark green and have an acrid odor. Daily drainage should be <500 ml.* • Observe and record color of urine and stool daily. *Bilirubin that has reentered circulation is excreted via renal and intestinal tracts; changes in stool/urine color may indicate abnormal bile/bilirubin excretion/drainage.* • Inspect wound for signs of infection. **THERAPEUTIC INTERVENTIONS** • Stabilize T tube securely with waterproof tape. *Dislodgment of T-tube may cause bile leakage into peritoneum, causing peritonitis, which results in markedly increased morbidity and mortality.* • Pin or tie T-tube collection device to patient's clothing *to allow movement, minimize tube dislodgment risk.* • Use sterile technique while changing dressing and manipulating T-tube insertion site. • Administer antibiotics and/or antipyretics as ordered.	Risk of infection is reduced.
Ineffective breathing pattern *Related to:* Painful surgical incision	**ONGOING ASSESSMENT** • Perform respiratory assessment; note rate, depth of respirations. • Assess degree to which decreased LOC and/or pain contributes to breathing pattern.	Effective breathing will be achieved.

NURSING DIAGNOSES / DEFINING CHARACTERISTICS	NURSING INTERVENTIONS / *RATIONALES*	EXPECTED OUTCOMES
Anxiety Decreased compliance secondary to general anesthesia Decreased diaphragmatic movement **DEFINING CHARACTERISTICS** Shallow respirations Poor coughing efforts Adventitious breath sounds Guarded respirations with splinting	**THERAPEUTIC INTERVENTIONS** · Explain importance of turning, coughing, and deep breathing. · Assess patient use of incentive spirometer. · Help patient change position in bed; assist with ambulation. · Administer pain medications and other relieving measures as needed *to facilitate coughing and deep breathing*. · Teach patient to splint own incision while deep breathing and coughing. · See Breathing pattern, ineffective, p. 8.	
Knowledge deficit *Related to:* Unfamiliarity with postoperative diet needs/plan Unfamiliarity with T-tube care **DEFINING CHARACTERISTICS** Patient/significant others unaware of need to alter diet after surgery Patient/significant others observed selecting fatty foods from menu Multiple questions from patient/significant others Observed patient/significant other's inability to care for T tube	**ONGOING ASSESSMENT** · Take diet history of fatty food intake. · Note food selected from menu. · Assess patient's/significant others' ability to understand T-tube and site care. · Assess patient's/significant others' willingness to care for T tube and site. **THERAPEUTIC INTERVENTIONS** · Advise patient to avoid excessive fatty food intake *(may stimulate increased bile production)*. · Advise patient/significant others that no special food preparation is required. · Encourage patient to maintain well-balanced diet, avoiding extremes. · Consult dietitian if necessary. · Explain purposes and location of T tube at level patient/significant others can understand. · Instruct patient/significant others to observe for jaundice, tea-colored urine, clay-colored stools, and signs/symptoms of peritonitis and notify physician if any of these occurs. · Teach patient/significant others to change dressing at site, using clean technique. *Risk of infection is minimal by time of discharge; compliance may be improved by use of clean versus sterile technique in home.* · Teach patient/significant others proper tube clamping if indicated. · Stress importance of follow-up care.	Patient/significant others verbalize and demonstrate appropriate dietary selection and T-tube care.

Originated by: Dorothy Lewis, RN,C BSN

Colon resection

(HEMICOLECTOMY)

Removal of the lower sigmoid or rectosigmoid portion of the rectum through a low midline incision in the abdomen. Continuity is established by an end-to-end anastomosis of the proximal colon and the rectum by sutures or a circular stapling device. This procedure is used to treat adenocarcinoma and polyposis of colon and/or rectum.

NURSING DIAGNOSES / DEFINING CHARACTERISTICS	NURSING INTERVENTIONS / *RATIONALES*	EXPECTED OUTCOMES
Preoperative or intraoperative anxiety *Related to:* Impending surgery Impending pathology results Possibility of ostomy Preoperative preparation **DEFINING CHARACTERISTICS** Nervous appearance Trembling Hand wringing Multiple questions/ lack of questions Increased BP, pulse, and respiratory rate	**ONGOING ASSESSMENT** · Assess knowledge and understanding of impending surgery. · Assess degree of anxiety. **THERAPEUTIC INTERVENTIONS** · Arrange for visit from operating room personnel. *Preoperative visit promotes confidence in operating room staff.* · Provide information about intraoperative care. *Knowledge of what to expect may relieve some anxiety.* · Document and communicate patient's concerns to others involved in care (i.e., recovery room personnel). · Inform patient that significant other will be allowed to wait with patient in preanesthesia care unit. · Maintain a quiet operating room environment. *Noise, traffic, hurried movements increase anxiety level.* · Remain with patient before and during induction of anesthesia. *Having someone close by at critical moment is very reassuring.* · See Anxiety, p. 4.	Anxiety will be managed.
Intraoperative potential for injury *Related to:* Urinary catheterization Lithotomy position during 5- to 6-hr procedure (pelvis higher than head) **DEFINING CHARACTERISTICS** Cloudy, foul-smelling urine Positive urine cultures Frequency, urgency, burning after catheter removal Pain in extremities Numbness, tingling of extremities Swelling of legs	**ONGOING ASSESSMENT** · Monitor catheterization procedure to ensure asepsis. · Assess patient's body alignment throughout procedure to: *Provide optimum access and exposure to operative site.* *Sustain circulatory and respiratory function.* *Guard against joint damage, muscle stretch, and strain.* **THERAPEUTIC INTERVENTIONS** · Position and tape urinary catheter securely *to prevent disconnection, traction, or kinking.* · Adjust and pad stirrups *to ensure symmetrical position and minimize pressure and venous pooling.* · Adjust arm boards properly *to prevent hyperextension, abduction, and damage to brachial plexus;* cover arms, hands, and fingers with drawsheet *for additional protection.* · Wrap each of lower extremities with ace bandage *(lessens pooling and may prevent thrombus formation).* · Raise and lower patient's legs simultaneously and slowly, supporting foot and knee. *Any change in body position affects hemodynamics; slow movements allow gradual circulation adjustment.* · Apply straps snugly across foot and lower leg *to keep leg in place.* · Remind surgical team not to lean on arms or legs during procedure.	Risk of injury during operation is reduced.
Potential ineffective thermoregulation *Related to:* Use of anesthetic agents	**ONGOING ASSESSMENT** · Monitor temperature throughout procedure. · Monitor vital signs. · Send specimen for ABGs and electrolyte analysis.	Appropriate body temperature will be maintained.

Colon resection— cont'd

NURSING DIAGNOSES / DEFINING CHARACTERISTICS	NURSING INTERVENTIONS / *RATIONALES*	EXPECTED OUTCOMES
Cool OR environment Exposure during preparation Prolonged visceral exposure Family history of hyperthermia during induction **DEFINING CHARACTERISTICS** *Hypothermia:* Decreased baseline temperature Decreased BP Arrhythmia Abnormal ABGs and electrolytes Postoperative shivering Skin pale and cold *Hyperthermia:* Increased baseline temperature Tachycardia Acidosis Electrolyte imbalance Hyperventilation Arrhythmia Muscular vesiculation	**THERAPEUTIC INTERVENTIONS** *To prevent hypothermia:* • Place a blanket-size aquamatic K pad on operating room bed; set to appropriate temperature before patient's arrival. *Device raises, lowers, or maintains body temperature through heat conduction or cold transfer between blanket and patient.* • Maintain adequate room temperature until draping completed. • Cover patient with warm blankets until ready for skin preparation and immediately after sterile drape removal *(allows minimal exposure and loss of body heat).* • Use warm irrigation and warm moist sponges to cover exposed abdominal organs *(warms circulating blood in abdominal cavity).* • Consult anesthesiologist about use of humidified air delivered via ventilator and warm IV solution via warmers. *To treat hyperthermia:* • Set aquamatic machine to desired temperature. • Assist anesthesiologist to discontinue anesthesia and administer emergency drugs. *This is a life-threatening complication of anesthesia that can be triggered by commonly used anesthetic agents (succinylcholine and halothane).* • Remove IV from warmer; hang cold IV fluids. • Place ice packs around patient. • Prepare for iced gastric lavage. • Assist surgical team to complete procedure as quickly as possible.	
Potential fluid volume deficit *Related to:* Blood loss in surgery Blood loss after surgery **DEFINING CHARACTERISTICS** *Intraoperative:* Decreased blood pressure Increased heart rate Decreased central venous pressure Decreasing Hct *Postoperative:* As above, plus Saturated dressings Large amount of blood from NG or other tubes Decreased urine output Restlessness Confusion	**ONGOING ASSESSMENT** *Intraoperative:* • Assess vital signs throughout procedure. *Early detection of symptoms will enable surgical team to institute treatment, prevent shock.* • Monitor and record I & O during procedure *to replace blood loss accurately.* • Observe for signs/symptoms of transfusion reaction if blood administered. *Postoperative:* • Assess vital signs per institution's postoperative protocol. • Monitor abdominal dressing for excess drainage. • Monitor Hb and Hct. • Monitor changes in LOC, differentiating changes related to hypovolemia/anesthesia. **THERAPEUTIC INTERVENTIONS** • Check availability of blood; have half sent to the operating room. Blood must be *accessible for immediate transfusion.* • Inform anesthesia of blood loss through sponges, suction, and drapes *to ensure appropriate fluid replacement.* • Administer IV fluids and/or blood/blood components as ordered. *Most patients can tolerate 500 ml to 1 L blood loss without difficulty. Blood replacement is necessary if blood loss exceeds this amount. Albumin, dextran, hydroxyethyl starch, and electrolyte solution can be used instead of blood.* • Report laboratory results to physician *so correct replacement of blood, fluid and electrolyte can be maintained.* • Administer O_2 if blood loss after procedure.	Normal fluid volume will be maintained.

Continued.

NURSING DIAGNOSES / DEFINING CHARACTERISTICS	NURSING INTERVENTIONS / *RATIONALES*	EXPECTED OUTCOMES
Potential infection *Related to:* Length of procedure, tissue exposure Leakage of bowel contents intraoperatively Insertion of circular staple gun through rectum to abdominal cavity Incomplete line of staples Postoperative wound contamination Incomplete suturing caused by staple gun malfunction or misfiring **DEFINING CHARACTERISTICS** Incisional redness Swelling, pain Foul-smelling wound drainage Fever Positive wound culture Elevated white blood count History of difficult anastomosis	**ONGOING ASSESSMENT** *Intraoperative:* • Assess aseptic technique throughout procedure. *Aseptic techniques exclude microorganisms in environment, prevent them from reaching operative wound, prevent infection, facilitate wound healing.* *Postoperative:* • Assess wound for redness, drainage, pain, swelling, or dehiscence. • Culture suspicious drainage. • Monitor temperature. • Monitor WBC. **THERAPEUTIC INTERVENTIONS** *Intraoperative:* • Clean and disinfect skin area of and around proposed incision site. • Shave operative site only as necessary and immediately before surgery. *Abraded, injured skin is very conducive to cutaneous bacteria proliferation, increasing chance of infection.* • Correct breaks in technique when observed. *Sterile members of surgical team not always aware of violations of asepsis while concentrating on the operative field.* • Irrigate and suction around rectum *to remove retained fluid from enema to keep rectosigmoid free of fluid and fecal material and prevent leakage into abdominal cavity.* • Keep instruments contacting GI mucosa separate from other instrument; remove entirely from field after anastomosis. • *Ensure availability and function of stapling devices by:* Having all sizes available at outset of procedure. Reviewing function of instrument with team. Assisting with use at appropriate time. • Have GI suture material ready *in case stapling is unsatisfactory.* • Irrigating abdominal wound with water to check for bubbles *(indicate anastomotic leak).* *Postoperative:* • Use aseptic technique for dressing changes. • Administer antibiotics and antipyretics as ordered. • If stoma present, isolate fecal drainage by maintaining good skin seal (See Fecal ostomy, p. 311).	Risk of infection will be reduced.
Postoperative pain *Related to:* Surgical incision Endotracheal intubation for anesthesia administration Tubes/drains present **DEFINING CHARACTERISTICS** Report of incisional pain Verbalization of sore throat Grimacing Reluctance to move, cough, or take deep breaths Protection of tubes/ drains	**ONGOING ASSESSMENT** • Assess pain: Location Intensity Duration Precipitating factors Quality • Assess degree to which pain interferes with ability to turn, cough, and deep breathe. **THERAPEUTIC INTERVENTIONS** • Anticipate need for analgesia *to prevent peak pain periods.* • Provide oral hygiene, lozenges, and throat spray *to ease sore throat.* • Teach patient to use hands or pillows to splint incision when deep breathing, coughing, or changing position. • Consider/recommend use of patient-controlled analgesia (PCA). • Secure all tubes/drains *to minimize movement and subsequent pain.* • See Pain, p. 39; Patient-controlled analgesia, p. 631; Surgical tube/drains, p. 322.	Pain will be relieved.

NURSING DIAGNOSES / DEFINING CHARACTERISTICS	NURSING INTERVENTIONS / *RATIONALES*	EXPECTED OUTCOMES
Altered bowel elimination: postoperative ileus *Related to:* General anesthesia Manipulation of bowel **DEFINING CHARACTERISTICS** Silent abdomen on auscultation No stooling Report of bloated feeling	**ONGOING ASSESSMENT** • Assess for bowel sounds every shift. • Note passage of first flatus, stool. *Postoperative ileus usually resolves within 96 hr after surgery.* **THERAPEUTIC INTERVENTIONS** • Maintain NPO status until bowel sounds return. • Ensure patency of NG tube *to keep stomach empty.* • Encourage/assist with ambulation *to hasten resolution of ileus.* • Assist patient with initial food/fluid selection *to minimize gaseous distention.* • Inform patient that stool pattern, consistency, frequency may not return to preoperative status, *depending on portion/length of colon resected.*	Bowel elimination will return to normal.
Altered nutrition: less than body requirements *Related to:* Increased metabolic demands (stress of surgery) NPO Primary diagnosis Fever **DEFINING CHARACTERISTICS** Weight loss Poor wound healing Low serum albumin Low energy level Low Hb, Hct	**ONGOING ASSESSMENT** • Assess postoperative weight; compare to preoperative weight. • Remain cognizant of length of NPO status. • Monitor vital signs, especially temperature. **THERAPEUTIC INTERVENTIONS** • Administer IV fluids as ordered: *1 L of 5% dextrose provides approximately 200 calories, which may achieve protein sparing for short time.* • If evidence of poor nutritional status and ileus has not resolved, consider peripheral or central hyperalimentation *to maintain anabolic state.* • Administer antipyretics *to control fever; for each 1°C above normal body temperature, metabolic need for calories increases by 7%.* • Plan activities *to allow adequate rest.* • See Nutrition, altered: less than body requirements, p. 37.	Adequate nutrition will be maintained.

Knowledge deficit *Related to:* Lack of previous experience with colon surgery Need for home management **DEFINING CHARACTERISTICS** Multiple questions Lack of questions Inability to provide self-care upon discharge	**ONGOING ASSESSMENT**
	• Assess readiness and ability to learn.
	• Determine diet, activity, and wound care needs.
	
	THERAPEUTIC INTERVENTIONS
	• Teach patient/significant other the following:
	  Importance of well-balanced diet based on food tolerances *to promote continued healing*
	  Bowel activity will stabilize over 6-8 wk *(normal time to adapt to shortened bowel)*
	  Importance of prescribed wound care
	  Need for follow-up appointments
	  Signs/symptoms to report: fever, loss of appetite, abdominal pain, change in appearance of wound, significant change in bowel elimination
	  Need for gradual return to preoperative activity level
	• Allow for return demonstration of wound care.
	• Document teaching done and patient's responses.
		Patient/significant other will verbalize and/or demonstrate home care.

Originated by: Jacqueline Monaco, RN
Sharon Canariato, RN, BSN

Enteral tube feeding

(ENTERAL HYPERALIMENTATION; G-TUBE; JEJUNOSTOMY; DUODENOSTOMY)

A method of providing nutrition using a nasogastric tube, a gastrostomy tube, or a tube placed in the duodenum or jejunum. Feedings may be continuous or intermittent (bolus).

NURSING DIAGNOSES / DEFINING CHARACTERISTICS	NURSING INTERVENTIONS / *RATIONALES*	EXPECTED OUTCOMES
Potential ineffective airway clearance *Related to:* Aspirations resulting from: Lack of gag reflex Poor positioning Overfeeding **DEFINING CHARACTERISTICS** Abnormal breath sounds Shortness of breath Coughing Diaphoresis Anxiety Restlessness Poor skin color	**ONGOING ASSESSMENT** • Assess correct position of tube before initiating feeding. • Assess presence of gag reflex before each feeding. • Assess LOC before administration of feeding. • Document patient's baseline respiratory status. Monitor patient's respiratory status throughout feeding. • Check tube placement before feeding by injecting air and listening over stomach *(gurgling sound indicates correct placement).* • Check for residual feeding before each feeding. • Document incorrect tube placement and amount of residual feeding obtained. • See Airway clearance, ineffective p. 3. **THERAPEUTIC INTERVENTIONS** • Elevate HOB up to 30 degrees for 30 min after feeding (unless contraindicated) *to facilitate gravity flow to stomach.* • In case of aspiration: Stop tube feeding. Monitor vital signs. Assess respiratory status. Notify physician. Keep HOB elevated. Suction as necessary. • Document time feeding was stopped, patient's appearance, and changes in respiratory status. *High-risk patients are comatose, have decreased gag reflex, or cannot tolerate elevated HOB. Nasoduodenal or gastroduodenal feedings are preferred for high-risk patients.*	Potential for aspiration will be reduced.
Altered nutrition: less than body requirements *Related to:* Mechanical problems during administration of feedings, such as: Clogging of tube Inaccurate flow rate Incorrect tube administration set for pump Defective tube administration set Long-term feeding (i.e., G-tube/J-tube) **DEFINING CHARACTERISTICS** Continued weight loss Persistent anergy	**ONGOING ASSESSMENT** • Monitor equipment for proper functioning. • Assess tubing for passage of formula. • Assess nitrogen balance as ordered. • See Nutrition, altered: less than body requirements, p. 37. **THERAPEUTIC INTERVENTIONS** • Care of tube: Flush tubing with 20 ml water after feedings *to reduce risk of clotting.* Crush medications and dilute with water; use elixir form when possible. Flush tube after medication administration. Check tubing connections. • Care of pump: Keep alarms on. Attach to outlet unless patient is walking.	Nutritional support will be maximized.
Potential diarrhea *Related to:* Intolerance to tube feeding because of: Hyperosmolarity Temperature of feeding	**ONGOING ASSESSMENT** • Assess bowel sounds q8h. • Assess number and character of stools. • See Diarrhea, p. 16. • Monitor I & O. • Record frequency and consistency of all stools.	Intolerance to feeding will be reduced.

Enteral tube feeding— cont'd

NURSING DIAGNOSES / DEFINING CHARACTERISTICS	NURSING INTERVENTIONS / *RATIONALES*	EXPECTED OUTCOMES
Rate of delivery Anxiety Bacterial contamination of feeding **DEFINING CHARACTERISTICS** Abdominal cramps Abdominal pain Frequency of stools Loose, liquid stools Urgency Hyperactive bowel sounds	**THERAPEUTIC INTERVENTIONS** Delivery of formula: · Begin feedings slowly; consider dilute solution. · Increase rate and strength to prescribed amount but not at same time. *High-rate feeding combined with high osmolality may precipitate diarrhea.* · Administer feedings at room temperature. *Cold stimulates peristalsis.* · Do not allow formula to hang longer than 8 hr at room temperature *to minimize risk of bacterial contamination.* · Change setup daily. · Administer feedings in calm, relaxed atmosphere. · Notify physician of any intolerance. Patient activity: · Encourage light activity after feeding. · Document activity tolerance.	
Potential fluid volume deficit *Related to:* Osmolarity of feeding formula **DEFINING CHARACTERISTICS** Dry mucous membrane Poor skin turgor Elevated temperature Changes in mental status Azotemia	**ONGOING ASSESSMENT** · Assess patient for change in mental status every shift. · See Fluid volume deficit, p. 20. · Document baseline mental status *(sensitive indicator of hyperosmolar states).* **THERAPEUTIC INTERVENTIONS** · Keep pitcher at bedside, unless medically restricted. · Document changes in mental status; notify physician. · See Fluid volume deficit, p. 20.	Fluid volume will be maintained.

Alteration in glucose and fat metabolism
Related to:
Continuous feeding, rather than physiologic intermittent bolus schedule
 	
DEFINING CHARACTERISTICS
Glucose >120, flushed skin, headache, nausea, vomiting, fatigue, fruity breath
Glucose <70, hunger, sweating, pallor, cold skin, tremor, blurry vision, fatigue, dizziness
Foul-smelling, greasy stools
	ONGOING ASSESSMENT
	· Review laboratory values:
	    Monitor blood glucose level by chemstick as ordered.
	    Monitor urine sugar/acetone qid; notify physician of changes.
	· Assess patient for mental status changes and other defining characteristics.
	· Assess stool for odor and greasiness.
	· Monitor bowel sounds q8h.
	· Monitor number and characteristics of stools
	
	THERAPEUTIC INTERVENTIONS
	· Administer hyperglycemic/antihyperglycemic agents as ordered.
	· Notify physician if feeding stopped for any reason.
	· Notify physician of any change in stools.
		Potential alteration in glucose and fat metabolism will be reduced.

Pain *Related to:* Dry mucous membranes and tape irritation	**ONGOING ASSESSMENT** · Assess mucous membranes. · Assess tube insertion site for reddened areas. · See Pain, p. 39.	Pain will be reduced or relieved.

Continued.

Enteral tube feeding— cont'd

NURSING DIAGNOSES / DEFINING CHARACTERISTICS	NURSING INTERVENTIONS / *RATIONALES*	EXPECTED OUTCOMES
Defining Characteristics Dry, cracked lips Soiled tape Reddened area where tube positioned Swallowing difficulty Verbalized discomfort	**Therapeutic Interventions** • Provide skin/mucous membrane care. Change position of tube at nares; re-tape q12h. • Provide mouth care q4h. • Allow hard candy or gum if permissible *(stimulate salivary secretion).*	
Social isolation *Related to:* Change in body image **Defining Characteristics** Patient stays in room and resists environmental changes Patient refuses visitors	**Ongoing Assessment** • Assess patient's behavior pattern during contact with significant others/staff. **Therapeutic Interventions** • Allow time for verbalization. *Reactions to changed body are normal.* • Arrange privacy for visits. • Encourage patient's/significant others' participation in daily care. • Encourage activity outside room if allowable.	Withdrawn behavior will be reduced.
Body image disturbance *Related to:* Change in body image: feeding tube extending from nose **Defining Characteristics** Patient verbalizes feelings of being unable to eat normally Patient will not look at tube Patient will not participate in daily hygiene	**Ongoing Assessment** • Assess patient's use of defense mechanisms in past crises. • Assess patient's support systems **Therapeutic Interventions** • Explain reason for tube feeding. • Allow patient time to express feelings, ask questions. • Allow patient/significant others to help with feedings. • Allow self-care to extent possible *to increase/reinforce patient's capabilities.*	Disturbances in self-concept will be reduced.
Knowledge deficit: need for nutritional support *Related to:* New procedure and treatment **Defining Characteristics** Patient verbalizes inaccurate information Patient exhibits inappropriate behavior Patient asks questions about tube feeding	**Ongoing Assessment** • Assess for prior experience with tube feeding. • Assess patient's knowledge of tube feeding. **Therapeutic Interventions** • Demonstrate feedings and tube care. • Allow return demonstration *so that necessary alteration in teaching plan can be undertaken.* • Document progress.	Patient will verbalize reasons for tube feedings and begin to participate in self-care.

Originated by: Mary Martinat, RN, BSN
                Frankie Harper, RN
                Susan Smalheiser, RN, MSN

Fecal ostomy

(COLOSTOMY; ILEOSTOMY; FECAL DIVERSION; STOMA)

A surgical procedure that results in an opening into small or large intestine for the purpose of diverting the fecal stream past an area of obstruction or disease, protecting a distal surgical anastomosis, or providing an outlet for stool in the absence of a functioning intact rectum.

NURSING DIAGNOSES / DEFINING CHARACTERISTICS	NURSING INTERVENTIONS / *RATIONALES*	EXPECTED OUTCOMES
Pre-operative knowledge deficit *Related to:* Lack of previous similar experience Need for additional information **DEFINING CHARACTERISTICS** Verbalized need for information Verbalized misinformation/misconceptions	**ONGOING ASSESSMENT** • Assess previous surgical experience. • Inquire as to information from surgeon about ostomy formation (i.e., purpose, site). • Ascertain (from chart, physician) whether stoma permanent or temporary. **THERAPEUTIC INTERVENTIONS** • Reinforce and re-explain proposed procedure. • Answer questions directly and honestly. • Use diagrams, pictures, and AV equipment to explain: 　Anatomy, physiology of GI tract 　Pathophysiology necessitating ostomy 　Proposed location of stoma • Explain need for pouch in terms of loss of sphincter. • Show patient actual pouch or one similar to his/hers. • Allow patient to wear pouch preoperatively. *Stoma site selection is facilitated by observing adhesive faceplate in situ.*	Patient will understand alteration in normal GI anatomy or physiology requiring surgical creation of the ostomy and understand that loss of sphincter will likely necessitate wearing a pouch.
Fear *Related to:* Proposed creation of ostomy Previous contact with poorly rehabilitated ostomate **DEFINING CHARACTERISTICS** Verbal expression of concern/anxiety Tense facial expression Restlessness Multiple questions Lack of questions	**ONGOING ASSESSMENT** • Assess patient's level of anxiety: note nonverbal signs. • Elicit from patient (or other source) normal coping strategies. **THERAPEUTIC INTERVENTIONS** • Ask patient to describe in detail what is causing fear/anxiety. • Correct misconceptions; fill in knowledge gaps. • Offer visit from rehabilitated ostomate. *Often, contact with another individual who has "been there" is more beneficial in decreasing fear/anxiety than factual information.* • See Anxiety, p. 4.	Level of anxiety will be decreased or manageable.
Anticipatory grief *Related to:* Proposed loss of fecal continence Anticipated loss of function, love, job, body image **DEFINING CHARACTERISTICS** Crying Rage Questioning Bargaining with self, God, health care professionals Withdrawal from usual relationships	**ONGOING ASSESSMENT** • Recognize the signs of anticipatory grief (see Defining Characteristics). • Assess perceived loss of: 　Life 　Function 　Social status 　Love 　Control 　Other **THERAPEUTIC INTERVENTIONS** • Encourage patient to verbalize feelings. • Assure patient such grief is real, expected, and appropriate. *Anticipatory grief facilitates postoperative grieving; and often follows patterns similar to actual grief patterns.*	Anticipatory grief will be recognized and facilitated.

Continued.

311

NURSING DIAGNOSES / DEFINING CHARACTERISTICS	NURSING INTERVENTIONS / *RATIONALES*	EXPECTED OUTCOMES
Altered bowel elimination *Related to:* Preoperative preparation for surgery **DEFINING CHARACTERISTICS** Orders for dietary restriction, cathartics, cleansing enemas	**ONGOING ASSESSMENT** • Assess preparedness of bowel for surgery: clear/near-clear returns on enemas. *Postoperative complications are decreased when surgical area properly emptied and cleansed.* • Observe for weakness, bradycardia, perianal discomfort. **THERAPEUTIC INTERVENTIONS** • Carry out necessary bowel preparation. • Explain necessity of bowel preparation. • Provide privacy during evacuation. • Allow rest periods between enemas.	Bowel will be sufficiently prepared for surgical procedure.
Potential toileting self care deficit *Related to:* Presence of stoma Presence of pouch **DEFINING CHARACTERISTICS** Presence of old abdominal scars Presence of bony prominences on anterior abdominal surface Presence of skinfolds over abdomen Extreme obesity Pendulous breasts	**ONGOING ASSESSMENT** • Assess abdominal surface for presence of: Old scars Bony prominences Skin folds Contour Visibility to patient **THERAPEUTIC INTERVENTIONS** • Indelibly mark proposed stoma site in area: Patient can easily see Patient can easily reach Scars, bony prominences, skinfolds are avoided Hip flexion does not change contour *Stoma location is a key factor in self-care. A poorly located stoma can delay/preclude self-care abilities.* • Note usual sites for stoma: *Ileostomy: lower right quadrant.* *Ascending colostomy: right upper or lower quadrant.* *Transverse colostomy: midwaist or just below midwaist.* *Descending and sigmoid colostomies: lower left quadrant.* • If possible, have patient wear pouch over proposed site; evaluate effectiveness 12-24 hr after applying pouch.	Potential for self-care deficit will be decreased.
Postoperative alteration in bowel elimination *Related to:* Surgical diversion of fecal stream **DEFINING CHARACTERISTICS** Structural or functional absence of anal sphincter Presence of stoma	**ONGOING ASSESSMENT** • Assess stoma q4h postoperatively for: Color Shape Size Presence of supportive device (rod, catheter) Function (flatus, stool) Drainage that is not stool **THERAPEUTIC INTERVENTIONS** • Apply pouch to stoma as soon as possible postoperatively *to protect other surgical sites from fecal contamination and protect peristomal skin.* • Notify physician if stoma appears dusky or blue. *Stoma (a piece of intestine) should be pink, moist, indicating good perfusion and adequate venous drainage.*	Bowel function via stoma will return within 8 hr (ileostomy) or 1-4 days (colostomy).
Body image disturbance *Related to:* Presence of stoma; loss of fecal continence	**ONGOING ASSESSMENT** • Assess perception of change in body structure and function. • Assess perceived impact of change. *Assigned importance of body part or importance major factor in impact.* • Note verbal references to stoma, altered bowel elimination.	Feelings about altered bowel function, stoma, and changes in self-concept will be acknowledged.

NURSING DIAGNOSES / DEFINING CHARACTERISTICS	NURSING INTERVENTIONS / *RATIONALES*	EXPECTED OUTCOMES
DEFINING CHARACTERISTICS Verbalized feelings about stoma and altered bowel elimination Refusal to discuss, acknowledge, touch, or care for stoma, pouch	**THERAPEUTIC INTERVENTIONS** • Acknowledge appropriateness of emotional response to perceived change in body structure and function. *Because control of elimination is skill/task of early childhood and socially private function, loss of control precipitates body image change and possible self-concept change.* • Assist patient in looking at, touching, and caring for stoma when ready. • Reoffer visit from rehabilitated ostomate. • See Body image disturbance, p. 6	
Knowledge deficit: ostomy self-care *Related to:* Presence of new stoma Lack of similar experience **DEFINING CHARACTERISTICS** Demonstrated inability to empty and change pouch Verbalized need for information about diet, odor, activity, hygiene, clothing, interpersonal relationships, equipment purchase, financial concerns	**ONGOING ASSESSMENT** • Assess: 　Ability to empty and change pouch 　Ability to care for peristomal skin and identify problems, potential problems 　Appropriateness in seeking assistance 　Knowledge of: 　　Diet 　　Activity 　　Hygiene 　　Clothing 　　Interpersonal relationships 　　Equipment purchase 　　Financial reimbursement for ostomy equipment **THERAPEUTIC INTERVENTIONS** • Build on information given preoperatively. • Plan and share teaching plan with patient. • Begin psychomotor teaching during first and subsequent applications of pouch. • Gradually transfer responsibility for pouch emptying and changing to patient. • Allow at least one opportunity for supervised return demonstration of pouch change before discharge. *Ostomy care requires both cognitive and psychomotor skills. Postoperatively, learning ability may be decreased, requiring repetition and opportunity of return demonstrations.* • Instruct patient on the following: 　Diet: 　　*For ileostomy:* balanced diet: special care in chewing high-fiber foods (popcorn, peanuts, coconut, vegetables, string beans, olives): increased fluid intake during hot weather, vigorous exercise. 　　*For colostomy:* balanced diet: no foods specifically contraindicated; certain foods (eggs, fish, green leafy vegetables, carbonated beverages) may increase flatus and fecal odor. 　Odor control: best achieved by eliminating odor-causing foods from diet: oral agents, deodorant available. 　Activity: should not be restricted because of stoma or pouch; direct forceful blows to stoma should be prevented.	Patient will be capable of ostomy self-care on discharge.
Pain *Related to:* Surgical incision(s) **DEFINING CHARACTERISTICS** Facial mask of pain Verbal complaints of pain	**ONGOING ASSESSMENT** • Assess level of comfort. • Elicit from patient possible sources of discomfort/recommendations for relief. **THERAPEUTIC INTERVENTIONS** • Institute pain relief measures, incorporating patient's suggestions when possible. *Patients who have undergone abdominal-perineal resection have both abdominal and perineal incisions and may need additional assistance achieving adequate pain relief.*	Pain will be reduced.

Continued.

Fecal ostomy— cont'd

NURSING DIAGNOSES / DEFINING CHARACTERISTICS	NURSING INTERVENTIONS / *RATIONALES*	EXPECTED OUTCOMES
Inability to turn, cough, deep breathe, get out of bed Decreased concentration	· See Pain, p. 39	

Originated by: Audrey Klopp, RN, PhD, ET
        Nola D. Johnson, RN

Gastrectomy

(BILLROTH I; BILLROTH II; SUBTOTAL GASTRECTOMY; TOTAL GASTRECTOMY)

Removal of all or a portion of the stomach, most commonly performed because of GI bleeding from ulcers or gastritis. A gastrectomy may also be done for stomach cancer.

NURSING DIAGNOSES / DEFINING CHARACTERISTICS	NURSING INTERVENTIONS / *RATIONALES*	EXPECTED OUTCOMES
Ineffective breathing pattern *Related to:* Upper abdominal incision pain Abdominal distention compromising lung expansion **DEFINING CHARACTERISTICS** Poor coughing effort Shallow breathing Splinting respirations Refusal to use incentive spirometer	**ONGOING ASSESSMENT** · Assess rate and depth of respirations. · Auscultate breath sounds. · Observe for splinting. · Assess ability to use incentive spirometer. **THERAPEUTIC INTERVENTIONS** · Provide analgesia per physician order. · Position patient with HOB elevated 30 degrees. · Encourage use of incentive spirometer. · Help patient splint abdominal incision by using hands or a pillow. *Splinting the incision eases the discomfort of coughing and taking deep breaths.* · Ambulate as tolerated.	Ability to breathe effectively and cough will be maximized.

Potential fluid volume deficit
Related to:
Nasogastric suctioning
Intestinal or space drains
Wound drainage
Blood loss in surgery
NPO status
Vomiting
 	
DEFINING CHARACTERISTICS
Decreased urine output
Concentrated urine
Dry mucous membranes
Hypotension
	ONGOING ASSESSMENT
	· Mark extension of drainage from incisions. *Outlining the stain on the surface of the dressing and indicating the time of the observation allow later staff to quantify amount of drainage.*
	· Assess hydration status:
	    Check CVP.
	    Monitor BP, heart rate.
	    Check mucous membranes for moisture.
	    Check skin turgor.
	· Monitor and record I & O, including urinary output, nasogastric (NG) tube output, surgical drains, and incisional drainage (check for leakage around drains).
	· Measure any emesis.
	· Check Hb and Hct as ordered.
	· Weigh patient daily.
	· See Fluid volume deficit, p. 20.
	
	THERAPEUTIC INTERVENTIONS
	· Administer IV fluids per order.
	· Secure all drains, tubes.
	· Ensure patency of drains, tubes.
		Normal fluid volume will be maintained.

NURSING DIAGNOSES / DEFINING CHARACTERISTICS	NURSING INTERVENTIONS / *RATIONALES*	EXPECTED OUTCOMES
	• Ensure function of suction machines (*protects gastric suture line from tension*).	
Pain *Related to:* Abdominal incision Presence of drains, tubes **DEFINING CHARACTERISTICS** Subjective complaint of pain Guarded movement	**ONGOING ASSESSMENT** • Assess nature of pain (location, quality, duration). • Monitor change in perception of pain associated with abdominal distention. • Check abdomen for rigidity and rebound tenderness (*may indicate peritonitis*). • See Pain, p. 39. **THERAPEUTIC INTERVENTIONS** • Assist patient to comfortable position. • Use nonpharmacologic measures to reduce perception of pain (distraction, relaxation). • Administer analgesics; maintain patient-controlled analgesia (PCA) as ordered. • Document patient's response to pain-relieving measures.	Pain will be relieved.
Altered nutrition: less than body requirements *Related to:* Postoperative restriction of food/fluid Diminish gastric capacity Disease process necessitating surgical procedures Dumping syndrome **DEFINING CHARACTERISTICS** Nausea Vomiting Diarrhea Anemia Weight loss	**ONGOING ASSESSMENT** • Weight patient daily. • Auscultate abdomen for return of bowel sounds. • Monitor intake of food/fluid. • Observe stool for steatorrhea. *Fatty, greasy stools indicate malabsorption.* • Monitor for early satiety. • Note regurgitation of food/fluid. • Monitor for signs of dumping syndrome: *rapid emptying of gastric contents into small intestine, causing diarrhea accompanied by weakness, palpitation, cold, clammy skin.* • See Nutrition, altered: less than body requirements, p. 37. **THERAPEUTIC INTERVENTIONS** • Administer parenteral fluid as ordered. • Provide mouth care q2h during NPO regimen. • Provide oral food/fluid when bowel sounds return. • Increase food/fluid per patient's tolerance. • Provide small, frequent low-carbohydrate, high-protein meals (*decrease dumping syndrome by slowing transit time through stomach and intestine*). • Encourage patient to rest after food/fluid ingestion. *Activity hastens emptying; resting decreases dumping syndrome.* • Replace vitamin B_{12} per order. *If stomach portion producing intrinsic factor removed, B_{12} cannot be absorbed and must be replaced to prevent anemia.*	Nutrition appropriate to body requirements/tolerance will be provided.
Potential for infection *Related to:* Abdominal incision Indwelling urinary catheter Venous access devices Impaired nutritional status Intra-abdominal abscess Anastomotic leaks	**ONGOING ASSESSMENT** • Assess wound for redness, drainage, separation, dehiscence, evisceration at each dressing change. • Monitor temperature. • Monitor CBC/WBC results. • Observe urine for clarity, odor. • Check all tubes and drains for leakage at exit site. **THERAPEUTIC INTERVENTIONS** • Maintain asepsis when changing dressings. • Provide IV site care per policy. • Provide daily meatal care. • Maintain all drains and tubes to closed drainage/suction; avoid opening systems whenever possible. *Interruption of closed systems allows pathogens to enter, increasing risk of intra-abdominal infection.*	Risk of infection will be reduced.

Continued.

Gastrectomy— cont'd

NURSING DIAGNOSES / DEFINING CHARACTERISTICS	NURSING INTERVENTIONS / *RATIONALES*	EXPECTED OUTCOMES
DEFINING CHARACTERISTICS Purulent wound drainage Evidence of fistula formation Increased temperature Increased WBC Cloudy, foul-smelling urine		
Constipation or diarrhea *Related to:* Gastrointestinal surgery General anesthesia Immobility Altered eating patterns **DEFINING CHARACTERISTICS** Frequent, loose bowel movements No bowel movements Abdominal discomfort Cramping Urgency Change in stool color Flatulence	**ONGOING ASSESSMENT** • Monitor patient for first bowel movement after surgery. • Note color, consistency, and frequency of stools. **THERAPEUTIC INTERVENTIONS** • Encourage routine time for bowel movement. • Provide privacy; assist as needed. • Provide perianal skin care. • Help patient identify foods/fluids that facilitate normal stooling. • Encourage ambulation. *Resolution of postoperative ileus facilitated by ambulation (helps fluid, gas move distally through bowel).*	Preoperative bowel elimination pattern will be achieved.

Knowledge deficit
Related to:
Lack of previous surgical experience
Need for dietary modification related to gastrectomy
 	
DEFINING CHARACTERISTICS
Multiple questions
Lack of questions
Verbalized misconceptions
Dietary indiscretion
	ONGOING ASSESSMENT
	• Assess patient's postoperative interest and ability to learn.
	• Assess patient's level of understanding of need for postoperative dietary modification related to gastrectomy.
	
	THERAPEUTIC INTERVENTIONS
	• Explain that physical activity increases bowel activity; rest inhibits it.
	• Explain food types and relation to rate of passes. *Carbohydrates are most easily digested, pass most quickly, and may stimulate dumping syndrome. Proteins and fats less easily digested, pass through the intestine more slowly.*
	• Encourage fluid restriction at mealtime.
	• Encourage small, frequent meals. *Bulk stimulates peristalsis.*
	• Instruct patient to seek medical follow-up for:
	    Emesis after meals
	    Feelings of distention
	    Hematemesis
	    Weakness
	    Weight loss
		Patient verbalizes relationship between ingestion patterns and elimination.

Originated by: Fannie Royster, RN,C

Gastric restrictive procedure for morbid obesity

One of several types of surgical procedures used to restrict gastric capacity in order to reduce caloric intake.

(GASTRIC STAPLING; GASTRIC BYPASS)

NURSING DIAGNOSES / DEFINING CHARACTERISTICS	NURSING INTERVENTIONS / *RATIONALES*	EXPECTED OUTCOMES
Body image disturbance *Related to:* Obesity Others' reaction(s) of to obesity **DEFINING CHARACTERISTICS** Statements of inferiority Negative comments relating to body size History of excessive weight gain concurrent with life crisis History of multiple diets, use of diet aids and clinics with weight fluctuations History of medical sequelae of obesity (e.g., glucose intolerance, respiratory and vascular insufficiency, hernias, hypertension) Body weight at least 100 lb above ideal weight adjusted for height, age, and sex established by Metropolitan Life Insurance Tables	**ONGOING ASSESSMENT** • Assess client's concept of self. • Determine facts concerning onset of obesity, diet habits, exercise, prior weight reduction efforts and results, and average caloric intake. • Assess client's perceptions of physical limitations and expectations from surgery. • Assess support system available to client. • Review medical history and inquire about current medical conditions. **THERAPEUTIC INTERVENTIONS** • Encourage verbalization of feelings. • Provide realistic goals for future weight loss. • Encourage use of support groups. • See Body image disturbance, p. 6.	Exploration of body image will be facilitated.
Anxiety *Related to:* OR environment Misconceptions about procedure **DEFINING CHARACTERISTICS** Multiple questions Extreme increase or decrease in attention to activities in environment Noncompliance with simple requests Verbalized nervousness	**ONGOING ASSESSMENT** • Assess changes in anxiety level. • Assess prior knowledge of surgical environments and events. • Assess knowledge of strict restrictive procedure and postoperative results. • Assess OR suite for proper preparation for gastric restrictive procedure; check supplies for proper size and functioning (*so patient does not misinterpret delays related to equipment problems as self-related*). **THERAPEUTIC INTERVENTIONS** • Minimize noise and traffic within OR suite. • Explain cause of delay and approximate duration. • Give client reasons for events and actions before they occur. • Stand by client and provide reassurance during induction. • Perform many preparatory procedures (e.g., catheterization) after client anesthetized.	Anxiety will be managed.

Continued.

NURSING DIAGNOSES / DEFINING CHARACTERISTICS	NURSING INTERVENTIONS / *RATIONALES*	EXPECTED OUTCOMES
Potential intraoperative injury *Related to:* Positioning during procedure Equipment use Patient's size **DEFINING CHARACTERISTICS** Electrical burns Bruises Skin abrasions Neurovascular impairment of extremities within 48 hr after surgery	**ONGOING ASSESSMENT** · Assess skin integrity, ROM. · Assess electrical equipment for safe functioning before procedure. **THERAPEUTIC INTERVENTIONS** · Apply cautery grounding pad on muscular and vascular body parts such as thighs, upper arms, buttocks, back, or abdomen *to prevent electrical burns.* Avoid bony prominences, open wounds, wet skin, areas with excessive hair, places where fluids might pool. · Pad bony prominences with foam or soft cloth. · Maintain proper body alignment. · Request sufficient help to move to and from OR table. · Apply padded foot plate. · Apply safety strap. · Document position of client, placement of padding, cautery grounding pad, safety strap, and medications.	Risk of injury is reduced.
Ineffective breathing pattern *Related to:* Obesity Postoperative pain Anesthetic agents **DEFINING CHARACTERISTICS** Dyspnea Wheezing Diminished breath sounds Increased respiratory rate Shallow excursion	**ONGOING ASSESSMENT** · Assess rate, depth, and quality of respirations. · Note operative complications *that could predispose to postoperative ineffective breathing pattern:* Difficult intubation Prolonged anesthesia time · Monitor ABGs. **THERAPEUTIC INTERVENTIONS** · Instruct patient in importance of: Coughing and deep breathing Splinting and incision during pulmonary exercise, before and after surgery · Administer O_2 as ordered. · Suction patient unable to clear secretions.	An effective breathing pattern will be maintained.
Potential hypothermia *Related to:* Exposure during operation Increased body mass **DEFINING CHARACTERISTICS** Drop of 2 to 3 °F in temperature Skin cool to touch Increase in heart rate	**ONGOING ASSESSMENT** · Assess intraoperative body temperature. · Assess length of exposure. **THERAPEUTIC INTERVENTIONS** · Place blanklet ol heating pad on OR bed before transfer; set at 110 °C. · Place temperature probe rectally. · Warm all solutions *to prevent conductive heat loss.* · Cover with warm blankets at end of case for transport. · See Hypothermia, p. 31.	Normal body temperature will be maintained.
Potential infection *Related to:* Inadequate skin preparation Surgical incision **DEFINING CHARACTERISTICS** Elevated temperature	**ONGOING ASSESSMENT** · Note intraoperative breaks in sterile technique. · Monitor body temperature, WBC after surgery. · Assess wound for redness, swelling, drainage **THERAPEUTIC INTERVENTIONS** · Observe sterile technique of surgical team, making known breaks in technique. · Document skin breaks observed before incision.	Risk of infection is reduced.

NURSING DIAGNOSES / DEFINING CHARACTERISTICS	NURSING INTERVENTIONS / *RATIONALES*	EXPECTED OUTCOMES
Wound red Purulent drainage Elevated WBC	• Remove excess hair from incisional area with minimal trauma to tissue. *Hair harbors bacteria*. • Clean skin and abdominal skin folds.	

Originated by: Kristine Alessandrini, RN, BSN
Audrey Klopp, RN, PhD, ET

Pancreaticoduodenectomy (Whipple's operation)

Removal of all or part of the pancreas, distal stomach, duodenum, and gallbladder. Remaining pancreas, stomach, and common bile duct are anastomosed to the jejunum. This procedure is most commonly performed for pancreatic cancer but may be performed for unrelenting severe chronic pancreatitis. When the procedure is performed because of cancer, postoperative mortality is 15% and 5-year survival rate is less than 10%.

NURSING DIAGNOSES / DEFINING CHARACTERISTICS	NURSING INTERVENTIONS / *RATIONALES*	EXPECTED OUTCOMES
Fear/anxiety *Related to:* Lack of previous surgical experience Unknown outcome/prognosis of surgery **DEFINING CHARACTERISTICS** Restlessness Expressed concern Facial tension	**ONGOING ASSESSMENT** • Assess level of fear/anxiety. • Elicit specific cause(s) of fear/anxiety, if known to patient. • Inquire about previous surgical experience. • Determine whether patient knows diagnosis/prognosis. **THERAPEUTIC INTERVENTIONS** • Encourage patient to verbalize fears/concerns. • Stay in room with patient when surgeons propose/explain necessary surgical intervention. *Patient may need further or simplified explanations or repeated explanations*. • Assist patient in identifying and using strategies for managing fear/anxiety. • Include family/support system in care plan. • See Fear, p. 18 and Anxiety, p. 4.	Fear/anxiety will be reduced.
Pain *Related to:* Abdominal incision Multiple tubes/drains Postoperative (adynamic) ileus **DEFINING CHARACTERISTICS** Moaning Guarding/splinting Self-imposed limitations on movement Verbalized pain Requests for pain medication Lack of bowel sounds	**ONGOING ASSESSMENT** • Assess location, quality of pain. • Assess for proper functioning of tubes/drains. *Increased intra-abdominal pressure(s) resulting from nonfunctional drains/tubes may aggravate incisional pain*. • Check bowel sounds every shift. *Postoperative ileus usually resolves 72-96 hr after surgery. Gas a common source of postoperative pain*. **THERAPEUTIC INTERVENTIONS** • Assist patient to comfortable position. • Help patient to splint wound with pillow or hands when moving, coughing, or taking deep breaths. • Encourage ambulation as soon as possible after surgery *to help resolve ileus and relieve gas pains*. • Provide distractions (telephone, television, newspapers, mail, conversation). • Encourage use of pain medication before peak pain periods. • See Pain, p. 39.	Pain will be relieved.

Continued.

NURSING DIAGNOSES / DEFINING CHARACTERISTICS	NURSING INTERVENTIONS / *RATIONALES*	EXPECTED OUTCOMES
Ineffective breathing pattern *Related to:* Residual anesthetic Abdominal pain **Defining Characteristics** Shallow respirations Rales Poor cough effort	**Ongoing Assessment** • Assess rate, rhythm, and depth of respirations. • Check breath sounds. • Determine whether rhonchi clear after cough. **Therapeutic Interventions** • Place patient in semi-Fowler's position *to facilitate diaphragmatic movement.* • Encourage use of splinting when taking deep breaths and/or coughing. • Teach and encourage incentive spirometer use. • Plan administration of analgesics around key times (coughing, deep breathing, use of incentive spirometry). • Administer O₂ as ordered. • See Breathing pattern, ineffective, p. 8.	Normal or adequate breathing pattern will be maintained.
Potential fluid volume deficit *Related to:* Hemorrhage Shifting of fluids from vascular space Drainage from tubes/ drains Drainage from biliary and/or pancreatic fistulae **Defining Characteristics** Decrease in blood pressure Increase in heart rate Dry mucous membranes Excessive drainage on dressing or from tubes/drains Peripheral edema Low urine output	**Ongoing Assessment** • Assess vital signs. • Monitor amount of drainage on dressings. • Record amount, color of drainage from tubes/drains; note significant amounts of drainage around tube/drain insertion sites. • Check extremities for presence of edema. • Weigh daily. • Check availability of blood products. • Record accurate I & O. • Monitor coagulation profile. **Therapeutic Interventions** • Administer oral and/or parenteral fluids as ordered. • Notify physician of significant wound or tube/drain, drainage increase or bloodiness. *Bloody incisional drainage usually superficial, indicating that uncauterized or unligated small vessels were cut. Bloody drainage from tubes/drains indicates intraluminal or space hemorrhage. Any blood drainage may indicate generalized coagulopathy.* • Be prepared to administer blood, blood products, or volume expanders if necessary. • See Fluid volume deficit, p. 20. • See also Site care: surgical drains/tubes, p. 322.	Normal fluid volume will be maintained.
Potential infection *Related to:* Existence of preoperative intra-abdominal infection(s) Postoperative fluid accumulation in abdominal spaces Inadequate or faulty abdominal drainage Abscess formation Wound contamination	**Ongoing Assessment** • Assess temperature q4h. • Note WBC results daily or as available. • Assess all drainage for purulent appearance or odor. • Check wound, rest of abdomen for swelling, redness, or tenderness. **Therapeutic Interventions** • Use sterile technique during dressing changes. • Minimize interruption of drainage. *Tubes/drains may be disconnected from suction devices for short periods at physician's discretion.* • Tape all drainage tubing connections *to reduce risk of inadvertent contamination.* • Administer antipyretics and antibiotics as ordered.	Risk of infection will be reduced.

NURSING DIAGNOSES / DEFINING CHARACTERISTICS	NURSING INTERVENTIONS / *RATIONALES*	EXPECTED OUTCOMES
DEFINING CHARACTERISTICS Elevated WBC Hyperthermia Purulent drainage on dressings or through tubes/drains Abdominal pain (not incisional) Localized swelling, redness		
Potential alteration in skin integrity *Related to:* Copious drainage Biliary or pancreatic fistulae drainage **DEFINING CHARACTERISTICS** Red, painful skin Weeping skin	**ONGOING ASSESSMENT** • Assess condition of abdominal skin, particularly noting areas: Around tubes/drains Beneath dressings Covered by tape That are constantly moist • Assess color, pH of the suspicious drainage. *Clear, colorless fluid with high (alkaline) pH may indicate pancreatic fistula. Green or golden yellow drainage may indicate biliary fistula. Both are extremely damaging to skin and cause chemical burns within 1 hr of contact.* **THERAPEUTIC INTERVENTIONS** • Change dressing as often as needed *so drainage-saturated dressings not in contact with skin.* • Protect skin with liquid barrier film beneath dressings and tapes, around tubes/drains. • Consider pouching any wound/area requiring dressing more often than q2h. • Use alternate methods of dressing stabilization (Montgomery straps, net panties) *to reduce adhesive use on skin.* • See Enterocutaneous fistula, p. 281. • See Skin integrity, impaired, p. 48.	Abdominal skin integrity will be maintained.
Potential altered skin integrity *Related to:* Jaundice **DEFINING CHARACTERISTICS** Yellow-tinged skin Yellow-tinged sclerae Itching Clay-colored stool Nonfunctional T-tube	**ONGOING ASSESSMENT** • Assess skin and sclerae for jaundice. • Monitor color of stool. • Assess for itching. • Check T-tube patency; record output accurately. **THERAPEUTIC INTERVENTIONS** • Keep skin clean and moist. • Remove irritants (lint, crumbs, starched linen) from environment (*may trigger itching*). • Remind patient not to scratch. • Put gloves on hands at night if necessary. • Keep T-tube drainage collector below level of insertion site *to facilitate drainage.*	Skin integrity will be maintained.
Altered nutrition: less than body requirements *Related to:* NPO status Preoperative nutritional deficit Infection Increased metabolic demand	**ONGOING ASSESSMENT** • Weigh patient daily. • Consult nutritionist to determine daily calorie needs. • Monitor fractional urine q4h. • Monitor blood glucose levels. • Check stools for greasiness, buoyancy. • Monitor fat-soluble vitamin assays.	Adequate nutrition will be provided.

Continued.

Pancreaticoduodenectomy (Whipple's operation)— cont'd

NURSING DIAGNOSES / DEFINING CHARACTERISTICS	NURSING INTERVENTIONS / *RATIONALES*	EXPECTED OUTCOMES
Reduced insulin production Altered digestive pathway Fistulae Reduced pancreatic exocrine function **DEFINING CHARACTERISTICS** Weight less than ideal body weight Poor wound healing Low energy levels Weakness Poor fat absorption	**THERAPEUTIC INTERVENTIONS** • Provide oral nutrition as appropriate. • Provide high-protein, high-calorie food patient prefers. • Divide feeding into small portions. • Assist patient with eating. • Provide hyperalimentation as ordered. • Provide insulin as necessary. • Administer vitamin K *(fat-soluble vitamin not absorbed from gut in adequate amount)* as ordered. • See Nutrition, altered: less than body requirements, p. 37.	

Knowledge deficit
Related to:
Lack of previous surgical experience
New, unfamiliar treatment
 	
DEFINING CHARACTERISTICS
Multiple questions
Lack of questions
Lack of participation in care
	ONGOING ASSESSMENT
	• Assess patient's cognitive ability and desire to learn.
	
	THERAPEUTIC INTERVENTIONS
	• Teach patient:
	  Consequences of surgical alterations on nutritional status
	  Need for endocrine support
	  Need for vitamin therapy
	• Instruct patient in insulin administration and blood glucose testing.
	• Refer to diabetes clinical nurse specialist.
	• Stress importance of follow-up care. *Prognosis is not good for patients with pancreatic cancer, but palliative care can improve quality of remaining life.*
		Patient will understand that nutrition and endocrine support will be necessary.

Originated by: Maretha Bryant, RN, C

Surgical tubes/drains

(GASTROSTOMY TUBE; JEJUNOSTOMY TUBE; DUODENOSTOMY TUBE; JACKSON-PRATT DRAIN; SUMP DRAINS; T-TUBES)

Tubes/drains may be placed into body cavities, surgical spaces, or the lumen of the gut for purposes of drainage, decompression, of feeding/administration of medication or irrigation

NURSING DIAGNOSES / DEFINING CHARACTERISTICS	NURSING INTERVENTIONS / *RATIONALES*	EXPECTED OUTCOMES

Potential impaired skin integrity
Related to:
Leakage of effluent around tube insertion site
Poor stabilization of tube/drain
Caustic nature of drainage around insertion site
Inadvertent tube/drain movement or migration
	ONGOING ASSESSMENT
	• Assess tube/drain insertion site daily for redness, pain, drainage.
	• Assess stability of tube/drain.
	• Assess degree to which leakage at insertion site interferes with intended purpose of tube/drain (e.g., lost enteral feedings).
	
	THERAPEUTIC INTERVENTIONS
	• Maintain tube/drain stability:
	  Tape securely.
	  Use commercially available drain/tube attachment device.
	  Inquire about possibility of suturing.
	• Apply a liquid film barrier to skin around insertion site *to prevent direct skin contact with caustic effluent.*
		Skin around drain/tube insertion site will remain intact.

Surgical tubes/drains— cont'd

NURSING DIAGNOSES / DEFINING CHARACTERISTICS	NURSING INTERVENTIONS / *RATIONALES*	EXPECTED OUTCOMES
DEFINING CHARACTERISTICS Redness around insertion site Pain around insertion site	• Change gauze or hydrocolloid-type dressing around insertion site as necessary. • Notify physician of leakage noted around drain/tube insertion site.	

Potential infection
Related to:
In-and-out movement of unstable drain/tube
Invasion by pathogens through impaired skin
Invasion by pathogens through purposely or inadvertently interrupted systems
 	
DEFINING CHARACTERISTICS
Fever
Localized pain
Elevated WBC
Purulent drainage from site of insertion
Purulent drainage from tube/drain
	ONGOING ASSESSMENT
	• Assess vital signs.
	• Monitor WBC.
	• Assess insertion site daily; observe for:
	  Redness
	  Purulent drainage
	  Pain
	• Note color, consistency, and odor of drainage from tube/drain.
	• Culture any drainage.
	
	THERAPEUTIC INTERVENTIONS
	• Use aseptic technique when manipulating tube/drain or changing dressing.
	• Ensure that system (tube and collection/suction device) remains intact; tape connections with waterproof tape.
	• Irrigate only per physician's order, using sterile technique *to prevent pathogen entry into body cavity.*
	• Administer antibiotics and antipyretics as ordered.
		Risk of infection will be reduced.

Body image disturbance *Related to:* Presence of tube/drain on body surface or from body cavity Difficulty concealing presence of tube/drain Presence of foul-smelling drainage from tube/drain **DEFINING CHARACTERISTICS** Patient unwilling to look at/care for tube/drain Patient verbalizes concern about appearance/odor of drain/tube Patient isolates self	**ONGOING ASSESSMENT** • Assess feelings/concerns about tubes/drains. **THERAPEUTIC INTERVENTIONS** • Reinforce normalcy of feelings/concerns. • Keep drain/tube site and dressing clean and dry *to minimize odor.* • Utilize room deodorants sparingly *(may reinforce, call attention to barely noticeable odors).* • Tape excess tubing in coiled fashion near body, beneath clothing (unless contraindicated). • See Body image disturbance, p. 6.	Body image will be enhanced.

Knowledge deficit
Related to:
No previous experience with tube/drain
	ONGOING ASSESSMENT
	• Assess readiness to learn tube/drain site care.
	• Assess barriers to learning:
	  Pain
	  Inability to visualize insertion site
	  Poor eyesight
	  Poor manual dexterity
		Patient/significant other verbalizes and demonstrates safe tube/drain site care.

Continued.

■ **Surgical tubes/drains— cont'd**

NURSING DIAGNOSES / DEFINING CHARACTERISTICS	NURSING INTERVENTIONS / RATIONALES	EXPECTED OUTCOMES

DEFINING CHARACTERISTICS
Multiple questions
Lack of questions
Demonstrated inability to provide tube/drain care
	THERAPEUTIC INTERVENTIONS
	• *Maximize teaching* by reducing/eliminating barriers to learning:
	    Provide analgesia.
	    Use mirrors.
	    Provide eyeglasses if appropriate.
	    Consider teaching willing significant other.
	• Teach patient the following:
	    Purpose of tube/drain; expected output
	    Site care
	    Care of collection devices
	    Need to notify health care professional if:
	        Tube/drain comes out (should not attempt reinsertion)
	        Nature/amount of drainage changes
	        Skin around insertion site painful, red, or has drainage
	        Fever
	        Pain not related to tube/drain insertion site	

Originated by: Carol Gawron, RN, MSN, ET

Total parenteral nutrition (TPN)

(INTRAVENOUS HYPERALIMENTATION)

Total parenteral nutrition (TPN) is the administration of concentrated glucose and amino acid solutions via a central or large-diameter pheripheral vein. TPN therapy is necessary when the gastrointestinal tract cannot be or is not used to meet the patient's nutritional needs. TPN solutions may contain 20 to 60% glucose and 3.5 to 10% protein (in the form of amino acids), in addition to various amounts of electrolytes, vitamins, minerals, and trace elements. These solutions can be modified, depending on the presence of organ system impairment and/or the specific nutritional needs of the patient.

NURSING DIAGNOSES / DEFINING CHARACTERISTICS	NURSING INTERVENTIONS / RATIONALES	EXPECTED OUTCOMES
Altered nutrition: less than body requirements, with need for TPN *Related to:* Prolonged NPO status Alterations in GI tract function (e.g., GI surgery, fistulas, bowel obstruction, esophageal injury/disease, dysphagia, stomatitis, nausea, vomiting, or diarrhea)	**ONGOING ASSESSMENT** • Perform a comprehensive nutritional assessment on admission and periodically thereafer and document findings. • Observe for metabolic/local complications of TPN (e.g., hyper- or hypoglycemia, infection, fluid and electrolyte imbalance, air embolism). • Assess response to nutritional support (e.g., daily weights, lab results: electrolytes, glucose, albumin, wound healing, skin condition). • Obtain accurate calorie counts and I & O. **THERAPEUTIC INTERVENTIONS** • Assist with insertion, maintenance of central or peripheral line. • Administer prescribed TPN solution, preferably via infusion pump *(to assure constant infusion rate)*. • Be familiar with additive content of TPN solution (glucose, amino acids, electrolytes, insulin, vitamins, and trace minerals). • Assist with oral intake if indicated. • Provide oral care at least q2h for patient or NPO program. • Refer to/collaborate with appropriate resources: nutritional support team, dietitian, pharmacy. • Refer to Nutrition, altered: less than body requirements, p. 37.	Nutritional status will be maximized.

Total parenteral nutrition— cont'd

NURSING DIAGNOSES / DEFINING CHARACTERISTICS	NURSING INTERVENTIONS / *RATIONALES*	EXPECTED OUTCOMES
High glucose concentration of TPN solution provides excellent microbial growth medium Pre-existing susceptibility to infection secondary to poor nutritional status **DEFINING CHARACTERISTICS** Inflammation, swelling, or drainage noted at catheter site Elevated temperature Elevated WBC count Positive culture results	**THERAPEUTIC INTERVENTIONS** · Assist with central line placement for TPN under sterile conditions. · Use sterile technique when caring for central line during dressing tubing and solution changes. · Change TPN tubing and filter q24h or according to hospital policy. · Maintain sterile, occlusive TPN dressing. Perform dressing changes under sterile technique q48h or according to hospital policy. · Change individual TPN bag after 24 hr or more often, as ordered. *(High glucose concentration of TPN provides excellent microbial growth medium).* · Keep TPN solutions refrigerated until needed. · Never use TPN line for medications, blood draws, or CVP readings *(to lessen risk of contamination of line).* · Do not place additives in prepared TPN solution. Return TPN solution to pharmacy if additives needed. *TPN is prepared in pharmacy under a laminar air flow hood to decrease risk of microbial contamination of fluid.* · Do not infuse TPN into pre-existing central lines or Swan-Ganz catheters. · If line-related infections are suspected, assist physician with reinsertion of central line at new site. Use new TPN solution, tubing, and filter. · If infection present, administer antibiotics as ordered.	
Potential for injury: air embolism *Related to:* Entry of air into vascular system via central TPN catheter **DEFINING CHARACTERISTICS** Shortness of breath Tachypnea Cyanosis Chest pain Mental status changes	**ONGOING ASSESSMENT** · Obtain vital signs, including respiratory rate, q4h. · Assess breath sounds every shift. · Monitor arterial blood gases as ordered. · Assess patient closely for signs of air embolism. · Monitor TPN infusion rate q1h. Do not let infusion run dry. **THERAPEUTIC INTERVENTIONS** · Use Luer-Lock tubings on TPN line and tape all connections securely. · Use infusion device that will detect presence of air in line. *Air will then be detected before reaching patient.* · If TPN infusion runs dry, clamp tubing, aspirate air from line, and remove all air from line before continuing infusion with new bag. · Have patient perform Valsalva maneuver during tubing changes *(prevents patient from taking breath, which would cause air to be sucked into an "open" central line).* · Use air elimination filter according to hospital policy. · If air embolus is suspected: 　Immediately turn patient on left side, in Trendelenberg's position. *If air has already traveled into heart, it will then stay on right side of RA or RV and away from pulmonic valve.* · Call physician stat. *This is a life-threatening emergency.* · Monitor vital signs and cardiac status closely. · Assist physician with aspiration of air through central line while patient performs Valsalva maneuver.	Air embolism will be prevented.
Potential for injury: pneumothorax/ hydrothorax *Related to:* Placement of central IV line **DEFINING CHARACTERISTICS** Decreased breath sounds on side of central line placement	**ONGOING ASSESSMENT** · Assess breath sounds before, after central line placement. · Assess for complaints of IV site pain or shoulder pain. · Assess for swelling near central line site. · Assess for subcutaneous emphysema and asymmetrical chest movement. · Obtain initial chest x-ray after line placement and monitor chest x-ray reports. **THERAPEUTIC INTERVENTIONS** · Properly position patient for placement of central line: 　Put head of bed flat. 　Place towel roll between shoulder blades *to allow shoulders to drop back, revealing correct anatomic placement of subclavian vein.*	Potential for injury from pneumothorax/ hydrothorax will be reduced.

Continued.

Total parenteral nutrition— cont'd

NURSING DIAGNOSES / DEFINING CHARACTERISTICS	NURSING INTERVENTIONS / *RATIONALES*	EXPECTED OUTCOMES
Continued complaints of pain after procedure Asymmetrical chest movement Subcutaneous emphysema Swelling near central line site	• After central line is started, infuse D_5W or $D_{10}W$ until x-ray report validates placement *(ensures TPN not inadvertently infused into pleural space)*. • Notify physician of signs of pneumothorax/hydrothorax.	
Anxiety/fear *Related to:* Knowledge deficit about TPN Dependence on TPN for nutritional intake with inability to eat normally and subsequent psychosocial ramifications Disease process necessitating TPN Change in body image related to central venous catheter **DEFINING CHARACTERISTICS** Patient/significant others verbalize fears, anxiety related to patient's condition and need for TPN	**ONGOING ASSESSMENT** • Recognize patient's/significant others' anxiety/fear level. • Assess patient's normal coping patterns. **THERAPEUTIC INTERVENTIONS** • Explain rationale for TPN method of delivery and need for related monitoring. • Encourage patient/significant others to verbalize questions, anxieties, and concerns. • Provide comfort measures and diversional activities. • Support realistic view of need for and duration of therapy. • Avoid depersonalizing patient by focusing on TPN line, dressing, infusion pump, or related "monitoring equipment" during care-giving activities. • See Anxiety, p. 4 and Fear, p. 18.	Reduction in patient's/ significant others' anxiety/fear level.

Originated by: Debbie Lazzara, RN, MS, CCRN

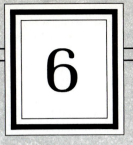

Renal Care Plans

DISORDERS
Coping with renal disease
End-stage renal disease (ESRD): out-
  patient on dialysis with fluid volume
  excess
Hypocalcemia and bone disease in
  end-stage renal disease
Nephrotic syndrome

Peritonitis related to peritoneal dialysis
Renal failure, acute

THERAPEUTIC INTERVENTIONS
Catheter for hemodialysis
External arteriovenous shunt for
  hemodialysis

Internal arteriovenous fistula for
  hemodialysis
Nephrostomy tube, percutaneous
Peritoneal dialysis
Renal transplant, postoperative

Coping with renal disease

The impact of end stage renal disease and the stresses of dialysis can be detrimental to one's ego and can place patients under severe mental and emotional stress. Depression is a common psychological occurrence in patients on hemodialysis. Although the patient is dependent on the machine, personnel, and treatment regimen, he/she is at the same time encouraged to be independent, work, and lead a "normal" life. This dependence/independence conflict may create conflicting feelings that are difficult or impossible to express

NURSING DIAGNOSES / DEFINING CHARACTERISTICS	NURSING INTERVENTIONS / *RATIONALES*	EXPECTED OUTCOMES
Self concept disturbance *Related to:* Loss of body function Altered body image Role changes Feelings of decreased control **DEFINING CHARACTERISTICS** Dependent behaviors Withdrawal Self-criticism Expression of helplessness, disappointment Ambivalence	**ONGOING ASSESSMENT** • Assess patient's self-concept. • Explore meaning of illness and treatment with patient. **THERAPEUTIC INTERVENTIONS** • Convey acceptance to patient. Reinforce that he/she is a worthwhile human being. • Assist patient in working through feelings of disappointment related to losses. See Grieving, p. 333. • Focus on patient's strengths when goal setting. • Discourage emphasis on failure *to prevent self-criticism*. • Avoid false praise. Offer positive reinforcement for actual accomplishments. • See Self-concept disturbance, p. 46.	Self-concept will be enhanced.
Body image disturbance *Related to:* Presence of hemodialysis access Failure to develop secondary sex characteristics in teenagers Gynecomastia in males **DEFINING CHARACTERISTICS** Hiding or overexposing parts of body with changes Negative feelings about body Feelings of helplessness/powerlessness Verbal preoccupation with body changes Change in social behavior	**ONGOING ASSESSMENT** • Assess patient's perception of change/lack of development. • Assess patient's behavior in terms of actual or perceived change/lack of development. **THERAPEUTIC INTERVENTIONS** • Encourage patient to verbalize feelings about change/lack of development. • Assist patient in identifying major areas of concern related to altered body image. Use problem-solving technique with patient to explore ways of minimizing these concerns. *The nurse-patient relationship can provide strong basis for implementing other strategies to assist patient/family with adaptation.* • Assist patient in incorporating changes into ADL, social life, interpersonal relationships, and occupational activities. • Encourage use of support groups. • See Body image disturbance, p. 6.	Body image will be enhanced.
Powerlessness *Related to:* Inability to perform role responsibilities	**ONGOING ASSESSMENT** • Assist patient in identifying feelings of powerlessness. • Identify factors contributing to sense of powerlessness. • Assess usual level of control and decision making.	Sense of control over condition/problem will be increased.

Coping with renal disease— cont'd

NURSING DIAGNOSES / DEFINING CHARACTERISTICS	NURSING INTERVENTIONS / *RATIONALES*	EXPECTED OUTCOMES
Knowledge deficit Perceived loss of control Chronic disease **DEFINING CHARACTERISTICS** Expressions of uncertainty Dependent behavior Apathy Depression Nonparticipation in care	**THERAPEUTIC INTERVENTIONS** · Help patient differentiate those situations that can be changed from those that cannot. · Encourage patient to recognize his/her potential. · Provide patient opportunities to make decisions. *When patients are involved in decisions about their care, they begin to feel more in control of situation, treatment, and life.* · Record patient's specific choices on care plan *to ensure staff adherence.* · Provide specific time to keep patient informed of his/her condition and progress. · See Powerlessness, p. 42.	
Anxiety/fear *Related to:* Altered self-concept Threat to role functioning Uncertainty of outcomes Unfamiliar treatment regimen Restriction of diet, medications, treatment Decreased feelings of control **DEFINING CHARACTERISTICS** Noncompliant behaviors Denial Irritability Nervousness Increased heart rate, blood pressure, and respirations Inability to concentrate	**ONGOING ASSESSMENT** · Assess patient's level of anxiety. · Ask patient to describe in detail what is causing fear/anxiety *(any previous negative experience may be basis).* · Determine particular stressor or, if generalized, nonspecific threats. **THERAPEUTIC INTERVENTIONS** · Acknowledge appropriateness of patient's feeling; correct any misinterpretations. · Maintain calm, nonthreatening manner. · Provide continuity of care as much as possible. · Be empathic. · Educate patient *so he/she will understand condition and treatment regimen.* · With patient, explore ways he/she can assume control. · If particular stressors identified, explore ways to minimize them. · For generalized, nonspecific threats provide feedback about reality of current situation.	Anxiety/fear will be reduced.

Grieving
Related to:
Loss of kidney function
Failure of access device
Loss of roles
Loss of relationships
 	
DEFINING CHARACTERISTICS
Expressions of:
Anger
Denial
Guilt
Crying
Withdrawn behavior
	ONGOING ASSESSMENT
	· Assess patient's expression of grief.
	· Explore with patient his/her perception of change ESRD has caused.
	
	THERAPEUTIC INTERVENTIONS
	· Assist patient throughout grieving process:
	  Denial phase:
	    Be genuine and honest about loss.
	    Acknowledge normalcy of denial.
	  Anger phase:
	    Be tolerant and patient; avoid defensiveness.
	    Allow patient to express anger constrictively and acceptably. *Patient may hesitate to cry or let go of feelings. Convey to patient that behaviors such as crying are acceptable.*
	    Explore feelings of guilt.
		Grief is expressed, acknowledged, and facilitated.

Continued.

NURSING DIAGNOSES / DEFINING CHARACTERISTICS	NURSING INTERVENTIONS / *RATIONALES*	EXPECTED OUTCOMES

	Realization phase:
	    Offer support and acceptance.
	    Encourage patient to share feelings with significant others.
	Acceptance phase:
	    Assist patient in formulating new goals.
	    Assist in adjusting life-style.
	• Provide/encourage discussions with other patients with renal failure *to share their responses to illness.*	

Noncompliance *Related to:* Knowledge deficit Lack of resources Side effects of treatment, diet, and medications Poor relationship with health care team Denial **DEFINING CHARACTERISTICS** Missed appointments Unused medications Abnormal laboratory values Acknowledgement of noncompliance Persistence of symptoms Suicidal gesture	**ONGOING ASSESSMENT** • Assess contributing factors to noncompliance. • Elicit patient's understanding of treatment regimen. • Explore with patient his/her feelings about illness and treatment. **THERAPEUTIC INTERVENTIONS** • Maintain consistency of care givers *(helps develop therapeutic relationship)*. • Promote decision making and ADL management; use social support systems. *Social support has been closely liked to compliance with dialysis; it is necessary to manage the role demands of daily living and especially important in coping with stressful life events and transitions.* • Explore alternatives with health care team to reduce side effects. • Contract with patient for behavioral changes. • Use social work department *to explore available resources.* • See Noncompliance, p. 36.	Noncompliant behavior will diminish.

Sexual dysfunction
Related to:
Effects of uremia on the endocrine system
Psychosocial effects of renal failure and its treatment
 	
DEFINING CHARACTERISTICS
Adults:
Amenorrhea, failure to ovulate, and decreased libido in females
Azoospermia, atrophy of testicles, impotence, decreased libido, and gynecomastia in males
Children:
Failure to achieve menarche in females
Failure to produce sperm in males
	ONGOING ASSESSMENT
	• Assess impact of changes in sexual function on patient.
	• Explore meaning of sexuality with patient.
	
	THERAPEUTIC INTERVENTIONS
	• Discuss alternate methods of sexual expression with patient/significant others. *Emphasize that intercourse not only method for satisfying sexual relationship.*
	• Emphasize importance of giving and receiving love and affection, as opposed to "performing".
	• Confer with physician about medical treatments and procedures that may alleviate some sexual dysfunction:
	    Discuss possibility of penile implant/prosthesis.
	    If patient has low zinc levels, discuss possible replacement for male patients.
	• See Sexuality patterns, altered, p. 47.
		Sexual functioning will be enhanced.

NURSING DIAGNOSES / DEFINING CHARACTERISTICS	NURSING INTERVENTIONS / *RATIONALES*	EXPECTED OUTCOMES
Failure to develop secondary sex characteristics in both sexes		

Originated by: Susan Pische, RN, BSN, MBA

End-stage renal disease (ESRD): outpatient on dialysis with fluid volume excess

End-stage renal disease (ESRD) is defined as irreversible kidney disease causing chronic abnormalities in the body's homeostasis and necessitating treatment with dialysis or renal transplantation for survival. Uremia or the uremic syndrome consists of the signs, symptoms, and physiologic changes that occur in renal failure. These changes are related to fluid and electrolyte abnormalities, accumulation of uremic toxins that cause physiologic changes and alter function of various organs, and regulatory function disorders (hypertension, renal osteodystrophy, anemia, and metastatic calcifications).

NURSING DIAGNOSES / DEFINING CHARACTERISTICS	NURSING INTERVENTIONS / *RATIONALES*	EXPECTED OUTCOMES
Fluid volume excess *Related to:* Excess fluid intake Excess sodium intake Compromised regulatory mechanisms **DEFINING CHARACTERISTICS** Edema BP elevated (above patient's normal BP) before dialysis Weight gain	**ONGOING ASSESSMENT** · Assess patient's vital signs q1h. · Assess amount of edema by palpating area over tibia, at ankles, sacrum, back, and assessing appearance of face. · Assess patient's compliance to dietary and fluid restrictions at home. **THERAPEUTIC INTERVENTIONS** · Weigh at every visit before and after dialysis (weight gain not to exceed 1 kg between visits). · Restrict fluid intake as required by patient's condition. · Restrict dietary sodium *(sodium intake produces feeling of thirst). By restricting sodium intake amount of fluid patient drinks can be reduced.* · Advise patient to elevate feet when sitting down *to prevent fluid accumulation in lower extremities.* · Instruct patient about necessity to follow prescribed fluid/dietary restriction. · Give antihypertensive medications if prescribed. · At initiation of treatment, run off normal saline in the lines and use patient's own blood as a prime *(will minimize fluid given to patient to least amount possible).*	Effects of fluid volume excess will be reduced.
Potential impaired gas exchange *Related to:* Pulmonary edema: Altered blood flow Alveolar-capillary membrane changes	**ONGOING ASSESSMENT** · Assess vital signs. · Auscultate for moist rales. · Check for distended neck veins. · Assess for cyanosis. · Assess breathing pattern. If abnormal, see Breathing pattern, ineffective, p. 8. **THERAPEUTIC INTERVENTIONS** · Maintain optimal positioning for air exchange. Have patient sit up if he/she complains of shortness of breath.	Optimal gas exchange will be maintained.

Continued.

End-stage renal disease: outpatient on dialysis with fluid volume excess— cont'd

NURSING DIAGNOSES / DEFINING CHARACTERISTICS	NURSING INTERVENTIONS / *RATIONALES*	EXPECTED OUTCOMES
DEFINING CHARACTERISTICS Shortness of breath Tachypnea Orthopnea Chest pain Tachycardia Restlessness Confusion	• Notify physician of signs of impaired gas exchange. • Perform ultrafiltration as ordered per physician *to remove fluid rapidly.*	
Potential impaired skin integrity *Related to:* Edema related to end-stage renal disease **DEFINING CHARACTERISTICS** Pitting of extremities on manipulation Low Hct Puffy eyelids Demarcation of clothing and shoes on patient's body	**ONGOING ASSESSMENT** • Assess skin integrity. • See Skin integrity, impaired, p. 48. **THERAPEUTIC INTERVENTIONS** • Instruct the patient to wear loose-fittting clothing when edema present. *Restrictive clothing can increase risk of skin breakdown.* • Teach patient factors important to skin integrity: Nutrition Mobility Hygiene Early recognition of skin breakdown	Optimal skin integrity will be maintained.
Self-concept disturbance *Related to:* Prolonged outpatient dialysis Loss of body function Financial cost of chronic dialysis Change in perceptions as autonomous and productive individual **DEFINING CHARACTERISTICS** Depression Expressed anger Withdrawal	**ONGOING ASSESSMENT** • Assess for presence of depression and withdrawal. • Allow patient time to voice concerns and express anger related to condition. **THERAPEUTIC INTERVENTIONS** • Talk with patient, significant others, and friends, if possible, about chronic outpatient dialysis. • Discuss problems and possible solutions with patient. • Explore strengths and resources with patient. • Have social workers see patients regularly as preventive measure. *Social worker can give psychological support and assist in financial arrangements.* • Refer to psychiatric consultant as necessary. *Most dialysis patients experience some degree of emotional imbalance. With professional psychiatric consultant, most can gradually accept changed self-concept.*	Disturbance in self-concept will be reduced.
Knowledge deficit *Related to:* Lack of interest in learning Unfamiliarity with disease process Information misinterpretation	**ONGOING ASSESSMENT** • Assess patient's understanding of end-stage renal disease. • Observe for dietary deviations and noncompliance when patient is on unit. **THERAPEUTIC INTERVENTIONS** • Instruct patient in methods to relieve dry mouth and maintain fluid restriction: Allow ice chips as needed. *One cup of ice equals only ½ cup of water. Sucking cup of ice takes much longer than drinking cup of water; patient can attain more satisfaction.* Suggest keeping hard candy on hand to alleviate dry mouth *(stimulates secretion of saliva and alleviates some mouth dryness).*	Patient will verbalize an understanding of necessary dietary restrictions.

NURSING DIAGNOSES / DEFINING CHARACTERISTICS	NURSING INTERVENTIONS / *RATIONALES*	EXPECTED OUTCOMES
DEFINING CHARACTERISTICS Verbalization of misconceptions Questioning Noncompliance Signs: fluid volume excess, edema, respiratory signs	Suggest frequent mouth rinses with ½ cup mouthwash mixed with ½ cup ice water. *Rinses can produce freshness in mouth and alleviate thirst temporarily.* • Instruct patient in dietary restrictions. • Use available resources (dietitian, pamphlets, books, dietary list) to aid instruction as necessary. • Involve significant others in instruction sessions on special diets and fluid restrictions. *They may prepare patient's food.* • Instruct patient in recognition of signs of fluid volume excess. *Patient can adjust sodium and water intake independently if they know how to assess for signs of fluid overload.*	

Originated by: Laura Watanabe, RN
      Dadi Ding, RN

Hypocalcemia and bone disease in end-stage renal disease

A syndrome consisting primarily of the effects of secondary hyperparathyroidism.

NURSING DIAGNOSES / DEFINING CHARACTERISTICS	NURSING INTERVENTIONS / *RATIONALES*	EXPECTED OUTCOMES
Altered fluid composition: hypocalcemia *Related to:* Increased phosphorus level Renal failure **DEFINING CHARACTERISTICS** Tingling sensations at the end of fingers Muscle cramps Tetany Convulsion	**ONGOING ASSESSMENT** • Assess for signs/symptoms of hypocalcemia: Tingling sensations at ends of fingers Muscle cramps and carpopedal spasms Tetany Convulsion • Observe for signs/symptoms of calcium-phosphorus imbalance: Pruritus Blurred vision Cardiac arrhythmias • Monitor calcium and phosphorus levels every week/month *to determine whether patient at risk of metastatic calcification from high-calcium and high-phosphate product.* **THERAPEUTIC INTERVENTIONS** • Administer phosphate-binding medications as ordered *so ingested phosphorus will not be absorbed but can bind with medication and be excreted via feces.* • Apply lotion for itchiness; recommend use of scratcher rather than fingernails.	Normal calcium level will be maintained.
Potential bone injury *Related to:* Decreased blood calcium level (demineralization of the bones makes bones brittle, porous, and thinner)	**ONGOING ASSESSMENT** • Assess for signs/symptoms of extreme pain and joint swelling. • Observe patient's gait. • Assess history for tendency to fracture easily. • Observe ambulation and movement of extremities.	Appropriate ambulation and safety measures will be followed.

Continued.

Hypocalcemia and bone disease in end-stage renal disease— cont'd

NURSING DIAGNOSES / DEFINING CHARACTERISTICS	NURSING INTERVENTIONS / *RATIONALES*	EXPECTED OUTCOMES

DEFINING CHARACTERISTICS
Change in bone structure
History of bones breaking easily
Severe pain
	THERAPEUTIC INTERVENTIONS
	• Provide safety measures:
	  Side rails
	  Uncluttered room
	  Orientation to surroundings
	  Proper lighting. *Bones becomes so fragile that they break easily even from mild trauma.*
	• Refer to rehabilitation medicine department as indicated for:
	  Use of crutches
	  Transport from wheelchair to chair or vice versa	

Body image disturbance *Related to:* Stunted growth Disfigured face, body, extremities Waddling gait **DEFINING CHARACTERISTICS** Verbalizes about appearance Verbalizes feeling of isolation Refuses to participate in social activities	**ONGOING ASSESSMENT** • Assess perception of body image. • Assess readiness for help. • Assess coping mechanisms. **THERAPEUTIC INTERVENTIONS** • Establish continuing one-to-one patient-nurse relationship *to promote optimal communication.* • Allow opportunity to verbalize feelings. • Accept patient's feelings. • Encourage patient to maintain ADL. • Include significant others in planning activities. • Use health team members from related disciplines (psychiatric liaison, social worker, etc.) for support.	Improvement in body image will be evidenced.
Knowledge deficit *Related to:* Unfamiliarity with disease process **DEFINING CHARACTERISTICS** Multiple questions Noncompliance with medications and diet	**ONGOING ASSESSMENT** • Assess knowledge of condition, readiness to learn, and ability to learn. • Assess knowledge of medication and diet. **THERAPEUTIC INTERVENTIONS** • Discuss causes and complications of hypocalcemia and bone disease *so patient will have full understanding of consequences of secondary hyperparathyroidism and bone disease.* • Teach patient/significant others to observe for signs/symptoms of hypocalcemia. Provide list of symptoms on discharge. • Discuss importance of taking prescribed medications. • Discuss thoroughly, before discharge, patient's medications, dosages, and side effects. • Explain need for special diet and adherence to it *so patient will understand how medication and diet work together to fight bone disease.* Use resources (list, pamphlet, dietitian) as appropriate. • Encourage significant others to verbalize feelings, insecurities, and other concerns before discharge. • Refer to other health members as indicated.	The patient will verbalize a general understanding of the disease, prevention of complications, dosage, side effects, and contraindications of medications.

Originated by: Ofelia Zafra, RN, BSN

Nephrotic syndrome

(GLOMERULAR NEPHRITIS; NEPHROSIS; RENAL INSUFFICIENCY)

Nephrotic syndrome comprises a group of symptoms (edema, proteinuria, hypoalbuminemia, hyperlipidemia) that result from the dumping of plasma proteins into the urine. This occurs when the glomerular capillary membrane becomes excessively permeable after membrane damage/injury. These symptoms may or may not become chronic, depending upon etiology.

NURSING DIAGNOSES / DEFINING CHARACTERISTICS	NURSING INTERVENTIONS / *RATIONALES*	EXPECTED OUTCOMES
Potential for injury: glomerular capillary membrane *Related to:* Glomerulonephritis (antigen-antibody reaction): Diabetes mellitus Systemic lupus erythematosus Renal vein thrombosis Nephrotoxins Congenital Idiopathic **DEFINING CHARACTERISTICS** Severe proteinuria Hypoalbuminemia Hyperlipidemia Edema	**ONGOING ASSESSMENT** • Obtain historical data (e.g., medications, drug use, recent illness, hereditary illness) that may help identify etiology. • Collect urinary specimens for renal function tests. • Assess lab results: Serum albumin, triglycerides Urinary protein, WBCs, RBCs **THERAPEUTIC INTERVENTIONS** • Administer steroids *(used to treat antigen-antibody and inflammatory reactions and decrease edema and protein loss).* • Prepare for needle biopsy of kidney *(necessary for definitive diagnosis).*	Effects of injury will be reduced.
Fluid volume excess *Related to:* Decreased renal filtering capacity Fluid loss into interstitial spaces **DEFINING CHARACTERISTICS** Total body edema Low BP Puffy eyelids Elevated BUN and creatinine levels Abnormal electrolytes Decreased Hb and Hct	**ONGOING ASSESSMENT** • Monitor temperature, pulse, respirations, and postural BP. • Monitor I & O. • Obtain weight; compare with estimated dry weight. • Check urine specific gravity and dipstick for protein, blood, pH. • Measure abdominal girth every day. • Monitor lab work: Hb Hct Electrolytes BUN/creatinine • Assess for signs of anemia: Stools for blood Pallor • Assess for signs of shock. **THERAPEUTIC INTERVENTIONS.** • Limit IV and PO fluid intake as prescribed. • Administer electrolytes as ordered. • Administer salt-poor albumin and diuretics as ordered. *Albumin causes shift of fluids into vascular system, enhancing diuretic effects.*	Optimal fluid balance will be achieved.
Potential impaired skin integrity *Related to:* Tissue edema	**ONGOING ASSESSMENT** • Assess dependent areas for skin breakdown. • Assess for pitting edema. • Observe open wounds for proper healing.	Optimal skin integrity will be maintained.

Continued.

NURSING DIAGNOSES / DEFINING CHARACTERISTICS	NURSING INTERVENTIONS / *RATIONALES*	EXPECTED OUTCOMES
DEFINING CHARACTERISTICS Poor skin turgor Skin tautness over bony areas Taut, shiny, thin skin at points of edema	**THERAPEUTIC INTERVENTIONS** · Change position frequently. · Use pillows for support when positioning *to relieve pressure areas and prevent tissue breakdown.* · Keep skin clean and dry. · Avoid tight clothing. · Elevate edematous extremities. · Provide pressure-relieving devices *as prophylactic measures.* · Refer to Skin integrity, impaired, p. 48.	

Altered nutrition: less than body requirements
Related to:
Impaired renal function and protein loss
Poor appetite
 	
DEFINING CHARACTERISTICS
Low serum protein
Proteinuria
Muscle wasting
Weight loss
	ONGOING ASSESSMENT
	· Monitor food intake.
	· Monitor proteinuria.
	
	THERAPEUTIC INTERVENTIONS
	· Obtain dietary consult.
	· Administer vitamin supplements.
	· Offer small, frequent meals of preferred foods.
	· Provide diet:
	    High in protein, calories (CHO), and potassium
	    Low in sodium, fat. *Protein is required for tissue growth, carbohydrates for protein sparing and for energy. Potassium is needed because of high loss with interstitial fluid shift and diuresis.*
		Adequate dietary requirements will be maintained.

Potential infection *Related to:* Immunosuppression of steroid therapy **DEFINING CHARACTERISTICS** Elevated temperature Elevated WBC Malaise Signs and symptoms of infection without fever	**ONGOING ASSESSMENT** · Assess for signs of infection. · Assess vital signs, especially temperature. · Observe visitors for obvious symptoms of infection. **THERAPEUTIC INTERVENTIONS** · Screen roommates or consider private room. · Limit visitors and staff contact. Screen visitors for infection. · Report signs of infection immediately *to ensure prompt treatment and prevent exacerbation of renal symptoms.*	Risk of infection will be reduced.

Knowledge deficit
Related to:
New diagnosis
Chronicity of disease
Long-term medical management
 	
DEFINING CHARACTERISTICS
Lack of questions
Excessive anxiety
Inability to talk about present status
	ONGOING ASSESSMENT
	· Assess knowledge base, readiness for learning.
	· Assess support system and ability to provide home/self-care.
	
	THERAPEUTIC INTERVENTIONS
	· Explain nephrotic syndrome, all tests and procedures.
	· Instruct to observe for increased edema by:
	    Daily weights
	    Periorbital edema
	    Abdominal distention
	    Ankle edema
	· Provide instruction:
	    On use of dipsticks for protein
	    On signs of infection
	    On dietary needs/restrictions
	    On medication therapy
	· Schedule follow-up appointments and encourage compliance.
		Patient/family will understand disease process and follow-up care.

Originated by: Kathy Alexander, RN

Peritonitis related to peritoneal dialysis

Inflammation of the peritoneum caused by introduction of bacteria or fungus by contamination (intraluminal), exit site infection (periluminal), fecal leak (transmural), or bacterial seeding of the peritoneum via the blood stream (hematogenous).

NURSING DIAGNOSES / DEFINING CHARACTERISTICS	NURSING INTERVENTIONS / *RATIONALES*	EXPECTED OUTCOMES

Actual infection
 Related to:
 Break in aseptic technique
 GI perforation
 Defective supplies
 	
 DEFINING CHARACTERISTICS
 Fever
 Generalized malaise
 Abdominal pain
 Nausea
 Vomiting
 Diarrhea
 Constipation
 Positive culture
 Elevated peritoneal WBCs
	ONGOING ASSESSMENT
	 • Assess patient for signs/symptoms of infection:
	   Vital signs
	   Abdominal pain
	   Cloudy effluent
	   Drainage at exit site
	 • Palpate abdomen for rebound tenderness and pain along catheter tunnel tract. *Rebound tenderness or pain along tunnel tract indicates inflammation.*
	 • Auscultate abdomen for bowel sounds. *Absent bowel sounds may indicate ileus from bacterial toxins.*
	
	 THERAPEUTIC INTERVENTIONS
	 • Completely drain effluent from peritoneal cavity:
	   Observe effluent for:
	     Cloudiness: *indicates increased WBC, chyle*
	     Volume: *decreased volume noted with increased peritoneal permeability*
	     Fibrin: *increased production noted with peritonitis*
	   Collect effluent for:
	     WBC with differential: *cell count >100 cells/cmm with >50 percent polys indicates peritonitis*
	     Culture/sensitivity with Gram's stain: *indicates need of appropriate antibiotic. Gram's stain may reveal fungus, which takes 5-7 days to grow.*
	 • Send any purulent drainage from exit site for culture and sensitivity.
	 • Change tubing per institutional policy *to assure asepsis of all connections and tubing.*
	 • Assist with peritoneal lavage per doctor's orders *to remove products of inflammation and relieve pain.*
	 • Administer antibiotics intraperitoneally per doctor's orders using shortened dwell periods for first 24 h *(puts medications at source of infection). Shortened dwell periods are used so dialysate reabsorption is decreased.*
	 • If aminoglycosides administered, send blood levels after 48 hrs. *Ototoxicity can occur with prolonged use.*
	 • Add heparin to dialysate, per physican orders, *to decrease fibrin production.*
	 • Perform exit site care per unit protocol.
		Resolution of peritonitis.

Fluid volume excess
 Related to:
 Failure to drain
 Increased peritoneal permeability to glucose, H$_2$O, protein
 	
 DEFINING CHARACTERISTICS
 Acute weight gain
 Elevated BP
 Pulmonary/peripheral edema
 Elevated serum glucose
	ONGOING ASSESSMENT
	 • Assess for fluid overload (see Defining Characteristics).
	 • Obtain history of estimated dry weight BP and dialysate solution used. *Elevated BP and weight gain can be caused by dialysate reabsorption.*
	 • Obtain baseline weight when peritoneal cavity is empty, then every day
	 • Measure inflow/outflow of dialysate with each exchange.
	 • Auscultate breath sounds q8h. *Increased fluid absorption can lead to pulmonary congestion.*
	 • Check for sacral and peripheral edema.
	 • Monitor I/Os every shift.
	 • Monitor:
	   Serum glucose *(glucose absorption may occur with dialysate).*
	   Use of hypertonic dialysate *(May lead to fluid volume deficit if not closely monitored).*
		Fluid volume excess will be reduced.

Continued.

Peritonitis related to peritoneal dialysis— cont'd

NURSING DIAGNOSES / DEFINING CHARACTERISTICS	NURSING INTERVENTIONS / *RATIONALES*	EXPECTED OUTCOMES
	THERAPEUTIC INTERVENTIONS · Administer insulin per physician orders *to control hyperglycemic episodes.* · Obtain dietary consultation *to help monitor protein loss and caloric intake.* · See Peritoneal dialysis, p. 355.	
Noncompliance with aseptic technique *Related to:* Patient value system: health beliefs, cultural influences, spiritual values Client-provider relationships Knowledge **DEFINING CHARACTERISTICS** Direct observation of behavior indicating failure to adhere to techniques Statement by patient/ significant other of failure to adhere to techniques Development of infection Repeated complications or persistence of symptoms	**ONGOING ASSESSMENT** · Determine patient's basic understanding of peritoneal dialysis procedure. · Determine reason for noncompliance to aseptic technique. **THERAPEUTIC INTERVENTIONS** · Have patient demonstrate CAPD procedure *to determine whether further training needed.* · Establish specific goals and objectives for learning, providing positive reinforcement when patient does well. · Provide patient/significant other detailed specific in appropriate techniques for CAPD *to clarify misconceptions* (see Knowledge Deficit). · Provide patient opportunity to verbalize feelings about illness and treatment regimen; refer to social service, psychiatry, or discussion group as needed.	Compliance will be maximized.

Knowledge deficit
Related to:
Unfamiliarity with peritoneal dialysis and its complications
 	
DEFINING CHARACTERISTICS
Verbalizes inaccurate information
Requests information
Acknowledges noncompliance
Expresses frustration/ confusion when performing task
Performs task incorrectly
	ONGOING ASSESSMENT
	· Identify existing misconceptions about peritoneal dialysis.
	· Assess ability to learn.
	· Assess ability to perform tasks.
	
	THERAPEUTIC INTERVENTIONS
	· Provide quiet uninterrupted atmosphere *to facilitate learning experience.*
	· Demonstrate and have patient perform return demonstration:
	  Appropriate handwashing techniques
	  Steps to peritoneal dialysis:
	    Assuring a clean work area
	    Using appropriate supplies
	    Checking dialysate for expiration date, dextrose concentration, correct volume, pinhold leaks, and foreign particles
	    Wearing mask during the procedure
	    Clamping tubing; using sterile technique when spiking or unspiking from dialysate
	· Describe signs/symptoms of infection/peritonitis, including basis of occurrence and when to call physician.
		Patient will become proficient at performing CAPD and able to verbalize signs/ symptoms of infection.

Originated by: Adrian Cooney, RN, BSN

Renal failure, acute

(ACUTE TUBULAR NECROSIS [ATN]; RENAL INSUFFICIENCY)

In acute renal failure, the kidneys are incapable of clearing the blood of the waste products of metabolism. This may occur as a single acute event with return of normal renal function or result in chronic renal insufficiency or chronic renal failure. During the period of loss of renal function, hemodialysis or peritoneal dialysis is used to clear the accumulated toxins from the blood. Renal failure can be divided into three major types: prerenal failure (resulting from a decrease in renal blood flow), postrenal failure (caused by an obstruction), and intrarenal failure (caused by a problem within the vascular system, the glomeruli, the interstitium, or the tubules). Hospital-"acquired" renal failure is most likely acute tubular necrosis (ATN) which results from nephrotoxins or an ischemic episode.

NURSING DIAGNOSES / DEFINING CHARACTERISTICS	NURSING INTERVENTIONS / *RATIONALES*	EXPECTED OUTCOMES

Urinary retention
Related to:
Severe renal ischemia secondary to sepsis, shock, or severe hypovolemia with hypotension (usually after surgery or trauma)
Nephrotoxic drugs or antibiotics such as amphotericin and gentamicin
Renal vascular occlusion
Hemolytic blood transfusion reaction
 	
Defining Characteristics
Increased BUN and creatinine
Urine specific gravity fixed at or near 1.010
Hematuria, proteinuria
Urine output <400 ml/24 hr (in absence of inadequate fluid intake or fluid losses by other route)
	Ongoing Assessment
	• Assess for alteration in urinary elimination.
	• Monitor and record I & O q1h; include all fluid losses (e.g., stool, emesis, and wound drainage).
	• Monitor urine specific gravity; check for protein and blood q4h.
	• Palpate bladder for distention.
	• Assess for patency of Foley catheter (if present).
	• Notify physician of urine output <30 ml/hr.
	• Monitor blood and urine chemistry as ordered:
	  Electrolytes (Na, K, Cl, Ca, P, Mg)
	  BUN, creatinine
	  Urinalysis, urine electrolytes (Notify physician of abnormalities.)
	• Obtain daily weights.
	
	Therapeutic Interventions
	• Administer fluids and diuretics as ordered; document response.
	• Maintain patency of Foley catheter. If urine output decreases, irrigate catheter with sterile saline *to ensure patency.*
	• When administering medications (e.g., antibiotics) metabolized by kidneys, remember that excretion of these drugs may be altered. *Dosages may require adjustment.*
		Optimal urine elimination will be maintained.

Fluid volume excess *Related to:* Inability to excrete fluid and electrolytes properly Excessive administration of oral/IV fluids during periods of decreased renal function	**Ongoing Assessment** • Assess for signs of circulatory overload, congestive heart failure, and pulmonary congestion. • Monitor heart rate, BP, CVP, and respiratory rate q1h. • Monitor and record I & O q1h. Include all stools, emesis, and drainage. • Weigh patient daily (before and after dialysis); record. • Auscultate breath sounds and heart sounds. Notify physician of abnormalities. • Monitor lab work (e.g., serum electrolytes and osmolality) as ordered.	Optimal fluid balance will be maintained.

Continued.

343

Renal failure, acute— cont'd

NURSING DIAGNOSES / DEFINING CHARACTERISTICS	NURSING INTERVENTIONS / *RATIONALES*	EXPECTED OUTCOMES
DEFINING CHARACTERISTICS Increased central venous pressure and BP Acute weight gain, edema Signs/symptoms of congestive heart failure (jugular vein distention, rales) Shortness of breath, dyspnea Pericarditis, friction rub	**THERAPEUTIC INTERVENTIONS** • Administer oral and IV fluids per orders *to replace sensible and insensible losses. Note: Not all patients enter oliguria phase of renal failure. If urine output remains high, volume replacement can be considerable.* • Administer medications (e.g., diuretics) per orders; document response. • Prepare patient for hemodialysis, ultrafiltration, or peritoneal dialysis if indicated *to clear body of excess fluid and waste products. Even when patient reaches diuretic phase of renal failure, dialysis is needed to clear solutes.* • If peripheral edema present, handle extremities/move patient gently *to prevent shearing.*	
Potential decreased cardiac output *Related to:* Arrhythmias caused by electrolyte imbalance from acute renal failure: *Primary hyperkalemia:* Decreased renal elimination of electrolytes: K, P, Mg, Na Metabolic acidosis (present with acute renal failure) exacerbates hyperkalemia by causing cellular shift of H^+ and K^+. Excess H ions traded intracellularly with K ions, causing increased extracellular K^+ *Hyponatremia* results from excessive extracellular fluid (dilutional effect), edema, and restricted IV or dietary intake *Hypocalcemia* can also occur; exact cause unknown	**ONGOING ASSESSMENT** • Assess for signs of decreased cardiac output and electrolyte disturbances. • Monitor vital signs, notify physician of abnormalities. • Monitor serum electrolytes as ordered. • Monitor cardiac rhythm; notify physician of abnormalities. Determine patient's hemodynamic response to arrhythmias. **THERAPEUTIC INTERVENTIONS** • Administer oral and IV fluids as ordered *to maintain optimal fluid balance;* note effects. • Administer medications (e.g., sodium bicarbonate [$NaHCO_3$], calcium salts, glucose/insulin, K^+ exchange resins) per order *to equilibrate electrolyte disturbances temporarily.* Note patient's response. • Maintain hemodynamic parameters (heart rate, BP, CVP, urine output) as indicated. • Administer O_2 as needed. • Provide calm environment with minimal stressors. • Restrict activity *to conserve* O_2. • Prepare patient for dialysis or ultrafiltration when indicated. • See Cardiac output, decreased, p. 9.	Optimal cardiac output will be maintained.
DEFINING CHARACTERISTICS *Decreased cardiac output:* Change in BP, heart rate, CVP, peripheral pulses		

Renal failure, acute— cont'd

NURSING DIAGNOSES / DEFINING CHARACTERISTICS	NURSING INTERVENTIONS / *RATIONALES*	EXPECTED OUTCOMES

Decreased urine output
Abnormal heart sounds
Arrhythmias
Anxiety/restlessness
Hyperkalemia (K > 5.5 mEq/L):
ECG changes:
  Widened QRS segment, increased T waves
  Prolonged PR interval
  Bradycardic arrhythmias, cardiac arrest
Hyponatremia (Na <115 mEq/L):
Nausea/vomiting
Lethargy, weakness
Seizures (with severe deficit)
Hypocalcemia (Ca <6.0 mg/dl):
Perioral paresthesia
Twitching, tetany, seizures
Cardiac arrhythmias		

Ineffective breathing pattern *Related to:* Volume overload leading to congestive heart failure/left ventricular failure Metabolic acidosis (caused by kidney's inability to excrete hydrogen ions properly) leading to hyperventilation as compensatory mechanism **DEFINING CHARACTERISTICS** Shortness of breath Rales, wheezes Dyspnea Hyperventilation Orthopnea	**ONGOING ASSESSMENT** • Assess rate and depth of respiration. • Auscultate breath sounds; document findings. Notify physician of adventitious sounds present. • Monitor ABGs as ordered and as needed; notify physician of abnormal results. • Monitor results of chest radiographs. **THERAPEUTIC INTERVENTIONS** • Encourage pulmonary toilet: turning, coughing, and deep breathing exercises q1h. • Use tracheal suction as needed *to clear airway*. • Maintain head of bed (HOB) at angle at least 30 degrees *to promote lung expansion*. • Administer O_2 as ordered. • Administer medications (e.g., diuretics, bronchodilators) as ordered. • For further interventions/assessment see Airway clearance, ineffective, p. 3; Breathing pattern, ineffective, p. 8.	Effective breathing pattern will be maintained.
Altered nutrition: less than body requirements *Related to:* Stomatitis	**ONGOING ASSESSMENT** • Assess for possible etiology of patient's decreased appetite or GI discomfort. • Assess actual oral intake; obtain calorie counts as necessary. • Monitor serum laboratory values (e.g., electrolytes, albumin level).	Nutritional state will be maximized.

Continued.

NURSING DIAGNOSES / DEFINING CHARACTERISTICS	NURSING INTERVENTIONS / *RATIONALES*	EXPECTED OUTCOMES
Anorexia, decreased appetite Nausea, vomiting Diarrhea Constipation Melena, hematemesis **DEFINING CHARACTERISTICS** Loss of weight Documented inadequate caloric intake Caloric intake inadequate to keep pace with abnormal disease/metabolic state	• Record emesis and stool output. Observe all stools/emesis for gross blood; test for occult blood. Report results to physician. • Assess weight gain pattern. **THERAPEUTIC INTERVENTIONS** • Administer small, frequent feedings as tolerated. • Consult dietitian *to assist in providing patient with a low-potassium, high-carbohydrate diet as indicated.* • Administer enteral/parental feedings as ordered. • Provide frequent oral hygiene *to freshen mouth.* • Offer ice chips/hard candy if not contraindicated. • Offer antiemetics (e.g., diphenhydramine [Benadryl] or dimenhydrinate [Dramamine]) as ordered. • See Nutrition, altered: less than body requirements, p. 37.	

Potential for injury: anemia
Related to:
Bone marrow suppression secondary to insufficient renal production of erythropoietic factor
Increased hemolysis leading to decreased life span of red blood cells secondary to abnormal chemical environment in plasma
Bleeding tendencies:
  Decreased platelets and defective platelet cohesion
  Inhibition of certain clotting factors
 	
DEFINING CHARACTERISTICS
Fatigue
Pallor
Dyspnea
Hct <30 percent
Prolonged PT/PTT
Bleeding tendencies, especially from GI tract
	ONGOING ASSESSMENT
	• Observe, document signs of fatigue, pallor, bleeding from puncture sites and incisions and bruising tendencies.
	• Monitor studies (Hb, Hct, platelets, coagulation studies) as ordered; report results to physician.
	• Check for guaiac in all stools and emesis. Report results to physician.
	• Observe for signs of fluid overload and adverse reactions during transfusion.
	
	THERAPEUTIC INTERVENTIONS
	• Administer O_2 as ordered *to maintain oxygenation.*
	• Administer blood transfusions as ordered.
	• If fluid overload a problem after transfusion, administer diuretics as ordered.
		Occurrence of anemia is reduced.

Actual or potential altered levels of consciousness *Related to:* Accumulation of toxic waste products of metabolism Electrolyte imbalances Hypoxia	**ONGOING ASSESSMENT** • Assess for alteration in level of consciousness (LOC), muscular weakness, and irritability. • Document patient's neurologic status. • Check electrolyte/ABG results for abnormalities *to determine cause of LOC change.*	Optimal state of consciousness will be maintained.

NURSING DIAGNOSES / DEFINING CHARACTERISTICS	NURSING INTERVENTIONS / *RATIONALES*	EXPECTED OUTCOMES
DEFINING CHARACTERISTICS Decreased concentration Apathy Confusion Lethargy leading to coma Neuromuscular irritability Asterixis	**THERAPEUTIC INTERVENTIONS** • Notify physician of LOC changes. • Reorient patient to environment as needed. • Maintain bed in low position with side rails up at all times *for safety.* • Keep call light within easy reach of patient. • Use seizure precautions for patient with decreased LOC; keep side rails padded. • See Consciousness, altered level of, p. 234.	
Potential for systemic or local infection *Related to:* Debilitated state with poor nutrition Poor skin integrity and wound healing Use of indwelling catheters, subclavian lines, Foley catheters, ET tubes, etc. **DEFINING CHARACTERISTICS** Increased temperature Decreased white blood cell count Local inflammation, redness, or abnormal drainage Positive culture results (blood, wound, sputum, or urine)	**ONGOING ASSESSMENT** • Assess for potential sites of infection: urinary, pulmonary, wound, or IV line. • Monitor temperature q4h; notify physician of temperature >38 °C. • Monitor WBC count. • Note signs of localized or systemic infection; report promptly. • If infection suspected, obtain specimens of blood, urine, sputum, etc., for culture and sensitivity as ordered. **THERAPEUTIC INTERVENTIONS** • Provide scrupulous perineal and catheter care. • Provide meticulous skin care *to prevent skin breakdown over pressure areas.* • Use aseptic technique during dressing changes, wound irrigations, catheter care, and suctioning. • Avoid use of indwelling catheters or IV lines whenever possible. • If indwelling catheters or IV lines mandatory, change them per unit/hospital policy. • Protect patient from exposure to other infected patients. • If infection present, administer antibiotics as ordered.	Potential for systemic/local infection will be reduced.
Knowledge deficit *Related to:* New condition New procedures **DEFINING CHARACTERISTICS** Verbalized confusion about treatment Lack of questions Request for information	**ONGOING ASSESSMENT** • Assess patient's/significant others' current knowledge, understanding of illness. **THERAPEUTIC INTERVENTIONS** • Encourage expression of feelings and questioning. • Discuss need for monitoring equipment and frequent assessment. • Explain all tests and procedures *before* they occur. Use terms the patient can understand; be clear and direct. • Explain purpose of fluid and dietary restrictions. • Explain need for dialysis and what to expect during procedure. • Instruct the patient to perform deep breathing and coughing exercises *to promote lung expansion and clearing.* • Involve the patient's family in care as much as possible (when appropriate). • Encourage family conferences with members of patient's health care team (e.g., physician, nurses, rehabilitation personnel, social workers) as necessary. *This will facilitate family involvement in multidisciplinary planning.* • Consult appropriate resource persons (e.g., rehabilitation personnel, physicians, social workers, psychologists, clergy, occupational therapists, and clinical specialists) as needed.	Patient/significant others will verbalize understanding of disease process and associated treatments.

Originated by: Deborah Lazzara, RN, MSN, CCRN
Susan Galanes, RN, MS, CCRN

Catheter for hemodialysis (subclavian, intrajugular, femoral)

Hemodialysis is a process of cleansing the blood of accumulated waste products. It is used for acutely ill patients who require short-term dialysis and for patients with end-stage renal failure. A rigid or semi-rigid catheter is inserted into the subclavian, intrajugular, or femoral vein. Sterile procedure is used and local anesthetic is injected subcutaneously. The catheter is inserted and sutured into place. This catheter may be either single- or double-lumen. A single-lumen catheter serves as the arterial source, and the venous return is made via a peripheral vein or by the use of an alternating flow device. A double-lumen catheter is used for both the arterial source and the venous return. Femoral catheters are used only with inpatients on a short-term basis, because of their location and low durability. The subclavian or intrajugular catheters can be used for weeks or even months on an outpatient basis.

NURSING DIAGNOSES / DEFINING CHARACTERISTICS	NURSING INTERVENTIONS / *RATIONALES*	EXPECTED OUTCOMES

Potential for infection
Related to:
Hemodialysis catheter
 	
DEFINING CHARACTERISTICS
Pain around the catheter site
Fever
Red, swollen, warm area around catheter exit site
Drainage from catheter exit site
	ONGOING ASSESSMENT
	• Assess hemodialysis catheter site for signs and symptoms of infection.
	• Obtain blood and catheter exit site culture if evidence of infection.
	• Visually inspect and palpate the areas around and over intact dressing each shift for phlebitis, tenderness, inflammation, and infiltration.
	
	THERAPEUTIC INRTERVENTION
	Subclavian and intrajugular catheters
	• Maintain asepsis with the subclavian/intrajugular catheters during dialysis:
	  Clean area with antiseptic. *Povidone-iodine (Betadine) solution is recommended.*
	  Change sterile dressing over catheter exit site before each dialysis treatment.
	  Use sterile technique when initiating or discontinuing dialysis.
	  Instill heparin into catheter and secure placement of catheter and caps after diaylsis.
	  Do not use catheter for any purpose but hemodialysis.
	• Explain to patient/significant others importance of maintaining asepsis with catheter. *Because of its location and long-term use, infection is almost inevitable. Infection may be localized at exit site, but septicemia can occur.*
	• *Instruct patient/significant others to keep the dressing clean and dry at all times. Meticulous care of catheter site and maintenance of dry intact dressing lessen infection risk.*
	  Protect catheter dressing during bathing.
	  Advise against swimming.
	  If dressing loosens, reinforce with tape.
	  If dressing comes off or becomes *wet,* go to dialysis unit as soon as possible for sterile catheter site care if incapable of performing at home.
	Femoral catheters:
	• Maintain asepsis with femoral catheter during dialysis:
	  Use sterile technique when initiating or discontinuing dialysis.
	  Instill heparin into catheter, secure placement of catheter end caps after dialysis.
	  If intravenous line cannot be started in peripheral vessel, femoral catheter may be used with extreme caution.
	• Maintain femoral catheter:
	  Change *all* dressings q48h or more often if soiled.
	  Notify physician if infection suspected.
	  Anticipate need to change femoral catheter q48-72h *to lessen infection risk.*
	  Maintain strict bed rest if patient has femoral catheter, *with cannulated leg flat to prevent kinking of intravenous catheter.*
		Potential for infection will be reduced.

Catheter for hemodialysis: subclavian, intrajugular, femoral— cont'd

NURSING DIAGNOSES / DEFINING CHARACTERISTICS	NURSING INTERVENTIONS / *RATIONALES*	EXPECTED OUTCOMES

Knowledge deficit
Related to:
Unfamiliarity with catheter insertion and maintenance
 	
DEFINING CHARACTERISTICS
Questions
Confusion about treatment
Inability to comply with treatment
Lack of questions
	ONGOING ASSESSMENT
	• Determine patient's/significant others' understanding of disease process, complications, and treatment.
	
	THERAPEUTIC INTERVENTIONS
	• Encourage patient/significant others to ask questions.
	• Instruct patient/significant others to inform physician or call dialysis unit *immediately* of signs/symptoms of infection:
	    Pain around catheter site
	    Fever
	    Wet dressing caused by blood or drainage (*Information given to patient/significant others on condition will increase patient's awareness and decrease anxiety about activities of daily living with renal failure.*)
	• Instruct patient/significant others if dressing comes off or becomes *wet* to go to dialysis unit as soon as possible for sterile catheter site care and to notify physician and/or dialysis staff.
		Patient/significant others will be able to verbalize concerns about intravenous catheter access, recognize signs and symptoms of infection, know how to notify the physician/dialysis staff if infection is suspected.

Originated by: Susan Pische, RN, BSN, MBA

External arteriovenous shunt for hemodialysis

(AV SHUNT)

Hemodialysis is a process of cleaning the blood of accumulated waste products. It is used for acutely ill patients who require short-term dialysis and for patients with end-stage renal failure. The objective of hemodialysis is to extract toxic nitrogenous substance from the blood and remove excess water. Access into the circulating blood flow is a requirement. The shunt is made surgically by using two rigid Teflon tips: one implanted into an artery and one into a vein. Silastic tubing is attached to the Teflon vessel tip and brought to the outside through puncture wounds in the skin. The Silastic tubes are connected to allow uninterrupted blood flow. Placement site depends on the availability of undamaged vessels of the proper size. The nondominant upper extremity (upper arm or forearm) is the preferred site, although shunts may be placed in the lower extremities: thigh or ankle. An external shunt is indicated (1) when immediate access to the circulation is needed in patients with acute renal failure and (2) while waiting for the A-V fistula or graft to mature. External shunts are not frequently used for acute renal failure or new end-stage renal failure patients because of the perfection of the subclavian catheter access.

NURSING DIAGNOSES / DEFINING CHARACTERISTICS	NURSING INTERVENTIONS / *RATIONALES*	EXPECTED OUTCOMES

Potential for infection
Related to:
Postoperative A-V shunt access
	ONGOING ASSESSMENT
	• Assess A-V shunt for signs/symptoms of infection.
	
	THERAPEUTIC INTERVENTION
	• Maintain asepsis with the A-V shunt during dialysis:
	    Clean area with antiseptics; povidone-iodine (Betadine) solution is recommended.
	    Apply providone-iodine ointment to exit site.
		Potential for infection will be reduced.

Continued.

External arteriovenous shunt for hemodialysis— cont'd

NURSING DIAGNOSES / DEFINING CHARACTERISTICS	NURSING INTERVENTIONS / *RATIONALES*	EXPECTED OUTCOMES
DEFINING CHARACTERISTICS Pain over access site Fever Red, swollen, warm area around site Drainage from access site	Dress arm/limb with sterile gauze; wrap with Kerlix dressing. Obtain specimen for culture if infection suspected. • Explain to patient/significant others importance of maintaining asepsis with A-V shunt: *infection almost inevitable complication of external shunt. Infection may be localized cellulitis, but septicemia can occur. Meticulous daily care and prevention of trauma to shunt lower infection risk.* • Instruct patient/significant others to keep dressing clean and dry: Protect shunt dressing while bathing. No swimming.	
Potential altered peripheral tissue perfusion *Related to:* Interruption in arteriovenous (A-V) shunt blood flow **DEFINING CHARACTERISTICS** Pain over access area Absence of pulse above venous site Absence of thrill over shunt area Absence of bruit over arterial site Decreased temperature of affected limb	**ONGOING ASSESSMENT** • Assess A-V shunt for signs/symptoms of inadequate blood flow. **THERAPEUTIC INTERVENTIONS** • Check for adequate blood flow: Palpate for pulse and thrill. Auscultate for bruit; "swishing" sound should be audible. *When artery is connected to vein, blood is "shunted" from artery into vein, causing turbulence. This may be palpated above venous side of shunt for "thrill" or buzzing.* • Promote following preventive measures to ensure adequate blood flow: Do not take blood pressure in cannulated limb. Do not draw blood specimens from cannulated limb. • Instruct patient/significant others to *avoid:* Sleeping on shunt limb Wearing tight clothing over limb with shunt Carrying handbags or packages over shunt arm Activities or sports that involve active use of cannulated limb *Thrombosis is common complication of external shunt, caused by thrombi (caused by venipunture), extrinsic pressure (by BP cuff, tourniquet, sleeping on limb or tight clothes), or cannula tip malalignment within vessel (caused by activities or sports that involve active use of cannulated limb).* • Maintain proper positioning of cannulated limb: it must be elevated *to reduce dependent edema.* If shunt placed in arm, use arm sling for support when patient is ambulatory/discharged home.	Patency of A-V shunt will be maintained.
Knowledge deficit *Related to:* Unfamiliarity with disease process and new procedure **DEFINING CHARACTERISTICS** Questions Confusion about treatment Inability to comply with treatment regimen Lack of questions	**ONGOING ASSESSMENT** • Determine patient's/significant others' understanding of disease process, complications, and treatment regimen. **THERAPEUTIC INTERVENTION** • Encourage patient/significant others to ask questions. • Teach patient/significant others to check for adequate blood flow: Arrange teaching sessions when participants are ready. Demonstrate how to feel for pulses and thrill. Designate specific areas to feel for pulses and thrill. Allow adequate time for return demonstration. • Instruct patient/significant others to inform physician or call dialysis unit *immediately* for any signs/symptoms of infection: Pain over access site Fever Red, swollen, warm access site Drainage from access • Teach patient/significant others how to manage accidental separation or dislodgment of shunt connections. *Information given to patient/significant others about medical condition and proper care of external shunt will increase patient's awareness of condition and decrease anxiety about living with renal failure.*	Patient/significant others will know how to check for adequate blood flow through shunt, when to call physician or dialysis unit, and how to manage accidental separation of shunt connections.

Originated by: Ofelia Mallari, RN
Susan Pische, RN, BSN, MBA

Internal arteriovenous fistula for hemodialysis

(AV FISTULA)

Hemodialysis is a process of cleansing the blood of accumulated waste products. It is used for acutely ill patients who require short-term dialysis and for patients with end-stage renal failure. The objective of hemodialysis is to extract toxic nitrogenous substance from the blood and remove excess water. Access into the circulating blood is required. Since hemodialysis requires a rapid blood flow rate, the patient's artery is chosen because of its capacity to deliver adequate blood flow. The fistula is made surgically by creating an anastomosis between an artery and a vein, thus allowing arterial blood to flow through the vein, causing engorgement and enlargement. Placement may be in either forearm, using the radial artery and cephalic vein or branchial artery and cephalic vein. The patient's own vessels are preferable to synthetic devices since they have lower clotting occurrences and infection rates than those of external A-V shunts.

NURSING DIAGNOSES / DEFINING CHARACTERISTICS	NURSING INTERVENTIONS / *RATIONALES*	EXPECTED OUTCOMES
Potential altered peripheral tissue perfusion *Related to:* Postoperative care of A-V fistula: Access creation Access revision **DEFINING CHARACTERISTICS** Absence of "bruit" over arterial site Decreased temperature of affected limb Cyanotic fingers with serosanguinous fluid around nail beds	**ONGOING ASSESSMENT** • Assess A-V fistula for signs/symptoms of inadequate blood flow. **THERAPEUTIC INTERVENTIONS** *First 24 hr:* • Note and mark drainage on outer bandage; reinforce dressing if necessary. • Observe and note edema to postoperative arm. Elevate on pillows or suspend arm from IV pole with stockinette. • Keep ace bandage in place for first 24 hr after surgery *to reduce bleeding and edema.* • Observe and note temprature, color, and sensation to fingers. • Notify surgeon if bleeding saturates bandage or if distal part of extremity becomes cyanotic. *24 hr to 10 days after surgery:* • Check for adequate blood flow: Palpate for thrill. Auscultate for bruit; "swishing" sound should be audible even through dressings. *When artery is connected to vein, blood is "shunted" from artery into vein, causing turbulence, which may be palpated at anastomosis as thrill or "buzzing".* • Observe for generalized edema: edematous, cyanotic fingers and serosanguineous fluid around nail beds. *To increase circulation:* Wrap arm in ace bandage when patient awake; start at fingers, end above operative area. Elevate arm on pillows or suspend on IV pole. When discharged, patient may wear arm in sling and position fingertips toward shoulder. *Wrapping with Ace bandage and elevating operative limb will help reduce dependent edema and promote circulation.* • Promote preventive measures *to ensure adequate blood flow:* Do not take blood pressure on cannulated limb. Do not draw blood specimens from cannulated limb. *Thrombosis of A-V fistula may result from: Extrinsic pressure, as from tight bandage Recent thrombi caused by venipuncture Hypovolemia or marked hypotension* • Recognize early signs of thrombosis, notify surgeon as soon as possible if they occur: Absence of bruit or thrill Poor or *no* blood flow from fistula. *Thrombosis is complication of A-V fistula. Diagnosis made by fistulogram. Treatment is surgical declotting or creation of other access. Declotting is more successful when procedure performed early.*	Potential for altered tissue perfusion will be reduced.

Continued.

Internal arteriovenous fistula for hemodialysis— cont'd

NURSING DIAGNOSES / DEFINING CHARACTERISTICS	NURSING INTERVENTIONS / *RATIONALES*	EXPECTED OUTCOMES
Potential for infection *Related to:* Care of A-V fistula after surgery: 24 hr through 10 days **DEFINING CHARACTERISTICS** Pain over access site Fever Red, swollen, warm area around site Drainage from access, suture line	**ONGOING ASSESSMENT** • Assess A-V fistula for signs/symptoms of infection: 　Red, swollen, warm area around access site 　Drainage from suture sites 　Edematous, cyanotic fingers and oozing of serosanguiness fluid around nail beds 　Extreme sensitivity to touch at access site **THERAPEUTIC INTERVENTIONS** • Obtain specimen for wound culture when infection suspected. • Notify surgeon *immediately* if infection suspected. • Cleanse area daily with antiseptic: povidone-iodine (Betadine) solution. *Daily cleansing of access will reduce potential of infection.* Dress limb with sterile gauze; wrap with Kerlix dressing.	Potential for infection will be reduced.
Knowledge deficit *Related to:* Unfamiliarity with disease process and new procedure **DEFINING CHARACTERISTICS** Questions Confusion about treatment Inability to comply with treatment Lack of questions	**ONGOING ASSESSMENT** • Determine patient's/significant others' understanding of disease process, complications, and treatment. **THERAPEUTIC INTERVENTIONS** • Encourage patient/significant others to ask questions. • Arrange teaching session when participants are ready. • Teach patient/significant others to check for adequate blood flow: 　Demonstrate how to feel for pulses and thrill. 　Designate specific areas to feel for pulses and thrill. 　Allow adequate time for return demonstration. • Instruct patient/significant others to inform physician or call dialysis unit *immediately* of signs of infection: 　Pain over access site 　Fever 　Red, swollen, warm access site 　Drainage from access site. *Information given to patient/significant others about medical condition and proper care of A-V fistula will increase patient's awareness of condition, also will help decrease anxiety about ADL with renal failure.* • Inform patient that A-V fistula maturation may be hastened by exercising: 　Resistance exercise may begin 10-14 days after surgery. 　Apply light tourniquet to upper arm to impede venous flow and distend forearm vessels; use care not to occlude blood flow with tourniquet; apply tightly enough to distend vessels. Instruct patient to open and close fist to pump arterial blood against venous resistance caused by tourniquet. Patient's squeezing rubber ball, tennis ball, hand grips, or rolled up pair of socks will help exert pressure. 　Repeat exercises for 5-10 min, 4-5 times/day. Patient may do exercises while watching TV. *Resistance exercises cause vessels to stretch and engorge with blood.*	Patient/signifciant others will be able to check for adequate blood flow by palpating for bruit and will recognize signs/symptoms of infection.

Originated by: Susan Pische, RN, BSN, MBA

Nephrostomy tube, percutaneous

(PYELOSTOMY TUBE)

A percutaneous nephrostomy tube is a rigid tube passed under fluoroscopic control through the skin and into the renal pelvis for drainage, for patients with an obstruction above the bladder, or with strictured or non-functional ureters.

NURSING DIAGNOSES / DEFINING CHARACTERISTICS	NURSING INTERVENTIONS / *RATIONALES*	EXPECTED OUTCOMES

Urinary retention
Related to:
Nephrostomy tube(s):
  Dislodgement
  Kinking
  Obstruction from sedimentation
 	
DEFINING CHARACTERISTICS
Decrease in urinary output
Increase in urine sediment
Kink in urine drainage tubing
	ONGOING ASSESSMENT
	• Monitor I & O.
	• Assess nephrostomy tube(s) patency, stability.
	
	THERPAUETIC INTERVENTIONS
	• Stabilize nephrostomy tubes according to policy *to prevent dislodgment.*
	• Encourage patient to drink water; 8-10 glasses/day, *to prevent stagnation and sedimentation formation.*
	• Position patient in bed so tubing is not kinked.
	• Gently roll tubing between fingers *to dislodge particles adherent to inner lumen.*
	• Use aseptic technique to irrigate nephrostomy tube as ordered.
		Adequate urinary elimination via nephrostomy tube(s) will be maintained.

Potential for infection *Related to:* Direct percutaneous opening to renal pelvis Long-term use of collection devices Alkaline urine **DEFINING CHARACTERISTICS** Cloudy, foul-smelling urine Fever Elevated WBC Percutaneous site drainage Positive urine cultures Urine pH > 6.0	**ONGOING ASSESSMENT** • Assess urine amount, color, clarity, odor. • Monitor vital signs, especially temperature. • Monitor WBC. • Assess nature of drainage on percutaneous site dressing(s). • Monitor urine cultures, pH. **THERAPEUTIC INTERVENTIONS** • Using aseptic technique, clean percutaneous site, dress with occlusive bandage *to exclude environmental pathogens and enable patient to shower/bathe.* • Clean or replace collection system and/or leg bag daily. • Administer antibiotics and antipyretics as ordered. • Encourage intake of cranberry juice (at least 3 glasses/day) *to maintain acidic urine. Cranberry juice yields hippicuric acid as it metabolizes; acidic urine is infected less often than alkaline urine.*	Risk of infection is reduced.

Potential altered skin integrity
Related to:
Drainage at percutaneous exit site(s)
Accumulation of moisture, perspiration beneath occlusive dressing(s)
Mechanical irritation related to inadvertent movement of tube(s)
 	
DEFINING CHARACTERISTICS
Redness at percutaneous exit site(s)
	ONGOING ASSESSMENT
	• Assess percutaneous exit site(s) for:
	  Redness
	  Excoriation
	• Ask patient whether area itches or burns.
	
	THERAPEUTIC INTERVENTION
	• Stabilizes tubes *to minimize inadvertent movement.*
	• Change dressing if moist.
	• Consider use of liquid skin barrier film.
	• See Skin integrity, impaired, p. 48.
		Percutaneous skin will remain intact.

Continued.

NURSING DIAGNOSES / DEFINING CHARACTERISTICS	NURSING INTERVENTIONS / *RATIONALES*	EXPECTED OUTCOMES
Excoriation around exit site(s) Itching, burning at exit site(s)		
Potential fluid volume deficit *Related to:* Hemorrhage from renal pelvis **DEFINING CHARACTERISTICS** Hematuria Decreased blood pressure Increased heart rate	**ONGOING ASSESSMENT** • Assess for hematuria visually or with dipstick. • Monitor vital signs. **THERAPEUTIC INTERVENTIONS** • Notify physician if hematuria present. • Administer IV fluids as ordered. • Prepare patient for return to surgery/x-ray department. • See Fluid volume deficit, p. 20.	Normal fluid volume will be maintained.

Knowledge deficit
Related to:
Lack of experience with percutaneous nephrostomy tube(s)
 	
DEFINING CHARACTERISTICS
Multiple questions
Lack of questions
Demonstrated inability to provide self-care
	ONGOING ASSESSMENT
	• Assess readiness for learning.
	• Assess ability to reach tube(s) site(s). *Many patients unable to reach or visualize flank sites.*
	
	THERAPEUTIC INTERVENTIONS
	• Teach patient/significant other:
	  Need for keeping sterile occlusive dressing in place
	  Need for changing wet or soiled dressing
	  Importance of maintaining high fluid intake and drinking cranberry juice *to maintain acidic urine.*
	  Importance of seeking health care for:
	    Blood in urine
	    Cloudy, foul-smelling urine
	    Decrease in urine output from nephrostomy tube(s)
	    Fever
	    Pain
	    Drainage at percutaneous site(s)
	• Document teaching and patient response.
		Patient/significant other demonstrates and verbalizes appropriate percutaneous nephrostomy tube(s) and site(s) care.

Originated by: Lacy Roach, RN

Peritoneal dialysis

[CONTINUOUS AMBULATORY PERITONEAL DIALYSIS [CAPD])

The diffusion of solute molecules, usually uremic toxins, and fluids across a semipermeable membrane. During dialysis, the peritoneum functions as the membrane by which molecules flow from the side of high concentration to the side of lower concentration. This procedure removes excess fluid and waste products from the blood during renal failure. Hemodialysis, peritoneal dialysis, or transplantation are necessary to maintain life in patients with no kidney function.

NURSING DIAGNOSES / DEFINING CHARACTERISTICS	NURSING INTERVENTIONS / *RATIONALE*	EXPECTED OUTCOMES
Fluid volume excess *Related to:* Renal insufficiency Malfunctioning peritoneal dialysis **DEFINING CHARACTERISTICS** Abdominal pain Complaints of fullness Shortness of breath Nausea Decreased urinary output Increased abdominal girth Weight gain	**ONGOING ASSESSMENT** • Obtain baseline vital signs and dry weight. • Monitor patient's BP q4h during dialysis. • Record fluid I & O. • Weigh patient bid (once before dialysis begins). • Measure abdominal girth daily at end of drain time. • Monitor patient for tachypnea, retractions, nasal flaring. • Auscultate breath sounds q4h. • Monitor patient's electrolytes, especially K^+. • Observe for nausea, vomiting, edema, or disorientation. • Monitor each exchange, checking that outflow is equal to or greater than inflow *as dialysis treatments can eliminate or markedly decrease end-stage renal disease manifestations.* • Check catheter for kinks. • Check catheter for fibrin or clots. • Assure proper functioning if using automatic cycler. **THERAPEUTIC INTERVENTIONS** • Change position at least q2h *to maximize drainage.* Put HOB at 45 degrees; turn patient on side. • Discontinue dialysis if signs of hypokalemia present. • Notify physician and change dialysate concentration when patient reaches dry weight *so as not to dehydrate patient by removing too much fluid.* • Stop dialysis if drainage inadequate. *Overinfusion causes pain, dyspnea, nausea, and electrolyte imbalance.*	Fluid volume will be maintained in normal range.
Potential for infection *Related to:* Contamination of peritoneal catether entry site **DEFINING CHARACTERISTICS** Complaints of abdominal pain, tenderness, warm feeling, chills Rigid abdominal wall Pericatheter site reddened with discharge Fever Cloudy returned dialysate Positive culture and sensitivity	**ONGOING ASSESSMENT** • Assess peritoneal drainage with each exchange (normal is clear). • Assess area around catheter site; should be clean with no signs of inflammation. • Assess patient for complaint of abdominal tenderness. • Assess vital signs q4h unless patient febrile, then q2h. • Ask patient to describe how he/she feels during exchanges. *Early detection and treatment of infection minimize complications of infection.* **THERAPEUTIC INTERVENTION** • Use strict aseptic technique when setting up dialysis and hooking up patient *(poor hygiene and improper technique during hook-up can lead to catheter site infection, the most common complication of peritoneal dialysis).* • Maintain drainage receptacle below level of peritoneum to prevent backflow of dialysate. • Maintain closed system whenever possible. • Notify physician of any signs of infection. • See Peritonitis related to peritoneal dialysis, p. 341.	Potential for infection will be reduced.
Pain *Related to:* Length of procedure	**ONGOING ASSESSMENT** • Assess patient continually for signs of discomfort. • See Pain, p. 39.	Pain relief will be maximized.

Continued.

NURSING DIAGNOSES / DEFINING CHARACTERISTICS	NURSING INTERVENTIONS / *RATIONALES*	EXPECTED OUTCOMES
Actual infusing of dialysate Distended abdomen **DEFINING CHARACTERISTICS** Complaints of abdominal pain during procedure Tossing about in bed Complaints of feeling full Crying Restlessness and irritability	**THERAPEUTIC INTERVENTIONS** ▪ Remain at bedside during initiation of dialysis. ▪ Allow/encourage family involvement during dialysis *to provide comfort.* ▪ Change patient position *to relieve discomfort during inflow.* ▪ Allow patient to ambulate if permitted. ▪ Provide diversional activities *to divert attention from procedure.* ▪ Refer to Diversional activity deficit, p. 17.	
Knowledge deficit *Related to:* New procedure **DEFINING CHARACTERISTICS** Anxiousness Restlessness Withdrawal Regression Frequent questions Frequent complaints Vague physical complaints	**ONGOING ASSESSMENT** ▪ Assess knowledge level. ▪ Assess ability to learn. ▪ Assess family interactions. **THERAPEUTIC INTERVENTIONS** ▪ Review patient diagnosis. ▪ Review peritoneal dialysis and rationale. ▪ Discuss dietary/fluid requirements and restrictions: low sodium, low potassium, adequate protein, high calories, free fluids. ▪ Arrange dietary consultation if necessary. ▪ Discuss medications and use. ▪ Demonstrate and request return demonstration of peritoneal catheter care. ▪ Discuss return appointments, follow-up care, emergency numbers. ▪ Arrange social service consultation if necessary. ▪ If dialysis long-term, consider referral to CAPD nurse.	Patient/significant other will be able to verbalize/demonstrate appropriate home care measures.

Originated by: Agnes Jones-Perry, RN

Renal transplant, postoperative

(KIDNEY TRANSPLANT)

Renal transplantation is the surgical implantation of a renal allograft from either a cadaver or live donor into a patient with end-stage renal failure. Most frequently transplant candidates are on chronic hemodialysis or peritoneal dialysis, exhibiting symptoms of azotemia, anemia, fluid overload, and oliguria. After a successful operative course, the renal transplant recipient recovers in the intensive care unit or stepdown unit, where fluid shifts and vital signs are monitored.

NURSING DIAGNOSES / DEFINING CHARACTERISTICS	NURSING INTERVENTIONS / *RATIONALES*	EXPECTED OUTCOMES
Potenial fluid volume deficit/excess *Related to:* Variable time for initial renal function: Immediately after renal transplantation patient may vacillate between fluid depletion and fluid overload Prolonged transport time causing ATN: patients may experience diuresis several days postoperatively **DEFINING CHARACTERISTICS** *Deficit:* Polyuria Weight loss Dry mucous membranes Weakness Thirst *Excess:* Edema Weight gain Shortness of breath, orthopnea Intake greater than output Abnormal breath sounds: rales (crackles)	**ONGOING ASSESSMENT** • Weigh daily. Use same scale *to prevent discrepancies in measuring device.* • Monitor I & O hourly in the ICU and q4h on general unit. • Note and document presence of peripheral or sacral edema. • Auscultate lungs q4h to assess for rales (crakles). • Assess skin turgor and hydration of mucous membranes. **THERAPEUTIC INTERVENTIONS** • Replace fluids cc per cc plus 30 cc/hr *to account for insensible loss or according to unit protocol (may vary among institutions). Acute tubular necrosis (ATN) patients may have diuresis several days after surgery, exceeding 200-400 cc/hr. Living-related transplant recipients have greater urine volumes in early postoperative period (may exceed 400-600 cc/hr). Fluid replacement must match output so patient does not dehydrate.* • Notify physician if urine output <30 cc/hr. • Administer diuretics and restrict fluids as indicated. • Encourage deep breathing, coughing, and turning *to prevent associated respiratory complications.* • Begin progressive ambulation *to facilitate adequate tissue perfusion to edematous body areas.*	Optimal fluid status will be maintained.
Potential urinary retention *Related to:* Obstructed Foley catheter **DEFINING CHARACTERISTICS** Bladder distention Small, frequent voiding	**ONGOING ASSESSMENT** • Obtain preoperative history of patient's pattern of urinating. *If patient was oliguric, urinary bladder may be atrophied and/or reduced in size.* • Assess urine for color, amount, sediment, and presence of clots. *Depending on volume of urine, bladder capacity, muscle tone, and degree of hematuria, indwelling catheter will remain in place 2-7 days.* • Assess for abdominal/bladder distention resulting from clotted Foley catheter or anastamosis leak. • Record accurate I & O (q1h in ICU or q4h on general unit). • After discontinuing Foley catheter, assess color, clarity, sediment, and blood in voided urine.	Urinary retention is prevented.

Continued.

Renal transplant, postoperative— cont'd

NURSING DIAGNOSES / DEFINING CHARACTERISTICS	NURSING INTERVENTIONS / *RATIONALES*	EXPECTED OUTCOMES
Absence of urine output Sensation of bladder fullness Dysuria	**THERAPEUTIC INTERVENTIONS** • Maintain Foley catheter drainage, preventing kinks which would *obstruct flow*. • If gross hematuria evident, strain urine for clots. Irrigate Foley catheter with physician approval. *Bleeding from anastomosis can cause clotted catheter.* • After discontinuing Foley catheter, ask patient to void q1-2h *to prevent urinary retention and urinary bladder overdistention. If bladder capacity significantly compromised, patient will need to empty bladder more often. Full bladder causes additional strain on ureteral anastomosis.* • Instruct patient to record daily urine output and notify transplant physician if output decreases or color, clarity, or consistency changes.	
Potential for local/ systemic infection *Related to:* Immunosuppression with antirejection medications (*decrease circulating lymphocytes and the ability to fight infectious organsism*) **DEFINING CHARACTERISTICS** Fever Wound infection Upper respiratory infection Positive cultures	**ONGOING ASSESSMENT** • Monitor temperature 1-3 times/day. • Inspect wound twice daily for local erythema, purulent drainage, or dehiscence; notify transplant physician if they occur. • Culture wound for aerobic organisms if drainage purulent, green, or foul-smelling. • Culture urine if patient febrile, dysuric or if urine turns cloudy. • Monitor all culture reports. **THERAPEUTIC INTERVENTIONS** • Wash hands before and after touching patient. *Bacteria, viruses, fungi, and protozoa indigenous in nontransplant populations may be infectious in immunosuppressed transplant patient. Patients do not require isolation, but private room recommended. Restrict visitors and flowers at transplant team's discretion.* • Administer antibiotics as ordered. • Teach patient/signifciant other about avoidance of infectious crowds, importance of good hygiene, signs/symptoms of infection. *Patient must understand increased infection risk and importance of calling transplant physician for signs of infection.*	Potential for infection will be reduced.
Pain *Related to:* Incisional pain Ineffective analgesia Pain exacerbated by straining and early ambulation **DEFINING CHARACTERISTICS** Facial mask of pain Crying/moaning Complaints of pain Guarding behavior Diaphoresis BP and pulse rate change Respiratory rate change	**ONGOING ASSESSMENT** • Assess for verbal and nonverbal pain symptoms. • Observe and record vital sign changes indicating increased pain. • Assess prescribed analgesia's effectiveness. **THERAPEUTIC INTERVENTIONS** • Reinforce relaxation techniques and position changes *to alleviate incisional or muscular pain, thereby reducing need for narcotic analgesia.* • Encourage patient to splint abdominal incision *to reduce pain.* • Titrate prescribed analgesia as needed. • Premedicate patient 20 min before ambulating, performing ADLs, or having large dressing changes *to minimize movement-induced pain.* • Assist with ambulation and ADLs until patient can resume self-care.	Pain will be reduced.
Anxiety/fear *Related to:* Change in health status: No longer on dialysis	**ONGOING ASSESSMENT** • Assessfor signs of anxiety/fear. • Assess patient's/family's dependent/independent behaviors. • Assess available support systems. • Assess functional coping mechanisms. • Assess patient's ability to accept self-care responsibility.	Anxiety/fear will be reduced.

NURSING DIAGNOSES / DEFINING CHARACTERISTICS	NURSING INTERVENTIONS / *RATIONALES*	EXPECTED OUTCOMES
Threat of rejection or infection Change in role functioning **DEFINING CHARACTERISTICS** Apprehension Feelings of inadequacy Facial tension Restlessness Fear Worry	**THERAPEUTIC INTERVENTIONS** • Allow patient time to ventilate fears and anxiety. *After surgery, transplant patient must maintain health and cannot rely on dialysis staff. Independence often frightening, especially with potential for rejection or infection.* • Assist with identifying available support systems. • Offer emotional support, consult social service staff if indicated. • Set limits for regressive and aggressive behavior.	

Knowledge deficit:
Related to:
New condition
 	
DEFINING CHARACTERISTICS
Verbalized confusion about treatment
Lack of questions
Request for information
	ONGOING ASSESSMENT
	• Assess patient's/family's readiness to discuss transplant surgery, postoperative course, and potential life-style changes. *Teaching begins before surgery. Patients often do not understand impact of transplant until several months after surgery. Thus teaching begins during dialysis; staff proceeds gradually, taking into account patient's learning style, educational level, and readiness to learn.*
	• Assess previous knowledge of transplant; clarify misconceptions.
	• Identify barriers to learning.
	• Assess ability to learn.
	• Assess appropriateness of teaching materials.
	
	THERAPEUTIC INTERVENTIONS
	• Prepare and use visual aids and logs for record keeping (e.g., medication charts, I & O sheets, vital sign log)
	• Develop and implement teaching plan:
	  Signs/symptoms of graft rejection
	  Medication teaching:
	    Instruct patient to take medication *every day* for life. *Immunosuppressive medications must be taken daily as long as patient has kidney transplant, to prevent rejection.*
	    Instruct patient to wear medical alert bracelet *stating that he/she uses antirejection medications and is transplant patient.*
	    Instruct and supervise medication self-administration at bedside, *to prepare for home self-administration.*
	  Signs/symptoms of local and systemic infection. *Transplant recipients at increased risk for developing infection because of immunosuppressive therapy.*
	  Diet restrictions, if any
	  Self-physical exam:
	    24 hr I & O
	    BP, pulse, temperature (twice/day)
	    Daily weight
	    Daily self-assessment for graft tenderness
	• Instruct patient on appropriate course of action for suspected rejection or infection.
		The patient/significant other will state an understanding of renal transplantation, including postoperative self-care.

Originated by: Gina Marie Petruzzelli, RN, BSN

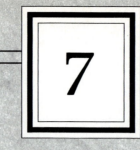

Genitourinary Care Plans

DISORDERS
Urinary tract infection

THERAPEUTIC INTERVENTIONS
Extracorporeal shock wave lithotripsy
Penile prosthesis
Prostatectomy

Urinary tract infection
(UTI; CYSTITIS; URETHRITIS)

Urinary tract infection (UTI) is an invasion of all or part of the urinary tract (kidneys, bladder, urethra) by pathogens causing infection.

NURSING DIAGNOSES / DEFINING CHARACTERISTICS	NURSING INTERVENTIONS / *RATIONALES*	EXPECTED OUTCOMES
Infection *Related to:* Instrumentation Indwelling catheter Improper toileting Pregnancy Chronically alkaline urine Stasis **DEFINING CHARACTERISTICS** Burning on urination Frequency of urination Fever Cloudy urine Elevated WBCs Low back pain Suprapubic tenderness Hematuria Bacteria in urine	**ONGOING ASSESSMENT** • Assess signs/symptoms of UTI (see Defining Characteristics). Note that patient may be asymptomatic, especially with recurrent infections. • Assess laboratory data: Urinalysis: hematuria, pyuria Urine culture: causative organism WBC: polymorphonuclear leukocytosis >11,000/ml • Assess for prior UTI history. **THERAPEUTIC INTERVENTIONS** • Encourage patient to drink extra fluid *to promote renal blood flow and flush bacteria from urinary tract.* • Instruct patient to void frequently (q2-3h during day) and empty bladder completely *to enhance bacterial clearance, reduce urine stasis, and prevent reinfection.* • Suggest cranberry or prune juice *to acidify urine.* • Give prescribed antibiotic; note effectiveness.	Urinary tract will be free of infection.
Pain *Related to:* Infection **DEFINING CHARACTERISTICS** Pain, cramps, or spasm in lower back and bladder area; dysuria; body malaise Facial mask of pain Guarding behavior Protective decreased physical activity	**ONGOING ASSESSMENT** • Solicit patient's description of pain. • Assess pain characteristics, including quality, severity, location, onset, and duration. **THERAPEUTIC INTERVENTIONS** • Apply heating pad to lower back *for back pain.* • Instruct patient in use of sitz bath *for perineal pain.* • Encourage adequate rest. • Administer analgesics and antispasmodics as ordered; note effectiveness. • Use distractions and relaxation techniques whenever appropriate. • See Pain, p. 39.	Pain is relieved.
Knowledge deficit *Related to:* Unfamiliarity with nature and treatment of UTI **DEFINING CHARACTERISTICS** Lack of questions Apparent confusion about events Expressed need for more information	**ONGOING ASSESSMENT** • Assess knowledge base about nature of UTI. • Assess preventive measures patient may currently use to minimize UTI. **THERAPEUTIC INTERVENTIONS** • Provide health teaching and discharge planning *to prevent recurrence of infection.* Instruct patient in: Having follow-up urine studies to determine whether asymptomatic infection present (thus marked tendency to recomence) Following hygienic measures *to decrease introital concentration of pathogens* by washing in shower or while standing in tub and washing perineum with soap and water from front to back after each bowel movement Voiding immediately after sexual intercourse Voiding at first urge *to prevent urinary distention* Changing underpants daily and wearing well-ventilated clothes (e.g., cotton underpants, cotton-crotched pantyhose) Taking medication for long-term antimicrobial therapy before bedtime *to ensure overnight concentration of drug*	Patient remains free of UTI.

Originated by: Caroline Sarmiento, RN, BSN

Extracorporeal shock wave lithotripsy (ESWL)

Extracorporeal shock wave lithotripsy (ESWL) is a painless, noninvasive procedure that uses ultrasound (electrically generated shock waves) delivered from outside the body to pulverize or break up kidney stones.

NURSING DIAGNOSES / DEFINING CHARACTERISTICS	NURSING INTERVENTIONS / *RATIONALES*	EXPECTED OUTCOMES
Knowledge deficit: ESWL *Related to:* Lack of experience with ESWL **DEFINING CHARACTERISTICS** Multiple questions Lack of questions Verbalized misconceptions	**ONGOING ASSESSMENT** · Assess knowledge of kidney stones and their management. · Assess understanding of ESWL and related care. **THERAPEUTIC INTERVENTIONS** · Teach patient/significant other: Preprocedure workup includes intravenous pyelogram (IVP), renal scan, ECG, coagulation studies, CBC, electrolyte profile, urinalysis, and urine culture. No incision made Coughing and deep breathing exercises important *to prevent atelectasis* Necessity of lying flat for 6 h after procedure if spinal anesthesia used Indwelling catheter in place and all urine strained *to monitor passage of stone fragments*. Hematuria normal at this point. Diagnostic studies may be repeated to assess effectiveness of ESWL. · Encourage questions. · Correct misconceptions. · Arrange tour of ESWL suite.	Patient/significant other will verbalize understanding of ESWL and nursing care.
Potential for injury *Related to:* History of bleeding tendency Drug/dye allergy History of cardiac arrhythmias OR environment Lithotomy position Large amount of irrigant instilled into bladder during procedure **DEFINING CHARACTERISTICS** Prolonged hematuria Allergic reaction during preprocedure diagnostic work-up Cardiac arrhythmias during procedure Hypothermia Numbness of extremities Generalized soreness	**ONGOING ASSESSMENT** · Assess for presence of Defining Characteristics before, during, and after ESWL. · Check pedal pulses after procedure. · Monitor body temperature throughout procedure. · Monitor cardiac rhythm; *lithotripter fires only while heart is depolarized to minimize risk of arrhythmias.* **THERAPEUTIC INTERVENTIONS** · *Prevent injury during procedure by*: Maintaining correct body alignment throughout procedure Padding stirrups to prevent pressure areas Moving legs to and from stirrups simultaneously and with adequate personnel Maintaining temperate OR environment and warming all fluids given to the patient *to decrease body heat loss through conduction* · See Cardiac dysrhythmias, p. 74; Skin integrity, impaired, p. 48; Hypothermia, p. 31; Routine perioperative care, p. 632.	Risk of injury during ESWL is reduced.
Potential anxiety *Related to:* Lack of experience with ESWL Relative newness of ESWL procedure in kidney stone management	**ONGOING ASSESSMENT** · Asses anxiety level. · Determine extent to which knowledge deficit triggers anxiety.	Anxiety will be managed.

Extracorporeal shock wave lithotripsy— cont'd

NURSING DIAGNOSES / DEFINING CHARACTERISTICS	NURSING INTERVENTIONS / *RATIONALES*	EXPECTED OUTCOMES
DEFINING CHARACTERISTICS Tense facial appearance Repeated questions Expressed need for more information about ESWL	**THERAPEUTIC INTERVENTIONS** · Encourage verbalization of concerns. · Explain all procedures before performance; repeat instructions when necessary. · During procedure, offer headphones *to minimize loud, repetitive shotgun-like sounds of the lithotripter's wave generator.* · Reassure patient that staff will be present at all times during ESWL. · See Anxiety, p. 4.	
Pain *Related to:* Shock wave bombardment of skin, soft tissue Passage of gravel with urine Instrumentation Passage of clots Distended bladder **DEFINING CHARACTERISTICS** Verbal complaints of pain, soreness Facial grimacing Altered sleep pattern Restlessness	**ONGOING ASSESSMENT** · Assess vital signs. · Check lower abdomen for bladder distention. · Assess pain: 　Location 　Quality 　Severity 　Precipitating factor(s) 　Duration · Assess patency of indwelling catheter and passage of clots, gravel. **THERAPEUTIC INTERVENTIONS** · Anticipate need for analgesics *to avoid peak periods of pain;* evaluate effectiveness. · Explore and use nonpharmacologic pain management methods successful for patient in past. · Minimize gross motor movement. · See Pain, p. 39.	Pain will be reduced.
Potential infection *Related to:* Instrumentation of urinary tract Urinary stasis Presence of gravel **DEFINING CHARACTERISTICS** Dysuria Frequency Hesitancy Retention Hematuria beyond expected stage Elevated WBC	**ONGOING ASSESSMENT** · Record I & O. · Note presence of clots, passage of gravel. *Retained clots/gravel provide bacterial growth medium.* · Observe for hematuria. · Monitor pattern of voiding after catheter removal. · Send urine/gravel for culture as indicated. · Monitor temperature. **THERAPEUTIC INTERVENTIONS** · While catheter is indwelling: 　Strain urine *to retrieve gravel for culture.* 　Instruct patient to report flank pain, chills. 　Encourage 2000-4000 cc/day fluid intake unless contraindicated *to flush stone fragments and other debris and prevent urine stasis.* 　Provide meatal care. 　Irrigate catheter by aseptic technique with 30 cc sterile water as ordered. 　Consider catheterization if patient fails to void 6 h after catheter removal. · After catheter removal: 　Encourage patient to continue to push fluids. 　Notify physician if patient has not voided within 6 h of catheter removal. 　Consider intermittent catheterization. 　See Urinary retention, p. 61. · If patient has nephrostomy tube(s), keep sterile dressings dry and intact; report pain or unusual drainage to physician. · See Urinary tract infection, p. 361. · See Nephrostomy tube, percutaneous, p. 353.	Risk of UTI will be reduced.

Continued.

Genitourinary Care Plans

NURSING DIAGNOSES / DEFINING CHARACTERISTICS	NURSING INTERVENTIONS / *RATIONALES*	EXPECTED OUTCOMES
Potential ineffective airway clearance *Related to:* Incomplete procedure preparation Anesthesia/analgesia Pain **DEFINING CHARACTERISTICS** Poor cough effort Abnormal breath sounds Change in rate, depth of respirations	**ONGOING ASSESSMENT** · Assess respirations; note rate, depth, quality. · Assess behavior changes consistent with O_2 deficit. **THERAPEUTIC INTERVENTIONS** Preprocedure: · Ensure NPO status after midnight on day of procedure *to minimize aspiration risk.* · Remove dentures before procedure. During procedure: · Keep suction equipment available. After procedure: · Encourage patient to turn, cough, and deep breathe at least q2h. · Encourage early ambulation. · Encourage use of incentive spirometer. · Suction if necessary.	Airway will remain patent.
Potential fluid volume deficit *Related to:* Postprocedure hemorrhage **DEFINING CHARACTERISTICS** Excessive hematuria (>12-24 hr) Clots in urine Hypotension Rapid pulse Restlessness Dry mucous membranes	**ONGOING ASSESSMENT** · Assess vital signs. · Assess amount of blood loss. **THERAPEUTIC INTERVENTIONS** · Administer IV fluids as ordered · Push oral fluids if tolerated. · Be prepared to administer blood/blood products as ordered. · See Fluid volume deficit, p. 20.	Risk of fluid volume deficit will be reduced.
Knowledge deficit: posthospitalization care *Related to:* First experience with ESWL Prolonged passage of gravel **DEFINING CHARACTERISTICS** Verbalized need for information Few questions Many questions	**ONGOING ASSESSMENT** · Assess readiness to learn posthospitalization care. **THERAPEUTIC INTERVENTIONS** · Teach patient/significant other: Importance of hydration: water 8-10 glasses/day *to keep urine dilute and flush out stone fragments* Antibiotic/antispasmodic drug schedule, expected actions, and untoward effects Important symptoms to report to urologist: Pain not relieved by medication Nausea, vomiting, chills Fever Hematuria Clots in urine Stone fragments may be passed several weeks after procedure. · Provide patient with resource phone numbers and follow-up appointment. · Document patient's understanding of discharge instructions.	Patient/significant other verbalize understanding of post-discharge care after ESWL.

Originated by: Therese Sineni, RN, C, BSN
Nancy Ruppman, RN, BSN, CURN

Penile prosthesis

The implantation of silicone into penile tissue to replace erectile tissue in the impotent man. These may be rigid, semirigid, or inflatable

NURSING DIAGNOSES / DEFINING CHARACTERISTICS	NURSING INTERVENTIONS / *RATIONALES*	EXPECTED OUTCOMES

Pain
Related to:
Penile incision
Postoperative edema
Indwelling catheter
Initial movement/
  inflation of prosthesis
 	
DEFINING CHARACTERISTICS
Verbalized pain
Guarded movement
Grimacing
Sleep disturbance
	ONGOING ASSESSMENT
	• Assess pain:
	  Location
	  Intensity
	  Duration
	  Precipitating factors
	• Monitor edema of penis and scrotal area.
	
	THERAPEUTIC INTERVENTIONS
	• Anticipate need for pain medications or patient-controlled analgesia (PCA).
	• Use bed cradle *to keep linens off operative area.*
	• Use nonadherent dressing (Telfa) *to prevent trauma to suture line.*
	• Postpone initial movement/inflation until edema subsides, usually 3-5 days after operation.
	• Tape indwelling catheter to abdomen *to keep penis perpendicular to body;* do not tape penis or prosthesis to bed cradles or other objects.
	• See Pain, p. 39; see Patient controlled analgesia, p. 631.
		Pain will be relieved.

Potential infection *Related to:* Implanted prosthesis **DEFINING CHARACTERISTICS** Redness, swelling, purulent drainage from incision Fever Elevated WBC	**ONGOING ASSESSMENT** • Assess condition of infrapubic, perineal, penile, or suprapubic incision; note redness, excessive swelling, or suspicious drainage. • Culture suspicious drainage. • Monitor temperature. • Monitor WBC. **THERAPEUTIC INTERVENTIONS** • Use aseptic technique for dressing changes. • Provide meticulous perineal care after bowel movements *to prevent fecal contamination of operative area.* • Provide daily or more frequent meatal care if indwelling catheter in place. • Administer antibiotics and antipyretics as ordered.	Risk of infection is reduced.
Body image disturbance *Related to:* Penile prosthesis Need for manipulation of genitalia **DEFINING CHARACTERISTICS** Verbalized feelings about prosthetic implant Focus on implant Refusal to look at or care for implant Embarrassment during implant care	**ONGOING ASSESSMENT** • Assess feelings about altered body part and function. • Assess degree to which patient's preoperative expectations met/unmet by surgical result. • Assess perceived impact of implant on significant relationships. **THERAPEUTIC INTERVENTIONS** • Encourage patient to discuss feelings; convey normalcy of both positive and negative feelings about implant. • Correct misconceptions; answer questions simply and honestly. • Include significant other in discussion when appropriate *so patient and partner accept changed body structure and function.* • See Body image disturbance, p. 6.	Resolution of body image issues is facilitated.
Altered sexuality *Related to:* Impotence Placement of prosthesis Expectations of self/partner after surgery	**ONGOING ASSESSMENT** • Assess preoperative impotence and impact on relationships and perceived sexuality. • Inquire about other methods of impotence therapy. • Ask patient/partner about expectations of implant.	Satisfactory sexual functioning will be achieved.

Continued.

Penile prothesis— cont'd

NURSING DIAGNOSES / DEFINING CHARACTERISTICS	NURSING INTERVENTIONS / *RATIONALES*	EXPECTED OUTCOMES
DEFINING CHARACTERISTICS Verbalized concern about sexual functioning Reported change in relationship with partner(s) Expressed increased or decreased satisfaction with sexual performance Inappropriate behavior or conversation related to sexual functioning	**THERAPEUTIC INTERVENTIONS** • Provide undisturbed private place/time to discuss altered sexuality with patient/partner. • Encourage patient/partner to verbalize concerns and feelings nonjudgmentally. • Help patient/partner differentiate concepts of erection, ejaculation, fertility, and orgasm. *Prosthetic implant restores erectile capability but has no impact on ejaculation, fertility, or orgasm.* • See Sexuality patterns, altered, p. 47.	

Knowledge deficit
Related to:
Postoperative care/ management of penile prosthesis
 	
DEFINING CHARACTERISTICS
Multiple questions
Lack of questions
Demonstrated inability to care for/ manipulate prosthetic device
	ONGOING ASSESSMENT
	• Assess knowledge and readiness to learn.
	
	THERAPEUTIC INTERVENTIONS
	• Teach patient type and name of prosthesis implanted. *Possible future need for genitourinary and/or prostatic procedures more difficult because of penile implants; patients need accurate, complete information.*
	• Inform patient that pain and edema expected for 5-14 days.
	• Teach perineal care to prevent infection.
	• Inform patient/partner about use of prosthesis:
	  Sexual activity may resume 6-8 wk after surgery unless pain present.
	  Lubricant should be used liberally *to prevent penile trauma, soft tissue perforation.*
	  Teach inflation/deflation of inflatable devices.
	• Offer to arrange talk with someone successfully functioning with implant.
	• Refer patient to sexual counseling if appropriate.
		Patient/significant other will verbalize knowledge of and demonstrate appropriate care/use of penile prosthesis.

Originated by: Dorothy Rhodes, RN
　　　　　　　Nancy Ruppman, RN, BSN, CURN

Prostatectomy

(TRANSURETHRAL RESECTION OF PROSTATE [TUR, TURP])

Surgical resection of the prostate gland, via a transurethral, retropubic, perineal, or suprapubic approach, is commonly performed for benign prostatic hypertrophy or for cancer of the prostate gland.

NURSING DIAGNOSES / DEFINING CHARACTERISTICS	NURSING INTERVENTIONS / *RATIONALES*	EXPECTED OUTCOMES
Altered patterns of urinary elimination *Related to:* Surgical resection Need for continuous intermittent bladder irrigation	**ONGOING ASSESSMENT** • Assess catheter for patency. • Observe urine for presence of clots bits of tissue. • Monitor color and viscosity of urine. • Record amount of instilled irrigant and urine output.	Normal patterns of urinary elimination will be achieved.

Prostatectomy— cont'd

NURSING DIAGNOSES / DEFINING CHARACTERISTICS	NURSING INTERVENTIONS / *RATIONALES*	EXPECTED OUTCOMES

DEFINING CHARACTERISTICS
Presence of indwelling catheter or suprapubic catheter
Urge incontinence after catheter removal
	THERAPEUTIC INTERVENTIONS
	• Position tubing and collection system in gravity-dependent fashion *to ensure drainage away from patient and prevent clotting.*
	• Perform irrigation (continuous or intermittent) as ordered.
	• Encourage 2000-3000 cc oral intake unless medically contraindicated *to keep urine dilute.*
	• When catheter removed (usually 5-7 days after surgery):
	    Encourage voiding schedule (reduces urge incontinence).
	    Encourage patient to stand *to facilitate voiding.*
	    Stimulate voiding by use of running water or inner thigh stimulation.
	    Replace catheter if patient unable to void or distention occurs.
	• See Urinary retention, p. 61.	

Potential fluid volume excess: dilutional hyponatremia *Related to:* Systemic absorption of bladder irrigant Clots in catheter (predispose to absorption of irrigant) **DEFINING CHARACTERISTICS** Decreased hematocrit Agitation Confusion Low serum sodium	**ONGOING ASSESSMENT** • Monitor amount of bladder irrigant instilled and returned. Note gross discrepancy. • Monitor hematocrit. • Monitor changes in level of consciousness (LOC). • Monitor serum sodium level. • Observe for clots or kinks in catheter or drainage system. **THERAPEUTIC INTERVENTIONS** • Ensure gravity drainage of irrigant. • Stop irrigation, report signs of fluid volume excess to physician *to prevent worsening of fluid volume excess.* • Use syringe to irrigate catheter manually *to break up clots and restore gravity drainage.*	Normal fluid volume will be maintained.
Potential for infection *Related to:* Surgical resection Instrumentation Open incision (except for transurethral procedure) Indwelling catheter Bladder irrigation Space drains Underlying malignancy **DEFINING CHARACTERISTICS** White blood cells in urine Fever Elevated WBC Redness, pain, swelling of incision Purulent drainage from incision	**ONGOING ASSESSMENT** • Monitor for signs of infection (see Defining Characteristics). • Monitor urinalysis report. • Observe dressings for suspicious drainage; culture apparently purulent drainage. • Monitor vital signs. **THERAPEUTIC INTERVENTIONS** • Maintain sterile, closed urinary drainage/irrigation system *to prevent bacterial invasion of compromised urinary tract.* • Change dressings by aseptic technique. • Provide and encourage intake of high-protein, high-calorie diet.	Risk of infection is reduced.

Pain
Related to:
Incision
Indwelling catheter(s)
Surgical drains
	ONGOING ASSESSMENT
	• Assess pain:
	    Location
	    Quality
	    Severity
		Pain will be relieved.

Continued.

NURSING DIAGNOSES / DEFINING CHARACTERISTICS	NURSING INTERVENTIONS / *RATIONALES*	EXPECTED OUTCOMES
Bladder spasms **DEFINING CHARACTERISTICS** Verbalized pain Facial mask of pain Guarding	Precipitating factors Methods of relief • Assess concurrence of irrigation or catheter care with pain onset. **THERAPEUTIC INTERVENTIONS** • Anticipate need for analgesics and antispasmodics *to prevent peak pain periods.* • Maintain traction on catheter *to prevent movement (can stimulate spasm).* • Teach and encourage use of splinting incision *to minimize incisional pain during movement and coughing.* • Stabilize other tubes/drains securely to minimize inadvertent movement. • See Pain, p. 39; Surgical drains/tubes, p. 322.	
Anxiety *Related to:* Possibility of incontinence Fear of sexual inability **DEFINING CHARACTERISTICS** Nervousness Increased questioning Inability to follow simple commands	**ONGOING ASSESSMENT** • Assess level of anxiety. • Determine specific cause of anxiety if possible. • Assess coping strategies. • Assess available support systems. **THERAPEUTIC INTERVENTIONS** • Encourage patient to verbalize concerns. • Provide clear, accurate information. • Correct misconceptions. *Urge incontinence may persist 2-3 wk after urethral catheter removal.* • See Anxiety, p. 4; Sexuality patterns, altered, p. 47; Urinary elimination, altered patterns, p. 58.	Anxiety will be reduced.

Knowledge deficit
Related to:
Lack of previous surgical experience
Need for postdischarge care
 	
DEFINING CHARACTERISTICS
 	
Multiple questions
Lack of questions
Verbalized misconceptions
	ONGOING ASSESSMENT
	
	• Assess readiness for learning.
	
	THERAPEUTIC INTERVENTIONS
	
	• Tell patient to avoid the following 4-6 wk after surgery:
	  Driving
	  Aggressive stair climbing
	  Heavy lifting
	  Sexual intercourse
	  Sports
	  Straining
	• Teach patient importance of finishing all antibiotic prescriptions. *Though they may feel well, postoperative risk of UTI exists and must be treated prophylactically.*
	• Instruct patient to notify physician of blood urine.
	• Instruct patient in importance of keeping follow-up appointments.
		Patient verbalizes understanding of postdischarge care.

Originated by: Nancy Ruppman, RN, BSN, CURN
             Encaracion Mendoza, RN, BSN

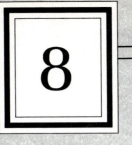

Endocrine and Metabolic Care Plans

DISORDERS
Adrenocortical insufficiency
Diabetes, insulin dependent
Diabetes insipidus
Diabetic ketoacidosis: acute
Diabetic patient with recurrent
  hypoglycemia/hyperglycemia

Excessive glucocorticoids
Hepatitis
Hypercalcemia
Hyperglycemic hyperosmotic nonketotic
  coma

Syndrome of inappropriate antidiuretic
  hormone

THERAPEUTIC INTERVENTIONS
Thyroidectomy

Adrenocortical insufficiency

(ADDISON'S DISEASE)

An abnormality of the adrenal glands with the destruction of the adrenal cortex and impairment of glucocorticoid and mineral corticoid production. Patients using steroids may also manifest adrenocortical insufficiency.

NURSING DIAGNOSES / DEFINING CHARACTERISTICS	NURSING INTERVENTIONS / *RATIONALES*	EXPECTED OUTCOMES
Decreased cardiac output *Related to:* Any situations requiring increased corticosteroids (e.g., stress, infection, GI upsets) may lead to shock or vascular collapse **DEFINING CHARACTERISTICS** Headache Listlessness and lethargy Physical weakness Nausea and vomiting Intractable abdominal pain Decreased BP Weak, thready pulse Decreased blood sugar Increased potassium Orthostatic hypotension Decreased sodium Increased temperature	**ONGOING ASSESSMENT** • Assess and record changes in mentation. • Monitor and record vital signs. • Assess for orthostatic hypotension by taking postural BP. • Assess for alteration in nervous system: weakness, paresthesia or paresis, and possible paralysis. • Assess patient's muscle strength and ability to ambulate. • Assess GI functioning. • Monitor and record I & O. • Monitor electrolytes. • Observe for signs of infection. *Fluid deficit puts patient at risk for poor skin turgor, which results in breakdown/infection.* • Closely monitor patient complaints of headache. • Monitor ABGs. **THERAPEUTIC INTERVENTIONS** • See Cardiac output, decreased, p. 9. • Minimize stressful situations. • Promote quiet environment. • Provide rest periods. • Explain all procedures; answer all questions. • Assist patient with activities as needed. • *Hypotension or shock may result from arrhythmias secondary to electrolyte imbalance.* See Cardiac dysrythmias, p. 74.	Optimal tissue perfusion will be maintained.
Altered nutrition: less than body requirements *Related to:* Decreased GI enzymes, causing loss of appetite and decreased oral intake tolerance Decreased gastric acid production Decreased urinary nitrogen excretion **DEFINING CHARACTERISTICS** Recent weight loss Decreased blood sugar Nausea/vomiting	**ONGOING ASSESSMENT** • Assess patient's general appearance. • Assess GI function. • Assess appetite. • Monitor and record weight daily. • Assess foods patient can tolerate. **THERAPEUTIC INTERVENTIONS** • Provide foods patient can tolerate. Prevent fasting. • Offer frequent small meals. *Inadequate caloric meals may precipitate hypoglycomia. Promotion of oral intake maintains adequate blood glucose levels and nutrition.* • Create environment conducive to eating. • Encourage rest periods. • Encourage high-protein, low-carbohydrate, high-sodium diet. • Explain need for diet supplements. *Patient tires because of inadequate production of the hepatic glucagon. Recommended diet prevents fatigue, hypoglycemia, and hyponatremia.*	Adequate nutritional status will be sustained.

NURSING DIAGNOSES / DEFINING CHARACTERISTICS	NURSING INTERVENTIONS / *RATIONALES*	EXPECTED OUTCOMES
Diarrhea Abdominal cramps Anorexia General malaise		

Knowledge deficit:
Related to:
Lack of experience with adrenocortical insufficiency
 	
DEFINING CHARACTERISTICS
Verbalized frustrations
Expressed need for further information
Denial of disease
Lack of compliance
	ONGOING ASSESSMENT
	• Assess feelings about disease.
	• Assess feelings about need for lifelong medication.
	• Assess available support systems.
	• Assess ability to comply with treatment.
	• Assess ability to identify/verbalize signs/symptoms that require physician consultation:
	  Fever
	  Nausea/vomiting
	  Weight gain
	  Diaphoresis
	  Progressive weakness
	  Dizziness
	
	THERAPEUTIC INTERVENTIONS
	• Instruct patient in self-administration of steroids, including expected effects, and dosage. *Steroidal replacement may be oral or IM. Knowledge of disease process and drug regimen will promote compliance.*
	• Offer information about need to adjust dosage when under stress.
	• Emphasize need for morning or evening dose. *Patient must identify personal stressors and learn to adjust steroidal drugs to compensate for stress response. Twice-daily dosing encouraged to prevent crisis.*
	• Stress importance of regular physician visits. *Drug levels may be adjusted to patient's requirements during visits.*
	• Discuss signs/symptoms requiring physician consultation.
	• Explain how to obtain medical identification tag and importance of wearing it.
	• Inform patient of availability of an injectable cortisol with sterile syringe. *Patients should carry a readily injectable syringe of cortisol at all times.*
		Patient will verbalize understanding of disease process and guidelines for replacement therapy.

Originated by: Cathy Croke, RN MSN
Charlotte Niznik, RN, BSN, CDE

Diabetes, insulin-dependent

(TYPE II DIABETES; JUVENILE DIABETES; DIABETES MELLITUS)

A pancreatic disorder in which the β cells of the islets of Langerhans do not secrete enough insulin, if any. Insulin, a hormone usually secreted after meals, facilitates glycogen storage in the liver and transport of glucose into muscle and fat cells and maintains blood glucose at normal levels. Inadequate insulin causes hyperglycemia and glycosuria, which lead to fluid and electrolyte imbalance. Gluconeogenesis (use of protein and fat stores) causes ketoacidosis, muscle wasting, and weight loss.

NURSING DIAGNOSES / DEFINING CHARACTERISTICS	NURSING INTERVENTIONS / *RATIONALES*	EXPECTED OUTCOMES
Altered nutrition: less than body requirements *Related to:* Decreased number or function of pancreatic islet cells Increased blood glucose level by poor cell uptake Glycosuria caused by exceeding renal tubular capacity limits **DEFINING CHARACTERISTICS** Polydipsia Polyphagia Polyuria Weight loss Increased blood glucose/abnormal glucose tolerance test	**ONGOING ASSESSMENT** • Assess for signs/symptoms of hyperglycemia or diabetic ketoacidosis: Assess vital signs q4h. Monitor strict I & O. Check urine for sugar and acetone at least every shift. Monitor blood lab results: Glucose (70-110 mg/dl) Na (136-147 mEq/L) Cl (95-110 mEq/L) CO_2 (21-32 mEq/L) **THERAPEUTIC INTERVENTIONS** • Administer insulin as ordered (progressively): Insulin drip (if condition warrants) Regular insulin subcutaneously preprandially Regular/NPH am and pm split-mixed dose when indicated. *Lifelong daily injections are necessary.* Rotate injection sites; document site of each injection *(sites rotated for optimal insulin absorption).* • Provide appropriate diet: Obtain dietary consultation. Reinforce need to consume all foods on tray, not save for later. Check each meal tray for proper identification. • Give all meals and snacks on time. *When individual cannot utilize insulin, metabolic state is altered.*	Nutritional requirements will be adequate while diabetic state is controlled.
Ineffective individual coping *Related to:* Diagnostic and treatment course New problem Chronic disease **DEFINING CHARACTERISTICS** Regressive behavior Anger/noncompliance with regimen Refusal to attempt procedures independently	**ONGOING ASSESSMENT** • Assess coping mechanisms for diagnosis and treatment. • Assess for noncompliance, anger, regressive behavior. • Assess patient/family relationship. • Assess past coping strategies. • Assess occupational interests, hobbies; identify potential stressors. **THERAPEUTIC INTERVENTIONS** • Perform all procedures calmly and unhurriedly. *Coping with chronic disease and mastering managerial skills are directly related to initial instruction.* • Encourage verbalization of feelings about diagnosis and chronicity. • Reinforce that anger and "mourning" loss of freedom are normal coping mechanisms. • Support and reinforce progress toward independence. • Answer any and all questions. • Obtain support services as needed:diabetes teaching service, psychiatric liaison.	Coping behaviors will be maximized.
Knowledge deficit *Related to:* Initial diagnosis of chronic disease	**ONGOING ASSESSMENT** • Assess willingness to learn. • Assess cognitive abilities. • Assess physical abilities. *Physical limitations (e.g., lack of motor control and poor vision) necessitate changes in teaching plan.*	Patient will demonstrate knowledge of and compliance with treatment regimen.

NURSING DIAGNOSES / DEFINING CHARACTERISTICS	NURSING INTERVENTIONS / *RATIONALES*	EXPECTED OUTCOMES

Multifaceted treatment involved in controlling diabetes and potential complications
 	
DEFINING CHARACTERISTICS
 	
Anxiety
Fear
Anger about chronicity
Many questions
Lack of questions
Noncompliance with dietary restrictions
Failure to attempt own insulin injections or blood glucose chemistry
	• Assess retention from one class session to next.
	
	THERAPEUTIC INTERVENTIONS
	• Contact diabetes teaching service.
	• Explain definition of diabetes, including signs/symptoms.
	• Reinforce that diabetes is chronic incurable condition that can be controlled by diet, insulin, and exercise.
	• Explain need for diet-controlled exchange system and importance of strict adherence.
	• Explain that daily exercise is important to lower blood sugar and allow normal socialization. *Exercise increases body's sensitivity to insulin and decreases serum cholesterol and triglyceride levels, decreasing the risk factors for developing cardiovascular complications of diabetes.*
	• Reinforce and encourage progress toward independence at blood glucose monitoring and insulin techniques.
	• Define insulin; discuss different types, action, duration, especially split-mixed insulin regimen.
	• Demonstrate accurate method of drawing up and administering insulin; explain rationale for rotating injection sites.
	• Explain that blood glucose monitoring necessary to diabetic control; normal glucose level is 70-110 mg/dl.
	• Demonstrate accurate method of obtaining and interpreting blood glucose Chemstrips.
	• Define hypoglycemia (blood glucose <40 mg/dl) and possible causes.
	• Discuss signs/symptoms of hypoglycemia:
	   Mild: Patient cool, sweaty, shaky, irritable, tired, weak; hungry; has personality changes; headache.
	   Moderate: Patient experiences nausea, sleepiness, disorientation, fainting, decreased LOC.
	   Severe: Patient has coma or convulsion.
	• Instruct in treatment for hypoglycemia symptoms (e.g., 4 oz orange juice, hard candy, sugar, candy bar)
	• Discuss use of glucagon for hypoglycemic coma.
	• Define hyperglycemia (serum glucose >140 mg/dl) and possible causes. Teach signs/ symptoms: glycosuria, polyuria (bed-wetting), polydipsia, polyphagia, acetone breath.
	• Discuss/define diabetic ketoacidosis and need for immediate medical attention. *Patient/family must learn basic survival skills of diabetes mellitus (DM) management to prevent complications.*
	• Discuss need for careful blood sugar monitoring during illness (may require insulin adjustment).
	• Reinforce need for regular follow-up care (e.g., of eyes, feet, and teeth) *to prevent microvascular complications of diabetes (e.g., reduced vision, blindness, foot problems, and renal failure).*
	• Encourage questioning for clarification and evaluation of effectiveness of teaching.	

Originated by: Linda Rosen-Walsh, RN, BSN
Charlotte Niznik, RN, BSN, CDE
Margaret A. Cunningham, RN, MS

Diabetes insipidus

(NEUROGENIC DIABETES)

Diabetes insipidus (DI), or neurogenic diabetes insipidus, is a disturbance of water metabolism caused by a failure of vasopressin (antidiuretic hormone [ADH]) synthesis or release resulting in the excretion of a large amount of dilute urine. Diabetes insipidus may also have a nephrogenic or psychogenic etiology.

NURSING DIAGNOSES / DEFINING CHARACTERISTICS	NURSING INTERVENTIONS / *RATIONALES*	EXPECTED OUTCOMES
Fluid volume deficit *Related to:* Compromised endocrine regulatory mechanism Neurohypophysial dysfunction Hypopituitarism Hypophysectomy **DEFINING CHARACTERISTICS** Polyuria Polydypsia Sudden weight loss Urine specific gravity <1.005 Poor hydration status Hypernatremia (Na^+ > 145 mEq/L)	**ONGOING ASSESSMENT** · Monitor I & O. · Report urine volume >200 ml for each of 2 consecutive hr or >500 ml in 2-hr period. · Monitor for increased thirst *(preference for cold or iced water hallmark of DI).* · Weigh daily *to detect excessive fluid loss, especially in incontinent patients with inaccurate I & O.* · Monitor urine specific gravity every shift *(may be as low as 1.005).* · Monitor for serum Na^+ levels >145 mEq/L. *Dehydration is hyperosmolar state in which serum Na^+ rises.* · Monitor for signs of hypovolemic shock (e.g., tachycardia, tachypnea, hypotension.) **THERAPEUTIC INTERVENTIONS** · Allow patient to drink at will. · Provide easily accessible fluid source. · If patient has decreased LOC or impaired thirst mechanism, obtain parenteral fluid orders. · Administer medication as ordered. If vasopressin given, monitor for water intoxication/rebound hyponatremia. · See Fluid volume deficit, p. 20.	Normal fluid volume will be achieved.
Discomfort: excessive thirst *Related to:* Large output Dehydration **DEFINING CHARACTERISTICS** Unquenchable thirst Preference for cold or iced water	**ONGOING ASSESSMENT** · Assess for polydypsia. · Continue to monitor state of hydration. **THERAPEUTIC INTERVENTIONS** · Provide frequent mouth care. · Provide fluids as desired. *Patients with intact thirst mechanisms may maintain fluid balance by drinking as much as they urinate.*	Thirst is satisfied.
Potential constipation *Related to:* Fluid volume deficit **DEFINING CHARACTERISTICS** Frequency and amount less than usual pattern Straining at stool Hard, formed stools	**ONGOING ASSESSMENT** · Assess usual bowel patterns and habits. · Assess for deviation from normal. · Assess characteristics of stool (color, consistency, amount). **THERAPEUTIC INTERVENTIONS** · See Constipation, p. 12.	Normal pattern of bowel elimination will be maintained.
Potential altered skin integrity *Related to:* Urinary frequency with potential incontinence	**ONGOING ASSESSMENT** · Inspect skin every shift; document condition and changes in status. *Early detection and intervention may prevent progression of impaired skin integrity.* · Assess for continence. · Assess other risks of patient's skin integrity (e.g. immobility, nutritional status).	Skin will remain intact.

NURSING DIAGNOSES / DEFINING CHARACTERISTICS	NURSING INTERVENTIONS / *RATIONALES*	EXPECTED OUTCOMES
DEFINING CHARACTERISTICS Polyuria, urinary incontinence Red, excoriated skin	**THERAPEUTIC INTERVENTIONS** • Provide easy access to bathroom/urinal/bedpan. • See Skin integrity, impaired, p. 48.	
Fear *Related to:* Unquenchable thirst Excessive urination Medications and treatments **DEFINING CHARACTERISTICS** Restlessness Increased questioning Withdrawal Excessive demands	**ONGOING ASSESSMENT** • Assess level of fear. • Assess usual coping strategies. **THERAPEUTIC INTERVENTIONS** • Encourage patient to verbalize feelings *(aids assessment of fear; provides patient awareness of feelings)*. • See Fear, p. 18.	Fear will be reduced.
Knowledge deficit *Related to:* Disease process Medications and treatments **DEFINING CHARACTERISTICS** Requests for more information Verbalized misconceptions/ misinterpretation	**ONGOING ASSESSMENT** • Assess level of knowledge of disease process. • Assess level of understanding of medications and treatments. **THERAPEUTIC INTERVENTIONS** • Explain condition and treatment(s) in simple, brief terms to patient/family/ significant others. • Ask patient/family/significant others to verbalize explanations of conditions/ treatments *(to indicate misconceptions or misinterpretations)*. • See Knowledge deficit, p. 33.	Patient will express understanding of disease and treatment.

Orginated by: Mary Ann Naccarato, RN, BSN

Diabetic ketoacidosis, acute (DKA)

(HYPERGLYCEMIA; DIABETES MELLITUS)

Diabetic ketoacidosis (DKA) is an acute, potentially life-threatening complication of diabetes mellitus. Normally the body metabolizes glucose for energy needs. In the diabetic, glucose metabolism does not occur because of absent or ineffective insulin that is necessary for migration of glucose into cells. Diabetes ketoacidosis (DKA) results from cellular metabolism of fat to produce energy. By-products of this metabolic process are ketone bodies (organic acids) that cause metabolic acidosis.

NURSING DIAGNOSES / DEFINING CHARACTERISTICS	NURSING INTERVENTIONS / *RATIONALES*	EXPECTED OUTCOMES
Potential for injury *Related to:* Ketoacidosis resulting from: Omission/reduction of insulin Inability of cells to recognize/use available insulin Initial onset of diabetes Infection/ intercurrent illness Acute pancreatitis Stress **DEFINING CHARACTERISTICS** *Clinical:* Polydipsia, polyuria Weakness, anorexia Abdominal pain Kussmaul respirations Acetone breath Blurred vision Nausea, vomiting Pallor, diaphoresis, dehydration *Laboratory:* Serum glucose >300 mg/dl and <900 mg/dl Serum ketones Decreased serum pH, phosphate, bicarbonate Normal/low/elevated serum potassium Urine glucose: 2 percent Urine acetone: large	**ONGOING ASSESSMENT** · Monitor and record urine ketone. *Presence of ketone denotes ketoacidotic state.* · Monitor blood glucose with Chemstrips as necessary. *Serum glucose levels decrease with appropriate IV fluid and insulin therapy.* · Monitor potassium level when therapy begins. *With metabolic and fluid correction, K^+ returns intracellularly and serum hypokalemia may result from K^+ loss with diuresis.* · Auscultate for bowel sounds. Assess for abdominal pain; check intensity and location of pain. Document and notify physician of any changes. *(Abdominal pain, nausea, vomiting result from ketoacidosis.)* · Monitor and record respiratory rate, depth, and presence of Kussmaul respirations; notify physician of deviations. *Deep, rapid respirations indicate increased acidic state. Carbon dioxide and acetone are blown off with each breath in an attempt to compensate acidosis.* · Monitor ABGs as ordered. Notify physician if abnormal. Maintain O_2 as ordered. · Monitor for hypoglycemia. Signs/symptoms include confusion, tremors, pallor, weakness, diaphoresis, serum glucose <60 mg/dl. **THERAPEUTIC INTERVENTIONS** · Administer and record IV fluids and additives as ordered: Use normal saline to correct volume depletion. *Restriction of glucose solutions is desired until blood glucose drops to 250 mg/dl.* Initiate K^+ therapy if indicated. · Administer sodium bicarbonate only in cases of severe, life-threatening acidosis. *Early or overzealous use of $NaHCO_3$ often causes rebound metabolic alkalosis when rehydration has occurred.* · Administer and record insulin injection, drip as ordered. Follow hospital/unit procedure for preparing insulin drip. *Short-acting insulin (IV infusion) allows glucose transport to cells and promotes fat/protein storage.* · If signs of hypoglycemia present, administer sugar under tongue if NPO or orange juice if patient tolerates oral fluids. Document and notify physician. *With decrease of blood glucose and IV infusion, patient at risk for hypoglycemia and cerebral edema.* · Document consistency and amount of emesis. Elevate head of bed (HOB) 30 degrees; prepare for possible nasogastric tube placement. · Administer antiemetics as ordered. · Maintain patient on complete bedrest.	Risk of injury caused by ketoacidosis will be reduced.
Fluid volume deficit *Related to:* Osmotic diuresis from hyperglycemia Vomiting Kussmaul respirations	**ONGOING ASSESSMENT** · Monitor vital signs q2h; notify physician of any abnormalities, especially heart rate, BP. *Severe hypotension and tachycardia precede hypovolemic shock.* · Assess skin turgor. · Monitor and record I & O. Notify physician if urine output <30 ml for 2 consecutive hr. *Urinary output should be at least 30 cc/hr. Lower output indicates decreased renal perfusion.*	Fluid volume deficit will be reduced.

Diabetic ketoacidosis, acute— cont'd

NURSING DIAGNOSES / DEFINING CHARACTERISTICS	NURSING INTERVENTIONS / *RATIONALES*	EXPECTED OUTCOMES
DEFINING CHARACTERISTICS Abdominal pain Hypotension, tachycardia Dilute urine Output greater than intake Increased serum values: WBC, Hb, Hct, glucose, BUN Increased sodium, creatinine Oliguria or anuria possible in severe dehydration and shock	- Monitor and record urine specific gravity (*early indicator of dehydration and/or electrolyte imbalance*). - Weigh patient daily; record. - Monitor serum Hct, Hb, osmolality, BUN, glucose, and urine laboratory values (*increased because of hemoconcentration*). **THERAPEUTIC INTERVENTIONS** - Administer isotonic IV fluid (saline) followed by glucose IV fluid when glucose levels drop. *Isotonic saline administered to increase volume quickly and maintain sodium balance. Restrict glucose only until serum glucose begins to drop to prevent hypoglycemia.* - Reassure patient during episodes of abdominal pain and vomiting. *These symptoms thought to be related to severe dehydration and electrolyte imbalance; should subside when fluid volume corrected.*	
Altered levels of consciousness *Related to:* Acid-base imbalance Ineffective breathing pattern Dehydration **DEFINING CHARACTERISTICS** Change in alertness, orientation, ability to respond verbally, decreased motor response, decreased pupillary reaction Kussmaul respirations Agitation Impaired judgment Lethargy Drowsiness Coma	**ONGOING ASSESSMENT** - Assess level of consciousness (LOC) by using coma scale on neurologic flow sheet. - Assess serum electrolytes, glucose, pH levels. - Monitor respiratory rate, tidal volume, quality. *Change in quality of respirations may lead to decreased sensorium, ultimate respiratory arrest.* **THERAPEUTIC INTERVENTIONS** - Maintain serial documentation on neurologic flow sheet. *Flow sheet documentation quickly identifies immediate changes in trends in patient's neurologic status.* - Correct serum electrolytes, fluid, glucose, and pH imbalance. - Ensure safety as necessary: side rails, restraints. - Explain all procedures as they are performed.	Normal LOC will be restored and maintained.

Potential decreased cardiac output
Related to:
Cardiac arrhythmias secondary to hyperkalemia/ hypokalemia
 	
DEFINING CHARACTERISTICS
Arrhythmias observed per ECG or cardiac monitor
Irregular pulse
Bradycardia
Low blood pressure
	ONGOING ASSESSMENT
	- Monitor ECG for early signs of potassium imbalance. *Electrolyte abnormalities exhibit specific ECG effects. Recognition of hyperkalemia/ hypokalemia can alert nurse to life-threatening situation.*
	  Progressive signs of hyperkalemia:
	    High-peaked T waves
	    Flat P waves
	    Prolonged PR interval
	    Atrial arrest
	    Prolonged QRS, slow ventricular rate
	    Ventricular fibrillation, asystole
	  Signs of hypokalemia:
	    Prolonged low-amplitude T waves
	    Prominant U waves
	    Ectopic beats
		Risk of cardiac complications is reduced.

Continued.

Diabetic ketoacidosis, acute— cont'd

NURSING DIAGNOSES / DEFINING CHARACTERISTICS	NURSING INTERVENTIONS / *RATIONALES*	EXPECTED OUTCOMES
Changes in mentation Dizziness Cool skin	· Monitor for changes in cardiac output; check B/P regularly. *BP and pulses reflect cardiac output.* **THERAPEUTIC INTERVENTIONS** · Provide accurate administration of fluids and electrolytes *to correct fluid, acid-base imbalance. Acidosis is associated with hyperkalemia, which causes slowed conduction. In contrast, aggressive treatment can cause hypokalemia, which causes ectopic cardiac rhythms.* · Place patient on cardiac monitor if indicated. *Patient in mild DKA may not require monitoring if clinically stable.*	
Altered nutrition: less than body requirements *Related to:* Lack of glucose metabolism caused by absence of effective insulin Use of fat/protein for energy needs *(Protein metabolism may occur but only when fat stores are depleted)* Protein loss caused by diuresis **DEFINING CHARACTERISTICS** Weight loss Ketoacidosis Hyperglycemia Abdominal discomfort Flushed skin Nausea/vomiting Diuresis	**ONGOING ASSESSMENTS** · Obtain weight; compare with usual weight if possible. · Assess skin condition, turgor. · Assess for muscle wasting, weakness. · Assess dietary habits, especially for new onset diabetic. · Monitor I & O. · Monitor urine for sugar and protein. · Monitor blood sugar routinely once DKA resolved. **THERAPEUTIC INTERVENTIONS** · Administer insulin (short-acting) *to enable glucose transport to cells. Glucose metabolism for energy requirements spares fat and protein for cell growth and maintenance and allows fat/protein storage.* · Notify physician when serum glucose has dropped to 250 to 300 mg/dl. *(At this time glucose IV should be administered and insulin therapy halted to prevent hypoglycemia and cerebral edema).* · Provide oral intaken when nausea and vomiting abate and LOC has stabilized. · Obtain dietary consultation. · Provide instruction on American Dietetic Association meal planning when oral nutrition tolerated and IV discontinued. · Continue to administer subcutaneous insulin on routine, daily basis to prevent recurrence of DKA. · Allow patient to test own blood sugar, self-administer insulin, and make menu selections when able. · See Diabetes, insulin-dependent, p. 372.	Optimal nutrition will be maintained.

Knowledge deficit
Related to:
Unfamiliarity with disease process and treatment
Noncompliance with medications, testing of urine and blood, and follow-up care
 	
DEFINING CHARACTERISTICS
Unawareness of factors leading to ketoacidosis
Verbalized lack of knowledge
Questions about ketoacidosis
	ONGOING ASSESSMENTS:
	· Assess understanding of causes and consequences of diabetic ketoacidosis.
	· Assess other factors that may contribute to inability to understand explanations:
	    Anxiety
	    Denial of illness
	
	THERAPEUTIC INTERVENTIONS
	· Explain to patient/significant others:
	    Symptoms of early acute diabetic ketoacidosis (drowsiness, nausea, vomiting, flushed skin, thirst, excessive urination, glycosuria, ketonuria). *Patient and family must identify signs/symptoms of impending hyperglycemia/ketoacidosis to prevent complications and future hospitalizations.*
	    Factors that predispose patient to diabetic ketoacidosis (illness, stress, infection, insufficient insulin, decreased activity and exercise).
	    Importance of balanced diet, routine exercise, weight control, accurate medication administration, regular urine ketone and blood testing, and follow-up care.
		Patient/significant others will demonstrate knowledge of disease process and importance of medications, urine and blood testings.

NURSING DIAGNOSES / DEFINING CHARACTERISTICS	NURSING INTERVENTIONS / *RATIONALES*	EXPECTED OUTCOMES

	Management of diabetes during other illness:
	    Importance of taking insulin even if feeling ill and not eating.
	    Appropriate diet and insulin dosage modifications.
	    Physician informed of status.
	    Frequent testing for ketonuria and hypoglycemia/hyperglycemia.
	Refer to Diabetes, insulin-dependent, p. 372.	

Originated by: Nola D. Johnson, RN
            Charlotte Niznik, RN, BSN, CDE

Diabetic patient with recurrent hypoglycemia/ hyperglycemia

(DIABETES MELLITUS)

Diabetes mellitus is a heterogenous group of clinical syndromes characterized by hyperglycemia, which is related to inadequate metabolism of glucose. The potential for development of hypoglycemia is related to an imbalance between insulin need and insulin dose. Both complications are beset with their own characteristics, symptoms, and management. When diabetes is successfully regulated, patients can successfully prevent these complications.

NURSING DIAGNOSES / DEFINING CHARACTERISTICS	NURSING INTERVENTIONS / *RATIONALES*	EXPECTED OUTCOMES

Altered health maintenance
Related to:
Altered or impaired communication
Perceptual/cognitive impairments
Complete/partial lack of necessary motor skills
Ineffective coping
Anxiety/fear
Lack of interest/ motivation
Lack of unfamiliarity with resources
 	
DEFINING CHARACTERISTICS
 	
Expressed lack of knowledge of basic health practices
Reported or observed inability to take/meet responsibility for health needs
Demonstrated lack of adaptive behaviors to environmental changes
	ONGOING ASSESSMENT
	▪ Assess all past patterns of health maintenance and health concepts.
	▪ Assess knowledge, perception, and management specific to diabetes mellitus.
	▪ Assess ability/willingness to learn about the condition:
	    Medications: oral agents versus insulin injections
	    Dietary management
	    Monitoring, control, and management of symptoms of acute/chronic complications
	
	THERAPEUTIC INTERVENTIONS
	▪ Offer guidance and support in realistic problem identification and solving.
	▪ Review past/present medical history *to identify need for maintenance and management of diabetes.*
	▪ Identify and assume appropriate responsibilities with regard to management of diabetes *to prevent hypoglycemic/hyperglycemic reactions.*
	▪ Encourage verbalization to allay fear and anxiety.
	▪ Provide appropriate guidelines for future health maintenance.
	▪ Facilitate referrals (e.g., financial counseling, social work staff, diabetes teaching service, visiting nurse) *to promote health maintenance. Some patients require psychological consults to work through denial, or self-destructive behavior.*
		Progress toward assumption of adequate health maintenance will be noted.

Continued.

NURSING DIAGNOSES / DEFINING CHARACTERISTICS	NURSING INTERVENTIONS / *RATIONALES*	EXPECTED OUTCOMES
Reported or observed lack of help-seeking behavior and/or impairment of personal support system Expressed need for outside resources		
Knowledge deficit *Related to:* Need for information about hyperglycemia/hypoglycemia **DEFINING CHARACTERISTICS** Expresses need for more information Lack of questions Confusion over signs and symptoms of hyperglycemia/hypoglycemia Inappropriate behavior (e.g., anger, hostility, withdrawal, apathy) Inadequate demonstration or absence of follow-through on previous instruction	**ONGOING ASSESSMENT** · Assess knowledge of diabetes mellitus, specifically hypoglycemia and hyperglycemia. · Observe for evidence of altered mental status/other impairments to learning. **THERAPEUTIC INTERVENTIONS** · Guide patient in performing blood glucose monitoring (BG Chemstrip). 　*Blood glucose monitoring tests must be performed with extreme accuracy. Manufacturer's instructions must be followed exactly because test results often determine dietary changes, need for oral hypoglycemic agent modification, and insulin dosage.* · Instruct patient in recognition of signs/symptoms of altered glucose metabolism: 　*Hypoglycemia:* hunger, sweating, pallor, tremor, feelings of nervousness or anxiety, lethargy, irritability, tingling or numbness in lips or tongue (early), blurred or double vision, mental dullness, change in behavior, fatigue, confusion, dizziness, slurred speech, slow or uncoordinated movement (gradual). 　*Hyperglycemia:* polydipsia, polyphagia, polyuria, nocturia, nausea, vomiting, dim or blurred vision, headache (early), abdominal pain, GI cramps, constipation, drowsiness, headache, weakness, flushed/dry skin, rapid labored or deep breathing, weak rapid pulse, elevated temperature, acetone breath odor, hypotension, coma (gradual). *Overall goal of patient care is to regulate glucose levels (to decrease risk of complications.) Secondary goal is to disrupt patient's life as little as possible with management regimens.* · Instruct patient/family about treatment regimen for altered glucose levels. 　Hypoglycemia: 　　10-15 g carbohydrate administered *to raise blood glucose levels to target range 70-110 mg/dl.* Source: 4 oz fruit juice, 2 tsp. honey, 5 life savers, or 1 glass soft drink. 　　If no response to treatment, oral carbohydrate may be repeated. 　　IV glucose source may be required. 　Hyperglycemia: 　　If patient conscious, sugar-free fluids taken; *water decreases hyperosmolar state.* 　　Blood specimens obtained *to monitor glucose functions.* 　　Parenteral fluids/insulin may be required *to decrease glucose levels and replace fluids. When diabetes successfully regulated, patient avoids complications of hyperglycemia/hypoglycemia.* 　　Reinforce information provided by diabetic teaching service/physician/other nursing staff. 　　Provide patient variety of resources in diabetes education as appropriate *to ensure health maintenance and diabetes control.*	Patient will understand hypoglycemia and hyperglycemia and can manage episodes effectively at home.

Originated by: Eileen Raebig, RN, C

Excessive glucocorticoids

(CUSHING'S SYNDROME)

The overproduction of cortisol, the primary glucocorticoid from the adrenal cortex. The numerous clinical features present in glucocorticoid excess are featured in Cushing's syndrome.

NURSING DIAGNOSES / DEFINING CHARACTERISTICS	NURSING INTERVENTIONS / *RATIONALES*	EXPECTED OUTCOMES
Potential fluid volume excess *Related to:* Retention of sodium and water caused by mineralocorticoid excess Depletion of potassium caused by mineralocorticoid excess **DEFINING CHARACTERISTICS** Hypertension Hypokalemia Cardiac arrhythmias Signs and symptoms of congestive heart failure (CHF): rales, jugular vein distention Elevated morning plasma cortisol levels with no normal decline as day proceeds Hypernatremia Impaired renal concentrating capacity	**ONGOING ASSESSMENTS** • Assess patient for signs of circulatory overload, CHF, and pulmonary congestion. • Monitor and record heart rate, BP, CVP, and respiratory rate. • Assess pulse for regularity. • Monitor and record I & O. • Assess patient for signs of muscle weakness. • Assess ECG for appearance of U wave. • Weigh patient daily and record. *Excessive corticoid secretion predisposes patient to fluid and sodium retention.* • Auscultate lungs and heart; notify physician of abnormalities. • Monitor lab work (especially potassium and sodium). **THERAPEUTIC INTERVENTIONS** • Encourage diet low in calories, carbohydrates, and sodium, with ample protein and potassium *to help control development of hyperglycemia, edema, and hyperkalemia.*	Fluid volume balance will be maintained.
Potential fluid volume deficit *Related to:* Glycosuria-induced diuresis, leading to intravascular depletion secondary to excessive secretion of glucocorticoids **DEFINING CHARACTERISTICS** Decreased urine output Increased urine specific gravity Urine output greater than input Sudden weight loss Hemoconcentration Increased serum sodium	**ONGOING ASSESSMENT** • Assess for presence of Defining Characteristics. **THERAPEUTIC INTERVENTIONS** • See Fluid volume deficit, p. 20.	Fluid volume and electrolyte balance will be maintained.

Continued.

NURSING DIAGNOSES / DEFINING CHARACTERISTICS	NURSING INTERVENTIONS / *RATIONALES*	EXPECTED OUTCOMES
Poor skin turgor Hypotension Dry mucous membranes		

NURSING DIAGNOSES / DEFINING CHARACTERISTICS	NURSING INTERVENTIONS / *RATIONALES*	EXPECTED OUTCOMES
Potential for infection *Related to:* Increased cortisol secretion keeping body in chronic stress state Increased cortisol suppresses leukocyte adherence to endothelial surface Increased cortisol decreases leukocyte accumulation at injury site Increased cortisol impairs WBC migration, antibody formation, and lymphocyte proliferation Increased cortisol increases protein breakdown **DEFINING CHARACTERISTICS** Increased temperature Increased white blood cells Local inflammation, redness, or abnormal drainage Positive culture results (blood, wound, sputum, or urine) Thin skin	**ONGOING ASSESSMENT** • Assess potential infection sites: urinary, pulmonary, wound or IV line. • Monitor and record temperature. • Monitor WBC count. • Note signs of localized or systemic infection, report promptly. • Assess for signs of skin breakdown. • Obtain specimens of blood, urine, serum, etc., for culture and sensitivity if infection suspected. **THERAPEUTIC INTERVENTIONS** • Use strict aseptic technique when performing dressing changes, wound irrigations, catheter care, or suctioning. • Avoid use of indwelling catheters or IV lines whenever possible. *Limited immune response predisposes patients to infection. Avoidance of catheters, IV lines decreases risk of potential infection.* • Protect patient from exposure to other patients with infections. • Administer antibiotics as ordered. • Protect patient from bumping and bruising. Change patient's position. *Protection from injury decreases susceptibility to infection.* • Pad bony prominences. *Protection/position changes promote peripheral tissue perfusion.* • Keep skin clean and dry. • If needed, see Skin integrity, impaired, p. 48.	Potential for injury will be reduced.
Potential for injury: fracture *Related to:* As protein catabolism increases, protein synthesis decreases, leading to osteoporosis from bone matrix wasting. In children can lead to retarded linear growth	**ONGOING ASSESSMENT** • Assess patient's ability to ambulate; observe gait. • Observe for loss of muscle mass and osteoporosis after minor trauma. • Assess patient for signs of kyphosis or height loss. • Assess fat distribution. • Measure actual height at time of admission; compare with past medical records. *Identifies possibility of minor fractures, disk or hip injury.* **THERAPEUTIC INTERVENTIONS** • Keep floor in patient's room clean, dry, and uncluttered to *decrease risk for injury.* • Encourage use of cane or walker if patient's gait unsteady. Provide necessary aids *to promote independence with mobility.*	Potential for fractures will be reduced.

NURSING DIAGNOSES / DEFINING CHARACTERISTICS	NURSING INTERVENTIONS / *RATIONALES*	EXPECTED OUTCOMES
Chronic cortisol hypersecretion redistributing body fat	• Encourage the patient to wear properly fitted low-heeled shoes. • Notify physician of even minor trauma.	
DEFINING CHARACTERISTICS Awkward, poorly coordinated movement Abnormal fat distribution: fat from arms and legs deposited on back, shoulder, trunk, and abdomen. *Chronic cortisol hypersecretion redistributes body fat* Kyphosis or height loss		
Body image disturbance *Related to:* Increased production of androgens may occur, giving rise to virilism in women; hirsutism (abnormal growth of hair) Disturbed protein metabolism results in muscle wasting, capillary fragility, and wasting of bone matrix: ecchymosis, osteoporosis, slender limbs, striae (usually purple) Abnormal fat distribution along with edema resulting in moon face, cervicodorsal fat (buffalo hump), trunk obesity	**ONGOING ASSESSMENT** • Assess for presence of Defining Characteristics. **THERAPEUTIC INTERVENTIONS** • See Body image disturbance, p. 6.	Body image will be enhanced.
DEFINING CHARACTERISTICS Verbal identification of feeling about altered body structure Verbal preoccupation with changed body Refusal to discuss or acknowledge change		

Continued.

NURSING DIAGNOSES / DEFINING CHARACTERISTICS	NURSING INTERVENTIONS / RATIONALES	EXPECTED OUTCOMES
Actual change in body structure Change in social behavior (withdrawal, isolation, flamboyancy) Compensatory use of concealing clothing, other devices		
Knowledge deficit *Related to:* Lack of experience with excessive glucocorticoids **DEFINING CHARACTERISTICS** Questioning, especially if repetitive Silence Anxiety Repeated hospital admissions for complications Verbalized misconceptions	**ONGOING ASSESSMENT** • Assess level of knowledge of Cushing's syndrome. • Assess patient's: 　Resources 　Strengths and weaknesses • Assess for Defining Characteristics. **THERAPEUTIC INTERVENTIONS** • Explain all tests to patient. *Patient/family must understand disease process and receive specific instructions related to treatment, methods to control symptoms, signs of infections, complications, and indicators of when to notify physician.* • Answer all questions honestly. • Explain methods, rationale, and expected effects of appropriate treatment: 　Surgery 　Radiation *(may be used to combat nonoperable tumors)* 　Drug therapy *(replacement may be temporary or permanent)* 　Diet restrictions	Patient will discuss treatment options and ask appropriate questions.

Originated by: Cathy Croke, RN, MSN
　　　　　　　 Charlotte Niznik, RN, BSN, CDE

Hepatitis

(HAV; HBV; SERUM HEPATITIS; INFECTIOUS HEPATITIS)

Inflammation of the liver caused by a virus. Type A (HAV) infectious hepatitis is commonly transmitted by fecal-oral route, poor sanitation, person-to-person contact, or contaminated food, water, or shellfish. Type B (HBV) serum hepatitis is commonly transmitted parenterally or by intimate contact with carriers; by blood, saliva, semen, and vaginal secretions; via contaminated needles and renal dialysis. Manifestations are more severe than those of type A. Administration of chemical substances that have damaging effects on the liver may result in hepatitislike syndrome.

NURSING DIAGNOSES / DEFINING CHARACTERISTICS	NURSING INTERVENTIONS / RATIONALES	EXPECTED OUTCOMES
Activity intolerance *Related to:* Decreased fat, carbohydrate, and protein metabolism and use	**ONGOING ASSESSMENTS** • Assess respiratory status before activity: 　Respiratory rate 　Use of accessory muscles 　Need for supplemental O_2	Activity tolerance will be maximized.

NURSING DIAGNOSES / DEFINING CHARACTERISTICS	NURSING INTERVENTIONS / *RATIONALES*	EXPECTED OUTCOMES

DEFINING CHARACTERISTICS
Patient report of fatigue and weakness
Abnormal respiratory responses to activity
Abnormal cardiac response to activity
	• Assess cardiac status before activity:
	    Pulse rate
	    Cardiac rhythm
	    BP
	    Skin color and perfusion
	• Assess need for ambulation aids.
	• Assess patient's/significant others' understanding of change in activity level and tolerance.
	• Monitor patient for signs of relapse precipitated by premature activity:
	    Increasing serum enzymes
	    Increasing anorexia
	    Increasing liver tenderness
	    These signs indicate poor healing or exacerbation of disease.
	
	THERAPEUTIC INTERVENTIONS
	• Maintain bed rest with bathroom privileges *so available energy is used for healing.*
	• Provide quiet environment *to promote rest and healing.*
	• Limit visitors.
	• Help patient learn relaxation.
	• Plan nursing care to *provide long rest periods.*
	• Medicate with sedatives or tranquilizers as ordered *to promote adequate rest.*
	• Increase activity levels as tolerated.	

Altered nutrition: less than body requirements
Related to:
Alteration in nutrient absorption
Alteration in nutrient metabolism
Decreased nutrient intake
 	
DEFINING CHARACTERISTICS
Loss of weight with or without adequate calorie intake
Documented inadequate calorie intake
Increased metabolic need not met by caloric intake
Anorexia
Nausea/vomiting
	ONGOING ASSESSMENTS
	• Document patient's actual weight.
	• Obtain nutritional history.
	• Obtain baseline laboratory values *to assess nutritional state:*
	    Serum protein
	    Serum albumin
	    Vitamin assays (as appropriate)
	    Mineral and trace element levels (as appropriate)
	    Serum osmolarity
	    Skin test for cellular immune response
	
	THERAPEUTIC INTERVENTIONS
	• Maintain bed rest *to decrease metabolic needs.*
	• Increase activity as patient tolerates.
	• Provide diet with:
	    High carbohydrates; fats and protein modified as patient tolerates. *Carbohydrates administered in anticipation of increased metabolic needs.*
	    Small meals *(large meals more difficult to tolerate with anorexia).*
	    Largest meal at breakfast *(anorexia often worsens during day).*
	• Give antiemetics before meals *to decrease nausea and increase food tolerance.*
	• Encourage patient to take fruit juice, carbonated beverages.
	• Avoid alcoholic beverages *(cause hepatic irritation).*
	• Administer vitamin supplements or parenteral nutrition as ordered.
	• See Nutrition, altered: less than body requirements, p. 37.
		Optimal nutritional status will be maintained.

Fluid volume deficit
Related to:
Vomiting
Diarrhea
Decreased dietary intake
	ONGOING ASSESSMENTS
	• Monitor I & O every shift.
	• Check weight daily. Note enteric losses of fluid (e.g., vomiting, diarrhea) *to determine fluid balance and plan for replacement.*
	• Monitor:
	    Serum sodium and osmolarity *to determine hydration status*
	    Total protein and serum albumin *to determine oncotic pressure*
	• Check for edema.
	• Monitor for signs/symptoms of dehydration.
		Fluid volume deficit will be reduced.

Continued.

NURSING DIAGNOSES / DEFINING CHARACTERISTICS	NURSING INTERVENTIONS / *RATIONALES*	EXPECTED OUTCOMES
DEFINING CHARACTERISTICS Decreased urine output Concentrated urine Hemoconcentration Increased serum sodium Thirst Edema Dry mucous membranes Decreased pulse pressure Increased heart rate	**THERAPEUTIC INTERVENTIONS** · Encourage oral intake of fluids. · Administer enteral and parenteral fluids as ordered *to supplement oral replacement and compensate for losses.* · See Fluid volume deficit, p. 20.	
Potential constipation/ diarrhea *Related to:* Alteration in dietary intake Alteration in digestive processes Decreased activity level **DEFINING CHARACTERISTICS** *Constipation:* Straining at stool Passage of liquid feces around impaction Abdominal distention Nausea/vomiting Fecal incontinence *Diarrhea:* Frequency of stool Loose/liquid stool Urgency Abdominal pain Hyperactive bowel sounds	**ONGOING ASSESSMENT** · Establish patient's history of elimination. · Determine whether patient uses medications to provide regular elimination. · Observe stool for color, consistency, frequency, amount. **THERAPEUTIC INTERVENTIONS** · Provide adequate dietary and fluid intake *to promote normal stool consistence.* · Administer medications for diarrhea or constipation as ordered. · See Diarrhea, p. 16, or Constipation, p. 12.	Normal bowel function will be maintained.

Impaired skin integrity
Related to:
Accumulation of bile salts in skin
Prolonged bed rest
Mechanical forces associated with bed rest (pressure, shearing)
Frequent diarrhea
Poor nutritional status
	ONGOING ASSESSMENT
	· Check skin for signs of breakdown or presence of lesions.
	· Assess nutritional status: diet, laboratory data, weight.
	
	THERAPEUTIC INTERVENTIONS
	· Position patient at least q2h *to prevent pressure lesions.*
	· Use pressure-relieving devices as necessary (see Skin integrity, impaired, p. 48).
	· For itching:
	    Encourage cool shower or bath with baking soda.
	    Use calamine lotion.
	    Administer antihistamines as ordered.
	    Keep fingernails short.
	    Provide patient with gloves *(prevent further injury from scratching).*
		Trauma to skin will be reduced.

NURSING DIAGNOSES / DEFINING CHARACTERISTICS	NURSING INTERVENTIONS / *RATIONALES*	EXPECTED OUTCOMES
DEFINING CHARACTERISTICS Itching Disruption of skin surface		
Potential diversional activity deficit *Related to:* Isolation **DEFINING CHARACTERISTICS** Verbal complaints of boredom Verbal reports of "feeling isolated" Pacing Daydreaming Excessive napping	**ONGOING ASSESSMENTS** • Assess tolerated activity level. • Solicit desire for activities/social contact. **THERAPEUTIC INTERVENTIONS** • Encourage expression of feelings about isolation. • Encourage use of radio, television, newspapers, telephone, calendar, photographs *to provide diversional activity.* • Plan nursing intervention *to provide contact throughout day.* • Encourage family members/friends to visit as tolerated.	Boredom and feelings of isolation will be reduced.
Knowledge deficit *Related to:* New condition Unfamiliartiy with treatment and disease course **DEFINING CHARACTERISTICS** Lack of questions Many questions Noncompliance with isolation procedure	**ONGOING ASSESSMENTS** • Determine patient's/significant others' understanding of disease process, complications, and treatment. • Determine understanding of disease transmission. • Assess understanding of information after teaching session. • Observe compliance with treatment regimen. • Observe compliance with isolation procedures *to determine level of understanding.* • Observe development of complications (e.g., exhaustion or relapse). **THERAPEUTIC INTERVENTIONS** • Give patient/significant others information about disease and isolation procedures. • Encourage patient/significant others to ask questions. • Assist patient in understanding need to avoid blood donation *to prevent disease transmission.* • See Knowledge deficit, p. 33.	Patient/significant others will demonstrate knowledge of and compliance with treatment regimen and isolation procedures.

Originated by: Martha Dickerson, RN, MS, CCRN

Hypercalcemia

An electrolyte imbalance that occurs when the bones release more calcium into the extracellular fluid than can be excreted in the urine. Hypercalcemia is often seen after bone destruction from an invasive metastasis. Other causes include multiple myeloma, sarcoidosis, tumor production of vitamin D-like substances, and hyperthyroidism.

NURSING DIAGNOSES / DEFINING CHARACTERISTICS	NURSING INTERVENTIONS / *RATIONALES*	EXPECTED OUTCOMES

Potential for injury *Related to:* Increased circulatory concentrations of calcium **DEFINING CHARACTERISTICS** *Central nervous system:* Depressed or absent deep tendon reflexes, drowsiness, lethargy, confusion, blurred vision, coma *Muscular system:* Fatigue, hypotonia, weakness, GI atony, anorexia, nausea, vomiting, abdominal pain *Skeletal system:* Bone pain, osteoporosis, pathologic fractures *Cardiovascular system:* Arrhythmias, bradycardia, shortened QT intervals, cardiac arrest	**ONGOING ASSESSMENTS**
	• Monitor laboratory values: calcium and other electrolytes (e.g., sodium, potassium, and magnesium, which are excreted with calcium).
	• Monitor renal status: BUN and creatinine levels.
	• Assess general appearance:
	  Level of consciousness (LOC)
	  Skin turgor
	  Activity and mobility levels
	  Appetite
	• Check patient's medical history related to cancer and drug therapy.
	• Monitor for drug therapy side effects.
	• Maintain accurate I & O.
	• Weigh daily.
	• Assess vital signs and neurologic status.
	
	THERAPEUTIC INTERVENTIONS
	• Reduce calcium by:
	  Promoting renal calcium excretion:
	    Saline hydration
	    Administration of loop diuretics (e.g., furosemide)
	    Use of acidic juices (e.g., cranberry and prune) *to dissolve calcium salts*
	  Decreasing calcium absorption:
	    Inhibit bone resorption through administration of glucocorticoids, cytotoxic antibiotics (e.g., plicamycin), calcitonin, decreased vitamin D intake. *For calcitonin therapy, keep epinephrine at bedside in case of anaphylactic reaction.*
	  Decreasing intestinal absorption of calcium:
	    Diets low or absent in calcium
	    Phosphate supplements
	• Administer IV fluids and drugs as ordered.
		Calcium balance will return to normal.

Potential fluid volume excess/deficit *Related to:* Fluid therapy Diuretic therapy **DEFINING CHARACTERISTICS** *Excess:* Acute weight gain Edema Moist rales upon lung auscultation Shortness of breath Puffy eyelids Decreased LOC, confusion *Deficit:* Acute weight loss Decreased body temperature	**ONGOING ASSESSMENTS** • Assess skin turgor; observe for dryness, swelling, or flushing. • Assess eyes for puffiness or dryness. • Monitor vital signs. • Assess lung sounds for rales *(indicate fluid overload)*. Observe character of respirations: rate, rhythm, depth, use of accessory muscles. • Palpate bladder for distention or urinary retention. Also observe for incontinence, pain, or increasing tenderness. • Monitor CVP. • Maintain I & O. • Check weight daily. • Monitor electrolytes, particularily potassium. • Assess for signs/symptoms of potassium deficiency/excess (e.g., anorexia, ileus, weakness, diarrhea, colic, intestinal irritability, and nausea). **THERAPEUTIC INTERVENTIONS** • Administer diuretic drugs to eliminate unnecessary fluid *which may cause cardiopulmonary complications.* • Insert Foley catheter *to assist in maintaining accurate I & O.* • Replace electrolytes with supplements. *Some electrolytes lost during diuretic therapy.* • See Fluid volume deficit, p. 20.	Hazards of fluid/ electrolyte imbalance will be reduced.

Hypercalcemia— cont'd

NURSING DIAGNOSES / DEFINING CHARACTERISTICS	NURSING INTERVENTIONS / *RATIONALES*	EXPECTED OUTCOMES
Dry skin and mucous membranes Longitudinal wrinkles Furrows of tongue Oliguria Anuria		
Potential altered levels of consciousness *Related to:* Hypercalcemia Fluid/electrolyte imbalance **DEFINING CHARACTERISTICS** Lethargy Restlessness Coma	**ONGOING ASSESSMENT** • Observe for changes in LOC. **THERAPEUTIC INTERVENTIONS** • Reassure patient during changes in LOC *to promote comfort and alleviate anxiety.* • See Consciousness, altered level of, p. 234.	Optimal LOC will be maintained.

Potential impaired physical mobility
Related to:
Decreased LOC
Bone pain
Hypotonia
 	
DEFINING CHARACTERISTICS
Presence of pain on movement
Stiffness of joints
Inability to perform active movements with or without assistance
Decreased intake of fluid and foods
	ONGOING ASSESSMENTS
	• Assess character, nature, and location of pain.
	• Assess skin, joint, and muscle integrity:
	  Check pressure areas for skin breakdown.
	  Check joints for ROM.
	  Check muscle for tone and loss of muscle mass.
	• Check patient's activity level.
	
	THERAPEUTIC INTERVENTIONS
	• Decrease bone pain:
	  Medicate with analgesics as needed; record response to medication.
	  Provide assistance and support if pain present on movement. *Pain restricts activity and decreases participation in therapy. Activity improves circulation and prevents pressure sores.*
	• Prevent contractures and decubitus ulcers by:
	  Providing assistance with ADL, ROM exercises, turning, ambulation.
	  Using assistive devices (e.g., pillows, footboards, air or water mattress, and Stryker boots) *to protect pressure points and reduce risk of decubitus.*
	• Keep side rails up, especially at night, *to protect against injury from falls.*
	• Leave small light on.
	• Use restraints as needed *to promote safety.*
	• Avoid backrubs *to prevent pathologic fractures.*
	• Establish and maintain regular turning schedule *to alleviate pressure points, improve tissue perfusion, and dislodge mucous stasis for mobilization.*
	• Refer patient to occupational therapy for follow-up *to allow optimal activity level.*
		Hazards of immobility will be reduced.

Potential ineffective airway clearance *Related to:* Decreased LOC Impaired mobility **DEFINING CHARACTERISTICS** Mucous plug or mucous stasis	**ONGOING ASSESSMENTS** • Auscultate lungs for presence of diminished breath sounds. • Observe and record character of respiratory rate/rhythm. • Assess LOC. • Assess pulse and blood pressure. **THERAPEUTIC INTERVENTIONS** • Prevent mucous stasis: Encourage increased fluid intake.	Airway will be free of secretions.

Continued.

Hypercalcemia— cont'd

NURSING DIAGNOSES / DEFINING CHARACTERISTICS	NURSING INTERVENTIONS / *RATIONALES*	EXPECTED OUTCOMES
Restlessness Tachycardia Use of accessory muscles Lethargy Buccal/nailbed cyanosis	Provide respiratory therapy (e.g., postural drainage, percussion, and vibration therapy) *to stimulate and mobilize secretions.* Help and supervise patient with regularly scheduled breathing exercises (e.g., diaphragmatic breathing and uses of spirometry *to increase mobility of secretions*). ▪ See Airway clearance, ineffective, p. 3.	
Knowledge deficit *Related to:* Unfamiliarity with cause of hypercalcemia **DEFINING CHARACTERISTICS** Questions from patient/significant others Demanding/ manipulative behavior Inability of patient/ significant others to describe diet or drug therapy	**ONGOING ASSESSMENT** ▪ Assess understanding of disease. ▪ Assess knowledge of therapy. ▪ Assess socioeconomic background. ▪ Assess support systems. **THERAPEUTIC INTERVENTIONS** ▪ Encourage patient/significant other to verbalize feelings/needs or problems: Establish trusting relationship. Maintain privacy during discussions. Show interest and willingness to listen. ▪ Provide health teaching and counseling: Provide information to patient/significant others based on identified needs or problems *to facilitate control of calcium balance.* Stress importance of following strict diet therapy, exercise, increased fluid intake, and drug therapy. Stress importance of keeping regular appointment to monitor/draw serum calcium levels *to prevent exacerbations and complications.* Encourage maximum participation of patient/significant others in total care (e.g., eating, mobility, ROM exercises, and performing ADLs) *to enhance independence, facilitate knowledge of disease process, and encourage calcium balance.*	Patient/family will understand importance of adhering to medical regimen to prevent recurrence of hypercalcemia.

Originated by: Bella Biag, RN, BSN
Charlotte Niznik, RN, BSN, CDE

Hyperglycemic hyperosmotic nonketotic coma (HHNC)

(DIABETIC COMA)

Hyperglycemic hyperosmotic nonketotic coma (HHNC) can be a complication of diabetes but may also result from hyperalimentation, dialysis, IV fluids, steroid therapy, diuretic administration, pancreatitis, diabetes insipidus, and severe burns. The severe hyperglycemia persists because of ineffective or inadequate insulin levels. The hyperglycemia results in osmotic diuresis and severe dehydration.

NURSING DIAGNOSES / DEFINING CHARACTERISTICS	NURSING INTERVENTIONS / *RATIONALES*	EXPECTED OUTCOMES
Fluid volume deficit *Related to:* Hyperglycemia Osmotic diuresis	**ONGOING ASSESSMENT** ▪ Assess for Defining Characteristics: Monitor electrolytes, glucose, I & O, weight, and CVP. Monitor vital signs, Hb, Hct, serum osmolarity, BUN, creatinine *to determine hemoconcentration and renal clearance.* Auscultate lungs for rhonchi, rales (*may result from circulatory overload caused by aggressive fluid therapy*).	Optimal fluid level will be maintained.

NURSING DIAGNOSES / DEFINING CHARACTERISTICS	NURSING INTERVENTIONS / *RATIONALES*	EXPECTED OUTCOMES
DEFINING CHARACTERISTICS Increased urine output Sudden weight loss Hemoconcentration Increased BUN/ creatinine Hypotension Thirst/dry skin and mucous membranes Poor skin turgor Decreased cardiac output Hypokalemia Hypernatremia Change in LOC Ventricular arrhythmias	**THERAPEUTIC INTERVENTIONS** • Administer isotonic IV fluids *to increase cardiac output and tissue perfusion along with correcting fluid imbalance.* • Administer insulin according to blood glucose levels. *Insulin therapy is essential to decrease serum glucose and osmolarity, allow extracellular fluid shift to intracellular fluid, alleviating intracellular dehydration.*	
Altered nutrition: less than body requirements *Related to:* Insulin deficiency Ineffective metabolism of available glucose **DEFINING CHARACTERISTICS** Weight loss Muscle weakness Hyperglycemia Abdominal pain	**ONGOING ASSESSMENT** • Monitor blood glucose levels. • Observe for abdominal pain. *Nausea and vomiting may result from fluid/ electrolyte imbalance as well as ketonemia. Ketonemia is not necessarily present until later in disease course.* **THERAPEUTIC INTERVENTIONS** • Administer continuous low-dose insulin infusion. *Rapid infusion of insulin may result in hypoglycemia.* • Promote nutrition. *When electrolyte and glucose imbalances corrected, appetite is restored.* • Provide fluids and progress diet as tolerated. • Obtain dietary consultation if needed.	Optimal nutrition will be maintained.

Altered level of consciousness
Related to:
Dehydration
Electrolyte imbalance
 	
DEFINING CHARACTERISTICS
Change in orientation, verbal response, motor response, pupillary action
Agitation
Impaired judgment
Seizure activity
Positive Babinski's sign
	ONGOING ASSESSMENT
	• Monitor LOC. Maintain neurologic flow sheet.
	• Monitor vital signs, fluid volume, and electrolyte balance.
	• Assess for potential for injury secondary to seizure activity.
	• See Consciousness, altered level of, p. 234.
	
	THERAPEUTIC INTERVENTIONS
	• Protect from injury caused by impaired neurologic function:
	  Keep side rails up and bed in low position at all times.
	  Maintain oral airway.
	  Reorient patient to surroundings as needed *(patient may be unaware of past events and limitations).*
	• Restore fluid volume. *As dehydration and hyperglycemia resolve, LOC improves.*
		Optimal LOC will be maintained.

Hypergylcemic hyperosmotic nonketotic coma— cont'd

NURSING DIAGNOSES / DEFINING CHARACTERISTICS	NURSING INTERVENTIONS / *RATIONALES*	EXPECTED OUTCOMES
Knowledge deficit *Related to:* Cognitive limitations Lack of interest New condition **DEFINING CHARACTERISTICS** Verbalized interest, questions Statement of misconception Request for information	**ONGOING ASSESSMENT** • Assess for predisposing factors and most current cause. • If patient diabetic, assess level of knowledge and home care practices *to identify factors interfering with health maintenance.* **THERAPEUTIC INTERVENTIONS** • Describe HHNC, its cause and treatment. Explain all procedures. • If the patient diabetic, review effective self-care practices and introduce new information/skills as necessary. *Note:* For more information on diabetes teaching, refer to Diabetes, insulin-dependent, p. 372. • Refer to Health maintenance, altered, p. 26.	Patient will understand current condition, treatment, and preventive measures.

Originated by: Charlotte Niznik, RN, BSN, CDE
     Michele Knoll Puzas, RN,C, MHPE

Syndrome of inappropriate antidiuretic hormone (SIADH)

(DILUTIONAL HYPONATREMIA)

A syndrome characterized by the continued synthesis and release of antidiuretic hormone (ADH) unrelated to plasma osmolarity; water retention and dilutional hyponatremia occur. Potential etiologies include head trauma, brain tumor, subarachnoid hemorrhage, and systemic cancer.

NURSING DIAGNOSES / DEFINING CHARACTERISTICS	NURSING INTERVENTIONS / *RATIONALES*	EXPECTED OUTCOMES
Fluid volume excess *Related to:* Compromised endocrine regulatory mechanisms Neurohypophysial dysfunction Inappropriate ADH syndrome Excessive fluid intake Renal failure Steroid therapy **DEFINING CHARACTERISTICS** Intake greatly exceeding output Sudden weight gain Cellular edema Absence of peripheral edema Cerebral edema	**ONGOING ASSESSMENT** • Carefully monitor intake and output and urine specific gravity. • Weigh daily: *a sudden weight gain of 2.2 lb can indicate retention of 1 L water. SIADH patients can retain 3-5 L.* • Assess patient for: Apprehension Confusion Muscle twitches Convulsions Nausea/vomiting Abdominal cramps • Assess for signs of cerebral edema: Headache Decreased mental status Seizures Vomiting • Check for fingerprint edema over sternum, reflecting cellular edema. *Peripheral edema absent because fluid not retained in interstitium.* • Monitor for symptoms of increased ICP (e.g., slow bounding pulse, increased pulse pressure).	Fluid volume and serum sodium and osmolarity are within normal limits.

NURSING DIAGNOSES / DEFINING CHARACTERISTICS	NURSING INTERVENTIONS / *RATIONALES*	EXPECTED OUTCOMES
Hyponatremia Water intoxication	• Monitor for symptoms of water intoxication (e.g., increase in mentation, confusion, incoordination). *Brain cells particularly sensitive to increased intracellular H_2O.* • Monitor serum Na^+ and serum osmolality. **THERAPEUTIC INTERVENTIONS** • Restrict fluid intake to 1-1.5 L/day. • Provide ice chips and frequent mouth care *to alleviate thirst.*	
Potential for injury *Related to:* Change in mentation secondary to water intoxication Seizure activity secondary to hyponatremia **DEFINING CHARACTERISTICS** Confusion Convulsions Lack of coordination	**ONGOING ASSESSMENT** • Assess LOC, orientation, and mental status. • Assess serum Na^+ levels *(normal: 135-145 mg/L).* When serum Na^+ level drops below 118, seizure activity may occur.* **THERAPEUTIC INTERVENTIONS** • Maintain bed in low position, side rails up. • Maintain Posey vest/soft restraints as indicated. • Provide assistance/supervision with ambulation. • See Seizure activity p. 263.	Potential for physical injury will be reduced.
Potential diarrhea *Related to:* Fluid volume excess **DEFINING CHARACTERISTICS** Loose, watery stools Increased stool frequency Increased bowel sounds Urgency	**ONGOING ASSESSMENT** • Assess usual bowel habits and patterns. • Assess for deviations from normal. • Assess characteristics of stool (i.e., color, consistency, amount). • Assess bowel sounds. • Include number of stools on I & O record. **THERAPEUTIC INTERVENTIONS** • Instruct patient to report episodes of diarrhea. • Administer medications as ordered; observe and report effectiveness. • Observe and report skin condition. *Frequent diarrhea stools may lead to irritation and excoriation.* • See Diarrhea, p. 16.	Bowel elimination will be established.
Potential constipation *Related to:* Fluid restriction Decreased motility secondary to hyponatremia **DEFINING CHARACTERISTICS** Frequency and volume less than usual pattern Straining at stool Hard, formed stools	**ONGOING ASSESSMENT** • Assess usual bowel habits and patterns. • Assess for deviations from normal. • Assess characteristics of stool, (i.e., color, consistency, amount). **THERAPEUTIC INTERVENTIONS** • Administer medications as ordered; observe and report effectiveness. • Provide adequate bulk in diet. • Encourage regular time for elimination. • See Constipation, p. 12.	Normal bowel elimination will be achieved.
Potential altered thought processes *Related to:* Severe hyponatremia	**ONGOING ASSESSMENT** • Monitor for LOC changes, confusion q2h. *This is early neurologic sign.* • Assess serum Na^+ levels. *Neurologic signs in patient with head injury may be caused by hyponatremia.*	Thought processes will return to normal.

Continued.

NURSING DIAGNOSES / DEFINING CHARACTERISTICS	NURSING INTERVENTIONS / *RATIONALES*	EXPECTED OUTCOMES
DEFINING CHARACTERISTICS If serum Na = 115-120 mg/L: Lethargy Personality changes If serum Na$^+$ <115 mg/L: Loss of reflexes Coma	• Monitor for disorientation, hostility, decreased deep tendon reflexes, drowsiness, lethargy, headache. **THERAPEUTIC INTERVENTIONS** • Administer hypertonic saline solution as ordered. • Reduce environmental stimuli that patient may find confusing. • Explain reasons for altered thought processes to family/significant others. • See Thought processes, altered, p. 52.	

Potential pain/ discomfort *Related to:* Stomach cramps secondary to hyponatremia Increased thirst secondary to fluid restriction Headache secondary to cerebral edema
 	
DEFINING CHARACTERISTICS Verbal/nonverbal communication of pain or discomfort Diaphoresis BP/pulse rate increased Pupillary dilation Increased/decreased respirations
	ONGOING ASSESSMENT
	• Assess characteristics of pain/discomfort: location, duration, quality, intensity.
	• Assess effective sources of relief for patient's pain/discomfort.
	
	THERAPEUTIC INTERVENTIONS
	• Alleviate etiologies of discomfort:
	   Continue measures to correct fluid volume excess and hyponatremia.
	   Offer ice chips and frequent mouth care *(help alleviate thirst)*.
	• See Pain, p. 39.
		Discomfort is relieved.

Altered nutrition: less than body requirements *Related to:* Anorexia Nausea Vomiting Abdominal cramps secondary to hyponatremia **DEFINING CHARACTERISTICS** Body weight 20 percent or more below ideal for height and frame Inadequate food intake	**ONGOING ASSESSMENT** • Assess nutritional intake. • Assess for nausea/vomiting. • Assess height, weight, and dietary needs. • Assess usual dietary pattern. • Assess food preferences. **THERAPEUTIC INTERVENTIONS** • Provide food preferences within prescribed diet limits. • If vomiting occurs, record amount and characteristics. • Refer to dietitian. *Collaboration increases effectiveness of dietary management.* • See Nutrition, altered: less than body requirements, p. 37.	Adequate nutritional intake.
Potential altered skin integrity *Related to:* Diarrhea Inadequate nutrition	**ONGOING ASSESSMENT** • Inspect skin every shift; document condition and changes. *Early detection and intervention may prevent further impairment.*	Skin integrity will be maintained.

NURSING DIAGNOSES / DEFINING CHARACTERISTICS	NURSING INTERVENTIONS / *RATIONALES*	EXPECTED OUTCOMES
DEFINING CHARACTERISTICS Frequent episodes of diarrhea Poor hygiene Inadequate access to BR/commode/bedpan Inadequate nutritional intake	• Assess frequency of diarrhea, need for hygiene, continence, proximity to BR/commode/bedpan. • Assess other risks to patient's skin integrity (e.g., immobility, urinary incontinence). **THERAPEUTIC INTERVENTIONS** • Provide easy access to BR/commode/bedpan. • Provide hygiene after every episode of diarrhea. • See Skin integrity, impaired, p. 48.	
Fear/anxiety *Related to:* Fluid restrictions Changes in mentation GI symptoms Medications and treatments **DEFINING CHARACTERISTICS** Restlessness Increased questioning Withdrawal Excessive demands	**ONGOING ASSESSMENT** • Assess level of anxiety/fear. • Assess usual coping strategies. **THERAPEUTIC INTERVENTIONS** • Encourage patient to verbalize feelings *to aid in assessment, make patient aware of own feelings.* • See Fear, p. 18, and Anxiety, p. 4.	Fear/anxiety is reduced.
Knowledge deficit *Related to:* New disease process Unfamiliarity with medications and treatments **DEFINING CHARACTERISTICS** Request for information Verbalized misconceptions/ misinterpretations	**ONGOING ASSESSMENT** • Assess level of knowledge of disease process. • Assess level of understanding of medications and treatments. **THERAPEUTIC INTERVENTIONS** • Explain patient's condition/treatments in simple, brief terms to patient/ family/significant others. • Ask patient/family/significant others to verbalize explanations of condition/ treatments *(will indicate misconceptions or misinterpretations)*. • See Knowledge deficit, p. 33.	Patient will understand disease process and rationale for medications and treatments.

Originated by: Mary Ann Naccarato, RN, BSN

Thyroidectomy

Surgical removal of the thyroid gland performed for benign or malignant tumor, hyperthyroidism, thyrotoxicosis, or thyroiditis.

NURSING DIAGNOSES / DEFINING CHARACTERISTICS	NURSING INTERVENTIONS / *RATIONALES*	EXPECTED OUTCOMES

Ineffective airway clearance *Related to:* Hematoma Laryngeal edema Vocal cord paralysis Tracheal collapse **DEFINING CHARACTERISTICS** Neck swelling, tightness Stridor, dyspnea, cyanosis Intercostal rib retraction during inspiration Voice normal, hoarse, or absent Immobility of vocal cord as visualized by laryngoscopy	**ONGOING ASSESSMENT**
	• Observe respiratory rate, rhythm.
	• Note voice quality.
	• Observe neck for swelling, tightness.
	• Examine wound for evidence of hematoma, oozing.
	• Observe for presence of stridor.
	
	THERAPEUTIC INTERVENTIONS
	• Keep tracheostomy tray at bedside. *If airway totally occluded, emergency tracheostomy may be necessary.*
	• Keep HOB elevated to 45 degrees.
	• Notify physician of change in:
	   Respiratory pattern
	   Voice quality
		Adequate airway clearance will be maintained.

Potential for injury: hypocalcemia *Related to:* Inadvertent surgical removal of parathyroid glands (hypoparathyroidism) Blood supply to parathyroids damaged (usually temporary but may be permanent) **DEFINING CHARACTERISTICS** Paresthesia of circumoral region, fingers, toes Total serum calcium level <7.7 mg/100 ml *indicating impending tetany (normal: 8.8-10.8 mg/ 100 ml)* Tetanic spasms Positive (+) Chvostek's sign Positive (+) Trousseau's sign Laryngeal stridor Seizure Lethargy Headache	**ONGOING ASSESSMENT** • Note circumoral and peripheral paresthesia. • Observe for tremors in extremities. • Check for presence of Chvostek's and Trousseau's signs. • Monitor serum calcium level. **THERAPEUTIC INTERVENTIONS** • Notify physician if Ca^+ <8.0 mg/100 ml. • Keep calcium gluconate and syringe at bedside *to treat dangerously low serum calcium levels.* • Maintain IV access. • Administer/monitor IV infusions of calcium gluconate; also administer oral calcium, vitamin D, as ordered. • See Seizure activity, p. 263.	Serum calcium level will remain within normal limits.

Thyroidectomy— cont'd

NURSING DIAGNOSES / DEFINING CHARACTERISTICS	NURSING INTERVENTIONS / *RATIONALES*	EXPECTED OUTCOMES
Potential for injury: wound dehiscence (low transverse anterior neck incision) *Related to:* Hematoma Excessive strain on suture line Improper positioning, movement Wound infection **DEFINING CHARACTERISTICS** Wound edges not approximated Drainage, swelling	**ONGOING ASSESSMENT** · Assess neck incision for approximated edges, redness, swelling, drainage, presence of staples/sutures. **THERAPEUTIC INTERVENTIONS** · Notify physician if wound edges not approximated. · Elevated HOB 45 degrees. · *Protect neck incision by instructing patient to:* Avoid neck flexion. Avoid rapid head movements. Support head with hands when rising.	Potential for wound dehiscence will be reduced.
Potential for injury: thyroid storm, hyperthyroidism *Related to:* Inadequate preoperative preparation (euthyroid state not achieved) Increased production of thyroid hormone leading to sensitivity to sympathetic nervous system **DEFINING CHARACTERISTICS** Increased pulse (up to 200 beats/min) Elevated temperature Increased BP Diaphoresis Nausea, vomiting, diarrhea, abdominal pain Tremor Restlessness, possibly delirium Arrhythmias	**ONGOING ASSESSMENT** · Assess for presence of Defining Characteristics. · Assess environment for excessive stimulation. · Assess anxiety level. · Monitor vital signs. **THERAPEUTIC INTERVENTIONS** · Provide quiet environment (control noise level). · Maintain IV infusion *for hydration, nutrition, electrolyte balance.* · Maintain adequate nutritional intake, especially protein, carbohdrates, vitamins; avoid caffeine. *Hypermetabolic states increase basal metabolic demand.* · Promote rest; administer sedatives as ordered; assist with ADL. · Protect patient from adverse effects of excess thyroid hormone: Lower temperature by keeping covers off; using hypothermia blanket, antipyretic agents; giving sponge bath. Administer antithyroid drug (iodine), β-receptor blocking agent (propranolol), adrenal corticosteroid as ordered.	Amount of circulating thyroid hormone will remain normal.
Knowledge deficit: home care *Related to:* Lack of previous experience	**ONGOING ASSESSMENT** · Assess ability and readiness to learn. · Assess knowledge of postoperative care. **THERAPEUTIC INTERVENTIONS** · Instruct patient to inform physician if the following develop: Circumoral, peripheral paresthesia; tremors *that may result from low serum calcium.* Signs of infection: Excessive or continual drainage from incisional line Incision open and/or red	Patient/significant other verbalize understanding of care upon discharge.

Continued.

NURSING DIAGNOSES / DEFINING CHARACTERISTICS	NURSING INTERVENTIONS / *RATIONALES*	EXPECTED OUTCOMES
DEFINING CHARACTERISTICS Multiple questions Lack of questions Demonstrated inability to provide home care	Difficulty in breathing Alteration in voice Sensation of pressure, tightness, fullness in neck Signs/symptoms of thyroid storm • Instruct patient to avoid abrupt head, neck movements. • Instruct patient to keep wound dry. May shower when approved by physician. • Instruct patient in dosage, schedule, desired effects, and side effects of medication(s) sent home.	

Originated by: Laura Vieceli-Brooks, RN, BSN

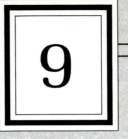

Musculoskeletal Care Plans

DISORDERS

Arthritis, rheumatoid
Osteoarthritis
Osteomyelitis
Osteoporosis
Systemic lupus erythematosus

THERAPEUTIC INTERVENTIONS

Amputation of a lower extremity, surgical
Arthroscopy of knee
Bunionectomy/hallux valgus repair
Extremity fracture
Laminectomy
Le Fort I osteotomy
Myelography

Partial anterior acromiectomy with or
  without rotator cuff repair
Scoliosis: spinal instrumentation
Skeletal traction to an extremity
Total hip arthroplasty/replacement
Total knee arthroplasty/replacement
Total shoulder arthroplasty/replacement

Arthritis, rheumatoid

A chronic, systemic, inflammatory disease that usually presents as symmetric synovitis primarily of the small joints of the body. Extra-articular manifestations may include rheumatoid nodules, pericarditis, scleritis, arteritis.

NURSING DIAGNOSES / DEFINING CHARACTERISTICS	NURSING INTERVENTIONS / *RATIONALES*	EXPECTED OUTCOMES

Joint pain
Related to:
Inflammation associated with increased disease activity
Degenerative changes secondary to long-standing inflammation
 	
DEFINING CHARACTERISTICS
Patient's/significant other's report of pain
Guarding on motion of affected joints
Facial mask of pain
Moaning or other sounds associated with pain
	ONGOING ASSESSMENT
	• Solicit patient's description of pain:
	    Quality
	    Severity
	    Location
	    Onset
	    Duration
	    Aggravating and alleviating factors
	• Assess for signs of joint inflammation (redness, warmth, swelling, decreased motion).
	• Determine past measures used to alleviate pain.
	• Assess interference with life-style.
	
	THERAPEUTIC INTERVENTIONS
	• Administer anti-inflammatory medication as prescribed. First dose of day should be given as early as possible, with small snack. Anti-inflammatory drugs should not be given on empty stomach *(can be very irritating to stomach lining and lead to ulcer disease).*
	• Use non-narcotic analgesic as necessary. *Narcotic analgesia appears to work better on mechanical as opposed to inflammatory types of pain. Narcotics can be habit-forming.*
	• Encourage patient to assume anatomically correct position. Do not use knee gatch or pillows to prop knees. Use small flat pillow under head.
	• Use hot (e.g., heating pad) or cold packs on painful, inflamed joints. Consult clinical specialist or physical/occupational therapist for suggestions. *Some individuals prefer heat to cold or vice versa. Patient may need to alternate. Try what works best at the time.*
	• Encourage use of ambulation aid(s) when pain related to weight bearing.
	• Apply bed cradle to keep pressure of bed covers off inflamed lower extremities.
	• Consult occupational therapist for proper splinting of affected joints.
	• See Pain, p. 39.
		Pain will be decreased.

Joint stiffness
Related to:
Inflammation associated with increased disease activity
Degenerative changes secondary to long-standing inflammation
 	
DEFINING CHARACTERISTICS
Patient's/significant other's complaint of joint stiffness
Guarding on motion of affected joints
Refusal to participate in usual self-care activities
	ONGOING ASSESSMENT
	• Solicit patient's description of stiffness:
	    Location: generalized or localized
	    Timing: morning, night, all day
	    Length of stiffness. Ask patient, "How long do you take to loosen up after you get out of bed?" Record in hours or fraction of hour.
	    Relationship to activities (aggravate/alleviate stiffness)
	• Determine past measures to alleviate stiffness.
	• Assess interference with life-style
	
	THERAPEUTIC INTERVENTIONS
	• Encourage patient to take 15-min warm shower or bath on rising. Localized heat (hand soaking) also useful.
	• Encourage patient to perform ROM exercises after shower or bath, two repetitions per joint.
	• Allow patient sufficient time for activities.
	• Avoid scheduling tests or treatments when stiffness present.
		Stiffness will be reduced.

NURSING DIAGNOSES / DEFINING CHARACTERISTICS	NURSING INTERVENTIONS / *RATIONALES*	EXPECTED OUTCOMES
Decreased functional ability	• Administer anti-inflammatory medications as prescribed. First dose of day as early in morning as possible, with a small snack. *The sooner patient takes the medication, the sooner stiffness will abate.* Many patients prefer to take these medications as early as 6 or 7 a.m. Ask patient about normal home medication schedule; try to continue it. *Anti-inflammatory drugs should not be given on empty stomach.* • Suggest use of elastic gloves (e.g., Isotoner) at night *to decrease hand stiffness.* • Remind patient to avoid prolonged periods of inactivity	

Fatigue
Related to:
Increased disease activity
Anemia of chronic disease
 	
DEFINING CHARACTERISTICS
Patient's/significant other's description of lack of energy, exhaustion, listlessness
Excessive sleeping
Decreased attention span
Facial expressions: yawning, sadness
Decreased functional capacity
	ONGOING ASSESSMENT
	• Solicit patient's description of fatigue:
	    Timing (afternoon or all day)
	    Relationship to activities
	    Aggravating and alleviating factors
	• Determine nighttime sleep pattern.
	• Assess interference with life-style.
	• Determine whether fatigue related to psychologic factors (stress, depression).
	• Determine past measures to alleviate fatigue.
	
	THERAPEUTIC INTERVENTIONS
	• Provide periods of uninterrupted rest throughout day (30 min 3-4 times/day). *Patients often have limited energy reserve.*
	• Reinforce principles of energy conservation taught by occupational therapist:
	    Pacing activities (alternating activity with rest). *Patient often uses more energy than others to complete same tasks.*
	    Adequate rest periods (throughout day and at night).
	    Organization of activities and environment.
	    Proper use of assistive/adaptive devices.
	• If fatigue related to interrupted sleep, see Sleep pattern disturbance, p. 50.
	• Consult clinical specialist if fatigue may be related to psychologic factors (see Nursing Diagnosis, Ineffective psychosocial adaptation, p. 403).
		Fatigue will be relieved.

Impaired physical mobility
Related to:
Pain
Stiffness
Fatigue
Psychosocial factors
Altered joint function
Muscle weakness
 	
DEFINING CHARACTERISTICS
Patient's/significant other's description of difficulty with purposeful movement
Decreased ability to transfer and ambulate
Reluctance to attempt movement
Decreased muscle strength
Decreased ROM
	ONGOING ASSESSMENT
	• Solicit patient's description of:
	    Aggravating and alleviating factors
	    Joint pain and stiffness
	    Interference with life-style
	• Observe patient's ability to:
	    Ambulate
	    Move all joints functionally
	• Assess need for analgesics before activity
	
	THERAPEUTIC INTERVENTIONS
	• Allow patient adequate time for all activities. *Patient may need more time than others to complete same tasks.*
	• Provide adaptive equipment (e.g., cane, walker) as necessary or ask significant other to bring them from home.
	• Reinforce proper use of ambulation devices as taught by physical therapist.
	• Encourage patient to wear proper footwear (well-fitting, with good support) when ambulating and avoid house slippers.
	• Assist with ambulation as necessary.
	• Reinforce techniques of therapeutic exercise (ROM and muscle strengthening) taught by physical therapist.
		Ability to move purposefully will be improved.

Continued.

NURSING DIAGNOSES / DEFINING CHARACTERISTICS	NURSING INTERVENTIONS / *RATIONALES*	EXPECTED OUTCOMES
	· Reinforce principles of joint protection taught by occupational therapist. · Reinforce proper body alignment when sitting, standing, walking, and lying down. *Improper body alignment can lead to unnecessary pain and contracture.*	

Self-care deficit
Related to:
Pain
Stiffness
Fatigue
Psychosocial factors
Altered joint functions
Muscle weakness
 	
DEFINING CHARACTERISTICS
Patient's/significant other's description of difficulty with self-care activities
Decreased functional ability of upper and/or lower extremities
	ONGOING ASSESSMENT
	· Observe patient's ability to:
	    Bathe
	    Carry out personal hygiene
	    Dress
	    Toilet
	    Eat
	· Assess impact of self-care deficit on life-style.
	· Determine assistive/adaptive devices used in self-care activities.
	· Assess need of home health care after discharge.
	
	THERAPEUTIC INTERVENTIONS
	· Encourage independence:
	    Assist only as necessary.
	    Provide necessary adaptive equipment (raised toilet seat, dressing aids, eating aids) or ask significant other to bring them from home.
	    Refer specialized needs to occupational therapy. *Patients' self-image improves when they can perform personal care independently.*
	· Allow patient adequate time for self-care activities.
	· Encourage a shower or bath rather than bed bath.
	· Do not schedule tests/activities during self-care time.
	· Offer patient guidance in pacing activities.
	· Reinforce self-care techniques taught by occupational therapist.
		Self-care activities will be maximized.

Knowledge deficit
Related to:
New disease/procedures
Unfamiliarity with treatment regimen
 	
DEFINING CHARACTERISTICS
Multiple questions
Lack of questions
Verbalized misconceptions
Verbalized lack of knowledge
	ONGOING ASSESSMENT
	· Assess patient's level of knowledge of rheumatoid arthritis and its treatment.
	· Identify priorities for patient education.
	· Assess patient's cognitive learning style (visual, verbal).
	· Assess degree to which discomfort will interfere with learning.
	
	THERAPEUTIC INTERVENTIONS
	· Provide private, quiet environment for patient education.
	· Schedule educational sessions when patient most comfortable. *Pain will distract patient; may lead to inability to absorb new information.*
	· Keep duration of sessions appropriate to attention span.
	· Teach patient according to cognitive style. *(Most effective to teach in manner in which patient learns best).*
	· Introduce/reinforce disease process information:
	    Unknown etiology
	    Chronicity of rheumatoid arthritis
	    Process of inflammation
	    Joint and other organ involvement
	    Remissions and exacerbations
	    Control versus cure
	· Introduce/reinforce information on drug therapy:
	    Name of drug
	    Purpose
	    Use of drug
	    Directions for administrations
	    Potential side effects
	    Other pertinent information (e.g., drug interactions)
	· Introduce/reinforce self-management techniques:
	    ROM exercises
	    Muscle strengthening exercises
		Patient will verbalize increased awareness of the disease and treatment.

NURSING DIAGNOSES / DEFINING CHARACTERISTICS	NURSING INTERVENTIONS / *RATIONALES*	EXPECTED OUTCOMES
	Pain management Joint protection Pacing activities Adequate rest Splinting Use of assistive devices · Introduce/reinforce nutritionally sound diet. · Stress importance of long-term follow-up. · Encourage patient to discuss new or over-the-counter treatments with health care worker.	
Ineffective psychosocial adaptation *Related to:* Altered body structure and function Biophysical factors Psychosocial factors Inadequate coping mechanism Inadequate support **DEFINING CHARACTERISTICS** *Grieving:* Anger, depression, withdrawal *Diminished self-concept:* Refusal to discuss limitations, altered body function, disparaging remarks about self, withdrawal from role responsibilities *Diminished coping:* Expressed hopelessness, prolonged denial of health status, verbalized inability to cope, altered behavior toward self or others *Sexual dysfunction:* Verbalization of problem, expression of dissatisfaction or change in sexual relationship *Diminished family coping:* Expressed hopelessness, limited involvement or noninvolvement with patient, verbalized inability to cope, prolonged denial of patient's health status	**ONGOING ASSESSMENT** · Identify behaviors that suggest grieving. · Assess behavioral patterns suggesting altered self-concept. · Identify behavioral cues suggesting ineffective individual coping. · Assess cues suggesting sexual dysfunction. · Identify behavioral cues suggesting ineffective family coping. **THERAPEUTIC INTERVENTIONS** · See Grief over long-term illness/disability, p. 618.	Psychosocial adaptation will be facilitated.

Continued.

403

NURSING DIAGNOSES / DEFINING CHARACTERISTICS	NURSING INTERVENTIONS / *RATIONALES*	EXPECTED OUTCOMES
Potential sleep pattern disturbance *Related to:* Pain Stiffness Psychosocial factors **DEFINING CHARACTERISTICS** Patient's/significant other's report of inability to fall asleep or frequent awakening at night Interrupted sleep pattern on several nights	**ONGOING ASSESSMENT** • Solicit patient's description of sleep pattern disturbance: Difficulty in falling asleep Frequent awakening through night Inhibition of sleep by pain/stiffness Aggravating and alleviating factors • Determine patient's nighttime rituals. • Assess need for special sleep devices (e.g., bed board, special pillow). • Determine whether sleep pattern disturbance related to psychologic factors (stress, depression). **THERAPEUTIC INTERVENTIONS** • Encourage warm shower or bath immediately before bedtime. *Warm water relaxes muscles, facilitating total body relaxation.* • Encourage gentle ROM exercises (after shower/bath) *to maximize effects of heat.* • Encourage patient to sleep in anatomically correct position (do not prop knees or head). Change positions frequently during night. • Suggest use of electric blanket (set at low temperature). • Provide quiet, and restful environment. Avoid wakening patient unnecessarily (routine vital signs). • Encourage patient to follow normal nighttime rituals. • Provide special sleep devices or ask family to bring them from home. *Familiar surroundings/items encourage relaxation.* • Avoid stimulating foods (caffeine) and activities before bedtime. • Encourage use of progressive muscle relaxation techniques. • Administer nighttime analgesic/long-acting anti-inflammatory drug as ordered. • Administer sleeping medication as ordered if requested by patient. • Consult clinical specialist if sleep pattern disturbance may be related to psychologic factors.	Sleep pattern will be maximized.
Altered nutrition: less than body requirements *Related to:* Loss of appetite related to chronic illness Psychosocial factors **DEFINING CHARACTERISTICS** Loss of weight with/without adequate caloric intake >10-20 percent below ideal body weight Documented inadequate caloric intake Caloric intake inadequate to keep pace with abnormal disease/metabolic state	**ONGOING ASSESSMENT** • Document patient's actual weight on admission (do not estimate). • Obtain nutritional history. • Obtain medication history. • Assess for functional deficits restricting ability to eat. • Assess for psychosocial factors affecting ability to eat. **THERAPEUTIC INTERVENTIONS** • Consult dietitian when appropriate. • Assist patient with meal setup as needed. • Encourage frequent oral ingestion of high-calorie/high-protein foods and fluids. *Small, frequent feedings may benefit patient with nausea.* • Reinforce dietary teaching.	Optimal caloric intake will be maintained.

Arthritis, rheumatoid— cont'd

NURSING DIAGNOSES / DEFINING CHARACTERISTICS	NURSING INTERVENTIONS / *RATIONALES*	EXPECTED OUTCOMES

Altered nutrition: more than body requirements *Related to* Inactivity Psychosocial factors
 	
 DEFINING CHARACTERISTICS Weight 10-20 percent above ideal for height and frame Reported or observed dysfunctional eating behavior
	ONGOING ASSESSMENT
	 • Document patient's actual weight on admission (do not estimate).
	 • Obtain nutritional history.
	 • Obtain medication.
	 • Assess for psychosocial factors affecting eating behaviors.
	
	 THERAPEUTIC INTERVENTIONS
	 • Consult dietician when appropriate.
	 • Assist patient in selecting appropriately from each food group.
	 • Encourage patient to be aware of eating behaviors:
	   Distinction between actual physical need and habitual eating.
	   Avoidance of diversional activities during mealtime.
	   Realization of pattern of rapid food ingestion.
	   Observation of cues that lead to overeating (e.g., odor, time, depression, and boredom).
	 • Encourage appropriate exercise. *Exercises that do not promote joint stress (e.g., aquatic aerobics or isometrics) beneficial to patient with arthritis.*
	 • Reinforce dietary teaching.
		Optimal nutrition will be maintained.

Originated by: Sue A. Conneighton, RN, MSN, Psy D Candidate
Linda Muzio, RN, MSN

Osteoarthritis
(DEGENERATIVE JOINT DISEASE [DJD])

Osteoarthritis is a common progressive degenerative joint disease that affects articular cartilage and subchondral bone.

NURSING DIAGNOSES / DEFINING CHARACTERISTICS	NURSING INTERVENTIONS / *RATIONALES*	EXPECTED OUTCOMES
Pain *Related to:* Joint degeneration Muscle spasm **DEFINING CHARACTERISTICS** Patient's/significant other's report of pain Facial grimaces Moaning, crying Protective, guarded behavior Restlessness Withdrawal Irritability	**ONGOING ASSESSMENT** • Assess description of pain. • Assess behavior and facial expressions. • Assess previous experiences with pain and pain relief. • Assess pain relief measure effectiveness. **THERAPEUTIC INTERVENTIONS** • Encourage patient to verbalize pain *so relief measures can be instituted.* • Respond immediately to complaints of pain. • Develop pain relief regimen based on patient's identified aggravating and relieving factors. • Encourage patient to verbalize emotional reaction to chronic pain. • Change patient's position while maintaining functional alignment (e.g., turning, adjusting pillows). • Administer analgesics and/or anti-inflammatory medication. • Apply hot or cold packs *to provide comfort.* • Encourage adequate rest periods. • Provide adaptive equipment (i.e., cane, walker) as necessary *to assist ambulation and reduce joint stress.* • Eliminate additional stressors. • Medicate for pain before activity and exercise therapy. • See Pain, p. 39.	Relief or reduction in pain will be achieved.

Continued.

Musculoskeletal Care Plans

NURSING DIAGNOSES / DEFINING CHARACTERISTICS	NURSING INTERVENTIONS / *RATIONALES*	EXPECTED OUTCOMES
Impaired physical mobility *Related to:* Pain Stiffness Fatigue Restrict joint movement Muscle weakness **DEFINING CHARACTERISTICS** Reluctance to move Limited ROM Decreased muscle strength Decreased ability to transfer and ambulate	**ONGOING ASSESSMENT** · Assess ROM. · Assess ability to perform ADLs. · Assess previous use of assistive ambulatory devices. **THERAPEUTIC INTERVENTIONS** · Assist patient with isometric, active, and passive ROM exercises to all extremities. *Muscular exertion through exercise promotes circulation and free joint mobility, strengthens muscle tone, develops coordination, and prevents nonfunctional contracture.* · Increase activity as indicated. Consult physical therapy (PT) staff. · Encourage patient to ambulate with assistive devices (i.e., crutches, walker, cane). · Provide adequate rest periods. · Allow patient adequate time for activities. · Maintain functional alignment. · Discuss environmental barriers to mobility. · See Mobility, impaired physical, p. 35.	Optimal mobility will be achieved.
Potential self-care deficit *Related to:* Pain Stiffness Fatigue Immobility Muscle weakness **DEFINING CHARACTERISTICS** Verbalized difficulty with self-care activities Decreased functional ability of upper/lower extremities Verbalized knowledge deficit for home care Increased anxiety as discharge approaches	**ONGOING ASSESSMENT** · Assess knowledge of required care upon discharge. · Assess ability to perform ADLs. · Assess family's/significant others' availability at home. · Assess home physical environment relating to mobility. · Assess interference of self-care deficit with life-style. **THERAPEUTIC INTERVENTIONS** · Encourage independence. · Provide necessary adaptive equipment. · Allow patient adequate time for self-care activities. · Reinforce all instructions given to patient. · Coordinate social services, PT, occupational therapy (OT) early *to provide adequate discharge planning.* · Encourage patient questions. · Instruct patient about discharge medications, exercises, and follow-up physician visits. *Adequate health knowledge increases person's ability to prevent further illness and increases awareness of current medical problem.* · Reinforce self-care techniques taught by OT.	Self-care deficits will be reduced.
Potential altered skin integrity *Related to:* Physical immobility **DEFINING CHARACTERISTICS** Stage I: redness, skin intact Stage II: blisters Stage III: necrosis Stage IV: necrosis involving bone and joints	**ONGOING ASSESSMENT** · Assess skin for breakdown; remove any splints or braces. **THERAPEUTIC INTERVENTIONS** · Turn patient q2h unless otherwise indicated. · Clean, dry, and moisturize skin every shift and prn as indicated. · Moisturize skin every shift, especially over bony prominences; massage *around* bony prominences. · Institute prophylactic use of antipressure devices as appropriate. · If actual skin breakdown occurs, see Skin integrity, impaired, p. 48.	Risk of skin breakdown will be reduced.

Osteoarthritis— cont'd

NURSING DIAGNOSES / DEFINING CHARACTERISTICS	NURSING INTERVENTIONS / *RATIONALES*	EXPECTED OUTCOMES

Potential knowledge deficit
Related to:
New disease/ procedures
Unfamiliarity with treatment regimen
 	
DEFINING CHARACTERISTICS
Multiple questions
Lack of questions
Verbalized misconceptions
Verbalized lack of knowledge
	ONGOING ASSESSMENT
	▪ Assess knowledge of osteoarthritis.
	▪ Assess previous hospital experiences.
	▪ Assess cognitive/intellectual level.
	▪ Assess existing medical problems.
	▪ Assess degree to which discomfort interferes with learning.
	
	THERAPEUTIC INTERVENTIONS
	▪ Provide private, quiet environment for patient education.
	▪ Schedule educational sessions when patient most comfortable.
	▪ Keep duration of sessions appropriate to attention span.
	▪ Introduce/reinforce disease process information. *Adequate health knowledge increases person's ability to understand health problem, prevent harm to self, and participate in care:*
	    Etiology
	    Mechanical factors contributing to disease process
	    Complication
	    Sites of involvement
	▪ Introduce/reinforce information on drug therapy.
	▪ Discuss use of exercise, diet, and relaxation techniques.
	▪ Stress importance of long-term follow-up.
		Patient will verbalize increased awareness of disease and treatment.

Originated by: Sandra Eungard, RN, MS

Osteomyelitis

Inflammation of the bone, especially the marrow, caused by a pathogenic organism, usually Staphylococcus, Streptococcus, Salmonella, or H-flu, and introduced via soft tissue trauma.

NURSING DIAGNOSES / DEFINING CHARACTERISTICS	NURSING INTERVENTIONS / *RATIONALES*	EXPECTED OUTCOMES

Bone infection
Related to:
Infection that has migrated to bone tissue
 	
DEFINING CHARACTERISTICS
Local inflammation of involved bone characterized by:
    Pain/guarding
    Edema
    Warmth
    Redness
	ONGOING ASSESSMENT
	▪ Assess affected area for signs/symptoms of infection:
	    Pain
	    Edema
	    Warmth
	    Redness (describe in detail)
	▪ Assess lab values, especially WBC and SED rate.
	▪ Assess x-ray or bone scan findings.
	▪ Obtain appropriate cultures and sensitivities:
	    Blood
	    Aspirate from bone abscess if present
	
	THERAPEUTIC INTERVENTIONS
	▪ Administer IV antibiotics as ordered.
	▪ Administer antipyretics.
	▪ Provide fluids *to prevent dehydration in febrile state.*
	▪ Cleanse area. *Sometimes primary soft tissue infection not found because healed when osteomyelitis evident.*
	▪ Apply warm compress or heating pad *to promote circulation to affected area.*
		Signs/symptoms of infection will be relieved.

Continued.

Osteomyelitis— cont'd

NURSING DIAGNOSES / DEFINING CHARACTERISTICS	NURSING INTERVENTIONS / *RATIONALES*	EXPECTED OUTCOMES
Pain *Related to:* Infection Inflammation **DEFINING CHARACTERISTICS** Verbalized bone pain with/without movement Nonverbal signs, cries, and grimaces Physical signs (e.g., increased heart rate, increased blood pressure, and diaphoresis)	**ONGOING ASSESSMENT** · Assess affected area for pain with movement. · Assess verbal and nonverbal signs of pain. · Assess analgesic effectiveness. · Monitor vital signs for signs/symptoms of pain. **THERAPEUTIC INTERVENTIONS** · Administer analgesics as ordered. · Immobilize limb. · Apply warm packs to affected area *(heat provides an alternate sensation to pain)*. · Encourage patient to use previous coping mechanisms. · Provide diversional activities (see Diversional activity deficit, p. 17).	Pain will be reduced.
Potential for injury *Related to:* Necrosis of bone Fragile bone **DEFINING CHARACTERISTICS** Pain of affected bone with movement Guarded movement of affected limb	**ONGOING ASSESSMENT** · Assess ROM. · Assess x-ray and bone scan findings for bone destruction. **THERAPEUTIC INTERVENTIONS** · Immobilize affected area. · Provide passive ROM as indicated. · Obtain PT consultation.	Chance of injury will be reduced.
Potential altered nutrition: less than body requirements *Related to:* Decreased intake caused by pain or change in diet Increased nutritional demands for healing **DEFINING CHARACTERISTICS** Poor appetite Decreased weight	**ONGOING ASSESSMENT** · Assess intake. · Assess appetite. **THERAPEUTIC INTERVENTIONS** · Provide desired foods. · Assist at mealtime as needed. *Poor intake may be caused by inability to feed self.* · Provide pain control before meals. *Appetite improves when patient pain-free.* · Refer to Nutrition, altered: less than body requirements, p. 37.	Adequate nutrition will be maintained.

Knowledge deficit
Related to:
Hospitalization and treatment
Lack of experience
 	
DEFINING CHARACTERISTICS
Verbalized lack of understanding
Questioning
	ONGOING ASSESSMENT
	· Assess readiness to learn and cognitive level.
	· Assess current status and ability to learn (e.g., *febrile or uncomfortable patient unable to listen and comprehend*).
	
	THERAPEUTIC INTERVENTIONS
	· Provide explanation:
	    Development of osteomyelitis
	    Importance of long-term IV therapy:
	        IV maintenance
	        Side effects of prescribed antibiotic
	· Explain necessity for tests (e.g., aspirations, blood culture and sensitivity, x-rays and scans).
	· Stress importance of continuing oral antibiotic after discharge.
	· Provide follow-up appointments, prescriptions, and home health services if home treatment possible.
		Patient will understand importance of tests, therapy, and follow-up.

Originated by: Susan Geoghegan, RN, BSN

Osteoporosis

A metabolic bone disease characterized by a decrease in mass resulting in porosity/brittleness. This leads to a greater risk for bone fractures and deformities. It is more common in women after menopause.

NURSING DIAGNOSES / DEFINING CHARACTERISTICS	NURSING INTERVENTIONS / *RATIONALES*	EXPECTED OUTCOMES

Impaired mobility
Related to:
Deformities
Fractures
Pain
 	
Defining Characteristics
Patient's/significant other's report of difficulty with purposeful movement
Decreased ability to transfer and ambulate
Reluctance to attempt movement
Decreased muscle strength
Decreased ROM
	Ongoing Assessment
	• Solicit patient's description of:
	    Aggravating and alleviating factors
	    Joint/bone pain and stiffness
	    Interference with life-style
	• Observe patient's ability to:
	    Ambulate
	    Move all body parts functionally
	
	Therapeutic Interventions
	• Promote mobility through physical therapy and exercise. Suggest moderate weight-bearing exercise (e.g., walking, bicycling, or dancing) for 30 min 3 times/wk. *Weight bearing stimulates osteoblastic activity and new bone growth.*
	• Reinforce techniques of therapeutic exercise (ROM and muscle strengthening) taught by physical therapist.
	• Assist with ambulation as necessary.
	• Provide adaptive equipment (e.g., cane, walker) as necessary to assist with ambulation.
		Patient will verbalize/ demonstrate increased ability to move purposefully.

Self-care deficit
Related to:
Deformities
Fractures
Pain
 	
Defining Characteristics
Patient's/significant other's report of difficulty with self-care activities
Decreased functional ability of upper/ lower extremities
	Ongoing Assessment
	• Observe patient's ability to:
	    Bathe.
	    Carry out personal hygiene.
	    Dress.
	    Use toilet.
	    Eat.
	• Assess interference with life-style.
	• Determine assistive/adaptive devices used in self-care activities.
	
	Therapeutic Interventions
	• Encourage independence.
	• Assist as necessary.
	• Provide necessary adaptive equipment (e.g. raised toilet seat, dressing aids, eating aids). Refer to OT for specialized needs. *Provision of necessary adaptive equipment promotes self-care.*
	• Allow patient adequate time for self-care activities.
	• Offer patient guidance in pacing activities.
	• Reinforce self-care techniques taught by occupational therapist.
		Self-care abilities will be maximized.

Potential for injury: fracture
Related to:
Falls
 	
Defining Characteristics
Pain
Immobility
	Ongoing Assessment
	• Assess environment for safety.
	• See Injury, potential for (high-risk fall status), p. 32.
	
	Therapeutic Interventions
	• Provide safe hospital environment:
	    Bed rails up
	    Bed in down position
	    Necessary items (e.g., telephone, call light, walker, cane) within reach
	    Adequate lighting
	    Grab bars in bathroom (if available)
	• Teach patient to create safe environment at home:
	    Remove or tack down throw rugs
	    Wear firm-soled shoes
		Potential for injury is reduced.

Continued.

Musculoskeletal Care Plans

NURSING DIAGNOSES / DEFINING CHARACTERISTICS	NURSING INTERVENTIONS / *RATIONALES*	EXPECTED OUTCOMES
	Install grab bars in bathroom Do not carry heavy objects *Safe home environment is necessary to prevent falls and potential fractures.*	
Pain *Related to:* Fracture Deformities **DEFINING CHARACTERISTICS** Patient's/significant other's report of pain Guarding on motion of affected area Facial mask of pain Moaning or other pain-associated sounds Autonomic responses (e.g., diaphoresis, change in BP, pulse, pupillary movement)	**ONGOING ASSESSMENT** · Solicit patient's description of pain. 　Quality 　Severity 　Location 　Onset 　Duration 　Aggravating and alleviating factors · Assess patient's response to pain medication or therapeutics aimed at abolishing/relieving pain. **THERAPEUTIC INTERVENTIONS** · Administer pain medications as necessary per order. · Encourage use of ambulation aid(s) for pain related to weight bearing. *Assistive devices can help support body weight that can add to pain in fractures of weight-bearing joints/bones.* · See Pain, p. 39.	Pain will be relieved.
Ineffective calcium utilization *Related to:* Dietary intake Hormonal changes **DEFINING CHARACTERISTICS** Patient's/significant other's report of dietary intake deficit in calcium and vitamin D Postmenopausal patient not having estrogen replacement therapy Insufficient dietary intake of calcium	**ONGOING ASSESSMENT** · Obtain history of calcium intake. Assess tobacco, alcohol, and exercise history. *Smoking, drinking alcohol, and having only minimal weight-bearing exercise are risk factors for development of osteoporosis.* · Assess for calcium supplementation. · Assess whether patient postmenopausal or has had hysterectomy with bilateral oophorectomy. · Assess serum calcium levels. · Assess whether patient taking medications that decrease calcium absorption. 　Cortisone 　Antacids 　Laxatives · Monitor calcium levels. *Elevated calcium levels indicate calcium malabsorption (may indicate need for vitamin D supplement to aid calcium absorption).* **THERAPEUTIC INTERVENTIONS** · Consult dietician when appropriate. · Encourage increased intake of calcium-rich foods: 　Skim milk/cheeses 　Whole-grain cereals 　Green leafy vegetables *Natural sources of calcium may provide more elemental or useful forms of calcium.* · Administer calcium supplementation/estrogen therapy as ordered. · Reinforce meal planning taught by dietitian.	Optimal calcium levels will be achieved.
Body image disturbance *Related to:* Deformities Fractures Use of assistive devices	**ONGOING ASSESSMENT** · Assess perception of change in body part structure/function. · Assess perceived impact of change on ADL, social behavior, personal relationships, occupational activities. · Note patient's behavior regarding actual or perceived changed body part/function or assistive device. · Note verbal references to actual or perceived change in body part/function.	Body image disturbance will be reduced.

NURSING DIAGNOSES / DEFINING CHARACTERISTICS	NURSING INTERVENTIONS / *RATIONALES*	EXPECTED OUTCOMES
DEFINING CHARACTERISTICS Verbalization of feelings about altered structure/function of body part or use of assistive devices Preoccupation with altered body part or function Refusal to use assistive devices	**THERAPEUTIC INTERVENTIONS** • Acknowledge normalcy of emotional response to actual or perceived change in body structure/function. • Help patient identify actual changes. • Assist patient in incorporating actual changes in ADL, social life, interpersonal relationships, occupational activities. • Encourage participation in support groups. *Allows for open, nonthreatening discussion of feelings with others with similar experiences.* • See Body image disturbance, p. 6.	

Knowledge deficit
Related to:
New disease
Unfamiliarity with treatment regimen
 	
DEFINING CHARACTERISTICS
Patient's/significant other's multiple questions, verbalized misconceptions, verbalized lack of knowledge
Lack of questions
	ONGOING ASSESSMENT
	• Assess patient's knowledge of osteoporosis and treatment.
	• Identify priorities for patient education.
	• Assess patient's style of learning (visual, verbal).
	• Assess degree to which discomfort will interfere with learning.
	
	THERAPEUTIC INTERVENTIONS
	• Provide quiet environment for patient education.
	• Schedule educational sessions when patient most comfortable. *Pain will distract patient and may lead to inability to absorb new information.*
	• Keep session duration appropriate to attention span and ability to integrate information.
	• Teach patient according to preferred style. *Most effective to teach in manner in which patient learns best*
	• Introduce/reinforce disease process information:
	    Causes
	    Risk factors
	    Process
	• Introduce/reinforce information on medications (calcium/vitamin D supplements and estrogen therapy):
	    Name of drug
	    Purpose
	    Use of drug
	    Directions for administration
	    Potential side effects
	    Other pertinent information (e.g., drug interactions)
	• Introduce/reinforce self-management techniques:
	    Exercise
	    Use of assistive devices
	    Pacing activity
	    Protection from injury/falls
	• Reinforce dietary teaching of increased calcium intake.
		Patient will verbalize increased awareness of the disease and treatment.

Originated by: Linda Muzio, RN, MSN

Systemic lupus erythematosus

(SLE; LUPUS)

A chronic, systemic inflammatory disease characterized by multisystem involvement. Mild disease can affect joints and skin. More severe disease can affect kidneys, heart, lung and central nervous system as well as joints and skin. Women are affected six times more often than men.

NURSING DIAGNOSES / DEFINING CHARACTERISTICS	NURSING INTERVENTIONS / *RATIONALES*	EXPECTED OUTCOMES

Altered skin integrity *Related to:* Inflammation Vasoconstriction
 	
DEFINING CHARACTERISTICS Change in skin and/or mucous membranes Redness Pain Tenderness Itching Skin breakdown Skin rash   Red   Nonraised   Tender   Malar rash   Oral/nasal ulcers
	ONGOING ASSESSMENT
	• Assess skin integrity:
	  Note color, moisture, texture, temperature.
	  Note any redness, swelling, or tenderness.
	  Note size of lesions, including oral, nasal, fingertip and leg ulcers.
	• Solicit patient's description of pain:
	  Quality
	  Severity
	  Location
	  Onset
	  Duration
	  Aggravating and alleviating factors.
	• Assess interference with life-style.
	• Assess interference with ADLs.
	
	THERAPEUTIC INTERVENTIONS
	• Clean, dry, and moisturize intact skin; use warm (not hot) water, especially over bony prominences, bid, using unscented lotion (Eucerin or Lubriderm). *Scented lotions may contain alcohol, which dries skin.*
	• Encourage adequate nutrition and hydration.
	• Provide prophylactic pressure-relieving devices (e.g., special mattress, elbow pads).
	• Administer analgesics before wound debridement as needed.
	• Assist with ADLs as needed.
	• Instruct patient to avoid ultraviolet light:
	  Wear maximum protection sunscreen (SPF 40) in sun.
	  Sunbathing: contraindicated.
	  Wear wide-brim hat and carry umbrella *to protect skin (sun can exacerbate skin rash)*.
	  Wear protective eyewear.
	• Introduce/reinforce information about use of hydroxychloroquine sulfate (Plaquenil Sulfate):
	  Purpose
	  Use
	  Potential side effects
	  Other pertinent information (e.g., toxicity to infants and children).
	• Inform patient of availability of special makeup (at large department stores) to cover rash, especially facial rash:
	  Covermark (Lydia O'Leary)
	  Dermablend
	• Instruct patient to rinse mouth with half-strength hydrogen peroxide tid when oral ulcers present. *Hydrogen peroxide helps keep oral ulcers clean.*
	• Instruct patient to avoid irritating foods (e.g., spicy or citric) when oral ulcers present.
	• Instruct patient to keep ulcerated skin clean and dry. Apply topical ointments as ordered.
	• Instruct patient to avoid contact with harsh chemicals (e.g., household cleaners, detergents).
	• Instruct patient to wear cotton-lined latex gloves when using harsh chemical *to protect skin.*
		Optimal skin integrity will be maintained.

NURSING DIAGNOSES / DEFINING CHARACTERISTICS	NURSING INTERVENTIONS / *RATIONALES*	EXPECTED OUTCOMES
Altered skin integrity: alopecia (scalp hair loss) *Related to:* Inflammation Exacerbation of disease process High-dose corticosteroid use Use of immunosuppressant drugs **Defining Characteristics** Diffuse hair loss areas Loss of discrete scalp hair patches Scalp hair loss may or may not be accompanied by scarring	**Ongoing Assessment** • Assess integrity of scalp hair: 　Note scalp hair loss amount and distribution. 　Note scarring in areas of scalp hair loss. • Assess degree to which symptom interferes with patient's life-style. **Therapeutic Interventions** • Instruct patient to avoid scalp contact with harsh chemicals (e.g., hair dye, permanent, curl relaxers): 　Use mild shampoo (e.g., P & S). 　Decrease frequency of shampooing. • Instruct patient that scalp hair loss occurs during exacerbation of disease activity: 　Scalp hair loss may be first sign of impending disease exacerbation. 　Scalp hair loss may not be permanent; *as disease activity subsides, scalp hair begins to regrow.* 　Short haircut useful during times of scalp hair loss. 　Regrown hair may have different texture, often finer. 　Hair will not regrow in areas of scarring. • Instruct patient that scalp hair loss may be caused by high-dose corticosteroids (prednisone) and/or immunosuppressant drugs. Hair will regrow as dose decreases. • Encourage patient to investigate ways *(scarfs, hats, wigs)* to conceal scalp hair loss, if interfering with life-style.	Hair loss will be reduced.
Fever *Related to:* Inflammation **Defining Characteristics** Temperature greater than 101°F (38.4°C) Chills Shaking chills (rigor) Diaphoresis Dehydration	**Ongoing Assessment** • Assess vital signs at least q2h. • Assess for chills, shaking, and diaphoresis. • Assess for dehydration signs: 　Decreased skin turgor 　Dry mucous membranes 　Decreased urine output • Monitor intake and output. **Therapeutic Interventions** • Administer antipyretics as ordered. If aspirin used, monitor patient for elevated liver enzymes. *Aspirin use by febrile lupus patients is documented to cause transient liver toxicity.* • Administer steroids in divided dose. • Encourage hydration. • If temperature remains above 103°F (39.5°C), apply cooling mattress. • See Hyperthermia, p. 31.	Optimal body temperature is maintained.
Altered peripheral tissue perfusion *Related to:* Vasospasm Structural changes **Defining Characteristics** Pain, numbness, cold sensation Triphasic color changes: white, blue, red	**Ongoing Assessment** • Assess hands and feet for color, temperature, and skin integrity. • Solicit description of pain, numbness, and cold sensations. • Assess interference with life-style. • Assess interference with ADLs. **Therapeutic Interventions** • Keep extremities warm (socks, blankets, gloves, mittens). • Remove vasoconstricting factors when possible. • Administer vasodilating medications (e.g., Nifedipine) as ordered. • Instruct patient to avoid undue cold exposure: 　Wear oven mitts for refrigerator or freezer. 　Wear multiple clothing layers (hat/cap, ear muffs, nose protector, mittens/gloves, socks) in cold environment.	Optimal tissue perfusion will be maintained.

Continued.

Systemic lupus erythematosus— cont'd

NURSING DIAGNOSES / DEFINING CHARACTERISTICS	NURSING INTERVENTIONS / *RATIONALES*	EXPECTED OUTCOMES

	Suggest wearing items made of wool, cotton, down, or thinsulate (*provide most protection from cold exposure*).
	 • Instruct patient to avoid caffeine and nicotine (*cause vasoconstriction*).
	 • Instruct patient in stress management (*stress can precipitate vasospasm*):
	   Identification of stressful situations
	   Identification of past coping mechanisms
	   Identification of new coping mechanisms
	   Instruction in techniques of progressive muscle relaxation, imagery, or biofeedback	

Joint pain *Related to:* Inflammation **DEFINING CHARACTERISTICS** Pain Guarding on motion of affected joints Facial mask of pain Moaning or other pain-associated sounds	**ONGOING ASSESSMENT** • Solicit description of pain. • Assess for signs of joint inflammation (redness, warmth, swelling, decreased motion). • Determine past measures used to alleviate pain. • Assess interference with life-style. **THERAPEUTIC INTERVENTIONS** • Administer anti-inflammatory medication as prescribed. First dose of day as early in morning as possible, with small snack. *Anti-inflammatory drugs should not be given on empty stomach (can be very irritating to stomach lining and lead to ulcer disease).* • Use non-narcotic analgesic as necessary. *Narcotic analgesia appears to work better on mechanical as opposed to inflammatory types of pain. Narcotics can be habit-forming.* • Encourage patient to assume anatomically correct position. Do not use knee gatch or pillow to prop knees; use small flat pillow under head. • Encourage use of ambulation aid(s) when pain related to weight bearing. • Apply bed cradle *to keep pressure of bed covers off inflamed lower extremities.* • Consult occupational therapist for proper splinting of affected joints. • See Pain, p. 39.	Pain will be reduced or relieved.

Joint stiffness
 Related to:
 Inflammation
 	
 DEFINING CHARACTERISTICS
 Verbalized complaint of joint stiffness
	ONGOING ASSESSMENT
	 • Solicit description of stiffness:
	   Location: generalized or localized
	   Timing: morning, night, all day
	   Length of stiffness. Ask patient: "How long do you take to loosen up after you get out of bed?" Record in hours or fraction of hour.
	   Relationship to activities
	   Aggravating/alleviating factors
	 • Determine past measures used to alleviate stiffness.
	 • Assess interference with life-style.
	
	 THERAPEUTIC INTERVENTIONS
	 • Encourage patient to take 15-min warm shower/bath on rising. *Water should be warm. Excessive heat may promote skin breakdown.*
	 • Encourage patient to perform ROM exercises after shower/bath, two repetitions per joint.
	 • Allow sufficient time for all activities.
	 • Avoid scheduling tests or treatments when stiffness present.
	 • Administer anti-inflammatory medication as prescribed. First dose of day as early in morning as possible, with small snack. *The sooner patient takes medication, the sooner stiffness will abate.* Many patients prefer to take medications as early as 6 or 7 a.m. Ask about normal home medication schedule and try to continue it. *Anti-inflammatory drugs should not be given on empty stomach.*
	 • Remind patient to avoid prolonged periods of inactivity.
		Stiffness will be reduced or eliminated.

Systemic lupus erythematosus— cont'd

NURSING DIAGNOSES / DEFINING CHARACTERISTICS	NURSING INTERVENTIONS / *RATIONALES*	EXPECTED OUTCOMES

Potential for injury
Related to:
Altered renal function
Inflammation and sclerosis of glomeruli
Side effects of connective tissue disease
 	
DEFINING CHARACTERISTICS
Increased BUN and creatine
Hematuria
Proteinuria
Peripheral edema
Altered LOC
Hypertension
Decreased cardiac output
Nausea
Vomiting
	ONGOING ASSESSMENT
	· Assess urinary output at least q2h.
	· Monitor fluid intake.
	· Obtain nutritional history.
	· Monitor electrolyte levels as drawn.
	· Monitor urine specific gravity, protein, and blood q2h.
	· Assess for edema, especially of lower extremities.
	· Assess vital signs at least q2h.
	· Assess for LOC changes.
	· Weigh daily.
	
	THERAPEUTIC INTERVENTIONS
	· Obtain dietary consultation as needed.
	· Administer immunosuppressant medications as ordered:
	    Methylprednisolone
	    Cyclophosphamide
	· Instruct patient of potential immunosuppressant medication side effects. See Potential for injury: side effects related to prednisone and immunosuppressant medications, p. 419.
	· See Renal failure, acute, p. 343; Hypertension, p. 95; Cardiac output, decreased, p. 9.
		Optimal renal function will be maintained.

Altered central nervous system: severe headaches, seizures, organic psychosis, organic brain syndrome
Related to:
Inflammation
Severe, active SLE (usually occurs early in disease course, often combined with increased disease activity in other organ systems)
Organic psychosis (may be caused by high-dose corticosteroids)
 	
DEFINING CHARACTERISTICS
Headaches, often severe and throbbing; usually accompanied by seizures or organic brain syndrome
Seizures, most often grand mal
Organic psychosis (see Ongoing Assessment)
Organic brain syndrome (see Ongoing Assessment)
	ONGOING ASSESSMENT
	· Assess for presence of headaches:
	    Location
	    Onset
	    Duration
	    Severity
	    Quality
	    Aggravating and alleviating factors
	· Assess for presence of seizure activity:
	    Aura
	    Type
	    Onset
	    Duration
	· Assess for presence of organic psychosis:
	    Impaired judgment
	    Inappropriate speech
	    Disorganized behavior
	    Disorientation
	    Impaired reality testing
	    Impaired comprehension
	    Decreased attention
	    Hallucinations
	· Assess for the presence of organic brain syndrome:
	    Impaired memory
	    Disorientation
	    Impaired judgment
	    Increased or decreased psychomotor activity
	    Loss of higher cortical functions (e.g., asphasia [language disorder], apraxis [motor disorder], agnosia [failure to recognize objects])
	    Personality changes
	
	THERAPEUTIC INTERVENTIONS
	· Provide quiet, restful environment during headaches.
	· Administer analgesics and corticosteroids as ordered for headaches.
		Optimal CNS function will be maintained.

Continued.

415

Systemic lupus erythematosus— cont'd

NURSING DIAGNOSES / DEFINING CHARACTERISTICS	NURSING INTERVENTIONS / *RATIONALES*	EXPECTED OUTCOMES

	· Instruct patient of potential immuno suppressant medication side effects. See Potential for injury: side effects related to prednisone and immunosuppressant medications, p. 419.
	· Provide quiet, safe environment during seizures. See Seizure activity, p. 263.
	· Administer neuroleptics, corticosteroids, and immunosuppressants as ordered.
	· Instruct patient in use, potential side effects of neuroleptic, prednisone, and immunosuppressants. See Seizures, p. 243.
	· Provide safe, structured, predictable environment when organic psychosis or organic brain syndrome present:
	    Same staff for daily care; one-to-one care may be necessary.
	    Decrease environmental stimuli. Keep patient in private room if necessary.
	    Remove potentially dangerous objects from room.
	    Orient patient to person, place, and time as necessary. Keep clock and calendar in room.
	    Provide clear, concise instructions.
	    Decrease ambiguity and confusion by offering limited choices.
	    Administer antipsychotic, corticosteroid, and immunosuppressant drugs as ordered.
	    Instruct patient in use, potential side effects of corticosteroids and immunosuppressants when patient able to comprehend.	

Potential impaired gas exchange *Related to:* Inflammation Pleuritis Pleural effusion Pulmonary infection Pleuritic chest pain **DEFINING CHARACTERISTICS** Shortness of breath Tachypnea Nasal flaring Respiratory depth changes Altered chest excursion Dyspnea on exertion Chest pain	**ONGOING ASSESSMENT** · Assess respiratory rate and depth by listening to breath sounds minimum of every shift. · Assess for dyspnea and quantify; relate dyspnea to precipitating factors. · Note use of breathing muscles (i.e, sternocleidomastoid, abdominal, diaphragmatic). · Assess position assumed for normal/easy breathing. · Assess for changes in orientation, restlessness. · Note changes in activity tolerance. · Assess interference with life-style. · Monitor changes in vital signs, especially breathing pattern. · Assess need for O$_2$ at home. **THERAPEUTIC INTERVENTIONS** · Pace and schedule activities *to prevent dyspnea caused by fatigue.* · Provide reassurance, allay anxiety by staying with patient during acute respiratory distress episodes. · Provide O$_2$ as ordered and as needed. · Instruct patient in environmental factors that may worsen pulmonary condition (e.g., pollen, smoking). · Instruct patient of "cold" symptoms and associated problems. · Assist patient with problem solving for manageable home environment. · Encourage patient to receive influenza vaccine every year and pneumococcal vaccine at some point. *CDC encourages all individuals with chronic illness or lung disease to immunize against flu.*	Optimal respiratory status within limits of disease will be achieved.
Potential decreased cardiac output *Related to:* Effusions Cardiac arrhythmias (atrial and ventricular)	**ONGOING ASSESSMENT** · Monitor heart for rate, rhythm, ectopy every shift. · Assess fluid status. · Assess mentation. · Assess energy level. **THERAPEUTIC INTERVENTIONS** · Administer antiarrhythmic medications as ordered. · If arrhythmia occurs, determine patient's response. Document and report if significant or symptomatic.	Optimal cardiac rhythm and output will be maintained.

NURSING DIAGNOSES / DEFINING CHARACTERISTICS	NURSING INTERVENTIONS / *RATIONALES*	EXPECTED OUTCOMES
DEFINING CHARACTERISTICS Patient report of palpitations Patient's/significant other/s report of fatigue or shortness of breath Irregular heart rate Tachycardia/ bradycardia Hypoxia	• Instruct patient in principles of energy conservation. See Nursing Diagnosis, Fatigue, below. • See Cardiac dysrhythmias, p. 74.	

Self-care deficit
Related to:
Pain
Stiffness
Fatigue
Psychosocial factors
Altered joint function
Muscle weakness
Joint contracture
 	
DEFINING CHARACTERISTICS
Patient's/significant other's report of difficulty with self-care activities
Decreased functional ability of upper/ lower extremities
	ONGOING ASSESSMENT
	• Observe patient's ability to:
	  Bathe
	  Carry out personal hygiene
	  Dress
	  Use toilet
	  Eat
	• Assess interference with life-style.
	• Determine assistive/adaptive devices used in self-care activities.
	• Assess need of home health care after discharge.
	
	THERAPEUTIC INTERVENTIONS
	• Encourage independence; assist only as necessary.
	• Provide necessary adaptive equipment (raised toilet seat, dressing aids, eating aids) or ask significant other to bring from home.
	• Refer specialized needs to occupational therapy. *Patients have improved self-image if able to perform personal care independently.*
	• Allow patient adequate time for self-care.
	• Encourage shower/bath rather than bed bath.
	• Do not schedule tests/activities during self-care time.
	• Offer patient guidance in pacing activities.
	• Reinforce self-care techniques taught by occupational therapist.
		Capabilities will be maximized.

Fatigue
Related to:
Increased disease activity
Anemia of chronic disease
 	
DEFINING CHARACTERISTICS
Lack of energy, exhaustion, listlessness
Excessive sleeping
Decreased attention span
Facial expressions: yawning, sadness
Decreased functional capacity
	ONGOING ASSESSMENT
	• Solicit patient's description of fatigue:
	  Timing (afternoon or all day)
	  Relationship to activities
	  Aggravating and alleviating factors
	• Determine night sleep pattern.
	• Assess interference with life-style.
	• Determine whether fatigue related to psychologic factors (stress, depression).
	• Determine past measures used to alleviate fatigue.
	
	THERAPEUTIC INTERVENTIONS
	• Provide periods of uninterrupted rest throughout day (30 min 3 to 4 times/ day). *Patients often have limited energy supply.*
	• Reinforce energy conservation principles taught by occupational therapist:
	  Pacing activities (alternating activity with rest). *Patient often needs more energy than others to complete same tasks.*
	  Adequate rest periods (throughout day/night)
	  Organization of activities and environment
	  Proper use of assistive/adaptive devices
		Fatigue will be decreased.

Continued.

NURSING DIAGNOSES / DEFINING CHARACTERISTICS	NURSING INTERVENTIONS / *RATIONALES*	EXPECTED OUTCOMES
	• If fatigue related to interrupted sleep, see Nursing Diagnosis, Sleep pattern disturbance, p. 421. • Consult clinical specialist if fatigue related to psychologic factors (see Ineffective psychosocial adaptation, p. 420).	
Impaired physical mobility *Related to:* Pain Stiffness Fatigue Psychosocial factors Altered joint function Muscle weakness Joint contractures **DEFINING CHARACTERISTICS** Patient's/significant other's report of difficulty with purposeful movement Decreased ability to transfer and ambulate Reluctance to attempt movement Decreased muscle strength Decreased ROM	**ONGOING ASSESSMENT** • Solicit patient's description of: Aggravating and alleviating factors Joint pain and stiffness Interference with life-style • Observe patient's ability to: Ambulate Move all joints functionally • Assess need for analgesics before activity. **THERAPEUTIC INTERVENTIONS** • Allow patient adequate time for all activities. *Patient often needs more time than others to complete same tasks.* • Provide adaptive equipment (e.g., cane, walker) as necessary or ask significant other to bring from home. • Reinforce proper use of ambulation devices as taught by physical therapist. • Encourage patient to wear proper footwear (well-fitting, with good support) for ambulation; avoid house slippers. • Assist with ambulation as necessary. • Reinforce techniques of therapeutic exercise (ROM and muscle strengthening) taught by physical therapist. • Reinforce principles of joint protection taught by occupational therapist. • Reinforce proper body alignment during sitting, standing, walking, and lying down. *Improper body alignment can lead to unnecessary pain, contractures.*	Physical mobility will be improved.
Knowledge deficit *Related to:* New disease/ procedures Unfamiliarity with treatment regime **DEFINING CHARACTERISTICS** Multiple questions Lack of questions Verbalized misconceptions Verbalized lack of knowledge	**ONGOING ASSESSMENT** • Assess knowledge of lupus and its treatment. • Identify priorities for education. • Assess cognitive learning styles (visual, verbal). • Assess degree to which discomfort interferes with learning **THERAPEUTIC INTERVENTIONS** • Provide private, quiet environment for patient education. • Schedule educational sessions when patient most comfortable. *Pain will distract patient and may lead to inability to absorb new information.* • Keep duration of sessions appropriate to patient's attention span and ability to integrate information. • Teach patient by using aids that facilitate learning. *Most effective to teach patient in manner in which patient learns best.* • Introduce/reinforce disease process information: Unknown etiology Chronicity of lupus Processes of inflammation and fibrosis Skin and other organ involvement Remissions and exacerbations Control versus cure • Introduce/reinforce information on drug therapy: Name of drug Purpose Use of drug Directions for administrations Potential side effects Other pertinent information (e.g., drug interactions)	Patient will verbalize increased awareness of disease and treatment.

NURSING DIAGNOSES / DEFINING CHARACTERISTICS	NURSING INTERVENTIONS / *RATIONALES*	EXPECTED OUTCOMES

	• Introduce/reinforce self-management techniques:
	  ROM exercises
	  Muscle strengthening exercises
	  Pain management
	  Joint protection
	  Pacing activities
	  Adequate rest
	  Splinting
	  Use of assistive devices
	  Skin care
	• Introduce/reinforce nutritionally sound diet.
	• Stress importance of long-term follow-up.
	• Discuss unproven remedies; encourage patient to verify/discuss new treatments before use.	

Potential for injury: side effects related to prednisone and immunosuppressant medication
Related to:
Long-term use
High dosage
 	
DEFINING CHARACTERISTICS
Prednisone:
  Facial puffiness
  "Buffalo" hump
  Hypertension
  Diabetes mellitus
  Osteoporosis
  Avascular necrosis
  Addisonian crisis
Immunosuppressants:
  Bone marrow suppression
  Sterility
  Cancer
	ONGOING ASSESSMENT
	• Assess facial contour. *If both ears not visible when patient viewed directly, patient considered cushingoid.*
	• Assess for fat pads on back (buffalo hump).
	• Assess blood pressure at least q4h.
	• Assess for lower extremity edema.
	• Monitor urine for sugar and acetone or monitor blood glucose at least once a day.
	• Monitor for spontaneous bone fractures.
	• Monitor for bone and joint pain, especially of hips and shoulders. *Avascular necrosis most prominent in femoral and humeral heads.*
	• Monitor CBC.
	• Monitor for blood in urine or pain, burning with urination *(signs of hemorrhagic cystitis).*
	
	THERAPEUTIC INTERVENTIONS
	• Instruct patient in potential side effects of long-term prednisone:
	  Facial puffiness
	  Buffalo hump
	  Diabetes mellitus
	  Osteoporosis
	  Avascular necrosis
	  Increased appetite
	  Increased infection risk
	• Instruct patient in potential side effects of immunosuppressant medications:
	  Increased infection risk *caused by bone marrow suppression*
	  Nausea/vomiting
	  Sterility
	  Hemorrhagic cystitis
	  Cancer
	• Instruct patient to wear Medic Alert tag stating use of prednisone at all times.
	• Instruct patient never to alter prednisone dose. Steroids must be tapered slowly after high-dose or long-term use. *Body produces the hormone cortisol in adrenal glands. After high-dose/long-term use of extraneous forms of steroids, body no longer produces cortisol. Increased cortisol levels needed in times of stress. Without supplementation, steroid-dependent person will enter Addisonian crisis.*
	• See Adrenocortical insufficiency, p. 370.
		Risk of injury related to medications is reduced.

Continued.

NURSING DIAGNOSES / DEFINING CHARACTERISTICS	NURSING INTERVENTIONS / *RATIONALES*	EXPECTED OUTCOMES
Altered nutrition: less than body requirements *Related to:* Loss of appetite related to chronic illness Psychosocial factors **DEFINING CHARACTERISTICS** Loss of weight with/ without adequate caloric intake >10-20% *below* ideal body weight Documented inadequate caloric intake Caloric intake inadequate to keep pace with abnormal disease/metabolic state	**ONGOING ASSESSMENT** • Document actual weight on admission (do not estimate). • Obtain nutritional history. • Obtain medication history. • Assess for functional deficits restricting ability to eat. • Assess for psychosocial factors affecting ability to eat. **THERAPEUTIC INTERVENTIONS** • Consult dietitian when appropriate. • Assist patient with meal setup as needed. • Encourage frequent oral ingestion of high-calorie/high-protein foods and fluids. *Small frequent feedings may benefit patient with nausea.* • Reinforce dietary teaching.	Optimal caloric intake will be maintained.
Altered nutrition: more than body requirements *Related to:* Inactivity Psychosocial factors **DEFINING CHARACTERISTICS** Weight 10-20% *above* ideal for height and frame Reported or observed dysfunctional eating behavior	**ONGOING ASSESSMENT** • Document actual weight on admission (do not estimate). • Obtain nutritional history. • Obtain medication history. • Assess for functional deficits restricting ability to eat. **THERAPEUTIC INTERVENTIONS** • Consult dietician when appropriate. • Assist with selection of appropriate foods from each group. • Encourage patient to be aware of eating behaviors: Distinction between actual physical need and habitual eating Avoidance of diversional activities at mealtime Realization of pattern of rapid food ingestion Observation of cues leading to overeating (e.g., odor, time, depression, and boredom)	Weight reduction over time will be achieved.
Potential ineffective psychosocial adaptation *Related to:* Altered body structure and function Biophysical Inadequate coping mechanism Inadequate support **DEFINING CHARACTERISTICS** Patient's/significant other's report of ineffective psychosocial adaptation to lupus *Grieving:* anger, depression, withdrawal	**ONGOING ASSESSMENT** • Identify behaviors suggesting grieving. • Assess behavioral patterns suggesting altered self-concept. • Identify behavioral cues suggesting ineffective individual coping. • Assess cues suggesting sexual dysfunction. • Identify behavioral cues suggesting ineffective family coping. **THERAPEUTIC INTERVENTIONS** • See Coping, ineffective individual, p. 15; Sexuality patterns, altered, p. 47; Grieving, anticipatory, p. 22.	Adaptation will be facilitated.

NURSING DIAGNOSES / DEFINING CHARACTERISTICS	NURSING INTERVENTIONS / *RATIONALES*	EXPECTED OUTCOMES
Diminished self-concept: refusal to discuss limitations/ altered body function, disparaging remarks about self, withdrawal from role responsibilities *Diminished coping:* expressed hopelessness, prolonged denial of health status, verbalized inability to cope, altered behavior toward self or others *Sexual dysfunction:* verbalization of problem, expressed dissatisfaction, change in sexual relationship *Diminished family coping:* expressed hopelessness, limited involvement or noninvolvement with patient, verbalized inability to cope, prolonged denial of patient's health status		

Potential sleep pattern disturbance
Related to:
Pain
Stiffness
Psychosocial factors
 	
DEFINING CHARACTERISTICS
Inability to fall asleep or frequent awakening
Interrupted sleep pattern on several nights
	ONGOING ASSESSMENT
	• Solicit description of sleep pattern disturbance:
	  Difficulty in falling asleep
	  Frequent awakening through night
	  Inhibition of sleep caused by pain/stiffness
	  Aggravating and alleviating factors
	• Determine patient's nighttime rituals.
	• Assess need for special sleep devices (e.g., bed board, special pillow).
	• Determine whether sleep pattern disturbances related to psychologic factors (stress, depression).
	
	THERAPEUTIC INTERVENTIONS
	• Encourage warm shower/bath immediately before bedtime. *Warm water relaxes muscles, facilitating total body relaxation; excessive heat may promote skin breakdown.*
	• Encourage gentle ROM exercises (after shower/bath) *to maximize warm bath/shower benefits.*
	• Encourage patient to sleep in anatomically correct position. Do not prop up affected joints. Change position frequently during night.
	• Suggest use of electric blanket (set at low temperature) when skin integrity intact.
	• Provide quiet, restful environment. Avoid unnecessary wakening (routine vital signs).
	• Encourage patient to follow normal nighttime rituals.
	• Provide special sleep devices or ask family to bring from home. *Familiar surroundings/items encourage relaxation.*
	• Avoid stimulating foods (caffeine), activities before bedtime.
	• Encourage use of progressive muscle relaxation techniques.
		Sleep patterns will be normalized.

Continued.

Systemic lupus erythematosus— cont'd

NURSING DIAGNOSES / DEFINING CHARACTERISTICS	NURSING INTERVENTIONS / *RATIONALES*	EXPECTED OUTCOMES
	· Administer nighttime analgesic and/or long-acting anti-inflammatory drug as ordered. · Administer sleeping medication as ordered if requested. · Consult clinical specialist if sleep pattern disturbance related to psychologic factors. · See Sleep pattern disturbance, p. 50.	

Originated by: Linda Muzio, RN, MSN
　　　　　　　Sue A. Conneighton, RN, MSN, Psy D Candidate

Amputation of a lower extremity, surgical

Removal of a lower limb for gangrene, which can result from circulatory disorders, diabetes mellitus, malignancy, or traumatic incidents. Medical amputation of a lower extremity is commonly performed before the surgical procedure to decrease the amount of anticipated bleeding and prevent the spread of infection. Dry ice is placed up to a predetermined marker (below the site of surgical amputation) to keep the affected extremity solidly frozen before removal. Surgical removal of the lower extremity is then performed. The most distal amputation level that will facilitate wound healing, maintain joint mobility, and create a stump appropriate for later prosthesis is selected.

NURSING DIAGNOSES / DEFINING CHARACTERISTICS	NURSING INTERVENTIONS / RATIONALES	EXPECTED OUTCOMES
Knowledge deficit *Related to:* Unfamiliarity with hospital routines, medical or surgical procedures **DEFINING CHARACTERISTICS** Increased anxiety level Questioning Verbalized misconceptions Fears about level of independence	**ONGOING ASSESSMENT** · Assess patient's understanding of hospitalization, routines associated with surgery, and the physical preparation of the extremity for the amputation. · Assess patient's level of readiness for learning. **THERAPEUTIC INTERVENTIONS** · Explain preoperative procedure: 　Consent for medical surgical amputation 　Preoperative tests 　Visit from anesthesia staff 　NPO after midnight 　Icing of extremity if applicable (refer to hospital policy). · Instruct patient in need to improve nutritional status *to facilitate wearing prosthesis.* · Instruct patient of the following *to prepare for smooth transition through recovery:* 　Postoperative care of residual limb 　Preparation for prosthesis 　Muscle strengthening exercises *to facilitate crutch walking* 　Phantom pain phenomena (sensations "felt" in amputated leg, which may persist for several weeks, months) 　Appropriate use of assistive devices (e.g., walker, crutches, cane, trapeze) · Teach prevention of postoperative complications (flexion abduction and external rotation of hip): 　Avoid sitting for long periods. 　Avoid use of pillows under residual limb.	Patient will be able to verbalize understanding of preoperative and postoperative routines, exercises, and activity regimen.

NURSING DIAGNOSES / DEFINING CHARACTERISTICS	NURSING INTERVENTIONS / *RATIONALES*	EXPECTED OUTCOMES
	Maintain proper alignment. Avoid flexing residual limb while sitting or lying. • If patient not candidate for prosthesis, instruct in self-care activities from amputee wheelchair. • Prepare patient to experience withdrawal and depression during adjustment period. *Rehabilitation period can be long and difficult. Avoid unrealistic goal setting.*	
Anxiety *Related to:* Anticipated loss of body part Fear of postoperative pain Change in body image **DEFINING CHARACTERISTICS** Increase in BP, pulse, respiration Increase in perspiration Nausea/vomiting Eating disturbances Body aches/pains Shakiness Restlessness Apprehension/tension Increased rate and quantity of verbalization Inability to focus or concentrate Irritability or withdrawal Verbal/physical aggressiveness	**ONGOING ASSESSMENT** • Recognize patient's anxiety level. • Assess patient's self-concept and health status. • Assess patient's conceptions and concerns about role, relationship changes. **THERAPEUTIC INTERVENTIONS** • Approach patient supportively and understandingly. • Provide information, including visual aids, *to promote patient's understanding of procedures and rehabilitation.* • Encourage verbalization of thoughts and feelings. Avoid misleading or unrealistic reassurances. • Identify support systems; mobilize if necessary.	Anxiety will be relieved.
Postoperative impaired physical mobility *Related to:* Change in center of gravity creating balance problems Activity limitations caused by loss of body part Difficulty in using assistive devices Pain upon mobility Fatigue	**ONGOING ASSESSMENT** • Assess level of understanding of mobility and restrictions. • Assess patient's understanding of postoperative activity and exercise program. • Assess proper positioning techniques; individualize to patient. • Assess activity tolerance. **THERAPEUTIC INTERVENTIONS** • Consult physician for orders for position and activity restrictions: Determine weight-bearing limitations (graded weight bearing starts 10 to 14 days after surgery). Have patient lie on back, keeping pelvis level and hip joint extended *to prevent contractions.* Maintain neutral rotation, abduction-adduction. Have patient lie prone with lower extremity in extension *to prevent deformities.* Encourage early ambulation (patient should be able to stand within 48 hr) to *promote confidence about regaining independence.* • Encourage use of assistive devices. • Refer to Mobility, impaired, physical, p. 35.	Optimal mobility within limitations is achieved.

Continued.

Musculoskeletal Care Plans

NURSING DIAGNOSES / DEFINING CHARACTERISTICS	NURSING INTERVENTIONS / RATIONALES	EXPECTED OUTCOMES
DEFINING CHARACTERISTICS Decreased muscle control Restricted mobility caused by postoperative protocol Resistance to movement		

Pain
Related to:
Phantom pain
Surgical procedure
Decreased mobility
 	
DEFINING CHARACTERISTICS
Verbal complaints
Facial expressions
Protection of stump
Crying, moaning
Restlessness
Withdrawal
Irritability
	ONGOING ASSESSMENT
	· Assess description of pain.
	· Assess for nonverbal signs of pain.
	· Assess previous pain experience and successful relief measures.
	· Assess understanding of occurrence/management of phantom limb pain. *Phantom limb sensations are normal and can last for months.*
	
	THERAPEUTIC INTERVENTIONS
	· Respond immediately to pain complaints. *Pain best relieved before too severe.*
	· Provide medications as ordered *for pain relief;* evaluate effectiveness.
	· Use additional comfort measures as appropriate:
	    Change in environment
	    Diversional activities
	    Relaxation techniques
	    ROM of stump
	    Position change
	    Application of pressure to residual limb
	    Heat lamp
	· Notify physician if interventions unsuccessful.
		Discomfort will be reduced or relieved.

Impaired skin integrity
Related to:
Surgical incision
Skin breakdown caused by immobility
Abnormal wound healing
 	
DEFINING CHARACTERISTICS
Redness
Pain
Edema
Drainage/discharge
	ONGOING ASSESSMENT
	· Assess wound for:
	    Normal healing
	    Bleeding/hemorrhage
	    Proper fit of cast or pressure dressing
	    Prolonged pressure on tissues associated with immobility
	· Assess nutritional status.
	
	THERAPEUTIC INTERVENTIONS
	· Reinforce dressing as needed; use aseptic technique; note drainage type, amount.
	· Instruct patient to report slippage of cast, rigid dressing, or compression dressing. *These appliances help prevent edema, minimize pain with movement, and facilitate shaping of stump for later prosthesis.*
	· Assist with stump wrapping; use elastic bandage when indicated (stump shrinker sometimes preferred).
	· Check stump for signs of impaired circulation (i.e., edema, pain).
	· Rewrap stump q3-4h or as needed for bunching or slippage. *Correct wrapping reduces swelling, promotes shaping of stump for prosthesis.*
	· Discuss weight-bearing limitations and their importance *to prevent skin breakdown and facilitate proper wound healing.*
	· For further interventions refer to Skin integrity, impaired, p. 48.
		Optimal wound healing will be achieved.

Potential for injury: falls *Related to:* Change in equilibrium from loss of limb	**ONGOING ASSESSMENT** · Assess mobility status. · Assess cognitive/intellectual level. · Assess knowledge of proper transfer/ambulation techniques.	Risk of injury is reduced.

Amputation of a lower extremity, surgical— cont'd

NURSING DIAGNOSES / DEFINING CHARACTERISTICS	NURSING INTERVENTIONS / *RATIONALES*	EXPECTED OUTCOMES
Inability to ambulate Pain **DEFINING CHARACTERISTICS** Reluctance to ask for assistance Failure to recognize limitations	**THERAPEUTIC INTERVENTIONS** ▪ Reinforce transfer and ambulation techniques taught by physical therapist. ▪ Clarify information given. ▪ Reinforce teaching of muscle strengthening and balancing exercises *to strengthen muscles and increase sense of balance*. ▪ Encourage patient to ask for needed assistance. ▪ Assist patient with transfers and ambulation until able to perform safely.	
Potential inefffective coping *Related to:* Loss of body part Change in body image and function Change in life-style **DEFINING CHARACTERISTICS** Depression/withdrawal Crying Irritability Changes in eating habits Insomnia Denial Noncompliance	**ONGOING ASSESSMENT** ▪ Assess patient's concept of loss of body part and its effect on future. ▪ Assess patient's ability to work through depression. **THERAPEUTIC INTERVENTIONS** ▪ Develop relationship of trust. ▪ Encourage verbalization of feelings about effect on future. *Allow patient time to work through grief stages*. ▪ Encourage family support. ▪ Help patient develop realistic goals. ▪ Identify misconceptions; provide information. ▪ Assist with referral to counseling services and support group as appropriate. *Provide mechanism for ongoing verbalization of feelings*. ▪ Identify and document negative behavioral changes (e.g., hysteria, excessive anger, suicidal tendencies).	Acceptance of changes in body and life-style is achieved.
Self-concept disturbance *Related to:* Change in body image Loss of independence Inability to maintain life-style **DEFINING CHARACTERISTICS** Depression/withdrawal Irritability Aggressiveness Anxiety	**ONGOING ASSESSMENT** ▪ Assess ability to adjust to loss of body part. ▪ Assess ability to use coping mechanisms. ▪ Assess need for support group. **THERAPEUTIC INTERVENTIONS** ▪ Listen and support verbalized feelings about life-style changes. ▪ Encourage participation in care of residual limb when able *to promote independence*. ▪ Explore successful past coping techniques. ▪ Encourage use of clothing *to enhance appearance*. ▪ Encourage patient to participate fully in therapy regime (*fosters sense of control*). ▪ Encourage family members to support patient and allow independence. ▪ Discuss use of prosthesis for cosmetic as well as ambulatory purposes. ▪ Consult social services for support groups. ▪ See also Self-concept disturbance, p. 46; Body image disturbance, p. 6.	Positive adaptation to change in life-style and body function is achieved.

Knowledge deficit: discharge instructions
Related to:
New role/life-style
New condition
	ONGOING ASSESSMENT
	▪ Assess knowledge of the following *to facilitate smooth transition from hospital to home:*
	  Care of residual limb
	  Phantom limb pain management
	  Signs/symptoms of circulatory problems
	  Prosthetic care
	  Follow-up appointments
	  Community resources
		Patient verbalizes understanding of limb, prosthetic, and follow-up care.

Continued.

Amputation of a lower extremity, surgical— cont'd

NURSING DIAGNOSES / DEFINING CHARACTERISTICS	NURSING INTERVENTIONS / RATIONALES	EXPECTED OUTCOMES
DEFINING CHARACTERISTICS Expressed concerns about home management Questions about medications/treatment	**THERAPEUTIC INTERVENTIONS** • Reinforce teaching for care of residual limb (e.g., stump wrapping, skin care, and weight-bearing limitations) *to promote optimal rehabilitation.* • Provide information for phantom limb pain/sensation management. • Discuss signs/symptoms of circulatory problems; encourage patient to report them to physician. • Reinforce teaching about care of prosthesis if applicable. • Inform of discharge medications, exercises, and follow-up appointments. • Coordinate social services, physical therapy, and occupational therapy *to provide adequate discharge planning and home treatments after discharge.* • Contact social services for information about community resources and support groups (i.e., visiting nurses, homemakers, outpatient therapy).	

Originated by: Sherry Weber, RN
              Carol Clark, RN

Arthroscopy of knee

A relatively painless endoscopic procedure that allows direct visualization of the joint area, including the synovium, articular surfaces, and menisci.

NURSING DIAGNOSES / DEFINING CHARACTERISTICS	NURSING INTERVENTIONS / *RATIONALES*	EXPECTED OUTCOMES

Impaired physical mobility
Related to:
Torn segment of meniscus
Loose body in knee joint
Degenerated or osteochondrotic knee areas
Internal knee derangement
Acute knee injuries
Ligamentous knee injuries
Patellar dislocation
 	
DEFINING CHARACTERISTICS
Complaints of pain, "locked knee," subsequent or intermittent buckling
Swelling
Aability to feel loose fragment
Loss of limited motion
Positive McMurray test ("click" heard with possible pain on flexion with rotation)
	ONGOING ASSESSMENT
	• Evaluate patient injury history/onset:
	   Mechanism of injury
	   Date of onset
	   Pertinent medical problems (e.g., osteoarthritis, hemophilia, vascular disease)
	• Assess preoperative and postoperative physical findings (see Defining Characteristics).
	• Monitor postoperatively:
	   Motor strength
	   Patient's tolerance to rehabilitation exercises
	   Possible hazards of immobility
	
	THERAPEUTIC INTERVENTIONS
	• Stage mobilization from lying to partial sitting, to sitting in chair, standing, then walking.
	• Demonstrate immediate postoperative exercises (e.g., quadriceps and hamstring strengthening, straight-leg raising, and walking with supportive devices such as a walker or crutches).
	• Assist with ambulation when initiated by physical therapy and with weight bearing as ordered.
		Optimal mobility will be achieved.

NURSING DIAGNOSES / DEFINING CHARACTERISTICS	NURSING INTERVENTIONS / *RATIONALES*	EXPECTED OUTCOMES
Altered tissue perfusion *Related to:* Compromised circulation Joint immobilization **DEFINING CHARACTERISTICS** Complaints of pain, feelings of severe numbness or coolness of affected extremity Swelling Sluggish/absent capillary refill Coldness Pallor Pulselessness Abnormal calf edema Unusual postoperative bleeding	**ONGOING ASSESSMENT** • Monitor and compare neurovascular status of both lower extremities before, after surgery. Include color, warmth, circulation, movement, sensation, pulses, and capillary refill. **THERAPEUTIC INTERVENTIONS** • Elevate affected extremity. • Apply ice packs *to decrease swelling.* • Maintain clean, snug-fitting but comfortable dressing *to absorb blood or fluid leakage but not compromise circulation.* • Document all signs/symptoms of neurovascular deficit; notify physician immediately *to prevent further complications.*	Adequate tissue perfusion (neurovascular function) will be maintained throughout postoperative course.
Pain *Related to:* Surgical pain and rehabilitation program **DEFINING CHARACTERISTICS** Complaints of pain Facial grimacing Moaning or crying Guarding behavior Limited movement Reluctance to move Irritability Restlessness Altered vital signs	**ONGOING ASSESSMENT** • Determine source of pain. • Assess degree and character of pain. • Determine patient's expectations of pain relief. **THERAPEUTIC INTERVENTIONS** • Anticipate and offer prescribed analgesics as needed *to implement relief measures.* • Encourage diversional activities. • Inform that overactivity may mimic pain. • Notify physician if pain persists after use of prescribed analgesics, rest, elevation of affected leg, and ice packs. • Document presence of pain, relief measures, and effectiveness.	Pain is relieved.

Potential for infection
Related to:
Incision
 	
DEFINING CHARACTERISTICS
Complaint of pain, chills, lethargy
Increased warmth of tissue surrounding wound
Temperature >37°C (100°F)
Erythema around wound
Purulent/foul-smelling drainage
Induration
Positive wound culture
	ONGOING ASSESSMENT
	• Perform assessment of:
	   Skin color and temperature
	   Absence/presence of fever
	   Character of any drainage present
	• Monitor laboratory results.
	
	THERAPEUTIC INTERVENTIONS
	• Administer antipyretics/antibiotics as prescribed.
	• Change bandage with sterile to clean technique as often as necessary *to prevent bacterial contamination.*
	• Encourage increased amounts of liquids.
		Risk of postoperative infection will be reduced.

Continued.

NURSING DIAGNOSES / DEFINING CHARACTERISTICS	NURSING INTERVENTIONS / *RATIONALES*	EXPECTED OUTCOMES
Potential knowledge deficit *Related to:* New condition New procedures **DEFINING CHARACTERISTICS** Verbalized misconception/lack of knowledge of hospitalization, surgical procedure, and rehabilitation program Lack of/abundance of questions and increased anxiety	**ONGOING ASSESSMENT** ▪ Assess patient's previous hospitalization/injury experience. ▪ Assess previous use of crutches or other supportive devices. ▪ Assess expectations of surgical outcome. ▪ Assess willingness to learn. **THERAPEUTIC INTERVENTIONS** *Preoperatively:* ▪ Describe surgical procedure in terms patient understands. *Postoperatively:* ▪ Provide instruction: 　Exercise essential *to strengthen structures supporting and stabilizing knee; must be performed routinely.* 　Increase activity as tolerated. Until first postoperative physician visit, leg should be elevated during sitting or lying down. 　Keep dressing clean and dry until first postoperative visit; shower within 48 hr if dressing kept dry. 　"Splashing" or "squashing" inside knee is normal; *residual liquid from surgery will be absorbed.* 　Bruises at puncture site will eventually disappear; apply no creams or lotions to incision. 　Use crutches safely: 　　Patient should wear flat-heeled, well-fitting shoes. 　　Crutches should be 1-1½ inch below axillae with arms slightly flexed. 　　Patient should look ahead, not down, when walking *to maintain balance.* 　　Tingling, numbness in upper torso may indicate incorrect use or wrong size crutches. 　　Crutches should have rubber tips and pads *to prevent slipping.* 　　Crutches used for support may be discontinued when patient able to walk without limp (generally after first 48 hr). 　Physician will give permission for return to work, sports, activities, etc. (generally 4-6 wk for running, jogging, or "stop-and-go" sports).	Patient will verbalize and demonstrate adequate knowledge of procedures and rehabilitation program prescribed before discharge.

Originated by: Lori Luke, RN
　　　　　　　Marilyn Magafas, RN,C, BSN, MBA

Bunionectomy/hallux valgus repair

Hallux valgus: *The great toe points toward the second toe but is rotated in the frontal plane so that the nail plate is facing away from the second toe.*
Bunion: *Localized enlargement at the first metatarsal head because of either malposition or overgrowth of bone.*
Bunionectomy: *A general class of many different operations that are designed to correct bunion deformity.*

NURSING DIAGNOSES / DEFINING CHARACTERISTICS	NURSING INTERVENTIONS / *RATIONALES*	EXPECTED OUTCOMES
Potential altered peripheral tissue perfusion *Related to:* Surgical procedure	**ONGOING ASSESSMENT** ▪ Assess and compare neurovascular status of both lower extremities, preoperatively and postoperatively. *Preoperative assessment will establish baseline data for subsequent comparisons.* 　Include: 　Color 　Warmth	Tissue perfusion will remain adequate.

NURSING DIAGNOSES / DEFINING CHARACTERISTICS	NURSING INTERVENTIONS / RATIONALES	EXPECTED OUTCOMES
DEFINING CHARACTERISTICS Pain, pallor, cyanosis, coolness, paresthesia, edema Sluggish, absent capillary refill noted in either or both lower extremities	Circulation Movement Sensation Pulses Capillary refill • Monitor neurovascular status q4h×48h immediately after surgery, then every shift if neurovascular status stable. *Circulation to operated extremity must be evaluated frequently since early recognition and treatment essential to prevent permanent damage.* **THERAPEUTIC INTERVENTIONS** • Report changes to surgeon immediately.	
Pain *Related to:* Surgical procedure Rehabilitation program **DEFINING CHARACTERISTICS** Complaint of discomfort or throbbing-type pain Decreased physical activity Guarded movement of lower extremities Altered vital signs Facial grimace Crying	**ONGOING ASSESSMENT** • Assess for presence of pain. • Elicit description of pain. • Assess which analgesics relieve pain most effectively. **THERAPEUTIC INTERVENTIONS** • Immediately after surgery, elevate operated foot on 3-4 pillows *to prevent/decrease swelling and help decrease throbbing sensation.* • Apply ice bags *to help promote comfort and prevent swelling.* • Administer medicine as needed for pain. Anticipate need for analgesics. Encourage patient to take medication before physical therapy. • Assist with repositioning foot/leg as needed. • Attach bedspan *to keep sheets off operated foot to decrease irritation and reduce pressure.* • Instruct patient to continue elevating foot after hospital discharge. *Increased swelling and discomfort are common when patient resumes more normal role at home.* • Instruct patient on action, dosage, and side effects of pain medication given upon discharge. • See Pain, p. 39.	Pain will be relieved or reduced.
Impaired physical mobility *Related to:* Surgical procedure Restricted movement caused by postoperative protocol **DEFINING CHARACTERISTICS** Inability to move about in bed, to transfer, and to ambulate Reluctance to move Decreased ROM Verbalized inability to perform	**ONGOING ASSESSMENT** • Assess patient's ability to carry out ADLs. • Assess weight-bearing ability, balance, and stability with ambulation. • Assess skin integrity, especially pressure points. Check for redness, tissue ischemia. **THERAPEUTIC INTERVENTIONS** • Teach and encourage leg exercises, quad sets, and ROM *to prevent thrombophlebitis and maintain muscle strength.* Instruct patient to continue exercises after discharge. • Assist with ambulation and appropriate use of assistive devices (including crutches, walkers). *Patients need encouragement to overcome hesitancy to walk on affected foot.* • Make sure patient has proper bunion shoe or boot. • Initiate/supervise progressive weight bearing as tolerated. Monitor balance and stability with ambulation. Use gait belt when initiating ambulation. • Instruct patient to continue protective ambulation (as tolerated) after discharge. • Arrange PT consultation.	Independence in ambulation and ADLs is achieved.
Potential for infection *Related to:* Surgical procedure	**ONGOING ASSESSMENT** • Assess incision site q4h×48h for signs/symptoms of infection. • Assess temperature q4h×48h, then every shift. Notify physician of temperature >38.5°C. • Assess lab values, especially WBC.	Risk of infection will be reduced.

Continued.

Bunionectomy/hallux valgus repair— cont'd

NURSING DIAGNOSES / DEFINING CHARACTERISTICS	NURSING INTERVENTIONS / *RATIONALES*	EXPECTED OUTCOMES
DEFINING CHARACTERISTICS Pain, swelling, redness at incision Increased WBC Increased temperature Drainage from incision	**THERAPEUTIC INTERVENTIONS** • Change incisional dressing as ordered using aseptic technique *to prevent wound contamination. Routine postoperative wound care critical to infection prevention.* • Document and notify physician of signs/symptoms of infection. • Administer antibiotics as ordered *(may be given as precautionary measure).*	

Knowledge deficit
 Related to:
 New condition and procedures
 	
 DEFINING CHARACTERISTICS
 Questions
 Lack of questions
 Confusion about treatment
	ONGOING ASSESSMENT
	 • Determine knowledge of postdischarge recovery guidelines. *Discharge information is necessary to facilitate follow-up care and help prevent complications.*
	
	 THERAPEUTIC INTERVENTIONS
	 • Instruct patient:
	     To ambulate as tolerated with walker, crutches, bunion shoes, etc., and protect operated foot from injury.
	     To keep operated foot/feet elevated. *Edema may not subside completely for weeks.*
	     To keep surgical dressings dry and clean.
	     To have frequent physician appointments for dressing changes.
	     To wear wide-toed shoes and sandals after dressings removed.
	     To notify physician if fever, drainage, increased pain, cyanosis, or calf pain appears.
	     To follow guidelines for proper foot care.
	     To continue foot-strengthening exercises.
		Patient will verbalize understanding of discharge instructions.

Originated by: Karen Peterson, RN, BSN
              Catherine Brown, RN

Extremity fracture

(CLOSED REDUCTION; OPEN REDUCTION; INTERNAL FIXATION; EXTERNAL FIXATION)

A fracture is a break or disruption in the continuity of a bone. Fractures occur when a bone is subjected to more stress than it can absorb. Fractures are treated by one or a combination of the following: closed reduction—alignment of bone fragments by manual manipulation without surgery; open reduction—alignment of bone fragments by surgery; internal fixation—immobilization of fracture site during surgery with rods, pins, plates, screws, wires, or other hardware; immobilization through use of casts, splints, traction, posterior molds, etc.; external fixation—immobilization of bone fragments with the use of rods/pins that extend from the incision externally and are fixed.

NURSING DIAGNOSES / DEFINING CHARACTERISTICS	NURSING INTERVENTIONS / *RATIONALES*	EXPECTED OUTCOMES

Pain
 Related to:
 Fracture and soft tissue injury
	ONGOING ASSESSMENT
	 • Assess for pain or discomfort.
	 • Assess pain characteristics:
	     Location
	     Quality/character
		Pain will be reduced.

Extremity fracture— cont'd

NURSING DIAGNOSES / DEFINING CHARACTERISTICS	NURSING INTERVENTIONS / *RATIONALES*	EXPECTED OUTCOMES
DEFINING CHARACTERISTICS Complaints of pain or discomfort Guarding behavior Muscle spasm Diaphoresis Increased pulse rate Increased blood pressure Increased or decreased respirations Pallor Crying, moaning Grimacing Anxiety Restlessness Withdrawal Irritability	Severity Onset Duration Precipitating factors Relieving factors • Determine past experience with pain and pain relief measures. **THERAPEUTIC INTERVENTIONS** • Maintain immobilization and support of affected part. *Immobility prevents further tissue damage and muscle spasm.* • Reposition and support unaffected parts as permitted *to promote general comfort.* • Elevate affected part *to decrease vasocongestion.* • Apply cold *to decrease swelling* (first 24-48 hr). Apply for 20-30 min q1-2h. • Anticipate need for analgesia. • Respond immediately to request for analgesia. Consider round-the-clock or continuous patient-controlled anesthesia (PCA). • Medicate 30 min before wound/pin care or PT *to decrease pain from movement.* • Teach relaxation techniques. • Administer muscle relaxants as necessary. • See Pain, p. 39.	
Potential fluid volume deficit *Related to:* Multiple fractures Long bone fractures Blood vessel damage with bleeding Third spacing of fluids caused by trauma **DEFINING CHARACTERISTICS** Weak, rapid pulse Cool, clammy skin Rapid, shallow respirations Decreased blood pressure Slow capillary refill Decreased urinary output Anxiety Altered LOC	**ONGOING ASSESSMENT** • Assess for symptoms of hypovolemia. • Assess amount of bleeding from external wounds. • Assess for third spacing or bleeding around fracture site. • Obtain circumference measurement of injured area q8h *to assess for further bleeding/third spacing fluid.* • Note amount of bleeding on cast. **THERAPEUTIC INTERVENTIONS** • Administer IV fluids and blood products as ordered. • Maintain alignment and immobility of fracture site *to prevent disruption of bone healing.* • See Fluid volume deficit, p. 20.	Fluid volume deficit will be reduced.

Potential altered peripheral tissue perfusion caused by neurovascular compromise
Related to:
Trauma
Surgery
Compartment syndrome
	ONGOING ASSESSMENT
	• Assess area distal to fracture site q2-4h×48h until stable, then q8h. Monitor:
	    Color
	    Sensation
	    Movement
	    Capillary refill
	    Swelling
	    Pulses (presence and quality)
	    Pain
	• Compare with opposite extremity.
		Neurovascular compromise is reduced.

Continued.

NURSING DIAGNOSES / DEFINING CHARACTERISTICS	NURSING INTERVENTIONS / *RATIONALES*	EXPECTED OUTCOMES
DEFINING CHARACTERISTICS *Distal to fracture site* Skin cool, cyanotic Diminished or absent pulse Slow/absent capillary refill Edema Hematoma Paresis Hypesthesia Numbness, tingling Pain (progressive and disproportional to injury) Pain on passive stretching of muscle Tightness of muscle compartment	**THERAPEUTIC INTERVENTIONS** · Remove restrictive clothing and/or jewelry from affected part. · Elevate affected part above level of heart on pillows or by suspension traction if ordered *to promote venous return and decrease edema.* Do not elevate *above* level of heart if compartment syndrome is suspected *so arterial blood flow is promoted.* · Encourage exercise of unaffected parts distal to site as allowed *to promote circulation.* · Report any neurovascular compromise to physician immediately. · Document all findings completely · Have cast cutter available for bivalving or removing cast if necessary. · Prepare patient for surgical intervention (i.e., fasciotomy) if compartment syndrome suspected. *Severe tissue swelling that decreases blood flow causes ischemia, may cause permanent motor and/or sensory damage.*	
Potential for infection *Related to:* Open fracture External fixation or traction pins Surgical intervention **DEFINING CHARACTERISTICS** *Local:* Pain/tenderness Redness Swelling Excess warmth Purulent drainage Delayed healing Loosening of pins *Systemic:* Increased pulse rate Fever Change in LOC Decreased urinary output Increased WBCs	**ONGOING ASSESSMENT** · Assess wound and/or pin site for: Local signs of infection Skin tension around pins Signs of developing gangrene: *vesicles filled with red watery fluid and gas bubbles from tissue* · Assess for systemic infection signs. · Monitor vital signs q2-4h×48h until stable, then q8h. · Assess for odors or drainage through immobilization devices that are not removed (i.e., casts, splints). **THERAPEUTIC INTERVENTIONS** · Maintain adequate hydration and nutritional status to promote wound healing. · Use sterile technique when changing wound dressings. · Keep dressing dry and intact. Give wound care as ordered. · Initiate wound precautions if purulent drainage present. · Document appearance of wound. · Administer antibiotics as ordered. · Administer tetanus toxoid and/or hypertet as indicated. · Provide skin care as ordered or use standard pin care protocol: Cleanse each pin site with H_2O_2 with sterile applicator; rinse with normal saline to remove crusting from pin site. Apply sterile dressing/ointment as ordered. Wipe off fixator with alcohol.	Risk of infection will be reduced.
Altered nutrition: less than body requirements *Related to:* Increased nutritional needs for wound and fracture healing Poor dietary selection	**ONGOING ASSESSMENT** · Monitor dietary intake and calorie count if indicated. · Assess patient preferences. · Assess lab values. **THERAPEUTIC INTERVENTIONS** · Encourage and teach importance of diet with adequate amounts of protein; calcium; vitamins C, D, and A; iron and calories *(essential for bone and tissue healing). Healing increases metabolism; caloric need increases to prevent protein breakdown.*	Healing of wound/ fracture will be maximized.

NURSING DIAGNOSES / DEFINING CHARACTERISTICS	NURSING INTERVENTIONS / *RATIONALES*	EXPECTED OUTCOMES
DEFINING CHARACTERISTICS Poor wound and fracture healing Delayed bone repair Decreased total protein, albumin, transferrin, lymphocyte levels	• Refer to clinical dietitian as needed. • Provide for adequate rest periods. *Rest conserves energy for cellular metabolism, which is necessary for tissue and bone repair and growth.*	
Impaired physical mobility *Related to:* Cast Fixation device Pain Surgical procedure **DEFINING CHARACTERISTICS** Reluctance to attempt movement Limited ROM Mechanical restriction of movement Decreased muscle strength and/or control Impaired coordination Inability to move purposefully within physical environment (bed mobility, transfer, ambulation)	**ONGOING ASSESSMENT** • Assess ROM of unaffected parts proximal and distal to immobilization device. • Assess ability to perform basic ADLs. • Assess ability to ambulate. • Assess present and preinjury mobility level. • Assess muscle strength in all extremities. **THERAPEUTIC INTERVENTIONS** • Encourage isometric, active, and resistive ROM exercises to all unaffected joints qid and as tolerated *to prevent muscle atrophy and maintain adequate muscle strength required in mobility.* • Apply splint to support foot in neutral position (applied to LE frames and traction) *to prevent foot drop.* • Perform flexion and extension exercises to proximal and distal joints of affected extremity when indicated. • Assist up to chair when ordered; teach transfer technique. • Lift extremity by external fixation frame if stable; avoid handling of injured soft tissue. • Reinforce crutch ambulation taught by physical therapist; use appropriate weight-bearing techniques. Assist with gait belt until gait stable. • See Injury, potential for (high-risk fall status), p. 32, as appropriate.	Maximum mobility within prescribed restrictions is achieved.
Potential altered breathing patterns *Related to:* Fat embolism Pulmonary embolus Type of immobilization device/site of fracture **DEFINING CHARACTERISTICS** Tachycardia Tachypnea Precordial chest pain Rales, wheezing Cough Dyspnea Shortness of breath Cyanosis Petechiae Altered LOC Abnormal blood gas values	**ONGOING ASSESSMENT** • Assess for symptoms of breathing pattern abnormality (see Defining Characteristics) **THERAPEUTIC INTERVENTIONS** • Encourage cough and deep breathing exercises *to promote adequate lung expansion.* • Position patient for maximum lung expansion. • Provide adequate hydration (IVs, PO fluids) *to mobilize secretions.* • Administer O_2 as ordered. • Alleviate anxiety caused by respiratory distress *to decrease O_2 demands.*	Breathing pattern will be maintained.

Continued.

NURSING DIAGNOSES / DEFINING CHARACTERISTICS	NURSING INTERVENTIONS / *RATIONALES*	EXPECTED OUTCOMES
Knowledge deficit: home management *Related to:* New procedures/ treatment New condition **DEFINING CHARACTERISTICS** Patient/family verbalizes inadequate knowledge of care/ use of immobilization device, mobility limitations, complications, and follow-up care Confusion; asking multiple questions Lack of questions Inaccurate follow-through of instruction Improper performance Inappropriate or exaggerated behaviors (i.e., hostile, agitated, hysterical, apathetic)	**ONGOING ASSESSMENT** · Encourage patient to verbalize questions. · Solicit current understanding of diagnosis, treatment, follow-up, etc. · Assess patient's/family's readiness and ability to assume care responsibility. **THERAPEUTIC INTERVENTIONS** · Instruct patient to: Elevate extremity above level of heart with pillows during reclining position *to prevent swelling;* prop affected leg on footstool or chair during sitting. Do prescribed exercises several times a day *to maintain muscle tone.* Use appropriate assistive device (walker, crutches) and maintain prescribed weight-bearing status. Identify and report to physician signs of neurovascular compromise of extremity: pain, numbness, tingling, burning, swelling, or discoloration. Use pain relief measures safely. Obtain proper nutrition *to promote bone/wound healing and prevent constipation.* Arrange for follow-up care. · Instruct patient in cast to: Notify physician: If cast cracks or breaks Of foul odor under cast Of fresh drainage through cast If anything gets inside cast Of areas of skin breakdown around cast Of pain or burning inside cast Of warm areas on cast Keep cast clean and dry; tub bath only if cast protected, not immersed. Inspect skin around cast edges for irritation. Do *not* put anything under cast, poke under cast, or put powder or lotion under cast. *This may abrade skin and cause infection.* · Instruct patient with surgical incision to observe incision for infection signs and notify physician if they develop. · Instruct patient with external fixation device to: Perform pin care. Perform wound care. Observe for loosening of pins. Cleanse device. · Involve patient/significant others in procedure. · Supervise those performing procedures. · Provide patient with own supplies as needed.	Patient/significant other verbalize understanding of treatment, possible complications, and follow-up care.
Potential altered skin integrity *Related to:* Presence of immobilization Improper immobilization device **DEFINING CHARACTERISTICS** Pain/tenderness/ burning Redness Swelling	**ONGOING ASSESSMENT** · Assess immobilized extremity for redness/breakdown. · If patient in cast, check cast edges for roughness. · Assess bony prominences for redness/breakdown. **THERAPEUTIC INTERVENTIONS** · Use antipressure devices (i.e., flotation devices, eggcrate mattress, air mattress) as appropriate. · Maintain adequate hydration and nutritional status. *Good nutrition necessary for tissue growth and repair.* · Reposition patient q2h. · Use bed cradle if necessary *to prevent pressure of sheets on toes.* · Trim and petal rough cast edges *to prevent irritation.* · Pad pin edges *to prevent injury to other areas.*	Skin integrity will be maintained.

NURSING DIAGNOSES / DEFINING CHARACTERISTICS	NURSING INTERVENTIONS / *RATIONALES*	EXPECTED OUTCOMES
Skin breakdown Foul smell, drainage, or warm area under cast	· Turn patient and provide skin care q2-4h. · See Skin integrity, impaired, p. 48.	
Body image disturbance *Related to:* Change in body part function Presence of stabilization devices **DEFINING CHARACTERISTICS** Refusal to participate in care Unrealistic perception of treatment course	**ONGOING ASSESSMENT** · Assess patient's/family's feelings/level of acceptance of injury and treatment method. **THERAPEUTIC INTERVENTIONS** · Perform preoperative teaching if time permits; use pictures of devices if necessary. · Explain procedures and treatment (show x-rays *to aid teaching*). · Encourage and permit patient to verbalize feelings. *Ventilation of feelings supports honesty and objectivity and promotes realistic perception.* · Encourage/support realistic assessment. · Avoid false reassurances. · Consult occupational therapist for clothing modification. · See Body image disturbance, p. 6.	Acceptance of injury and method of treatment is facilitated.
Self-esteem disturbance *Related to:* Loss of body function Inability to meet role responsibilities Loss of control **DEFINING CHARACTERISTICS** Withdrawal behavior Demanding behavior Inability to solve problems Anger Denial Hostility Noncompliance	**ONGOING ASSESSMENT** · Assess coping mechanism used by patient or family. **THERAPEUTIC INTERVENTIONS** · Help patient identify previous stress situations and ways of dealing with them. · Identify and reinforce patient's strengths. · Support continued significant roles with family/friends; provide for visits, phone calls, written work, etc., as tolerated. · Encourage patient to plan, participate in care activities. Adapt care to patient's routines and needs. · Provide opportunities for independent activities. *Independence facilitates coping.* · Arrange environment to promote independent use of materials needed for ADLs. *To develop self-esteem, patient/significant others must participate actively in rehabilitation.* · Continually teach and inform patient/family about physical status, treatment plan, etc. · See also Diversional activity deficit, p. 17. · Make social service referral early in hospitalization for financial and resource counseling as needed.	Positive expressions, feelings, and reactions about self and situation are expressed.
Potential for injury *Related to:* Loss of continuity of cast **DEFINING CHARACTERISTICS** Pain Malalignment on x-rays Skin breakdown inside cast Neurovascular impairment	**ONGOING ASSESSMENT** · Assess cast for cracks, weakened areas, indentations, softened or wet areas. **THERAPEUTIC INTERVENTIONS** · Leave cast open to air until completely dry. *Drying takes 24-48 hr. Air drying promotes drying from inside out to ensure stable cast.* · Prevent indenting cast by moving it with palms of hands and supporting it on nonplastic pillows until dry. *Plastic traps heat released during application.* · Reposition patient and cast q2h *to allow drying.* · Keep cast clean and dry. Prevent soiling from urine/feces.	Risk of injury is reduced.

Originated by: Marilyn Magafas, RN, BSN, MBA
　　　　　　　 Joanne Shearer, RN, MSN

Laminectomy

(HEMILAMINECTOMY; DISKECTOMY;
FASCETECTOMY; SPINAL FUSION)

Laminectomy: *A surgical procedure in which part or all of the lamina of a lumbar vertebra is removed to relieve posterior compression of the spinal cord. Also called decompressive lumbar laminectomy.*
Hemilaminectomy: *The excision of only the right or left lamina.*
Diskectomy: *The removal of the nucleus pulposus when nerve compression is associated with bulging, herniation, or extrusion.*
Fascetectomy: *Partial or complete removal of the fascet joint (one of the joints in the vertebral column).*
Spinal fusion: *Means of stabilizing the spine by surgically inducing a bony mass formed between one or more vertebra used for spondylosis, trauma, and extensive decompression.*

NURSING DIAGNOSES / DEFINING CHARACTERISTICS	NURSING INTERVENTIONS / *RATIONALES*	EXPECTED OUTCOMES
Potential fear/ anxiety: impending surgery *Related to:* Knowledge deficit Loss of control of activity Possible complications Lack of success **DEFINING CHARACTERISTICS** Withdrawn behavior Verbal cues: crying, hostility, negative expectations Avoidance of subject of surgery Obsession with possible complications Obsession with ideal of failure Physical manifestations: Tachycardia Increased BP Headache Backache	**ONGOING ASSESSMENT** · Assess knowledge of surgery. · Assess need for additional information: Exhibits anxiety with increased information Avoids receiving information Asks questions/seeks information · Assess understanding of information about surgery: Can repeat information in own words Can explain instructions to significant others accurately Can perform return demonstrations correctly Can state rationale for each instruction **THERAPEUTIC INTERVENTIONS** · Encourage patient to verbalize concerns. · Encourage patient to verbalize understanding of surgical procedure. · Approach patient calmly, nonjudgmentally. *Nurse's approach may increase or reduce anxiety.* · Review with patient purpose and general procedure. · Give patient pamphlets or slide show/movie if available. *Teaching aids enhance learning process.* · Inform patient of postoperative therapy: Use of incentive spirometer Practice in coughing and deep breathing Practice in log rolling from side to side/onto bedpan IV fluids Analgesic for discomfort Use of pain scale Use of sequential compression sleeves TED hose Foley catheter Hemovac drains Frequent checks by nurses Probable length of bed rest 1 to 3 days Positive aspects of surgery · Encourage significant others to support patient.	Fear/anxiety will be eliminated or reduced.
Pain *Related to:* Surgical incision Limited mobility Stiffness/soreness Muscle spasms Physical rehabilitation program	**ONGOING ASSESSMENT** · Assess for signs/symptoms of discomfort. · Assess description of pain. Encourage patient to describe discomfort: character, location, intensity, radiation, precipitating factor. Encourage patient to rate discomfort on pain scale. *Information must be specific to determine best management.* · Assess experiences with pain and relief measures. *Past experiences may increase or decrease perception of pain.* · Assess effect of analgesic. · Assess effect of repositioning.	Discomfort is relieved or reduced.

NURSING DIAGNOSES / DEFINING CHARACTERISTICS	NURSING INTERVENTIONS / *RATIONALES*	EXPECTED OUTCOMES

DEFINING CHARACTERISTICS
 	
Restlessness
Facial expressions
Body rigidity
Frequent use of nurse's light
Frequent requests for position changes
Guarded, protective behavior
Verbalized pain
	THERAPEUTIC INTERVENTIONS
	
	• Encourage patient to request analgesic or muscle relaxant at earliest sign of discomfort.
	• Encourage use of analgesics 30 min before physical therapy. *Pain diminishes tolerance and increases fatigue.*
	• Offer analgesic as ordered.
	• Instruct patient to evaluate effect of analgesic in relieving discomfort, using pain scale.
	• Encourage quiet environment.
	• Eliminate additional stressors; encourage divisional activity. *Diverting attention from pain may reduce perceived pain.*
	• Maintain correct body alignment at all times.
	• Log roll patient side to side q2h *(promotes comfort and reduces chance of skin breakdown).*
	• Maintain pillows behind back, hips; between legs; and under upper arms.
	• *Prevent strain on back muscles by:*
	    Maintaining HOB flat unless otherwise indicated.
	    Flexing upper legs with pillows when supine, or use knee gatch (avoid flexing knees with pillows directly under popliteal space).
	• When log rolling, place essential items (call light, emesis basin) within reach.
	• Gently massage back and extremities with lotion.
	• Offer cold compress/cloth to apply to face/forehead.
	• Instruct patient *to prevent soreness/stiffness* by:
	    ROM of ankles
	    Bending and extending of knees
	    Flexion and extension exercises of arms	

Potential altered lower extremity tissue perfusion: (neurovascular status)
Related to:
Surgical procedure
Immobility
 	
DEFINING CHARACTERISTICS
 	
Numbness/tingling
Absent or diminished reflexes
Absent or faint pedal pulse
Absent or sluggish capillary refill
Pallor
Coolness
Edema
Unrelieved pain
	ONGOING ASSESSMENT
	
	• Assess neurologic and circulatory status. *Potential for nerve and vascular damage is associated with orthopedic surgery.*
	    Check peripheral pulses: posterior tibial and dorsalis pedis.
	      If finding pulses difficult, mark location with felt pen *(promotes accuracy in subsequent data collection).*
	    Compare pulses bilaterally.
	    Assess for paresthesia:
	      Sharp versus dull sensation
	      Bilateral versus unilateral
	    Assess for pallor or cyanosis:
	      Check skin temperature and color.
	      Check capillary refill.
	    Assess for paralysis.
	    Assess for pain *(increases with edema from secondary nerve compression):*
	      Determine exact location.
	      Determine whether worsening or diminishing.
	    Assess mobility and muscle strength in lower extremities:
	      Active ROM
	      Passive ROM
	    Assess for deep vein thrombosis: Homan's sign.
	• Check sequential compression sleeves (if ordered) for:
	    Correct position (space for knees)
	    Tightness
	    Looseness
	    Excessive warmth
	• Remove sequential compression sleeves every shift and perform neurovascular assessment.
	• Check TED hose (if applicable) for:
	    Correct position
	    Constriction at thighs, ankles
	• Remove TED hose every shift and perform neurovascular assessment.
		Neurovascular status of lower extremities will remain unchanged from preoperative condition.

Musculoskeletal Care Plans

NURSING DIAGNOSES / DEFINING CHARACTERISTICS	NURSING INTERVENTIONS / *RATIONALES*	EXPECTED OUTCOMES
	THERAPEUTIC INTERVENTIONS • Encourage patient to perform ankle ROM exercises *to promote venous blood return*. • Reposition (log roll) q2h and as needed. • Apply sequential compression sleeves as ordered.	
Potential ineffective breathing pattern *Related to:* Anesthesia Immobility Inability to cough and deep breathe adequately Atelectasis Embolism **DEFINING CHARACTERISTICS** Increased respirations >24/min Decreased respirations <10/min Complaints of shortness of breath or dyspnea Decreased breath sounds Auscultation of wheezes, rhonchi, congestion Altered character of respiration: shallow, retractions Production of sputum from coughing	**ONGOING ASSESSMENT** • Assess rate, rhythm, depth, quality of respirations. • Assess ability to cough and deep breathe. • Assess type and duration of anesthesia used during surgery. • Monitor for temperature >38.5°C (101°F) **THERAPEUTIC INTERVENTIONS** • Encourage patient to use incentive spirometer. • Encourage patient to cough and deep breathe. • Log roll patient from side to side q2h *to prevent secretion pooling*. • Encourage patient to notify nurse or physician of shortness of breath or dyspnea. • Maintain proper hydration through oral and IV fluid administration.	Optimal respiratory status will be maintained.

Impaired physical mobility
Related to:
Surgical procedure
Bed rest activity
Discomfort
 	
DEFINING CHARACTERISTICS
Requests for assistance in movement
Verbalized difficulty in moving
Request for analgesic before movement
	ONGOING ASSESSMENT
	• Assess ability to reposition self in bed:
	  Independence
	  Assistance required
	  Poor coordination
	  Poor use of body mechanics
	• Assess muscular strength:
	  Strong
	  Weak/flaccid
	  Stiff
	• Assess ability to follow instructions.
	• Assess tolerance to activity:
	  No complaints
	  Easily tired
	  Verbalized discomfort:
	    Immediate
	    Within minutes
	  Requests for additional or progressive activity
	• Assess ability to perform ADL.
		Independence or minimal assistance with mobility will be achieved.

NURSING DIAGNOSES / DEFINING CHARACTERISTICS	NURSING INTERVENTIONS / *RATIONALES*	EXPECTED OUTCOMES
	THERAPEUTIC INTERVENTIONS	
	• Encourage active ROM of extremities in bed.	
	• Offer analgesic before activity.	

	• Assist patient to dangle at side of bed (when approved by physician).
	    Patient must be in side-lying position, near edge of bed, with knees bent.
	    Elevate HOB.
	    Use hands (patient's) to push up upper torso and pivot buttocks to sitting position with straight back.	

	• Dangle for 3-5 min:
	    Check for signs of lightheadedness, fainting, dizziness, or sweating *(signs of orthostatic hypotension)*.
	    During dangling, have patient flex each foot up and down. *Pumping action of leg muscles supports venous return.*	

	• When ambulating, provide slipper or nonskid shoes *to provide friction force to prevent slipping*.	

	• Ambulate patient as tolerated:
	    Patient uses hands/arms to push up hips from bed.
	    Patient stands for few minutes.
	    Patient uses assistance first time.	

	• Progress ambulation as tolerated. Use assistive devices as needed.	

	• Instruct patient in sitting:
	    Use straight-back chair.
	    Bend knees *(prevents stress on lumbar spine)*.
	    Support weight with arms.
	    Elevate feet with one pillow on floor *(relaxes back muscles)*.	

	• Instruct patient to ambulate or sit while wearing corset (if prescribed).	
	• Instruct patient not to sleep with corset on.	
	• Instruct patient to sit no longer than 10-15 min (first time) and progress as tolerated. No prolonged sitting	

Potential altered nutrition: less than body requirements
Related to:
Anesthesia
Constipation
Abdominal distention
Nausea/vomiting
Absent bowel sounds
NPO status
 	
DEFINING CHARACTERISTICS
Documented intake less than required
	ONGOING ASSESSMENT
	• Assess bowel sounds:
	    Absent
	    Hypoactive
	    Active
	• Assess tolerance to fluids. *Patient may be nauseated or vomit after surgery*.
	• Assess abdominal girth.
	• Monitor I & O.
	
	THERAPEUTIC INTERVENTIONS
	• If patient nauseated after surgery, encourage slow, deep breaths.
	• Avoid abrupt movement *(may aggravate nausea)*. *Log rolling may be postponed until nausea subsides.*
	• If vomiting occurs, offer oral hygiene immediately.
	• If postoperative bowel sounds absent, maintain patient NPO.
	• When bowel sounds return, increase diet as tolerated.
	• If patient has no bowel movement within 2 days of resuming regular diet:
	    Notify physician.
	    Administer laxative (if ordered).
	    Push oral fluids (e.g., prune juice).
	    Encourage bulk, fiber, and roughage.
	    Increase activity, especially ambulation.
		Optimal nutritional satus will be maintained.

Potential for infection *Related to:* Surgical procedure Dressing changes	**ONGOING ASSESSMENT** • Assess surgical incision every shift for appearance and drainage: color, odor, amount. • Assess urine for color, odor, specific gravity, consistency. • Monitor temperature.	Risk of infection will be reduced.

Continued.

NURSING DIAGNOSES / DEFINING CHARACTERISTICS	NURSING INTERVENTIONS / *RATIONALES*	EXPECTED OUTCOMES

Foley catheter
Surgical evacuating device (such as Hemovac)
 	
DEFINING CHARACTERISTICS
Elevated temperature >38.5°C (101°F)
Purulent drainage from incision
Elevated WBC
Signs/symptoms of wound infection
	• Monitor WBC.
	• Obtain samples for urinalysis, culture, and sensitivity if signs/symptoms of urinary tract infection.
	
	THERAPEUTIC INTERVENTIONS
	• Maintain dressing:
	    Use sterile technique during dressing changes.
	    Change or reinforce dressing when indicated.
	• Maintain patency and integrity of surgical evacuating device.
	• Perform Foley catheter care every day.
	• Encourage patient to drink adequate fluids.
	• Provide adequate nutrition *to promote wound healing.*	

Knowledge deficit: discharge
Related to:
New condition and procedures
 	
DEFINING CHARACTERISTICS
Questions
Lack of questions
Confusion with treatment
	ONGOING ASSESSMENT
	• Determine knowledge of postdischarge recovery guidelines.
	
	THERAPEUTIC INTERVENTIONS
	Ride home:
	• Lie on backseat with pillow.
	• Sit with pillow behind back, buttocks to back of seat, knees slightly elevated on book *to reduce stress on back muscles*
	Sleep:
	• Maintain correct body alignment.
	• Use firm mattress. Place board under soft mattress *to increase support.*
	• Sleep on side, with knees and hips flexed (*preferable to sleep on back or abdomen*)
	Activities:
	• Ambulate as tolerated with or without corset (per physician's instructions).
	• Perform exercises (if indicated) as instructed by physical therapist. Allow frequent rest periods.
	• Sit for short periods; may increase as tolerated. Sit in high straight-back chair. If chair too low, place pillow on seat.
	• Avoid lifting or carrying heavy objects. Lift objects at waist level.
	• Avoid reaching/stretching to pick up object. Raise to level required.
	• Sexual activity: recommended abstinence as instructed by physician. Some recommended positions: Assuming underlying position with pillow under buttocks or side-lying position.
	• Take showers; avoid tub baths. If baths a must, avoid flexing lower back when getting in or out.
	• Resume driving per physician order.
	• Return to work per physician order.
	Home treatments:
	• Avoid using heating pad for prolonged periods. Do not set on "high" or use all night.
	• If pain increases with heat application, apply ice for short periods.
	• Take only prescribed analgesics and muscle relaxants, not over-the-counter drugs unless physician recommends. *Drug reactions may result from certain combinations of medications.*
	Complications:
	• Notify your physician if:
	    Pain persists.
	    No treatment method relieves pain.
	    Pain begins to radiate elsewhere.
	    Weakness in extremities increases.
	    Bowel or bladder incontinence occurs.
	    Fever presents.
		Patient will verbalize understanding of discharge instructions.

Originated by: Linda M. Jones, RN, BSN
                 Lisa Berti, RN

Le Fort I osteotomy

(WIRED JAWS)

A surgical procedure in which bone is cut away to correct jaw deformities or repair traumatic injuries.

NURSING DIAGNOSES / DEFINING CHARACTERISTICS	NURSING INTERVENTIONS / *RATIONALES*	EXPECTED OUTCOMES
Ineffective breathing patterns *Related to:* Wired jaws Possible nasal or pharyngeal swelling Possible laryngeal edema caused by prolonged endotracheal intubation **DEFINING CHARACTERISTICS** Elevated respiratory rate Labored respirations Nasal breathing	**ONGOING ASSESSMENT** · Assess rate and rhythm of respirations. · Assess nasal airway for patency. · Auscultate breath sounds. **THERAPEUTIC INTERVENTIONS** · Keep HOB elevated at all times *to prevent aspiration, minimize edema.* · Have wire cutters taped to wall at HOB. · Have aspirator with Yankaeur suction at bedside. · Instruct patient on oral suctioning with Yankaeur suction tube. · Clean nasal airway with normal saline as appropriate. · Maintain humidified air per face tent. · Administer decongestants as ordered per physician. · Instruct patient about to vomit to sit up and turn head to side. Nurse should be prepared to suction out secretions *to prevent aspiration.*	Normal breathing pattern will be maintained.
Altered nutrition: less than body requirements *Related to:* Wire jaws Change in dietary habits Nausea **DEFINING CHARACTERISTICS** Weight loss Documented inadequate caloric intake	**ONGOING ASSESSMENT** · Monitor I & O every shift. · Determine dietary preferences. · Assess patient's weight. **THERAPEUTIC INTERVENTIONS** · Arrange dietary consultation for patient/significant other. · Keep HOB elevated. · Instruct patient on proper use of feeding syringes. · Instruct patient not to attempt to open mouth. · Provide patient with antiemetics as ordered. · Provide patient with diet high in calories, protein, and vitamin C. · Provide liquids and soft or blenderized foods *that require no chewing.* · Have dietary supplements at bedside. · Maintain IV fluids as ordered. Push oral fluids.	Optimal nutrition will be achieved.

Potential for infection
Related to:
Inadequate oral hygiene
 	
DEFINING CHARACTERISTICS
Elevated temperature
Excessive oral secretions
Foul odor from mouth
Increased facial swelling
Excessive drainage on head and face dressing
	ONGOING ASSESSMENT
	· Check head and face dressing for excessive drainage; note color, amount, presence of foul odor.
	· Monitor temperature.
	· Observe for increased facial swelling; loosen dressings as needed.
	
	THERAPEUTIC INTERVENTIONS
	· Administer IV antibiotics as ordered.
	· Administer corticosteroids as ordered.
	· Apply ice packs to both sides of face *to minimize edema.*
	· Instruct patient on proper mouth care *to remove particles of food providing medium for bacterial growth:*
	  Normal saline rinses after meals, at bedtime.
	  Brushing teeth with a child-size, soft toothbrush after meals, at bedtime, beginning 48 hr after surgery
		Potential for intraoral infection will be reduced.

Continued.

Le Fort I osteotomy— cont'd

NURSING DIAGNOSES / DEFINING CHARACTERISTICS	NURSING INTERVENTIONS / *RATIONALES*	EXPECTED OUTCOMES
Impaired verbal communication *Related to:* Wired jaws Increased facial swelling **DEFINING CHARACTERISTICS** Difficulty understanding patient speech	**ONGOING ASSESSMENT** · Determine whether patient can speak so understood by others. · Determine whether patient can write. **THERAPEUTIC INTERVENTIONS** · Have call light within patient's reach. · Provide paper and pen at bedside. · Instruct patient that opening mouth is not possible *with jaws wired closed.* · Inform patient that wires usually removed in 6-8 weeks. · Offer patient support and reassurance. · See Communication, impaired verbal p. 11.	Alternate means of communication will be established.
Knowledge deficit related to home care *Related to:* Lack of similar experiences **DEFINING CHARACTERISTICS** Repeated questions Lack of questions Patient unable to perform return demonstrations on proper use of feeding syringes and proper oral hygiene maintenance	**ONGOING ASSESSMENT** · Determine whether patient has questions. · Determine whether patient can use feeding syringes and perform proper oral hygiene with ease. **THERAPEUTIC INTERVENTIONS** · Inform patient/significant others of the following: Wire cutters provided *for emergency wire removal* Correct way to cut wires Dietary instructions provided per dietitian, with syringes and suction catheters for home use Proper cleaning of feeding syringes after each use Avoidance of alcohol *to minimize vomiting/loss of control of secretions* Best position to assume for vomiting Importance of maintaining proper oral hygiene Facial swelling usually gone in 1 wk	Patient will demonstrate and verbalize appropriate, safe self-care.

Orginated by: Patricia A. Hannon, RN

Myelography

(SPINAL X-RAY)

A radiologic exam that allows visualization of the spinal cord after a radiopaque dye is injected. It assists in the determination of spinal cord deficits.

NURSING DIAGNOSES / DEFINING CHARACTERISTICS	NURSING INTERVENTIONS / *RATIONALES*	EXPECTED OUTCOMES
Knowledge deficit *Related to:* Unfamiliar procedure **DEFINING CHARACTERISTICS** Verbalized lack of knowledge of procedure Lack of questions Multiple questions	**ONGOING ASSESSMENT** · Assess patient's previous experience with myelography. **THERAPEUTIC INTERVENTIONS** · Teach patient: Reason/need for myelography Premyelography care Elements of procedure Postprocedure care (transfer by cart, HOB elevated 40 degrees, restricted gross motor movements 10-12 hr after procedure, pushing of fluids, and administration of phenobarbital q6h *to prevent seizures.* · Document teaching and client's understanding. · Encourage and answer questions. · Include significant others in teaching as appropriate.	Patient will verbalize understanding of procedure and postprocedure care.

Myelography— cont'd

NURSING DIAGNOSES / DEFINING CHARACTERISTICS	NURSING INTERVENTIONS / *RATIONALES*	EXPECTED OUTCOMES

Pain
Related to:
Use of radiopaque dye
Postprocedure restrictions
 	
Defining Characteristics
Complaints of headache, backache, leg pain, numbness, tingling of extremities
Head holding
Reluctance to move
	Ongoing Assessment
	• Assess experiences with pain/analgesic use.
	• Assess pain:
	  Location
	  Intensity
	  Quality
	  Precipitating factors
	
	Therapeutic Interventions
	• Anticipate need for and administer analgesics. Use non-phenothiazine-derived narcotic potentiators and antiemetics. *Phenothiazine-derived narcotic potentiators, antiemetics may lower seizure threshold.*
	• Administer IV fluids as ordered *to facilitate dye excretion.*
	• *Prevent upward migration of dye by:*
	  Keeping HOB elevated.
	  Restricting gross motor movements.
	• Maintain bed rest as ordered.
		Pain will be relieved.

Potential for injury *Related to:* Presence of dye in spinal column **Defining Characteristics** Seizure activity	**Ongoing Assessment** • Assess history of drug use that may have lowered seizure threshold (e.g., phenothiazides, tricycle antidepressants, amphetamines, MAO inhibitors). • Assess previous seizure history. • Assess seizure activity; report immediately. **Therapeutic Interventions** • Administer phenobarbital as ordered. • Administer IV and oral fluids as ordered *to facilitate dye excretion.* • See Seizure activity, p. 263.	Seizures will be prevented.

Originated by: Lori Luke, RN

Partial anterior acromiectomy with or without rotator cuff repair

(BANKART REPAIR; PUTTI-PLATT OPERATION; BRISTOW REPAIR)

Decompression of the subacromial space by osteotomy of the anterior/inferior margin of the acromion and trans-section of the coracoacromial ligament, with examination of rotator cuff muscles and repair of defect if indicated.

NURSING DIAGNOSES / DEFINING CHARACTERISTICS	NURSING INTERVENTIONS / *RATIONALES*	EXPECTED OUTCOMES
Potential knowledge deficit related to surgical procedure *Related to:* New procedures Unfamiliarity with surgical routines	**Ongoing Assessment** • Assess previous hospital experiences. • Assess cognitive/intellectual level. • Assess existing medical problem. • Assess knowledge of present problem and recommended treatment. **Therapeutic Interventions** • Obtain complete nursing history. • Verbally review operative protocol.	Patient will demonstrate/verbalize understanding of preoperative instructions and postoperative care.

Continued.

Musculoskeletal Care Plans

NURSING DIAGNOSES / DEFINING CHARACTERISTICS	NURSING INTERVENTIONS / *RATIONALES*	EXPECTED OUTCOMES

DEFINING CHARACTERISTICS
 	
Many questions
Lack of questions
Increased anxiety level
Verbalized misconceptions
	· Instruct patient:
	    About hospital educational television with general pre-, intra- and post-operative information
	    In preoperative routines
	    On preop strength testing (Cybex testing) if necessary
	    On immediate postoperative routines (e.g., closed wound suction, drains, IV, diet, pain management)
	    On coughing and deep breathing exercises
	    On exercises and mobility limitations
	· Encourage questions; answer fully. *Knowledge increases patient's ability to understand health problem, reduces postoperative complications, and reduces postoperative pain.*	

Potential for infection *Related to:* Surgical procedure Incision **DEFINING CHARACTERISTICS** Increased warmth Redness Swelling Tenderness at incision site Increased WBC count Increased temperature	**ONGOING ASSESSMENT** · Assess patient for signs/symptoms of infection. · Monitor vital signs; notify physician of abnormalities. **THERAPEUTIC INTERVENTIONS** · Administer antibiotics as ordered. · Encourage fluid intake. *Body must maintain adequate fluid levels to support metabolism necessary for microbial defense.* · Maintain strict aseptic technique for dressing changes *to prevent contamination of wound.* · Maintain wound suction; use aseptic technique.	Risk of infection will be reduced.
Potential ineffective breathing pattern *Related to:* Immobility Fatigue **DEFINING CHARACTERISTICS** Increased temperature Adventitious breath sounds Chest pain Abnormal ABGs Increased anxiety Tachypnea Dyspnea Tachycardia Cyanosis	**ONGOING ASSESSMENT** · Monitor respiratory rate and rhythm. · Assess breath sounds. · Assess signs/symptoms of respiratory compromise/pulmonary embolus. **THERAPEUTIC INTERVENTIONS** · Instruct patient on incentive spirometer use, coughing and deep breathing exercises before surgery. · Encourage patient to use incentive spirometer q1-2h while awake. *Lung expansion facilitates gas exchange.* · Turn q2h as tolerated. · Encourage mobility (i.e., sit in chair; ambulate) *to promote greater lung expansion.* · Encourage fluid intake *to prevent thickening of lung secretions.*	Optimal breathing pattern is achieved.
Pain *Related to:* Surgical procedure **DEFINING CHARACTERISTICS** Patient's/significant other's report of pain Facial grimaces Moaning, crying Protective, guarded behavior	**ONGOING ASSESSMENT** · Assess description of pain. · Assess behavior and facial expressions. · Assess previous experiences with pain and pain relief. · Assess pain relief measure effectiveness. **THERAPEUTIC INTERVENTIONS** · Respond immediately to pain complaints. · Give analgesics as ordered; evaluate effectiveness. · Alter patient's position (turn to nonoperative side, adjust pillows to support affected shoulder, seat in chair or bed).	Pain is reduced or relieved.

Partial anterior acromiectomy with or without rotator cuff repair— cont'd

NURSING DIAGNOSES / DEFINING CHARACTERISTICS	NURSING INTERVENTIONS / *RATIONALES*	EXPECTED OUTCOMES
Restlessness Withdrawal Irritability	· Encourage appropriate rest periods. *Rest conserves energy necessary for cellular metabolism needed for tissue healing.* · Eliminate additional stressors, encourage diversional activity. · Instruct patient to report pain *so relief measures can be implemented.* · See Pain, p. 39 and Patient-controlled anesthesia, p. 631.	
Potential altered peripheral tissue perfusion to affected extremity *Related to:* Surgical procedure Restricted movement Swelling **DEFINING CHARACTERISTICS** Coldness Pallor Pain Edema Sluggish or absent capillary refill Pressure within muscle compartment	**ONGOING ASSESSMENT** · Use preoperative neurovascular assessment to establish baseline status for postoperative comparison. · Assess upper extremities; compare temperature, color, sensation, movement, edema, pulse, and capillary refill q4h×24h, then q8hr when stable. · Assess for increasing pain in affected extremity. **THERAPEUTIC INTERVENTIONS** · Notify physician of neurovascular status changes. *Diminished tissue oxygenation results from impaired circulation, which increases potential for tissue necrosis.*	Tissue perfusion will be maintained.
Ineffective individual coping *Related to:* Disability **DEFINING CHARACTERISTICS** Verbalized feelings related to temporary disability Fear Anger	**ONGOING ASSESSMENT** · Assess description of disability. · Assess normal coping patterns. · Assess support systems. **THERAPEUTIC INTERVENTIONS** · Encourage patient to verbalize feelings/thoughts on disability and work life. *Ventilation of feelings supports honesty and objectivity, promotes realistic perception.* · Assist patient to identify activities that do *not* involve use of operative shoulder. · Encourage maximum independence within limitations.	Optimal coping strategies will be facilitated.
Self-care deficit *Related to:* Restricted movement of extremity by immobilizer, sling, shoulder spica cast **DEFINING CHARACTERISTICS** Inability to perform ADL independently Bathing/hygiene Dressing/grooming Toileting Feeding	**ONGOING ASSESSMENT** · Assess preoperative and postoperative ability to perform ADLs. · Assess available home support systems. · Assess need for OT for ADL training. *Immobilization of upper extremity demands alternative methods of performing ADL.* **THERAPEUTIC INTERVENTIONS** · Assist in ADL training. · Reinforce OT and use of assistive devices if ordered. · Request social service consultation for home needs	Self-care activities are performed.
Knowledge deficit: home management *Related to:* Unfamiliarity with postoperative activity	**ONGOING ASSESSMENT** · Assess knowledge of postoperative activity. *Knowledge increases patient's ability to understand health problems.* · Assess cognitive/intellectual level.	Patient will demonstrate/verbalize understanding of home management.

Continued.

Partial anterior acromiectomy with or without rotator cuff repair— cont'd

NURSING DIAGNOSES / DEFINING CHARACTERISTICS	NURSING INTERVENTIONS / *RATIONALES*	EXPECTED OUTCOMES

DEFINING CHARACTERISTICS
Many questions
Increased anxiety about impending discharge
	THERAPEUTIC INTERVENTIONS
	• Emphasize importance of maintaining position in shoulder immobilizer, sling, or cast 3-6 wk.
	• Educate patient to put nothing under cast or immobilizer.
	• Instruct on:
	  Positions to avoid (abduction, lifting, etc.)
	  Need to keep incision dry and clean
	  Need to inspect skin around immobilizer or cast for irritation
	• Instruct patient to notify physician of:
	  Pain, numbness, tingling, edema, or discoloration of fingers
	  Pain, redness, drainage from incision
	  Persistent fever
	  Cracking or softened areas in cast
	  Pain, numbness, drainage, foul odors, or warm areas under cast
	  Anything inside cast
	  Areas of skin breakdown around cast or immobilizer
	• Discuss courses of rehabilitation:
	  PT starts in 3-6 wk
	  Complete rehabilitation take 6 mon to 1 yr
	• Give patient instructions for follow-up physician visit.	

Originated by: Sandra Eungard, RN, MS
                Kevin Walsh, MD
                Kevin Tetsworth, MD

Scoliosis: spinal instrumentation

(HARRINGTON ROD; LUQUE RODS; DWYER PROCEDURE)

Spinal instrumentation for severe scoliosis involves surgical fixation and correction of scoliosis that is progressive and not responsive to bracing and exercise. Correction is accomplished with Harrington, Luque, or Dwyer instrumentation, each of which uses a different kind of fixator. Differences in fixator dictate postoperative care. The Harrington rod is somewhat less stable and requires a longer period of postoperative immobility.

NURSING DIAGNOSES/ DEFINING CHARACTERISTICS	NURSING INTERVENTIONS / *RATIONALES*	EXPECTED OUTCOMES

Anxiety/fear
Related to:
Anticipation of physical harm or psychologic threat (e.g., impending surgery)
Forced adaptation to changed health status
 	
DEFINING CHARACTERISTICS
Mild
  Restlessness
  Increased awareness
  Increased questioning
Moderate to severe
  Avoidance of looking at equipment
	ONGOING ASSESSMENT
	• Recognize level of anxiety (mild, severe). Note signs/symptoms, especially nonverbal communication.
	• Assess normal coping patterns (interview patient/family/significant others/physician).
	• Assess knowledge levels, reasons for hospitalization, scoliosis, body image, anatomy involved, and postoperative expectations (e.g., ICU, frame).
	• See Anxiety, p. 4, and Fear, p. 18.
	
	THERAPEUTIC INTERVENTIONS
	• Orient to environment.
	• Display confident, calm manner and understanding attitude.
	• Establish rapport through continuity of care.
	• Explain preoperative and postoperative procedures/routines.
	• Encourage ventilation of feelings.
	• Provide quite environment; reduce distracting stimuli.
	• Encourage questions to clear up misconceptions.
	• Encourage family visits.
		Anxiety/fear will be reduced.

NURSING DIAGNOSES / DEFINING CHARACTERISTICS	NURSING INTERVENTIONS / *RATIONALES*	EXPECTED OUTCOMES
Little movement in bed Withdrawal Tense/anxious appearance	· Use other supportive measures (e.g., medications and psychiatric liaison). · Provide diversional measures. · Introduce to ICU staff before surgery. · Practice aspects of anticipated therapy (e.g., deep breathing, spirometer, leg exercises, use of frame, fracture bedpan). *Sometimes knowing what to expect lessens fear/anxiety, facilitates postoperative compliance.*	
Impaired physical mobility *Related to:* Required immobilization caused by nature of surgery Prolonged immobilization Surgery proximal to spinal cord and nerve roots Development of edema, infection, hematoma at surgical site with nerve root/cord compression **DEFINING CHARACTERISTICS** Inability to move purposefully within physical environment Weakness in leg, foot, or toes Reluctance to attempt mobility, limited ROM, decreased muscle strength and control Increased back pain Signs/symptoms of cord compression: Radiating pain in distal nerve root (thigh, calf, foot) Asymmetric lower extremity reflexes Change in sensory function	**ONGOING ASSESSMENT** · Assess for impaired mobility, cord compression: Use verbal commands; ask to do simple tasks (e.g., wiggle toes and dorsiflex feet) *to assess motor function.* Use light touch and pain to check sensations. · See Mobility, impaired physical p. 35. **THERAPEUTIC INTERVENTIONS** · Explain progressive physical activity. · Encourage early ADL when possible. · Turn patient on frame as scheduled. · Encourage appropriate use of assistive devices. · Maintain patient's body in good alignment. · Use antipressure devices prophylactically as ordered/indicated. · Perform *passive* ROM while patient on bed rest/frame *to minimize risk of injury that may be related to active ROM.*	Consequences of immobility will be reduced.
Pain *Related to:* Surgical procedure Immobility Bone harvesting (rib or iliac) **DEFINING CHARACTERISTICS** Guarding behavior Self-focus, withdrawal Crying Moaning	**ONGOING ASSESSMENT** · Assess for signs/symptoms of discomfort. *Postoperative pain is expected but should diminish over time. Sudden onset or increase in pain should be investigated as potential complication symptom.* **THERAPEUTIC INTERVENTIONS** · Anticipate need for analgesia. Consider PCA, around-the-clock injections, or continuous infusion to control immediate postoperative pain. · See Pain, p. 39.	Pain will be relieved or reduced.

Continued.

NURSING DIAGNOSES/ DEFINING CHARACTERISTICS	NURSING INTERVENTIONS / *RATIONALES*	EXPECTED OUTCOMES
Restlessness Irritability Facial mask of pain Altered muscle tone Changes in vital signs, respiration, color Altered sleep pattern Verbalized discomfort		
Potential altered tissue perfusion *Related to:* Immobility with venous stasis *(preventing normal blood flow and facilitating clot formation)* Reactions to anesthesia and medications Blood loss Lengthy surgical procedure **DEFINING CHARACTERISTICS** Ischemic pain Increased coldness, numbness, loss of hair, trophic skin changes, pallor, or rubor Swelling of lower extremities Changes in BP Delayed healing of lesions Venous distention in lower extremities Pulmonary embolism: Dyspnea Tachycardia Chest pain Fever Neck vein distention Cyanosis Restlessness Hypoxemia Hemoptysis	**ONGOING ASSESSMENT** · Observe skin over extremities for color, pallor, rubor, hair distribution. · Inspect for distention of superficial vessels of lower extremities. · Monitor vital signs. · Assess circulation, mobility, and sensation of all extremities. Compare temperature of extremities; palpate pulses (radial, femoral, pedal); compare symmetry. Palpate extremities for edema. · Assess for development of thrombophlebitis: leg swelling, redness, pain on dorsiflexion. Measure calves and thighs if symptoms of deep vein thrombosis present. · Assess for pulmonary embolism (see Defining Characteristics). Encourage patient to report pain, shortness of breath, or hemoptysis. **THERAPEUTIC INTERVENTIONS** · Maintain body alignment. · Apply TED hose. · Turn frequently or as ordered. · Encourage coughing and deep breathing. · Demonstrate and encourage leg exercises. · Administer anticoagulant therapy if ordered. *Not all patients will require anticoagulants, depending on type of surgery and age and condition of patient.* · Refer to Pulmonary thromboembolism, p. 200.	Optimal tissue perfusion will be maintained.
Potential impaired gas exchange *Related to:* Hypostatic pneumonia related to prolonged anesthesia	**ONGOING ASSESSMENT** · Assess respiratory rate, rhythm, amplitude. Auscultate breath sounds. · Monitor ABGs. · Obtain sputum for culture and sensitivity *if infection suspected.* · Note chest pain, shortness of breath, or hemoptysis.	Optimal gas exchange will be maintained.

NURSING DIAGNOSES / DEFINING CHARACTERISTICS	NURSING INTERVENTIONS / *RATIONALES*	EXPECTED OUTCOMES
Immobilization in OR and on frame **DEFINING CHARACTERISTICS** Sudden onset of shaking chills Fever Flushed skin Productive cough (pink-tinged) Sharp chest pain, increased on inspiration Headache Rales/rhonchi Tachypnea Decreased breath sounds over affected lung area Hypoxemia	**THERAPEUTIC INTERVENTIONS** · Turn on frame as scheduled. · Demonstrate breathing exercises and encourage use of spirometer (blow bottles, glove) *to prevent hypostatic pneumonia.* · Administer antibiotics, if ordered. · Perform chest percussion and postural drainage as necessary. · Administer humidified air or O_2 as ordered. · Encourage fluids *to decrease secretion viscosity.*	
Potential fluid volume deficit/excess *Related to:* Rapid blood loss or excess fluid loss (through fever, diarrhea, nasogastric drainage, diaphoresis, and inadequate fluid intake) Aggressive fluid therapy in OR **DEFINING CHARACTERISTICS** *Deficit:* Specific gravity >1.025 Decreased urine output Sudden weight loss Hypotension Thirst Tachycardia Decreased skin turgor Dry mucous membranes Weakness *Excess:* Specific gravity <1.010 Facial/peripheral edema Increased urine output	**ONGOING ASSESSMENT** · Monitor hydration status: 　Skin turgor 　Mucous membranes 　I & O 　Urine specific gravity 　Serum lytes 　*Note: Expect facial edema caused by positioning in OR.* · Monitor vital signs (including CVP) during initial postoperative course. · Monitor drainage from Hemovacs. **THERAPEUTIC INTERVENTIONS** · Administer IV fluids as prescribed. · Encourage oral liquid intake when patient able. · Notify physician of changes in hydration or excessive Hemovac/other drainage.	Fluid volume and electrolyte balance will be maintained.

Continued.

449

NURSING DIAGNOSES/ DEFINING CHARACTERISTICS	NURSING INTERVENTIONS / *RATIONALES*	EXPECTED OUTCOMES
Potential urinary retention *Related to:* Obstructive uropathy Recent anesthesia Medications Obstructed catheter Spinal cord compression, neurogenic bladder **DEFINING CHARACTERISTICS** Complaints of lower abdominal pain or discomfort Desire but inability to urinate Paresthesia Decreased (<30 ml/hr) or absent urinary output for 2 consecutive hr Frequency Hesitancy Urgency Lower abdomen distention Restlessness	**ONGOING ASSESSMENTS** • Assess for symptoms of urinary retention. • Evaluate medications, especially morphine or derivatives, for possible side effects. • Assess for decreased neurologic function, paresthesia of lower extremities, decreased bowel sounds. **THERAPEUTIC INTERVENTIONS** • Maintain patency of urinary catheter. • Notify physician if patient does not void within 4 hr after catheter removal. • If cord compression suspected, prepare for surgical intervention. • See Urinary retention, p. 61.	Optimal urinary elimination will be maintained.

Potential constipation/ impaction
Related to:
Anesthesia
Inadequate fluid or food intake
Decreased mobility
Analgesics
Spinal cord or nerve root compression or damage
 	
DEFINING CHARACTERISTICS
Feeling of fullness
Cramping pain
Tender abdomen
Headache
Nausea
Anorexia
Abdominal distention
Gurgling, decreased, or absent bowel sounds
Hard masses of stool on examination or expelled
	ONGOING ASSESSMENT
	• Monitor GI activity and fluid balance.
	• Monitor for signs of neurologic impairment that may accompany bowel elimination problem:
	    Paresthesia (numbness, tingling of extremities)
	    Absent or decreased reflexes (nerve root) or increased reflexes (spinal cord).
	
	THERAPEUTIC INTERVENTIONS
	• Notify physician of abnormal signs.
	• See Constipation, p. 12.
		Optimal bowel elimination will be maintained.

NURSING DIAGNOSES/ DEFINING CHARACTERISTICS	NURSING INTERVENTIONS / *RATIONALES*	EXPECTED OUTCOMES
Flatulence Dehydration Vomiting		

Potential for infection
Related to:
Surgical incision
 	
DEFINING CHARACTERISTICS
Fever
Increased WBC
Surgical incision:
  Swelling
  Hematoma
  Redness
  Odor
  Burning/itching
  Pain
  Numbness
	ONGOING ASSESSMENT
	• Assess surgical site:
	  Note color, moisture, texture, and temperature.
	  Assess incision line and dressing.
	  Check incision for cleanliness, approximation, swelling, hematoma, redness, odor.
	  Ask about burning or itching.
	• Assess nutritional status.
	• See Skin integrity, impaired, p. 48.
	
	THERAPEUTIC INTERVENTIONS
	• Keep dressing dry and intact.
	• Maintain Steri-strips to incision until significant healing, then remove all that have not fallen off before cast is applied.
	• Clean and dry skin with each turning.
	• Report any changes (redness, swelling, drainage, or heat) at incisional area.
	• *Prevent pressure on incisional area:*
	  Turn patient as scheduled on frame.
	  Use prophylactic antipressure devices.
	  Maintain proper body alignment.
	• Encourage adequate nutrition and hydration.
		Risk of infection is reduced.

Potential for injury
Related to:
Postoperative placement on Foster or Stryker frame
Unstable condition of spine
 	
DEFINING CHARACTERISTICS
Attempt to get up
Brakes not on bed
Improper lifting
Improper turning
	ONGOING ASSESSMENT
	• Assess environment for safety hazards.
	• Assess all equipment for proper working conditions (e.g., safety straps, brakes, screws in place).
	• Assess type of spinal instrumentation for expected limitations.
	
	THERAPEUTIC INTERVENTIONS
	• Provide safe environment.
	• Avoid jolting frame, especially in turning.
	• Place safety straps on all patients on turning frames.
	• Use proper turning/lifting techniques *to prevent displacement of spinal instrument:*
	  Turn frames smoothly, quickly, without jolting.
	  Turn in bed by log roll technique. Obtain assistance when necessary.
		Injury will be prevented.

Potential body image disturbance/self-concept disturbance *Related to:* Body image changes Body cast Lack of privacy Separation from family/significant others/peers **DEFINING CHARACTERISTICS** Dependence Depression Denial/grief Withdrawal	**ONGOING ASSESSMENT** • Assess patient's perception of self and expectations of surgery and casting. *Female adolescents are the most frequently seen patients with scoliosis requiring surgical correction and casting. Adolescents particularly concerned with self-concept and body image; require sensitive nursing care.* **THERAPEUTIC INTERVENTIONS** • Encourage verbalization of concerns. • Be sensitive to concerns about body image; intervene appropriately. • Provide mirrors so body can be visualized. • Assist with self-care activities, especially hair care, makeup. • Provide most privacy possible, especially during bathing and toileting. • Decorate body cast as desired. • Let continue normal activities as possible (e.g., ADL, schooling). • Provide diversionary activities (e.g., telephone, television, friends); establish schedules.	Body image/self-concept disturbance will be reduced.

Continued.

Scoliosis: spinal instrumentation— cont'd

NURSING DIAGNOSES/ DEFINING CHARACTERISTICS	NURSING INTERVENTIONS / *RATIONALES*	EXPECTED OUTCOMES
Restlessness Regression Anger Sadness Frequent questions Frequent complaints Negative attitude Crying/irritability Distorted self-image Expressed self-doubt Verbalized discontent with body		

Knowledge deficit
Related to:
Surgical procedure
Postoperative care
Casting and cast care
 	
DEFINING CHARACTERISTICS
Frequent questions
Frequent complaints
Vague physical complaints
Anxiousness
Restlessness
Withdrawal
Regression
	ONGOING ASSESSMENT
	• Assess current understanding of spinal instrumentation, postoperative care.
	• Assess knowledge of home care needs, ability to perform self-care.
	• Assess readiness for learning.
	
	THERAPEUTIC INTERVENTIONS
	• Provide information appropriate to type of surgery.
	• Provide information about:
	    Skin care
	    Cast care
	    Nutrition
	    Physical limitations
	    Medications
	• Arrange follow-up appointments; provide emergency phone number.
		Patient will verbalize understanding of surgery and demonstrate home/self-care measures.

Originated by: Denise Birkner, RN, BSN

Skeletal traction to an extremity

Traction is the application of a pulling force to an area of the body or to an extremity. Skeletal traction is applied directly through the bone via Steinman pins or Kirscher wires.

NURSING DIAGNOSES / DEFINING CHARACTERISTICS	NURSING INTERVENTIONS / *RATIONALES*	EXPECTED OUTCOMES
Knowledge deficit *Related to:* Lack of experience with traction **DEFINING CHARACTERISTICS** High anxiety level Multitude of questions Lack of questions Patient/family verbalized lack of knowledge of traction	**ONGOING ASSESSMENT** • Assess cognitive/intellectual level. • Assess previous hospital experiences. • Assess knowledge of traction. **THERAPEUTIC INTERVENTIONS** • Encourage patient to verbalize questions and concerns. • Explain purpose of traction as related to injury and healing process. *Providing information helps alleviate anxiety, enables patient to absorb, retain further information and instructions.* • Explain traction apparatus. • Teach patient prevention of possible injury- and traction-related complications (e.g., pain, malalignment).	Patient verbalizes understanding of purpose and application of traction.

NURSING DIAGNOSES / DEFINING CHARACTERISTICS	NURSING INTERVENTIONS / *RATIONALES*	EXPECTED OUTCOMES
	· Explain pin insertion procedure. · Explain pin and traction removal procedure and application of cast/brace as appropriate.	

Pain
Related to:
Fractured limb
Skeletal pins (pain at insertion site)
 	
DEFINING CHARACTERISTICS
Patient-verbalized pain
Irritability
Restlessness
Crying/moaning
Facial grimaces
Altered vital signs: increased pulses, blood pressure, and respirations
Withdrawal
Unwillingness to change position
Inability to sleep
	ONGOING ASSESSMENT
	· Solicit subjective information about pain.
	· Assess for signs/symptoms of pain.
	· Assess pain characteristics:
	   Location
	   Quality
	   Severity
	   Onset
	   Duration
	   Precipitating factors
	· Assess experience with pain and relief measures.
	· Assess present pain relief measures' effectiveness.
	· Assess for correct positioning of traction and alignment of affected extremity. *Incorrect positioning and malalignment can cause pain.*
	· Assess types of activity that increase pain.
	
	THERAPEUTIC INTERVENTIONS
	· Instruct patient to request analgesics at early sign of pain.
	· Respond immediately to pain complaint.
	· Anticipate need for analgesics.
	· Give analgesics as ordered; evaluate effectiveness *to determine whether effective.*
	· Eliminate additional stressors or sources of pain/discomfort with comfort measures:
	   Relaxation techniques
	   Diversionary activity: age-appropriate activities (books, games, television, sewing, radio)
	   Heat or cold application
	   Position changes
	   Verbal and physical reassurance
	   Touch (back rubs, holding)
	Directing attention from pain or to other body areas decreases pain perception.
	· Explain pain management regimen to patient/family.
	· Explore other possible causes of pain.
	· See Pain, p. 39.
		Pain will be reduced.

Potential altered tissue perfusion (neurovascular function)
Related to:
Fractured limb
Immobility imposed by traction
Insertion of skeletal pin
 	
DEFINING CHARACTERISTICS
Edema
Pale, cool extremity
Sluggish/absent capillary refill
Numbness and tingling
	ONGOING ASSESSMENT
	· Assess neurovascular status immediately after injury, after traction application, then q2-4h for 48 hr; every shift when stable:
	   Color
	   Capillary refill
	   Pulses above and below injury
	   Temperature
	   Sensation
	   Motion
	   Edema
	Baseline data useful to determining absence, presence, or extent of neurovascular compromise.
	· Assess degree of pain with passive motion.
	· Assess for positive Homan's sign.
	
	THERAPEUTIC INTERVENTIONS
	· Elevate extremity by suspension traction. *Elevation enhances venous blood return, which enhances circulation to area.*
	· Provide foot board or wrist splints as needed.
		Neurovascular function will be preserved.

Continued.

NURSING DIAGNOSES / DEFINING CHARACTERISTICS	NURSING INTERVENTIONS / *RATIONALES*	EXPECTED OUTCOMES
Diminished/absent pulses distal to injury Cyanosis Pain Altered sensation	· Instruct, encourage exercises for affected and unaffected extremities as allowed. · Apply antiembolic stockings or sequential compression devices as ordered; remove regularly for skin inspection. · Report neurovascular compromise to physician. · Inform patient/family of complications/warning signs of impaired circulation, methods to prevent complications.	
Potential altered tissue perfusion: compartment syndrome *Related to:* Severe tissue swelling that decreases blood flow, causes ischemia, and may cause permanent motor/sensory damage **DEFINING CHARACTERISTICS** Pain upon passive stretch of involved muscles Progressive pain disproportionate to expectations Pallor or cyanosis distal to injury site Edema of limb distal to injury Decreased active and passive muscle movement to injury site Numbness/tingling Tightness of compartment	**ONGOING ASSESSMENT** · Assess affected extremity for signs/symptoms. · Compare affected extremity to unaffected and to previous assessments. · Perform assessments of muscular strength with neurovascular checks. **THERAPEUTIC INTERVENTIONS** · Report complaints of increased pain to physician. · Remove constrictive dressings, straps, or equipment as indicated. *Constrictive forces may cause or worsen existing compartment syndrome.*	Risk of motor/sensory loss will be reduced.
Potential fluid volume deficit *Related to:* Multiple fractures Blood vessel damage **DEFINING CHARACTERISTICS** Weak, rapid pulse Cool, moist skin Decreased blood pressure Anxiety Slow capillary refill Decreased urinary output	**ONGOING ASSESSMENT** · Assess amount of bleeding. · Assess for symptoms of hypovolemia. *Amount of bleeding evaluated in relation to blood pressure, pulse rate, and other hemorrhage signs.* · Monitor vital signs. · Monitor lab values: Hb/Hct. · Record I & O. *Urinary output is sensitive indicator of fluid volume status.* **THERAPEUTIC INTERVENTIONS** · Apply pressure to bleeding areas. · Administer IV fluids and blood as ordered. · See: Fluid volume deficit, p. 20.	Risk of fluid volume deficit will be reduced.

Skeletal traction to an extremity— cont'd

NURSING DIAGNOSES / DEFINING CHARACTERISTICS	NURSING INTERVENTIONS / *RATIONALES*	EXPECTED OUTCOMES
Poential for infection: pin sites/open wounds *Related to:* Interrupted first line of defense Interruption of bone structure **DEFINING CHARACTERISTICS** Redness Swelling Purulent drainage Odor Tenderness/pain Warmth at affected site Elevated temperature Increased WBCs	**ONGOING ASSESSMENT** • Assess pin sites/open wounds for infection signs every shift: Drainage Odor Warmth Excessive pain/tenderness • Assess for skin tension at pin sites. • Assess vital signs (especially temperature) q4h. • Monitor lab values (WBC). **THERAPEUTIC INTERVENTIONS** • Perform pin care q8h as ordered. • Use aseptic technique to perform pin care, change dressings. • Document appearance of pin sites, wounds. • Administer antibiotics as ordered. • Instruct patient/family on purpose of pin care and infection signs/symptoms. • Encourage foods high in protein and vitamin C. *Vitamin C facilitates wound healing.* • Notify physician of infection or skin tension at pin sites.	Risk of infection will be reduced.
Impaired physical mobility *Related to:* Fractured limb Restrictions imposed by traction and injury **DEFINING CHARACTERISTICS** Reluctance to move Inability to move Limited ROM and muscle strength	**ONGOING ASSESSMENT** • Assess patient's ability to perform ADLs. • Assess present and preinjury mobility levels. • Assess ROM of unaffected extremity. • Assess muscle strength. **THERAPEUTIC INTERVENTIONS** • Encourage independence within limitation. • Instruct in use of assistive devices (overhead trapeze and siderails). • Teach isometric and other exercises to affected extremity as appropriate. *Quad sets, ankle pumps, straight leg raises, gluteal sets, push ups, heel slides, and abductor sets help prevent development of stiff joints and muscle atrophy.* • Assist with repositioning. Maintain body in functional alignment. • Initiate exercise program consultation. • Instruct patient/family on complications of immobility and preventive measures.	Optimal mobility will be maintained.
Potential for injury *Related to:* Improper positioning of traction **DEFINING CHARACTERISTICS** Verbalized pain or discomfort at traction site	**ONGOING ASSESSMENT** • Assess traction apparatus every shift: Weight Knots Ropes • Assess patient's position in traction. • Assess that ropes not frayed or stretched. • Assess that spreader bars, foot plate, or splints do not touch foot of bed. • Assess that bed linens not interfering with traction. **THERAPEUTIC INTERVENTIONS** • Maintain affected extremity in functional traction. • Tighten all traction equipment. • Secure all knots with tape. • Keep weights hanging freely. *Deviations alter amount of traction applied, thus therapeutic effect.* • Maintain continuous traction at all times. • Maintain rope in center of pulley.	Desired position and alignment will be maintained.

Continued.

Skeletal traction to an extremity— cont'd

NURSING DIAGNOSES / DEFINING CHARACTERISTICS	NURSING INTERVENTIONS / *RATIONALES*	EXPECTED OUTCOMES
	• Maintain adequate countertraction. Avoid elevating HOB > 30 degrees except during meals, for patients in lower extremity skeletal traction. *Countertraction necessary for effective traction.* • Provide foot plate or wrist splint *to maintain proper position of affected extremity.*	

Potential altered skin integrity
Related to:
Immobility
Prolonged bed rest
Contact with traction apparatus
Countertraction (patient's body weight)
 	
DEFINING CHARACTERISTICS
Redness
Blanching
Irritation
Excoriation
	ONGOING ASSESSMENT
	• Examine skin for pre-existing breakdown or potential problems.
	• Assess for pre-existing skin breakdown risk factors:
	    Physical conditions
	    Age
	    Mental state
	    Mobility
	• Inspect skin (especially affected extremity) at least q8h.
	
	THERAPEUTIC INTERVENTIONS
	• Clean, dry, and moisturize skin daily.
	• Massage bony prominences (never massage reddened areas).
	• Maintain correct padding for affected extremity in traction. *Pressure areas and skin irritation can develop under or at the edge of the traction device and/or other equipment.*
	• Keep bed linen wrinkle free and dry.
	• Apply eggcrate or water mattress to bed.
	• Encourage adequate hydration and teach the importance of balanced diet.
	• For actual skin breakdown, see Skin integrity, impaired, p. 48.
		Skin integrity will be maintained.

Potential ineffective breathing pattern *Related to:* Immobility Pulmonary embolus Fat embolism Pneumonia **DEFINING CHARACTERISTICS** Tachypnea Tachycardia Wheezing, rales Cough Dyspnea Shortness of breath Pleuritic chest pain Anxiety Restlessness and irritability Petechiae Altered LOC Hemoptysis Productive cough	**ONGOING ASSESSMENT** • Assess respiratory rate and depth of least once/shift. • Assess breathing pattern. • Assess past history of breathing problems. • Assess present history for pre-existing problems that may lead to breathing difficulties. • Assess mental status. • Monitor ABG results. **THERAPEUTIC INTERVENTIONS** • Encourage patient to perform cough and deep breathing exercises (*effective means of bronchial hygiene*). • Encourage frequent incentive spirometer use. • Use antiembolic devices as ordered. • Administer O_2 as ordered. • Report ineffective breathing pattern signs/symptoms to physician immediately. • See Breathing pattern, ineffective, p. 8.	Risk of ineffective breathing patterns will be reduced.
Potential constipation *Related to:* Immobility Medications	**ONGOING ASSESSMENT** • Assess bowel patterns before hospitalization. • Assess dietary habits. • Assess passage of flatus/stool. • Record bowel movements. • Assess medication and their contribution to constipation.	Normal bowel elimination is maintained.

NURSING DIAGNOSES / DEFINING CHARACTERISTICS	NURSING INTERVENTIONS / *RATIONALES*	EXPECTED OUTCOMES
DEFINING CHARACTERISTICS Straining at stool Passage of hard stool Distended abdomen Nausea/vomiting Complaint of no stool for several days Decreased appetite Complaint of abdominal pain/fullness	**THERAPEUTIC INTERVENTIONS** · Encourage diet high in roughage, bulk. *Bulk encourages regularity, facilitates easy evacuation.* · Encourage fluids. · Give stool softeners and laxatives as ordered. · Provide privacy during elimination. *Voluntary overriding of defecation reflex can cause severe constipation/impaction.* · Inform patient of possible medication-induced constipation.	

Potential altered urinary elimination
Related to:
Immobility
Presence of catheter
 	
DEFINING CHARACTERISTICS
Retention:
  Bladder distention
  Frequency
  Decreased output
  Inability to urinate
  Dribbling
Urinary tract infection (UTI):
  Burning/pain on urination
  Increased temperature
  Increased WBC
	ONGOING ASSESSMENT
	· Assess previous patterns of voiding.
	· Palpate bladder for distention.
	· Evaluate intervals between voiding. *Establishment of routine pattern minimizes complication risk.*
	· Assess frequency, amount, and character of urine.
	· Assess for retention signs/symptoms.
	· Assess for UTI signs/symptoms.
	
	THERAPEUTIC INTERVENTIONS
	· Initiate methods to encourage voiding.
	· Encourage fluids (preferred drinks or foods with high water content).
	· Encourage cranberry/prune juice *to keep urine acidic. Bacteria less active in acidic environment.*
	· Provide privacy.
	· Record intake and output.
	· Insert Foley catheter or intermittent catheterization as ordered.
	· Medicate with antibiotics as ordered *for UTI prophylaxis and treatment.*
		Normal urinary elimination pattern is maintained.

Potential for injury *Related to:* Pin migration **DEFINING CHARACTERISTICS** Pain at pin sites Movement at pin sites	**ONGOING ASSESSMENT** · Assess pin sites every shift for migration. · Assess skin around pin for tears. · Assess for pain at pin sites. **THERAPEUTIC INTERVENTIONS** · Report signs of pin migration to physician. · Cover pin with cork or adhesive tape *to protect from accidental injuries.*	Pins will be maintained in proper position.

Potential ineffective coping
Related to:
Restricted activity
 	
DEFINING CHARACTERISTICS
Verbalized frustration
Anger
High anxiety level
Verbalized concerns about sex
Lack of expression
Complaints of boredome and loneliness
	ONGOING ASSESSMENT
	· Assess psychosocial status before hospitalization and traction:
	  Age
	  LOC
	  Life-style
	· Assess level of dependence.
	· Assess for evidence of behavior change.
	· Assess support systems (family/significant others, etc.)
	· Assess emotional/sexual behavior and needs.
	
	THERAPEUTIC INTERVENTIONS
	· Provide time for talking and listening to patient's concerns. *Ventilation of feelings supports honesty and objectivity and promotes realistic perception.*
	· Listen supportively.
	· Provide privacy as needed.
		Acceptance of limitations that result from prolonged bed rest and traction is verbalized.

Continued.

NURSING DIAGNOSES / DEFINING CHARACTERISTICS	NURSING INTERVENTIONS / *RATIONALES*	EXPECTED OUTCOMES
Increase in daytime sleep periods	• Allow patient as much control over environment as possible. *Independence facilitates coping.* • Provide appropriate diversionary activities. • Allow patient to personalize environment. • Provide compatible roommate, if possible. • Stress positive aspects of cure and condition. • Initiate social service referrals as needed. • Introduce patient to others who have successfully dealt with similar situations. • Allow flexibility in visiting hours *to facilitate contact with support systems.* • Discourage inappropriate sexual behavior.	

Originated/Revised by: Catherine Brown, RN
Mary P. Knoezer, RN, BSN
Eileen Kringle, RPT
Kevin Walsh, MD
Ruth Novitt-Schumacher, RN, MSN

Total hip arthroplasty/ replacement

(HIP HEMIARTHROPLASTY; TOTAL HIP SURFACE ARTHROPLASTY; CUP/MOLD ARTHROPLASTY)

Total hip arthroplasty (THA)/replacement: *a total joint replacement by surgical removal of the diseased hip joint, including the femoral neck and head, as well as the acetabulum. The femoral canal is reamed to accept a metal component placed into the femoral shaft, replacing the femoral head and neck. A polyethylene cup replaces the reamed acetabulum.*

Hip hemiarthroplasty *(also known as Austin Moore, Bateman, Bipolar, or Leinbach hemiarthroplasty): surgical removal of the femoral head and neck and replacement with metal component.*

Total hip surface arthroplasty: *reaming out the acetabulum and implanting an acetabular cup while the femoral head is only reamed down to accept a metal femoral head.*

Cup/mold arthroplasty: *the acetabulum and head of the femur are reamed down to an untraumatized surface, and an appropriate sized metal cup is fitted over the head of the femur*

NURSING DIAGNOSES / DEFINING CHARACTERISTICS	NURSING INTERVENTIONS / *RATIONALES*	EXPECTED OUTCOMES
Potential knowledge deficit *Related to:* New procedures **DEFINING CHARACTERISTICS** Verbalized lack of knowledge of hospitalization and surgical regimen	**ONGOING ASSESSMENT** • Assess experience with hospitalizations. • Assess pre-existing medical problems. • Assess level of knowledge of present hospitalization, surgical procedures, etc. (include patient's desire for information). **THERAPEUTIC INTERVENTIONS** • Review/explain procedure and preoperative, perioperative, and postoperative events. • Instruct patient to watch slide/tape presentation "Total Joint Replacement: A Preoperative Teaching Program." *Well-informed patient has reduced anxiety, decreased recovery time, and fewer postoperative complications.*	Patient will recall instructions given preoperatively.

Total hip arthroplasty/replacement— cont'd

NURSING DIAGNOSES / DEFINING CHARACTERISTICS	NURSING INTERVENTIONS / *RATIONALES*	EXPECTED OUTCOMES
Increased anxiety level Lack of/multitude of questions	· Include family members/significant others in preoperative teaching. · Instruct in: Need to maintain legs abduction Avoidance of hip flexion >90 degrees Neutral/external rotation of legs	
Pain *Related to:* *Preoperative:* arthritic pain necessitating surgery *Postoperative:* Hip incisional pain related to bone and soft tissue trauma caused by surgery Hip pain related to intense physical therapy/ rehabilitation program **DEFINING CHARACTERISTICS** Complaint of pain Facial grimaces, guarding behavior, crying, anxiety, withdrawal, restlessness, irritability, altered vital signs	**ONGOING ASSESSMENT** · Assess experience of pain and analgesia. · Assess description of pain. *First step in alleviating pain is assessing location, severity, and degree of both physical and emotional pain.* · Assess mental and physical ability to use PCA versus IM/PO analgesics. · Assess what aggravates/intensifies pain and relieves pain. · Assess effectiveness of pain-relieving interventions. · Document all assessments. **THERAPEUTIC INTERVENTIONS** · Explain analgesic therapy, including medication, dose, schedule. If patient PCA candidate, explain concept and routine. · Administer analgesics as ordered and per hospital policy/procedure. Respond quickly to pain complaints. Instruct patient to request analgesic before pain severe. *Cycle of pain must be broken to be relieved. If pain too severe before analgesics/therapy instituted, relief takes longer.* · Encourage use of analgesics 30 to 45 min before therapy. *Unrelieved pain hinders rehabilitation progress.* · Provide egg crate mattress. · Change position (within hip precautions) q2h. · Document all responses to pain relief.	Pain will be relieved or reduced.
Potential for injury: hip dislocation *Related to:* Improper hip joint positioning Dislocation when hip joint articular surfaces out of anatomic position **DEFINING CHARACTERISTICS** Increased pain in affected hip joint. Position of legs in internal rotation or adduction Change in hip joint contour (dislocated hip may be palpated) Change in length of affected extremity (leg may appear shortened) X-ray confirmation of dislocation	**ONGOING ASSESSMENT** · Assess knowledge of proper position after total hip arthroplasty (THA): Abduction of legs Hip flexion <90 degrees Neutral/external rotation of affected leg · Assess leg position in bed, in chair, and during ambulation. · Assess transfer techniques during position changes. · Assess complaint of sharp hip pain after position changes and transfer. **THERAPEUTIC INTERVENTIONS** · Frequently instruct/reinforce hip positions: Abduction of legs Flexion of hip <90 degrees Neutral or external rotation of affected leg *Constant practice of precautions essential to prevent dislocation of new hip joint. Dislocation can occur easily, necessitating further hospitalization and possible surgery.* · Maintain abduction of legs and abduction splint (in and out of bed). *Abduction splint between patient's legs prevents adduction of legs.* · Instruct patient on use of raised toilet seat (*prevents hip flexion >90 degrees*). · Turn patient side to side in bed with abduction splint between legs (may turn on to affected hip unless contraindicated by physician).	Proper positioning of hip joint will be maintained at all times.

Continued.

Total hip arthroplasty/replacement— cont'd

NURSING DIAGNOSES / DEFINING CHARACTERISTICS	NURSING INTERVENTIONS / *RATIONALES*	EXPECTED OUTCOMES
Potential altered tissue perfusion *Related to:* Surgery Immobility **DEFINING CHARACTERISTICS** *Deep vein thrombosis:* +Homan's sign Swelling, tenderness, redness in calf Palpable cords Abnormal blood flow studies *Pulmonary embolism:* Abnormal ABGs Abnormal ventilation-perfusion scan Tachypnea DVT signs/symptoms Chest pain Dyspnea Tachycardia Hemoptysis Cyanosis Anxiety *Fat embolism* (usually second day after surgery): *Pulmonary:* Dyspnea Tachypnea Cyanosis *Cerebral:* Headache Irritability Delirium Stupor Coma *Cardiac:* Tachycardia Decreased BP Petechial hemorrhage of upper chest, axillae, conjunctiva Fat globules in urine	**ONGOING ASSESSMENT** • Assess rate, rhythm, depth, and quality of respirations. • Assess mobility. • Assess mental status. • Assess for signs/symptoms of deep vein thrombosis (DVT), pulmonary embolism (PE), and fat embolus (see Defining Characteristics). **THERAPEUTIC INTERVENTIONS** • Encourage patient to be out of bed as soon as ordered. Maintain THA precautions and weight bearing status. • Encourage incentive spirometry q1h while awake *to increase lung expansion and prevent atelectasis, hypoxemia, pneumonia, PE.* • Institute antiembolic devices as ordered (sequential compression device or TED hose). *Antiembolic devices increase venous blood flow to heart and decrease risk of DVT, PE.* • Encourage leg exercises, including quad sets, gluteal sets, active ankle ROM.	Risk of DVT, PE, and fat embolism will be reduced.
Impaired physical mobility *Related to:* Surgical procedure Discomfort	**ONGOING ASSESSMENT** • Assess fear/anxiety of transferring/ambulating. • Assess level of understanding of THA precautions. • Assess knowledge of PT role in rehabilitation. • Assess understanding of pain management during therapy.	Independence in mobility within limitations is achieved.

NURSING DIAGNOSES / DEFINING CHARACTERISTICS	NURSING INTERVENTIONS / *RATIONALES*	EXPECTED OUTCOMES
DEFINING CHARACTERISTICS Limited ability to ambulate or move in bed	**THERAPEUTIC INTERVENTIONS** · Encourage ROM in bed with all unaffected extremities. · Encourage use of analgesic before PT position changes. *Decreased or controlled pain allows better performance during therapy.* · Instruct patient on maintaining THA precautions during position changes *to prevent hip dislocation.* · Dangle patient at bedside several minutes before changing positions. · Reinforce physical therapist's instructions for exercises, ambulation techniques and devices. Maintain weight-bearing status on affected extremity as prescribed. *Consistent instructions from interdisciplinary team members promote safe, secure rehabilitation environment.* · Keep abduction pillow between legs while turning in bed. May turn onto operative side unless otherwise specified. · Use trapeze in bed *to assist in mobility.*	
Potential altered tissue perfusion to lower extremities (neurovascular) *Related to:* Surgical procedure Improper position of abduction splint straps Immobility **DEFINING CHARACTERISTICS** Pain Pallor Cyanosis Pulselessness Paresthesia Paralysis Edema Sluggish/absent capillary refill noted in one or both lower extremities Foot drop	**ONGOING ASSESSMENT** · Assess and compare neurovascular status of both lower extremities pre- and postoperatively. *Assessment must include unaffected and affected extremity to monitor for neurovascular status improvement or worsening.* · Assess lower extremities for neurovascular damage (see Defining Characteristics). · Assess for peroneal nerve palsy secondary to improper positioning or abduction splint straps. *Compression of peroneal nerve by abduction splint straps can cause peroneal nerve palsy.* · Check sequential compression device/TED stocking for extreme tightness *(produces tourniquet effect on extremity).* **THERAPEUTIC INTERVENTIONS** · Prevent abduction splint straps fom pressing against fibular head at proximal lateral aspect of lower leg *to prevent peroneal nerve palsy.*	Tissue perfusion will remain adequate throughout postoperative course.
Potential for infection *Related to:* Surgical incision **DEFINING CHARACTERISTICS** Increased redness at incision Increased WBC Increased temperature Increased drainage from incision (may be cloudy and foul-smelling) Increased warmth Increased tenderness	**ONGOING ASSESSMENT** · Assess incisional area for infection signs (see Defining Characteristics). · Assess vital signs, especially temperature (recommend q4h×72h, then every shift if stable). Notify if over 38.5°C. · Assess lab values, especially WBC. · Assess bladder/bowel habits, especially incontinence. · Assess nutritional intake. **THERAPEUTIC INTERVENTIONS** · Change incisional dressing daily (after initial dressing changed). Change more frequently if drainage noted. *Infection of surgical incision can lead to infection in new joint, which is very serious. If prosthesis is removed because of infection it can never be replaced.* · Administer antibiotics as ordered. · Clean incontinent patient *(proximity of urine and stool to surgical incision).* · Encourage high-protein, high-calories diet (unless otherwise restricted).	Risk of infection will be reduced.

Continued.

NURSING DIAGNOSES / DEFINING CHARACTERISTICS	NURSING INTERVENTIONS / *RATIONALES*	EXPECTED OUTCOMES
Potential altered skin integrity *Related to:* Immobility caused by surgery Shearing forces Friction Maceration **DEFINING CHARACTERISTICS** *Actual breakdown:* Stage I: skin intact, red Stage II: blisters Stage III: necrosis Stage IV: necrosis of bone and joints	**ONGOING ASSESSMENT** • Assess skin, especially over bony prominence (at admission). Note skin breaks or existing decubitus. • Inspect skin frequently. Remove splints and antiembolic devices to inspect skin. *Skin breakdown and decubitus pose risk of infection and delay rehabilitation.* **THERAPEUTIC INTERVENTIONS** • Turn patient q2h during bed rest (may turn to operated side unless otherwise specified by physician). Maintain abduction of legs with splint. *Frequent position changes decrease pressure on skin and prevent breakdown.* • Massage around bony prominences. • Initiate prophylactic antipressure devices. • Encourage patient to sit in chair and ambulate as soon as ordered. • For actual skin breakdown, see Skin integrity, impaired, p. 48.	Optimal skin integrity will be maintained.
Constipation *Related to:* Immobility Use of narcotics **DEFINING CHARACTERISTICS** Passage of small, hard, dry stool Absence of stool Distended hard abdomen. Complaint of full feeling, "no bowel movement in days"	**ONGOING ASSESSMENT** • Assess bowel habits before hospitalization. • Assess bowel sounds postoperatively. • Assess complaint of pressure in rectum or lower abdomen. • Assess dietary intake. • Assess use of narcotics. • Assess for signs/symptoms of constipation (see Defining Characteristics). **THERAPEUTIC INTERVENTIONS** • Encourage fluids. • Increase roughage in diet. • Encourage ambulation as soon as ordered. • Use laxative/stool softeners as ordered. • Offer bedpan regularly; encourage ambulation to bathroom. • Explain effect of analgesics on elimination. *Narcotic analgesics extremely constipating, especially on immobile patient.*	Regular bowel elimination will occur.

Knowledge deficit: discharge *Related to:* New condition **DEFINING CHARACTERISTICS** Lack of/multitude of questions Confusion about THA precautions	**ONGOING ASSESSMENT**
	• Assess understanding of discharge instructions.
	• Assess home support systems.
	THERAPEUTIC INTERVENTIONS
	• Review THA precautions:
	   Maintain abduction with ABD splint.
	   Always keep legs externally or neutrally rotated.
	   Avoid hip flexion >90 degrees.
	• Ambulate (weight bearing as instructed) with assistive device (walker/crutches).
	• Do not shower/tub bathe until all Steri-Strips on incision off (usually 4-5 days after application).
	• Resume sexual activity as long as THA precautions observed(best positions supine and side-lying).
	• Continue to use raised toilet seat.
	• Use ABD splint at home, especially at night, until next physician appointment.
	• Build up low chairs with firm pillow *to prevent hip flexion >90 degrees.*
	• Call physician immediately if sharp pain, "popping" of affected extremity, hip feeling "out of socket".
	• Continue exercise program of physical therapist. Home physical therapist will visit 3 times/wk for 1 mon to continue rehabilitation.
		Patient will verbalize understanding of discharge instructions.

NURSING DIAGNOSES / DEFINING CHARACTERISTICS	NURSING INTERVENTIONS / *RATIONALES*	EXPECTED OUTCOMES
	· Notify physician of complaints: Fever Drainage from incision Decreased sensation, numbness in toes Calf tenderness · Refer to handout "THA Home Discharge Instruction Sheet." · Ask social worker to arrange home physical therapy and homemaker (if needed).	

Originated by: Hope Hlinka, RN

Total knee arthroplasty/replacement

(KNEE HEMIARTHROPLASTY)

Replacement of deteriorated femoral, tibial, and patellar articular surfaces with prosthetic metal and plastic components.

NURSING DIAGNOSES / DEFINING CHARACTERISTICS	NURSING INTERVENTIONS / *RATIONALES*	EXPECTED OUTCOMES
Potential knowledge deficit: surgical procedure *Related to:* New procedures Unfamiliarity with surgical routines **DEFINING CHARACTERISTICS** Many questions Lack of questions Increased anxiety level Verbalized misconceptions	**ONGOING ASSESSMENT** · Assess previous hospital experience. · Assess intellectual level. · Assess existing medical problems. · Assess knowledge of anticipated surgical procedure. *Adequate health knowledge increases ability to understand treatment and management plan.* **THERAPEUTIC INTERVENTIONS** · Encourage questions; answer fully. · Review surgical protocol. · Inform of hospital educational TV for general pre-, intra-, and postoperative information. · Instruct in preoperative routines. · Inform of immediate postop routines (e.g., J-Vac, IV, diet, activity level, medications, Foley catheter). · Instruct on postoperative use of continuous passive motion (CPM) machine; inform of purpose and usage. · Instruct on leg exercises (quad sets, gluteal sets, and active ankle ROM). Encourage patient to practice preoperatively *to increase compliance.* · Instruct on coughing and deep-breathing exercises. Encourage practice. · Give TKA handout *(provides material for review of confused or forgotten information).* · Use available audiovisual materials on total joint replacement.	Patient will demonstrate or verbalize understanding of preoperative instructions.
Pain *Related to:* Surgical procedure Rehabilitation program	**ONGOING ASSESSMENT** · Obtain description of pain. · Assess behavior and facial expressions. · Assess experience of pain and pain relief. · Assess pain relief measure effectiveness.	Relief of pain.

Continued.

Total knee arthroplasty/replacement— cont'd

NURSING DIAGNOSES / DEFINING CHARACTERISTICS	NURSING INTERVENTIONS / *RATIONALES*	EXPECTED OUTCOMES
DEFINING CHARACTERISTICS Verbal report of pain Facial grimaces Moaning, crying Protective, guarding behavior Restlessness Withdrawal Irritability	**THERAPEUTIC INTERVENTIONS** • Give analgesics as ordered; evaluate effectiveness. • Alter patient's position (turning, adjusting pillows, etc.). • Respond immediately to pain complaints. • Encourage use of analgesic 30 min before PT *to facilitate patient's participation in exercise session.* • Encourage appropriate rest periods. • Eliminate additional stressors; encourage diversional activity. • Instruct patient to report pain *so relief measures can be started.* • Apply ice to knee 20-30 min, q2h and after exercising *to decrease edema.* • See Pain, p. 39; Patient-controlled anesthesia, p. 631.	

Impaired physical mobility
Related to:
Movement restricted by postoperative protocol
Surgical procedure
 	
DEFINING CHARACTERISTICS
Decreased muscle strength, control, and coordination
Reluctance to move
	ONGOING ASSESSMENT
	• Assess ability to carry out ADLs.
	• Assess ROM.
	• Assess knowledge of CPM.
	• Assess knowledge of early ambulation and physical therapy.
	• Assess experience with use of crutches or walker.
	• Assess underlying disease process for planning care.
	
	THERAPEUTIC INTERVENTIONS
	• If ordered, apply CPM to affected leg at prescribed degrees. *CPM enhances ROM, promotes wound healing, and prevents formation of adhesions to operative knee.*
	• Maintain proper position in CPM:
	  Maintain leg in neutral position.
	  Adjust CPM so knee joint corresponds to bend in CPM machine.
	  Adjust foot plate so foot in neutral position in boot.
	  Instruct patient to keep opposite leg away from machine *to prevent injury by moving parts.*
	• Assist and encourage to perform quad sets, gluteal sets, and ROM to both legs.
	• Reinforce ROM (extension/flexion) and muscle strengthening exercises taught by physical therapist *to optimize return of full knee extension.*
	• Elevate leg on pillow when not in CPM. Place pillow under calf *to promote full leg extension.*
	• Encourage and assist patient to sit in chair on first and second postoperative days. Instruct to sit with legs dependent several times a day *to promote flexion of knee.*
	• Initiate weight bearing as prescribed. *Weight-bearing status:*
	  For cemented prosthesis: as tolerated
	  For partially or fully uncemented prosthesis: toe-touch to partial weight bearing
	Protective weight bearing is required for 6 wk with uncemented prosthesis to allow bony ingrowth into prosthesis
	• Encourage ambulation with walker or canes after initiated by PT.
	• Encourage use of assistive devices provided by OT *to carry out ADLs* (reacher, sock aid, long-handled sponge, long-handled shoehorn).
	• At discharge, instruct in need to continue progressive exercises *to improve ROM and strengthen muscles.*
		Independence in ambulation and ADLs is achieved.

Potential altered peripheral tissue perfusion *Related to:* Surgical procedure Restricted movement Swelling	**ONGOING ASSESSMENT** • Use preoperative neurovascular assessment to establish baseline status for postoperative comparison of lower extremities. • Assess lower extremities, compare temperature, color, sensation, movement, pulses, edema, and capillary refill. • Remove antiembolic devices every shift *to inspect skin.* • Assess for increased pain to affected extremity. • Monitor sequential compression devices (SCDs).	Tissue perfusion will be maintained.

NURSING DIAGNOSES / DEFINING CHARACTERISTICS	NURSING INTERVENTIONS / *RATIONALES*	EXPECTED OUTCOMES
DEFINING CHARACTERISTICS Coldness Pallor Pain Pulselessness Edema Sluggish or absent capillary refill	**THERAPEUTIC INTERVENTIONS** • Maintain functional alignment. • Instruct to perform ROM exercises *to increase venous return and decrease probability of DVT.* • Apply TED hose and/or sequential compression devices as prescribed. • If signs of altered tissue perfusion noted, notify physician immediately. • See Tissue perfusion, altered, p. 56.	
Potential for infection *Related to:* Surgical procedure Incision **DEFINING CHARACTERISTICS** Increased warmth Redness Swelling Tenderness at incision site Increased WBC count Increased temperature	**ONGOING ASSESSMENT** • Assess for signs/symptoms of infection. • Monitor vital signs; notify physican of abnormalities. **THERAPEUTIC INTERVENTIONS** • Administer antibiotics as ordered. • Encourage fluid intake. • Maintain strict aseptic technique for dressing changes *to prevent wound contamination.*	Risk of infection will be reduced.
Potential altered skin integrity *Related to:* Physical immobility and/or contact with CPM **DEFINING CHARACTERISTICS** Stage I: redness, skin intact Stage II: blisters Stage III: necrosis Stage IV: necrosis involving bone and joints	**ONGOING ASSESSMENT** • Inspect skin q4h; remove TED hose/SCDs q8h; reapply. • Inspect leg, especially knee and thigh (medial, lateral, and posterior), in CPM for pressure points. **THERAPEUTIC INTERVENTIONS** • Turn and position q2h unless otherwise indicated. • Clean, dry, and moisturize skin q8h or as indicated by incontinence. • Moisturize skin q8h, massage around bony prominences. *Skin stimulation, especially around bony prominences, promotes circulation (thus prevents tissue damage).* • Pad areas resting on hard parts of CPM. • Apply egg crate mattress to bed. • If skin breakdown occurs, see Skin integrity, impaired, p. 48.	Skin will remain intact.
Potential constipation *Related to:* Immobility Medications Altered nutrition **DEFINING CHARACTERISTICS** Hard stools Straining for stool Abdominal distention Frequent attempts to defecate Nausea/vomiting	**ONGOING ASSESSMENT** • Compare preoperative, postoperative stool patterns. • Assess preoperative laxative use. • Assess dietary habits. • Assess activity level. • Assess current medications and their contribution to constipation. **THERAPEUTIC INTERVENTIONS** • Encourage increased dietary bulk *(improves intestinal muscle tone, promotes comfortable elimination).* • Encourage fluid intake. • Encourage ambulation; assist as needed. • Give laxatives and stool softeners as prescribed. • Provide privacy during defecation.	Normal bowel pattern will be maintained.

Continued.

Total knee arthroplasty/replacement— cont'd

NURSING DIAGNOSES / DEFINING CHARACTERISTICS	NURSING INTERVENTIONS / RATIONALES	EXPECTED OUTCOMES
Potential ineffective breathing pattern *Related to:* Immobility Fatigue **DEFINING CHARACTERISTICS** Increased temperature Adventitious breath sounds Chest pains Abnormal ABGs Increased anxiety Tachypnea Dyspnea Tachycardia, cyanosis	**ONGOING ASSESSMENT** • Assess respiratory rate and rhythm. • Auscultate breath sounds. • Assess for signs/symptoms of respiratory compromise/PE. **THERAPEUTIC INTERVENTIONS** • Preoperatively instruct in use of incentive spirometer, coughing and deep-breathing exercises. • Postoperatively encourage use of incentive spirometer 10 times q1-2h while awake. • Turn q2h as tolerated. • If pulmonary embolus signs noted, call physician and institute treatment for Pulmonary thromboembolism, p. 200.	Risk of respiratory compromise is reduced.
Potential/actual self-care deficit *Related to:* Postoperative condition/recovery process **DEFINING CHARACTERISTICS** Verbalized knowledge deficit in home care Increased anxiety as discharge approaches	**ONGOING ASSESSMENT** • Assess knowledge of home care requirements. *Adequate health knowledge increases ability to prevent complications.* • Assess home situation for family's/significant others' availability. • Assess home physical environment relating to mobility. **THERAPEUTIC INTERVENTIONS** • Reinforce all instructions to patient. Provide written materials *to improve retention.* • Coordinate social service, PT, OT early *to provide adequate discharge planning.* • Encourage patient to ask questions. • Instruct about discharge medications, exercises, and follow-up physician visits.	Patient verbalizes readiness for discharge.

Originated by: Sandra Eungard, RN, MS

Total shoulder arthroplasty/ replacement

(SHOULDER HEMIARTHROPLASTY)

Total shoulder arthroplasty is the surgical removal of the head of the humerus and the glenoid cavity of the scapula, with replacement by an articulating prosthesis. Shoulder hemiarthroplasty is the surgical removal of the head of the humerus with replacement by a prosthesis.

NURSING DIAGNOSES / DEFINING CHARACTERISTICS	NURSING INTERVENTIONS / RATIONALES	EXPECTED OUTCOMES
Knowledge deficit *Related to:* Lack of information about surgical procedures	**ONGOING ASSESSMENT** • Question patient/significant others about procedures and surgical events. • Assess patient/significant others for subjective response to questions/fears about surgery.	Patient will verbalize understanding of surgical procedure.

Total shoulder arthroplasty/replacement— cont'd

NURSING DIAGNOSES / DEFINING CHARACTERISTICS	NURSING INTERVENTIONS / *RATIONALES*	EXPECTED OUTCOMES

DEFINING CHARACTERISTICS
 	
Patient expresses lack of familiarity with exact nature of procedure
 	
Apparent confusion about events
 	
Lack of questions
	THERAPEUTIC INTERVENTIONS
	• Encourage/answer questions before and after surgery. *Well-informed patient has reduced anxiety, decreased recovery time, and fewer postoperative complications.*
	• Review procedure and perioperative events:
	   Purpose of surgery
	   Actual procedure in terms suited to intellectual/cognitive level of patient
	   Postoperative events and care, with emphasis on exercise
	• Inform patient about, encourage use of other teaching resources:
	   Hospital TV channel for perioperative events and care
	   Ancillary departments (e.g., PT, OT)
	• Review information after teaching session.
	• Document questions/concerns and instruction given.	

Potential for injury: altered neurovascular status *Related to:* Surgical procedures Edema with compression **DEFINING CHARACTERISTICS** Cool, cyanotic, or pulseless extremity Altered sensation or movement of extremity Sluggish/absent capillary refill Edema	**ONGOING ASSESSMENT** • Assess color, peripheral pulses, sensation (including numbness and paresthesias), and motor function postoperatively; compare to preoperative status. • Monitor and document neurovascular assessment *(allows early detection of compromised perfusion of arm/nerve compressions within arm).* Recommended frequency: q1h for first 4 hr postoperatively, then q2-4h for 24 hr, then q8h if status stable. • Measure extremity *to detect increased circumference or presence of edema.* Notify physician if circumference increase noted. **THERAPEUTIC INTERVENTIONS** • Report change in neurovascular status to physician immediately.	Optimal neurovascular status will be maintained.
Impaired physical mobility *Related to:* *Preoperative:* adhesions/pain *Postoperative:* pain, spasm, other factors **DEFINING CHARACTERISTICS** *Preoperative:* may have limited ROM of affected extremity *Postoperative:* initially will have limitations in flexion, abduction, and extension	**ONGOING ASSESSMENT** • Assess preoperative full ROM of affected extremity; document. • Assess postoperative ROM; document improvement/failure to progress. • Assess/document performance of ADL. **THERAPEUTIC INTERVENTIONS** • Maintain arm in shoulder immobilizer 1-2 days or as ordered. • After immobilizer removed (with physician's order), apply sling. • Begin ROM exercises (extension, abduction, flexion) of hand, elbow, and wrist in conjunction with PT personnel. *Passive ROM helps prevent development of adhesions yet does not strain tissues. Achieving increasing mobility is prime goal of surgery along with elimination of pain.* • Reinforce/assist with shoulder exercises after initiation/demonstration in PT department. • Encourage and assist patient in performing basic ADL: self-feeding, brushing teeth, combing hair.	Full ROM will be maintained.
Pain *Related to:* Surgical pain and PT treatment	**ONGOING ASSESSMENT** • Assess patient/significant others for subjective complaints of pain or discomfort. • Assess patient for objective symptoms of pain or discomfort. • Assess the vital signs q4h for first 48 hr postoperatively; q8h thereafter if vital signs stable and within normal limits. • Document observations. • Assess effectiveness of intervention(s) in relieving pain/discomfort.	Pain will be relieved or reduced.

Continued.

Total shoulder arthroplasty/replacement— cont'd

NURSING DIAGNOSES / DEFINING CHARACTERISTICS	NURSING INTERVENTIONS / *RATIONALES*	EXPECTED OUTCOMES

DEFINING CHARACTERISTICS
Patient's/significant others' complaint of pain or discomfort
Withdrawal, guarding behavior, crying, moaning, grimacing, anxiety, rigidity, tachycardia, diaphoresis
	THERAPEUTIC INTERVENTIONS
	· Give analgesics as ordered and as needed. Encourage patient to take medications before pain becomes severe or, if patient has PCA device, operate according to policy/procedures and physician orders. *Pain management very important to prevent vicious cycle of pain-tension-anxiety that breeds more pain and, equally important, prevents participation in PT and self-care activities. Many patients are unprepared for level of immediate post-operative pain experienced.*
	· Offer analgesia 30-45 min before PT.
	· Try other measures *to relieve pain/discomfort:*
	   Heat or ice pack to shoulder after exercise as needed (with physician's order).
	   Reposition patient q1-2h. Avoid positioning on operative side. Elevate HOB to 45-60 degrees or as tolerated. Place pillow under affected elbow.
	· Evaluate/document effectiveness of pain relief.	

Knowledge deficit
Related to
Unfamiliarity with postdischarge activity and self-care
 	
DEFINING CHARACTERISTICS
Multiple questions
Lack of questions
	ONGOING ASSESSMENT
	· Ask patient to verbalize questions related to activities/limitations after shoulder arthroplasty *so better able to adapt to stress of gradual progress (as long as 1 yr before full power, strength, and function restored).*
	· If patient has limited or poor cognitive ability, involve significant others/guardian in discharge teaching.
	· Observe and document ability to perform usual ADLs (dressing, transferring, positioning, eating, bathing).
	
	THERAPEUTIC INTERVENTIONS
	· Instruct patient/significant others at discharge:
	   Perform only passive ROM exercises for first 25 days. Thereafter, active exercises may be started.
	   Avoid activities such as heavy lifting, pulling, pushing.
	   Avoid activities that involve exaggerated external rotation and abduction (e.g., push-ups, golf, volleyball).
	   Avoid activity in which affected extremity is required to support body weight or if collisions or falls likely (contact sports and skiing).
	   Inform physician of infection signs (increased edema, tenderness, warmth along incision line, temperature above 38.3°C (101°F), increased pain).
		Patient will verbalize activities that may cause dislocation of the affected extremity or disruption of the surgical repair and demonstrate ability to perform usual ADLs.

Potential altered pulmonary function *Related to:* Surgery Immobility Pain Anesthesia Fat embolus **DEFINING CHARACTERISTICS** Abnormal breath sounds, respirations Abnormal ABGs Symptoms of early respiratory insufficiency/failure Inability to cough productively	**ONGOING ASSESSMENT** · Assess respiratory system; document and reporting significant abnormalities. Recommended frequency: q2-4h for first 24-48 h, then q8h if stable and no abnormalities. · If respiratory abnormalities develop, send urine for fat analysis; notify physician (fat embolus most likely to develop on second postoperative day). *Early detection of fat emboli (produced during surgery) can prevent unconsciousness and death.* · Monitor vital signs q1h for first 4 hr postoperatively, then q2-4h for 24 hr, then q8h if stable. **THERAPEUTIC INTERVENTIONS** · Encourage patient to use spirometer, to cough, and to turn to nonoperative side q2-4h *to prevent hypoxemia, pulmonary emboli, atelectasis, and pneumonia.* · Assist patient with ambulation per physician's order. · Document signs/symptoms of systemic manifestation of fat or pulmonary emboli; report immediately to physician. · Administer pain medication *to assist patient to cough, turn, and deep breathe more effectively.*	Optimal pulmonary function will be maintained.

NURSING DIAGNOSES / DEFINING CHARACTERISTICS	NURSING INTERVENTIONS / *RATIONALES*	EXPECTED OUTCOMES
Signs/symptoms of fat embolus: *Respiratory:* insufficiency/failure *CNS manifestations:* headache, irritability, delirium, progression to marked alteration in LOC *Cardiovascular:* Early: tachycardia, mild drop in BP; Late: shock symptoms *Renal:* Fat globules in urine *Integument:* Petechial hemorrhages on torso, axillae, conjunctiva		
Potential for infection Related to: Interruption of skin integrity secondary to surgical incision **DEFINING CHARACTERISTICS** Inability of wound to heal Abnormal appearance of wound, drainage Elevated temperature Left shift in differential WBC count (including polymorphonuclear cells, bands) Complaints of severe pain Incision warm to touch, edematous	**ONGOING ASSESSMENT** • Monitor incision for redness, pus, bulging, dehiscence. *Early detection may prevent spread to prosthesis and surrounding structures and prevent osteomyelitis (all serious and difficult to treat).* • Assess vital signs q4h; take temperature q4h; notify physician if temperature exceeds 38°C. • Assess laboratory values for WBC differential; document and report abnormal left shift. • Obtain culture, sensitivity, and Gram's stain per physician's order if infection suspected. **THERAPEUTIC INTERVENTIONS** • Administer preoperative scrub to area per physician's order. • Use sterile/aseptic technique for dressing changes and during wound inspection. • Administer appropriate antibiotics as ordered. • Notify appropriate personnel; document signs/symptoms of infection.	Risk for infection will be reduced.

Originated by: Cynthia Gordon, RN, BSN
Janet I. Linder, RPT

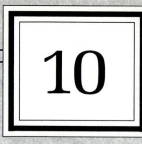

Integumentary Care Plans

Eczema/atopic dermatitis
Psoriasis

Scleroderma
Shingles

Skin loss, full thickness: comparable to
burn injury

Eczema/atopic dermatitis

A superficial, noninfectious inflammatory disease, whose most prominent feature is intense pruritus. These patients are usually managed as outpatients but may also present as inpatients with other problems and need for eczema care.

NURSING DIAGNOSES / DEFINING CHARACTERISTICS	NURSING INTERVENTIONS / *RATIONALES*	EXPECTED OUTCOMES

Impaired skin integrity
Related to:
History of:
Predisposition to eczema
Personal or family history of asthma or hay fever
Hypersensitivity to:
Protein
Rapid temperature changes
Sweating
Irritating or occlusive clothing
Detergents
Oil
Inhalants
Environmental allergies
Emotional, physical stress
Rhinitis
Eye edema
Conjunctivitis
 	
DEFINING CHARACTERISTICS
Dry, itchy skin
Blisters that develop into itchy, thickened patches
Evidence of other allergies/intolerances
	ONGOING ASSESSMENT
	• Assess for presence of lesions, noting:
	    Size
	    Shape
	    Color
	    Texture
	    Temperature
	    Distribution
	    Typical locations
	      Children: face, extensor surfaces of arms and legs
	      Adults: flexion points (neck, antecubital fossa popliteal space)
	    Distribution may also indicate nature of irritant.
	• Inquire about related factors *(their presence aids diagnosis).*
	
	THERAPEUTIC INTERVENTIONS
	• Document complete description of lesions and history given by patient.
	• Prevent irritation of lesions:
	    Avoid rubbing.
	    Avoid extreme temperatures.
	• Administer pharmaceuticals as ordered.
	    Corticosteroid ointments/creams (Avoid fluorinated preparations on face, *where skin thinner, more sensitive; or where skin touches skin [e.g., armpits] and may overabsorb fluorinated products.)*
	    Coal tar preparations
	    Other occlusives (e.g., petroleum jelly or vegetable shortening)
	• Avoid use of topical steroids if infection suspected.
	• Maintain skin in clean, moist condition:
	    During height of exacerbation, hydrate skin by soaking (or applying wet dressings to) affected area in warm—not hot—water and immediately applying occlusive preparation to damp skin *to enhance water absorption and seal in moisture.*
	    When condition under control, bathe at least once a day with mild soap; use occlusives or moisturizers. Avoid scented lotions or other known hyperallergenic products *(may contain perfumes that may trigger itching).*
	• Reduce irritation from bed linen.
	    Use old, soft sheets, if possible.
	    Avoid use of plastic linen protectors *(promote heat reactions and sweating).*
	    Use bed cradle *to prevent linens from rubbing.*
		Skin will be maintained in best possible condition.

Itching
Related to:
Increased histamine release resulting from lesions/patches
Increased itching resulting from scratching
 	
DEFINING CHARACTERISTICS
Reports of itching
Scratching
	ONGOING ASSESSMENT
	• Solicit verbal description of itchiness:
	    Location
	    Pattern (continuous, intermittent)
	    Factors believed by patient to cause or stop itching
	• Observe skin for evidence of scratching.
	
	THERAPEUTIC INTERVENTIONS
	• Discourage scratching *(increases itching).*
	• Use cloth mitts/gloves on children or adults who cannot cooperate.
	• Administer antihistamines as ordered.
	• Add soothing agents to soaks, baths (e.g., Burrow's solution, corn starch, oatmeal powder). Bath oils not recommended: *actually poor lubricants, which make bathtub dangerously slippery).*
		Itching/scratching will be decreased.

Continued.

Eczema/atopic dermatitis—cont'd

NURSING DIAGNOSES / DEFINING CHARACTERISTICS	NURSING INTERVENTIONS / *RATIONALES*	EXPECTED OUTCOMES
Presence of scratch marks Restlessness	• Keep linens free of irritating particles (crumbs, hair) *that may trigger further itching.*	
Potential for infection *Related to:* Exposure to pathogens from lesions, scratching **DEFINING CHARACTERISTICS** Open lesions Drainage from lesions Redness Swelling Pain Fever Elevated WBC	**ONGOING ASSESSMENT** • Assess lesions for openness, drainage. • Assess for signs of localized infection. • Check vital signs and temperature q4h. **THERAPEUTIC INTERVENTIONS** • Trim fingernails. • Discourage scratching *(opens lesions, introduces pathogens).* • Obtain culture and sensitivity from lesions that appear infected. • Initiate local wound isolation. • Administer topical/systemic antibiotic therapy as ordered.	Infection will be prevented.
Body image disturbance *Related to:* Lesions Patches Draining lesions Others' response to lesions **DEFINING CHARACTERISTICS** Ignoring *or* focusing on lesions Verbal preoccupation with lesions or their care Negative comments about physical self Withdrawal from social behavior	**ONGOING ASSESSMENT** • Assess patient's perception of physical self. • Note verbal and nonverbal references to lesions, general appearance. • Evaluate patient's participation in own care. *Nonparticipation may indicate altered body image.* **THERAPEUTIC INTERVENTIONS** • Encourage verbalization about appearance. • Acknowledge normalcy of concern about appearance. • Help patient identify ways to deal with altered appearance (use of concealing clothing, hats). • Remind patient that lesions will heal. • See Body image disturbance, p. 6.	Body image will be enhanced.
Knowledge deficit *Related to:* Lack of experience with eczema/dermatitis Misconceptions about cause/management **DEFINING CHARACTERISTICS** Multiple questions Lack of questions Verbalized misconceptions Frequent repeated exacerbations or complications	**ONGOING ASSESSMENT** • Assess patient's knowledge of cause and managment of eczema/dermatitis. **THERAPEUTIC INTERVENTIONS** • Explain causes of eczema and dermatitis. • Help patient identify and avoid those potential exacerbators. • Explain causes of pruritis. • Reinforce importance of not scratching lesions *so more itching and potential for infection minimized.* • Teach patient pharmacologic action of prescribed soaks, medications. • Encourage patient to seek health care if eczema/dermatitis exacerbated. • Remind patient that frequency/severity of exacerbations minimized by appropriate actions (avoidance of etiologic factors, use of prescribed therapies).	Patient will verbalize understanding of etiologic factors, management, and personal role in controlling eczema/dermatitis.

Originated by: Marie Lindsey, RN,C, MS, FNP

Psoriasis

A chronic, familial, noninfectious skin disease marked by a recurrent, inflammatory rash with epidermal proliferation. Although psoriasis is generally treated on an outpatient basis, chronic recalcitrant cases unresponsive to traditional therapy may require hospitalization to employ special treatment protocols.

NURSING DIAGNOSES / DEFINING CHARACTERISTICS	NURSING INTERVENTIONS / *RATIONALES*	EXPECTED OUTCOMES
Impaired skin integrity *Related to:* Familial predisposition Previous episode of eruptions Exacerbations in cold weather Recent episode of trauma or stress Strep throat in previous 7-10 days Generalized psoriasis possibly associated with fever, chills, malaises Psoriatic arthritis in approximately 4 percent of patients **DEFINING CHARACTERISTICS** Well-demarcated red plaques with loosely adherent silvery scales Pinpoint bleeding noted when scales removed with fingernail (Auspitz's sign) Pitting of fingernails and, rarely, toenails Rarely, pustules on palms, feet, and sometimes generalized areas	**ONGOING ASSESSMENT** • Assess for presence of lesions, noting: Size Shape Color Texture Temperature Distribution *Common plaque distribution: elbows, knees, scalp, genitalia, upper gluteal folds. Lesions may also form at sites of surgical wounds or scratch marks (Köbner's phenomenon).* • Inquire about related factors. • Check skin daily for increased thinning, redness, inflammation, or pustules *(all treatments potentially irritating).* **THERAPEUTIC INTERVENTIONS** • Document complete description of lesions and history given by patient. • Administer treatments/pharmaceuticals as ordered: Calamine lotion or starch baths Low-dose (10 percent) coal tar preparations Exposure to sunlight or ultraviolet light (black light) until skin slightly erythematous Corticosteroid ointments/creams *(Avoid stronger, fluorinated preparations on face, where skin thinner, more sensitive, and may overabsorb corticosteroid products/cause rosacea).* Remind patient to avoid touching eyes with corticosteroid preparation *(may cause cataract formation).* Occlusive dressings (e.g., Saran Wrap or other nonpermeable products) may be applied over steroid ointments. Coal tar prepartations and anthralin paste cause fabric staining; old pajamas and bed linens recommended. Anthralin may also temporarily discolor white or gray hair. Remove previously applied preparations and psoriatic scales by bathing with soap and water. (Aveeno Powder recommended; also mineral oil.) *All treatments enhanced by removal of old preparations and scales.* • Treat very severe cases with: Oral methotrexate PUVA: oral Psoralen (P) combined with long-wave ultraviolet light (UVA) therapy Etretinate	Skin will be maintained in best possible condition.
Itching and pain *Related to:* Increased histamine release which results from lesions/patches Increased itching which results from scratching Environmental temperature, especially cold	**ONGOING ASSESSMENT** • Solicit verbal description of itchiness: Location Pattern (continuous, intermittent) Factors believed by patient to cause or stop itching • Observe skin for evidence of scratching. **THERAPEUTIC INTERVENTIONS** • Discourage scratching *(increases itching).* • Administer pharmacuetical treatment as ordered. • Administer antihistamines as ordered. • Add oatmeal powder to soaks and baths *(soothing).*	Itching/scratching will be reduced.

Continued.

NURSING DIAGNOSES / DEFINING CHARACTERISTICS	NURSING INTERVENTIONS / *RATIONALES*	EXPECTED OUTCOMES
DEFINING CHARACTERISTICS Reports of itching Scratching Presence of scratch marks Restlessness		
Potential for infection *Related to:* Exposure to pathogens from lesions, scratching Irritation from treatments **DEFINING CHARACTERISTICS** Open lesions Drainage from lesions Redness Swelling Pain Fever Elevated WBC	**ONGOING ASSESSMENT** · Assess lesions for openness, drainage. · Assess for signs of localized infection. · Check vital signs and temperature q4h. · Obtain culture and sensitivity from lesions that appear infected. **THERAPEUTIC INTERVENTIONS** · Trim fingernails. · Discourage scratching *(opens lesions and introduces pathogens).* · Initiate local wound isolation. · Administer topical/systemic antibiotic therapy as ordered.	Infection will be prevented.
Body image disturbance *Related to:* Lesions Patches Draining lesions Others' response to lesions **DEFINING CHARACTERISTICS** Ignoring or focusing on lesions Verbal preoccupation with lesions or their care Negative comments about physical self Withdrawal from social behavior	**ONGOING ASSESSMENT** · Assess patient's perception of physical self. · Note verbal and nonverbal references to lesions, general appearance. · Evalute patient's participation in own care. *Nonparticipation may indicate altered body image.* **THERAPEUTIC INTERVENTIONS** · Encourage verbalization about appearance. · Acknowledge normalcy of concern over appearance. · Help patient identify ways to deal with altered appearances (concealing clothing, hats). · Urge patient to comply with treatment. · See Body image disturbance, p. 6.	Body image will be enhanced.
Potential impaired physical mobility *Related to:* Psoriatic arthritis Pain **DEFINING CHARACTERISTICS** Stiffness of joints, especially of fingers, toes; some sacroiliac spondylitis	**ONGOING ASSESSMENT** · Assess for stiffness. · Assess degree of mobility limitation. **THERAPEUTIC INTERVENTIONS** · See Arthritis, rheumatoid, p. 400; Mobility, impaired physical, p. 35.	Mobility will be maximized.

Psoriasis—cont'd

NURSING DIAGNOSES / DEFINING CHARACTERISTICS	NURSING INTERVENTIONS / *RATIONALES*	EXPECTED OUTCOMES
Inconsistent correlation of arthritic symptoms to cutaneous manifestations		
Knowledge deficit Lack of experience with psoriasis **DEFINING CHARACTERISTICS** Multiple questions No questions Verbalized misconceptions Frequent repeated exacerbations	**ONGOING ASSESSMENT** ▪ Assess patient's knowledge of cause and management of psoriasis. **THERAPEUTIC INTERVENTIONS** ▪ Explain that cause unknown but disease treatable. ▪ Teach importance of conscientious application of medications and treatments *to attain best results and minimize side effects.* ▪ Teach that expected course includes exacerbations and remissions.	Patient will verbalize understanding of management and personal role.

Originated by: Marie Lindsey, RN,C, MS, FNP

Scleroderma

(PROGRESSIVE SYSTEMIC SCLEROSIS [PSS]; CREST SYNDROME)

A chronic, inflammatory disease characterized by fibrous and degenerative changes in the skin, digital arteries, and internal organs, such as the esophagus, intestinal tract, lungs, kidneys, and heart. It can be a systemic disease or limited to a skin disease.

NURSING DIAGNOSES / DEFINING CHARACTERISTICS	NURSING INTERVENTIONS / *RATIONALES*	EXPECTED OUTCOMES

Altered skin integrity
Related to:
Inflammation
Vasoconstriction
Calcium deposition
Fibrosis
 	
DEFINING CHARACTERISTICS
Change in:
Skin texture
Redness
Swelling
Tenderness
Skin breakdown
Lack of:
Skin elasticity in affected areas
Redness
Swelling
Tenderness
Ulceration
	ONGOING ASSESSMENT
	▪ Assess skin integrity:
	  Note color, moisture, texture, temperature.
	  Note redness, swelling, or tenderness.
	  Note size of ulcers, including drainage and amount of dry necrotic tissue.
	▪ Solicit patient's description of pain:
	  Quality
	  Severity
	  Location
	  Onset
	  Duration
	  Aggravating and alleviating factors
	▪ Assess interference with life-style.
	▪ Assess interference with ADLs.
	
	THERAPEUTIC INTERVENTIONS
	▪ Provide prophylactic pressure-relieving devices (e.g., special mattresses, elbow pads).
	▪ Maintain functional body alignment.
	▪ Clean, dry, and moisturize intact skin with warm (not hot) water, especially over bony prominences, bid; use unscented lotion (e.g., Eucerin or unscented Lubriderm). *Scented lotions contain alcohol, which dries skin.*
		Optimal skin integrity will be maintained.

Continued.

NURSING DIAGNOSES / DEFINING CHARACTERISTICS	NURSING INTERVENTIONS / *RATIONALES*	EXPECTED OUTCOMES
Drainage Necrotic tissue Pain	• Encourage adequate nutrition and hydration. • Administer analgesics before wound debridement and as needed. • Use nonaffected skin areas for injections and infusion of IV solution. *Affected skin difficult to penetrate; once penetrated, allows further skin damage.* • Assist with ADLs as needed. • Instruct patient to avoid contact with harsh chemicals (e.g., household cleaners, detergents). • Instruct patient to wear cotton-lined latex gloves when using harsh chemicals.	

Altered peripheral tissue perfusion
Related to:
Vasospasm
Structural changes
 	
DEFINING CHARACTERISTICS
Pain, numbness, cold sensations
Triphasic color changes: white, blue, red
	ONGOING ASSESSMENT
	• Assess hands and feet for color, temperature, and skin integrity.
	• Solicit patient's description of pain, numbness, and cold sensations.
	• Assess interference with life-style.
	• Assess interference with ADLs.
	
	THERAPEUTIC INTERVENTIONS
	• Keep extremities warm (socks, blankets, gloves, mittens).
	• Remove vasoconstricting factors when possible.
	• Administer vasodilating medications (e.g., Nifedipine) as ordered.
	• Instruct patient to avoid undue cold exposure:
	  Wear oven mitts for refrigerator or freezer.
	  Wear multiple layers of clothing (hat/cap, ear muffs, nose protector, mittens/gloves, socks) in cold environment.
	  Suggest wearing items made of wool, cotton, down, or thinsulate (*provide most protection from cold exposure*).
	• Instruct patient to avoid caffeine and nicotine (*cause vasoconstriction*).
	• Instruct patient in stress management (*stress can precipitate vasospasm*):
	  Identification of stressful situations
	  Identification of past coping mechanisms
	  Identification of new coping mechanisms
	  Use of progressive muscle relaxation techniques, imagery, or biofeedback
		Optimal tissue perfusion will be maintained.

Joint pain *Related to:* Inflammation early in disease **DEFINING CHARACTERISTICS** Pain Guarding on motion of affected joints Facial mask of pain Moaning or other pain-associated sounds	**ONGOING ASSESSMENT** • Solicit patient's description of pain. • Assess for signs of joint inflammation (redness, warmth, swelling, decreased motion). • Determine past pain-relief measures. • Assess interference with life-style. **THERAPEUTIC INTERVENTIONS** • Administer anti-inflammatory medication as prescribed. *Suggest first dose of day as early in morning as possible, with small snack. Anti-inflammatory drugs should not be given on empty stomach (can be very irritating to stomach lining and lead to ulcer disease).* • Use non-narcotic analgesic as necessary. *Narcotic analgesia appears to work better on mechanical than inflammatory types of pain and can be habit-forming.* • Encourage anatomically correct position. Do not use knee gatch or pillows to prop knees. Use a small flat pillow under head. • Encourage use of ambulation aid(s) when pain related to weight bearing. • Apply bed cradle *to keep pressure of bed covers off inflamed lower extremities.* • Consult occupational therapist for proper splinting of affected joints. • See Pain, p. 39.	Pain will be reduced.

NURSING DIAGNOSES / DEFINING CHARACTERISTICS	NURSING INTERVENTIONS / *RATIONALES*	EXPECTED OUTCOMES

Stiffness
Related to:
Inflammation with early disease; contractures with advancing disease
 	
DEFINING CHARACTERISTICS
Verbalized complaint of joint stiffness
	ONGOING ASSESSMENT
	· Solicit patient's description of stiffness:
	  Location: generalized or localized
	  Timing: morning, night, all day
	  Length of stiffness: Ask patient, "How long do you take to loosen up after you get out of bed?" Record in hours or fraction of hour.
	  Relationship to activities
	  Aggravating/alleviating factor
	· Determine past measures to alleviate stiffness.
	· Assess interference with life-style.
	
	THERAPEUTIC INTERVENTIONS
	· Encourage patient to take 15-min warm shower/bath on rising. *Water should be tepid. Excessive heat may promote skin breakdown.*
	· Encourage patient to perform ROM exercises after shower/bath, two repetitions for each joint.
	· Allow sufficient time for all activities.
	· Avoid scheduling tests or treatments when stiffness present.
	· Administer anti-inflammatory medication as prescribed. *Suggest first dose of day as early in morning as possible, with small snack. The sooner patient takes medication, the sooner stiffness will abate. Many patients prefer to take medications as early as 6 or 7 a.m. Ask about normal home medication schedule; try to continue it. Anti-inflammory drugs should not be given on empty stomach.*
	· Remind patient to avoid prolonged inactivity.
		Stiffness will be reduced.

Altered gastrointestinal tract function:
Related to:
Inflammation
Stricture
Hypomotility
Atrophy
 	
DEFINING CHARACTERISTICS
Reports:
  Discomfort
  Pain
  Burning
  Regurgitation
  Constipation
  Diarrhea
  Loss of appetite
Weight loss
Low serum proteins
	ONGOING ASSESSMENT
	· Solicit patient's description of discomfort: pain, burning, regurgitation, constipation, diarrhea, and loss of appetite:
	  Quality
	  Severity
	  Location
	  Onset
	  Duration
	  Precipitating factors
	  Relieving factors
	· Document patient's actual weight at admission (do not estimate).
	
	THERAPEUTIC INTERVENTIONS
	· Prevent reflux by:
	  Elevating HOB at least 30 degrees
	  Applying shock blocks to HOB
	  Using pillows behind back for support
	· Administer medication (e.g., Zantac or Tagament) *to block gastric acid production and relieve burning/pain.*
	· Administer antibiotics as ordered. *Small doses used to treat symptoms of malabsorption; also help manage constipation/diarrhea.*
	· See Nutrition, altered: less than body requirements, p. 37.
	· See Constipation, p. 12; Diarrhea, p. 16.
		Relief of gastrointestinal symptoms will be realized.

Potential altered dental hygiene
Related to:
Microstomia
Sjögren's syndrome
	ONGOING ASSESSMENT
	· Assess patient's ability to open mouth wide.
	· Assess for obvious dental abnormalities.
	· Assess for gum bleeding.
	· Assess all mucous membranes for moisture.
	· Assess for salivary pools.
	  Have patient open mouth as wide as possible.
	  With mouth open, patient puts tip of tongue to roof of mouth.
	  Look under tongue for signs of moisture.
	· Assess lip moisture.
		Dental hygiene will be maintained.

Continued.

NURSING DIAGNOSES / DEFINING CHARACTERISTICS	NURSING INTERVENTIONS / *RATIONALES*	EXPECTED OUTCOMES
DEFINING CHARACTERISTICS Dry mouth Narrowed oral opening Dental caries Bleeding gums	**THERAPEUTIC INTERVENTIONS** · Encourage frequent hydration. · Provide lip moisturizer (e.g., petroleum jelly). · Instruct patient to brush teeth after every meal. *Water pick may be beneficial.* · Instruct patient to avoid high-sugar beverages and foods. Suggest sugar-free candy or beverages to moisten mouth *(may stimulate further salivary function). Saliva protects teeth from dental caries.* · Instruct patient to inspect oral cavity daily. · Instruct patient in ROM mouth exercises to increase oral opening. · Suggest frequent visits to dentist familiar with scleroderma. · Initiate dental consultation as appropriate.	

Altered nutrition: less than body requirements
Related to:
Loss of appetite related to chronic illness
Esophagitis
Malabsorption of nutrients
Microstomia
Psychosocial barriers to eating
 	
DEFINING CHARACTERISTICS
Loss of weight with/without adequate caloric intake ≥10-20% below ideal body weight
Documented inadequate caloric intake
Caloric intake inadequate to keep pace with abnormal disease/metabolic state
	ONGOING ASSESSMENT
	· Document patient's actual weight on admission (do not estimate).
	· Obtain nutritional history.
	· Obtain medication history.
	· Assess for functional deficits restricting ability to eat.
	· Assess for psychosocial factors affecting ability to eat.
	· Assess bowel habits.
	· Assess dental status.
	· Document foods known to cause symptoms.
	
	THERAPEUTIC INTERVENTIONS
	· Consult dietitian when appropriate.
	· Order bland diet.
	· Assist patient with meal setup as needed.
	· Instruct patient:
	    To eat frequent, small meals
	    To avoid eating minimum of 2 hr before lying down
	    To eat slowly
	· Instruct patient to avoid spicy foods, fruit juices, alcohol, bedtime snacks, coffee, any other *foods that produce symptoms of esophagitis.*
	· Administer vitamin/mineral supplements as ordered.
	· Reinforce dietary teaching.
		Optimal caloric intake will be maintained.

Hypertension secondary to potential altered renal function *Related to:* Constriction of renal vessels Scleroderma renal crisis Usually found in patients with diffuse, rapidly progressive skin thickening **DEFINING CHARACTERISTICS** Edema of ankles and feet	**ONGOING ASSESSMENT** · Solicit patient's description of edema, headaches, visual disturbances, fatigue, seizures. · Initially assess blood pressure in both arms while patient lying and sitting. · Assess impact of visual disturbances on life-style (especially safety). · Monitor and record I & O at least every shift. · Weigh daily and record. · Monitor blood and urine chemistries (BUN, creatinine, protein, electrolytes). Notify physician of abnormalities. See Renal failure, acute, p. 343. · Document seizure activity: frequency, type. Notify physician. *Scleroderma renal crisis may progress into renal failure and require dialysis.* · Monitor blood pressure, respiratory rate, and heart rate at least q4h. See Hypertensive crisis, p. 98. *Hypertension commonly accompanies scleroderma renal crisis.* **THERAPEUTIC INTERVENTIONS** · Introduce/reinforce information on use of Captopril: Purpose	Maintenance/improvement in renal function will be achieved.

NURSING DIAGNOSES / DEFINING CHARACTERISTICS	NURSING INTERVENTIONS / *RATIONALES*	EXPECTED OUTCOMES

Severe headaches
Visual disturbances
Fatigue
Increased skin thickening
Seizures
Elevated blood pressure (>140/90)
Decreased urine output (<600 ml/24 hr)
Proteinuria
Hematuria
Elevated BUN and creatinine
	Use
	  Directions for administration (empty stomach)
	  Potential side effects
	  Other pertinent information
	• Administer other antihypertension medication as ordered. Monitor blood pressure 30 min after administration of each dose. *Angiotensin-converting enzyme inhibitors (e.g., Captopril) are rapid-acting agents used to treat both renal failure and hypertension.*
	• Provide uninterrupted rest periods throughout day (30 min 3-4 times/day) *to reduce blood pressure.*
	• If visual disturbances related to hypertension present, provide assistance *to promote safety.*
	• Provide safe, quiet, restful environment.
	• Instruct patient in accurate blood pressure measurement:
	  Purchase a sphygmomanometer for home use to give valid, reliable measurement.
	  Demonstrate correct use of patient's own BP monitoring equipment. Obtain return demonstrations until patient demonstrates correct technique and verbalizes confidence with skill level.
	  Patient should monitor accuracy of own equipment q6mo (can be done by comparing reading from home equipment with reading from standardized, calibrated in-hospital equipment).
	• Instruct patient about the symptoms of scleroderma renal crisis:
	  Edema of ankles/feet
	  Severe headaches
	  Visual difficulties
	  Fatigue
	  Seizures
	• See Hypertension, p. 95; Renal failure, acute, p. 343.	

Potential impaired gas exchange *Related to:* Interstitial fibrosis Pulmonary hypertension **DEFINING CHARACTERISTICS** Shortness of breath Tachypnea Nasal flaring Respiratory depth changes Altered chest excursion Dyspnea on exertion	**ONGOING ASSESSMENT** • Assess respiratory rate and depth by listening to breath sounds a minimum of every shift. • Assess for dyspnea and quantify; relate dyspnea to precipitating factors. • Note use of breathing muscles (i.e., sternocleidomastoid, abdominal, diaphragmatic). • Assess position assumed for normal/easy breathing. • Assess for changes in orientation, restlessness. • Note changes in activity tolerance. • Assess interference with life-style. • Monitor changes in vital signs, especially breathing pattern. • Assess need for home O_2. **THERAPEUTIC INTERVENTIONS** • Pace and schedule activities *to prevent dyspnea resulting from fatigue.* • *Provide reassurance and allay anxiety* by staying with patient during acute episodes of respiratory distress. • Provide O_2 as ordered and as needed. • Instruct patient in environmental factors that may worsen pulmonary condition (e.g., pollen, smoking). • Instruct patient on "cold" symptoms and impending problems. • Assist patient with problem solving for manageable home environment. • Encourage patient to receive influenza vaccine every year, pneumococcal vaccine at some point. *CDC encourages all individuals with chronic illness or lung disease to immunize against flu.*	Optimal respiratory status within limits of disease will be achieved.

Continued.

Scleroderma—cont'd

Integumentary Care Plans

NURSING DIAGNOSES / DEFINING CHARACTERISTICS	NURSING INTERVENTIONS / *RATIONALES*	EXPECTED OUTCOMES
Potential decreased cardiac output *Related to:* Effusions Cardiac arrhythmias (atrial and ventricular) **Defining Characteristics** Patient reports palpitations Patient's/significant other's report of fatigue or shortness of breath Irregular heart rate Tachycardia/ bradycardia Hypoxia	**Ongoing Assessment** • Monitor heart for rate, rhythm, and ectopy every shift. • Assess fluid status. • Assess mentation. • Assess level of energy. **Therapeutic Interventions** • Administer antiarrhythmic medications as ordered. • If arrhythmia occurs, determine patient's response; document and report if significant or symptomatic. • Instruct patient in principles of energy conservation. • See Cardiac dysrhythmias, p. 74.	Optimal cardiac rhythm and cardiac output will be maintained.

Self-care deficit *Related to:* Pain Stiffness Fatigue Psychosocial factors Altered joint functions Muscle weakness Joint contractures **Defining Characteristics** Patient's/significant other's report of difficulty with self-care activities Decreased functional ability to upper/lower extremities	**Ongoing Assessment**
	• Observe patient's ability to:
	  Bathe
	  Carry out personal hygiene
	  Dress
	  Toilet
	  Eat
	• Assess interference with life-style.
	• Determine assistive/adaptive devices used in self-care activities.
	• Assess for need of home health care after discharge.
	
	Therapeutic Interventions
	• Encourage independence:
	  Assist only as necessary.
	  Provide necessary adaptive equipment (raised toilet seat, dressing aids, eating aids) or ask significant other to bring from home.
	  Refer to OT for specialized needs. *Patients have improved self-image if able to perform personal care independently.*
	• Allow patient adequate time for self-care.
	• Encourage patient to take a shower/bath rather than bed bath.
	• Refrain from scheduling tests/activities during self-care.
	• Offer guidance in pacing activities.
	• Reinforce self-care techniques taught by occupational therapist.
		Capabilities will be maximized.

Fatigue *Related to:* Increased disease activity Anemia of chronic disease **Defining Characteristics** Lack of energy, exhaustion, listlessness Excessive sleeping Decreased attention span	**Ongoing Assessment**
	• Solicit patient's description of fatigue:
	  Timing (afternoon or all day)
	  Relationship to activities
	  Aggravating and alleviating factors
	• Determine night sleep pattern.
	• Assess interference with life-style.
	• Determine whether fatigue related to psychologic factors (stress, depression).
	• Determine past measures to alleviate fatigue.
	
	Therapeutic Interventions
	• Provide uninterrupted rest periods throughout day (30 min 3-4 times/day). *Patients often have limited energy supply.*
		Fatigue will be decreased.

480

Scleroderma—cont'd

NURSING DIAGNOSES / DEFINING CHARACTERISTICS	NURSING INTERVENTIONS / *RATIONALES*	EXPECTED OUTCOMES
Facial expressions: yawning, sadness Decreased functional capacity	• Reinforce principles of energy conservation taught by occupational therapist. 　Pacing activities (alternating activity with rest). *Patient often uses more energy than others to complete same tasks.* 　Adequate periods of rest (throughout day and at night) 　Organization of activities and environment 　Proper use of assistive/adaptive devices • If fatigue related to interrupted sleep, see Sleep pattern disturbance, p. 483. • Consult clinical specialist if fatigue may be related to psychologic factors (see Ineffective psychosocial adaptation, p. 482).	
Impaired physical mobility *Related to:* Pain Stiffness Fatigue Psychosocial factors Altered joint function Muscle weakness Joint contractures **DEFINING CHARACTERISTICS** Patient's/significant other's report of difficulty with purposeful movement Decreased ability to transfer and ambulate Reluctance to attempt movement Decreased muscle strength Decreased ROM	**ONGOING ASSESSMENT** • Solicit patient's description of: 　Aggravating and alleviating factors 　Joint pain and stiffness 　Interference with life-style • Observe patient's ability to: 　Ambulate 　Move all joints functionally • Assess need for analgesics before activity. **THERAPEUTIC INTERVENTIONS** • Allow patient adequate time for all activities. *Patient often needs more time than others for same tasks.* • Provide adaptive equipment (e.g., cane, walker) as necessary or ask significant other to bring from home. • Reinforce proper use of ambulation devices taught by physical therapist. • Encourage patient to wear proper footwear (well-fitting, with good support) when ambulating; avoid house slippers. • Assist with ambulation as necessary. • Reinforce techniques of therapeutic exercise (ROM and muscle strengthing) taught by physical therapist. • Reinforce principles of joint protection taught by occupational therapist. • Reinforce proper body alignment when sitting, standing, walking, and lying down. *Improper body alignment can lead to unnecessary pain and contractures.*	Physical mobility will be improved.
Knowledge deficit *Related to:* New disease/ procedures Unfamiliarity with treatment regime **DEFINING CHARACTERISTICS** Multiple questions Lack of questions Verbalized misconceptions Verbalized lack of knowledge	**ONGOING ASSESSMENT** • Assess knowledge of scleroderma and its treatment. • Identify priorities for education. • Assess cognitive style of learning (visual, verbal). • Assess degree to which discomfort interferes with learning. **THERAPEUTIC INTERVENTIONS** • Provide private, quiet environment for patient education. • Schedule educational sessions when patient most comfortable. *Pain distracts patient and may lead to inability to absorb new information.* • Keep session duration appropriate to patient's attention span and ability to integrate information. • Teach patient according to cognitive style (*most effective to teach in manner in which patient learns best*). • Introduce/reinforce disease process information: 　Unknown etiology 　Chronicity of scleroderma 　Processes of inflammation and fibrosis 　Skin and other organ involvement 　Remissions and exacerbations 　Control versus cure	Patient will verbalize increased awareness of disease and treatment.

Continued.

481

Integumentary Care Plans

NURSING DIAGNOSES / DEFINING CHARACTERISTICS	NURSING INTERVENTIONS / *RATIONALES*	EXPECTED OUTCOMES

	• Introduce/reinforce information on drug therapy:
	    Name of drug
	    Purpose
	    Use of drug
	    Directions for administration
	    Potential side effects
	    Other pertinent information (e.g., drug interactions)
	• Introduce/reinforce self-management techniques:
	    ROM exercises
	    Muscle strengthening exercises
	    Pain management
	    Joint protection
	    Pacing activities
	    Adequate rest
	    Splinting
	    Use of assistive devices
	    Skin care
	    Dental hygiene
	• Introduce/reinforce nutritionally sound diet.
	• Stress importance of long-term follow-up.
	• Discuss unproven remedies; encourage to verify/discuss new treatments before use.	

Potential ineffective psychosocial adaptation *Related to:* Altered body structure and function Biophysical Inadequate coping mechanism Inadequate support **DEFINING CHARACTERISTICS** Patient's/significant other's report of ineffective psychosocial adaptation to scleroderma *Grieving:* anger, depression, withdrawal *Diminished self-concept:* refusal to discuss limitations/ altered body function, disparaging remarks about self, withdrawal from role responsibilities *Diminished coping:* expressed hopelessness, prolonged denial of health status, verbalized inability to cope, altered behavior toward self or others	**ONGOING ASSESSMENT** • Identify behaviors suggesting grieving. • Assess behavioral patterns suggesting altered self-concept. • Identify behavioral cues suggesting ineffective individual coping. • Assess cues suggesting sexual dysfunction. • Identify behavioral cues suggesting ineffective family coping. **THERAPEUTIC INTERVENTIONS** • See Coping, inffective individual p. 15; Sexuality patterns, altered, p. 47; Self-concept disturbance, p. 46; Grieving, anticipatory, p. 22.	Adaptation will be facilitated.

NURSING DIAGNOSES / DEFINING CHARACTERISTICS	NURSING INTERVENTIONS / *RATIONALES*	EXPECTED OUTCOMES
Sexual dysfunction: verbalization of problem, expression of dissatisfaction, change in sexual relationship *Diminished family coping:* expressed hopelessness, limited involvement/ noninvolvement with patient, verbalized inability to cope, prolonged denial of patient's health status		
Potential sleep pattern disturbance *Related to:* Pain Stiffness Psychosocial factors **DEFINING CHARACTERISTICS** Inability to fall asleep or frequent awakening Interrupted sleep pattern on several nights	**ONGOING ASSESSMENT** - Solicit description of sleep pattern disturbance: Difficulty in falling asleep Frequent awakening Inhibition of sleep by pain/stiffness Aggravating/alleviating factors - Determine patient's nighttime rituals. - Assess need for special sleep devices (e.g., bed board, special pillow). - Determine whether sleep pattern disturbance related to psychologic factors (stress, depression). **THERAPEUTIC INTERVENTIONS** - Encourage warm shower/bath immediately before bedtime. *Warm water relaxes muscles, facilitates total body relaxation; excessive heat may promote skin breakdown.* - Encourage gentle ROM exercises (after shower/bath) *to maximize benefits of warm bath/shower.* - Encourage patient to sleep in anatomically correct position. Do not prop up affected joints. Change positions frequently during night. - Suggest use of electric blanket (set at low temperature) when skin integrity intact. - Provide quiet, restful environment. Avoid unnecessary wakening (e.g., routine vital signs). - Encourage patient to follow normal nighttime rituals. - Provide special sleep devices or ask family to bring from home. *Familiar surroundings/items encourage relaxation.* - Avoid stimulating foods (caffeine), activities before bedtime. - Encourage use of progressive muscle relaxation technqiues. - Administer nighttime analgesic/long-acting anti-inflammatory drug as ordered. - Administer sleeping medications as ordered if requested by patient. - Consult clinical specialist if sleep pattern disturbance related to psychologic factors. - See Sleep pattern disturbance, p. 50.	Sleep patterns will be normalized.

Originated by: Linda Muzio, RN, MSN
Sue A. Conneighton, RN, MSN, Psy D Candidate

Shingles

(HERPES ZOSTER)

An infectious viral condition caused by a reactivation of latent varicella virus (the agent that causes chicken pox) in a partially immune person. It produces a painful vesicular eruption along the peripheral distribution of nerves from posterior ganglia and is usually unilateral. It is felt to be infectious only for the first 2 to 3 days after eruptions occur. Incubation period is from 7 to 21 days. Total course of the disease is 10 days to 5 weeks from onset to full recovery.

NURSING DIAGNOSES / DEFINING CHARACTERISTICS	NURSING INTERVENTIONS / *RATIONALES*	EXPECTED OUTCOMES
Potential for secondary infection *Related to:* Skin lesions: papules, vesicles, pustules, and crusts **DEFINING CHARACTERISTICS** Itching of lesions Redness and discharge from lesions	**ONGOING ASSESSMENT** • Assess for presence of skin lesions, defining type, description, and location. • Assess for itching or irritation from lesions. • Assess for signs of localized infection: redness and discharge. **THERAPEUTIC INTERVENTIONS** • Discourage scratching of lesions *to prevent inadvertent opening of lesions and cross contamination.* • Remind patient not to scratch. • Trim fingernails. • Use gauze *to separate lesions in skin folds* (e.g., breasts, axilla, fingers, toes). • Implement appropriate isolation precautions: Wound and skin precautions for localized infection Strict isolation for disseminated infection • Do not use topical steroids if secondary infection suspected *because of anti-inflammatory effect.* • Obtain culture and sensitivity of suspected secondary infected lesions as ordered *to indicate appropriate antibiotic treatment.*	Secondary infection will be prevented.
Pain *Related to:* Nerve pain, most commonly thoracic (55 percent), cervical (20 percent), lumbar and sacral (15 percent), ophthalmic division of trigeminal nerve **DEFINING CHARACTERISTICS** Complaints of pain localized to affected nerve Complaints of sharp, burning, or dull pain Facial mask of pain Alteration in muscle tone	**ONGOING ASSESSMENT** • Solicit patient's description of pain/discomfort, including characteristics: Quality Severity Location Onset Duration Precipitating/relieving factors • Assess for nonverbal signs of pain/discomfort. **THERAPEUTIC INTERVENTIONS** • Apply cool, wet dressing to pruritic lesions. • Use appropriate pharmaceuticals per physician's order: Corticosteroids *(anti-inflammatory effect)* Topical steroid ointment (e.g., triamcinolone acetonide [Kenalog]) Vidarabine (Vira-A) *(halts new vesicle formation; provides rapid pain relief)* Antihistamine: *(relief of itching)* • *Prevent irritation of lesions:* Avoid rubbing of skin or lesion. Avoid extreme temperatures. Avoid pressure against skin; use loose, nonrestricting clothing.	Discomfort will be relieved.
Potential anxiety *Related to:* Isolation Possibility of underlying disease in those past middle age	**ONGOING ASSESSMENT** • Assess for signs of anxiety or expressed fear. • Assess patient's coping patterns.	Anxiety will be relieved/reduced.

NURSING DIAGNOSES / DEFINING CHARACTERISTICS	NURSING INTERVENTIONS/ *RATIONALES*	EXPECTED OUTCOMES

DEFINING CHARACTERISTICS
Restlessness
Insomnia
Facial tension
Overexcitment/
jitteriness
Expressed concern
	THERAPEUTIC INTERVENTIONS
	• *Allay fears of isolation* by describing:
	   Necessity for isolation
	   Isolation techniques
	   Possible duration of isolation
	• Support patient undergoing diagnostic studies to investigate the presence of internal disease (Hodgkin's disease, lymphosarcoma, malignancy). *Patient may be anxious about test results.*
	• Display confident, calm manner and understanding attitude.
	• Establish rapport with patient.
	• Encourage ventilation of feelings.
	• Refer to Anxiety, p. 4.	

Potential altered levels of consciousness
Related to:
CNS inflammation
 	
DEFINING CHARACTERISTICS
Change in alertness
Change in orientation
Memory impairment
Impaired judgment
Irritability
	ONGOING ASSESSMENT
	• Assess level of consciousness (LOC).
	• Determine factors contributing to LOC change:
	   Medications
	   Awakening from sound sleep
	   Not understanding question
	
	THERAPEUTIC INTERVENTIONS
	• Refer to Consciousness, alteration in level of, p. 234.
		Alteration in LOC will be reduced.

Potential ineffective breathing pattern *Related to:* Varicella pneumonia (present in 15 percent of adults with herpes zoster) **DEFINING CHARACTERISTICS** Dyspnea Shortness of breath Cough Tachypnea	**ONGOING ASSESSMENT** • Assess respiratory rate and depth q4h. • Assess breath sounds. **THERAPEUTIC INTERVENTIONS** • See Pneumonia, p. 196.	Regular and unlabored breathing pattern will be maintained.
Potential body image disturbance *Related to:* Skin lesions **DEFININT CHARACTERISTICS** Verbal preoccupation with lesions Focusing behavior on lesion Refusal to look at/ participate in care of skin lesions	**ONGOING ASSESSMENT** • Assess perception of changed appearance. • Note verbal references to skin lesions. **THERAPEUTIC INTERVENTIONS** • See Body image disturbance, p. 6.	Feelings about skin lesions will be acknowledged.

Continued.

Shingles—cont'd

NURSING DIAGNOSES / DEFINING CHARACTERISTICS	NURSING INTERVENTIONS / *RATIONALES*	EXPECTED OUTCOMES

Knowledge deficit
Related to:
New condition and procedures
 	
DEFINING CHARACTERISTICS
Questions
Confusion about treatment
Inability to comply with treatment regimen
Lack of questions
	ONGOING ASSESSMENT
	· Determine patient's/significant other's understanding of disease process, complications, and treatment regimen.
	
	THERAPEUTIC INTERVENTIONS
	· Encourage patient/significant others to ask questions *so concerns can be addressed.*
	· Provide necessary information to patient/significant others:
	    Description of herpes zoster, including spread of disease
	    Explanation of need for isolation, including correct isolation procedures
	    Need to prevent scratching or irritation of lesions
	    Need to notify health professionals of signs of CNS inflammation or pneumonia
	· Evaluate understanding of information after teaching session *to be sure it is understood.*
	· Observe for compliance with treatment regimen.
		Patient/signifciant other will verbalize needed information about disease, treatment, and complications of herpes zoster.

Originated by: Susan Galanes, RN, MS, CCRN

Skin loss, full-thickness: comparable to burn injury

Full thickness skin loss involves destruction of the skin and structures underneath the skin with possible destruction of epithelium, fat, muscle, blood vessels, and bone. A variety of conditions/disorders can cause this destruction: perfusion disorders; disseminated intravascular coagulation (DIC); burns, or traumatic events, such as automobile/motorcycle accidents, falls, and crushing injuries.

NURSING DIAGNOSES / DEFINING CHARACTERISTICS	NURSING INTERVENTIONS / *RATIONALES*	EXPECTED OUTCOMES
Impaired skin integrity *Related to:* Burns Crushing injuries Thrombocytopenia purpura **DEFINING CHARACTERISTICS** Blancing of skin Redness Leathery appearance Skin color changes: brown to black Blistering, weeping skin Pain/absence of pain	**ONGOING ASSESSMENT** · Check color, texture, turgor, and depth of wound. · Check for blisters, large open wounds, blanching. · Assess degree of pain. · Assess for any odors. · Assess for adherent debris/hair. **THERAPEUTIC INTERVENTIONS** · Use burn pack or nonadherent sheeting *to prevent sticking.* · Use hydrotherapy tub as ordered *to aid in cleansing and loosening slough, exudate, eschar.* · Apply topical bacteriostatic substances as directed. *Use extreme care when removing topical ointments during dressing change to prevent removal of granulating skin.* · Elevate extremities, if possible, *to prevent swelling.*	Optimal skin integrity will be maintained.
Potential for infection *Related to:* Altered skin integrity Invasive therapies	**ONGOING ASSESSMENT** · Review laboratory data for any abrupt changes. · Monitor and record vital signs; notify physician if out of range. · Observe potential sites of infection: Assess odor and wound appearance at each dressing change.	The risk for infection will be reduced.

Skin loss, full thickness: comparable to burn injury—cont'd

NURSING DIAGNOSES / DEFINING CHARACTERISTICS	NURSING INTERVENTIONS / *RATIONALES*	EXPECTED OUTCOMES
DEFINING CHARACTERISTICS Elevated WBCs Elevated temperature Presence of positive cultures Wound sepsis: abdominal distention, ileus, disorientation	Routinely assess IV line sites, Foley catheter, and other invasive sites for infection. • Monitor topical agent's effectiveness via wound cultures as ordered. **THERAPEUTIC INTERVENTIONS** • Maintain aseptic technique: wear mask and sterile gloves for physical contact *to prevent iatrogenic contamination.* • Keep area clean. • Promote personal hygiene. • Administer antibiotics on schedule as ordered.	
Potential fluid volume deficit *Related to:* *Note:* Fluid volume deficit directly proportional to extent, depth of "burn" injury because of increased capillary permeability Massive fluid shifting and circulating volume loss *result in fluid accumulation in tissue with blister formation* Hemorrhage: stress ulcer (Curling's ulcer) **DEFINING CHARACTERISTICS** Altered mental status Tachycardia Hypotension Thirst Skin pale and cool, dusty-looking in dark skinned person Oliguria Restlessness Hypoxia Alteration in electrolytes, especially hyperkalemia Alteration in acid-base balance Catabolism (outpouring of K^+ and nitrogen) Coffee-ground emesis Bright-red blood emesis via nasogastric tube Melena stools	**ONGOING ASSESSMENT** • Assess for signs/symptoms of fluid volume deficit (see Defining Characteristics). • Monitor vital signs and hemodynamic status; report to physician if out of range. • Monitor urine specific gravity q4h. • Monitor I & O q2h; report urine output <30 ml/hr to physician. • Obtain daily weight. • Observe for cardiac arrhythmias associated with hyperkalemia. • Observe for coffee-ground emesis, bloody emesis, melena stools, abdominal distention, and epigastric pain. **THERAPEUTIC INTERVENTIONS** • Administer IV fluids as ordered *to prevent dehydration.* • See Fluid volume deficit, p. 20. • Administer antacids/H_2-receptor antagonist prophylactically *to minimize potential for bleeding.* • See Gastrointestinal bleeding, p. 284, as needed.	Fluid volume deficit will be reduced.

Continued.

NURSING DIAGNOSES / DEFINING CHARACTERISTICS	NURSING INTERVENTIONS / *RATIONALES*	EXPECTED OUTCOMES
Potential ineffective breathing pattern *Related to:* Massive injury Acidosis **Defining Characteristics** Dyspnea Shortness of breath Tachypnea Use of accessory muscles Cough Cyanosis Alterations in ABGs	**Ongoing Assessment** • Assess respiratory rate, rhythm, and depth. • Assess for dyspnea, shortness of breath, use of accessory muscles, cough, and presence of cyanosis. • Monitor ABGs. **Therapeutic Interventions** • Position patient with proper body alignment *for optimal breathing and lung expansion*. • Maintain O_2 delivery, as required. • See Breathing pattern, ineffective, p. 8.	Optimal breathing pattern will be maintained.
Potential altered peripheral tissue perfusion *Related to:* Blockage of microcirculation Blood loss Compartment syndrome (edema restricting circulation) Decreased platelets **Defining Characteristics** Weak, thready pulses Pallor Extremities cool to touch Pain Numbness Prolonged PT/PTT	**Ongoing Assessment** • Check pulses of all extremities. • Monitor vital signs (BP, heart rate, and respiratory rate) for abrupt changes. • Assess color and temperature of extremities. • Check for pain, numbness, or swelling of extremities. • Monitor laboratory data; report findings (e.g., platelets, PT/PTT) to physician. **Therapeutic Interventions** • Maintain good alignment of extremities *to allow adequate blood flow without compression on arteries*. • Notify physician immediately of noted alteration in perfusion. • Administer blood products as ordered.	Optimal tissue perfusion will be maintained.
Potential altered nutrition *Related to:* Excessive metabolic demands resulting from prolonged interference of ability to ingest or digest food Increased basal metabolic rate **Defining Characteristics** Increased ketones Decreased albumin Generalized weakness Negative nitrogen balance (hypoproteinemia)	**Ongoing Assessment** • Closely monitor caloric intake. • Monitor urine, serum glucose, and ketone levels. • Assess for muscle weakness. • Montior serum and urine electrolytes and BUN. • Check for bowel sounds. • Monitor gastric pH. **Therapeutic Interventions** • See Nutrition, altered: less than body requirements, p. 37. • Consult dietitian *to assist in meeting nutritional needs*. • See Enteral tube feeding, p. 308; Total parenteral nutrition, p. 324, as appropriate.	Alteration in nutrition will be reduced.

Skin loss, full thickness: comparable to burn injury—cont'd

NURSING DIAGNOSES / DEFINING CHARACTERISTICS	NURSING INTERVENTIONS / *RATIONALES*	EXPECTED OUTCOMES
Increased BUN Alteration in fluid and electrolyte status		

Pain
Related to:
Injury
 	
DEFINING CHARACTERISTICS
Complaints of pain
Increased restlessness
Alterations in sleep pattern
Irritability
Facial grimaces
Guarding
	ONGOING ASSESSMENT
	· Assess pain characteristics:
	    Quality
	    Severity
	    Location
	    Onset
	    Duration
	    Precipitating factors
	
	THERAPEUTIC INTERVENTIONS
	· Administer sedatives and analgesics prescribed for pain (via IV while patient critical).
	· Position patient *to promote comfort.*
	· Alleviate all unnecesary stressors or discomfort sources.
	· Allay fears and anxiety.
	· Turn patient *to help relieve pressure points.*
	· Use distraction/relaxation techniques as indicated.
		Pain will be relieved or reduced.

Anxiety *Related to:* Change in body image Anticipation of pain Questionable outcome **DEFINING CHARACTERISTICS** Restlessness Combativeness Tachypnea Tachycardia	**ONGOING ASSESSMENT** · Observe for signs of anxiety. · Identify normal level of coping. **THERAPEUTIC INTERVENTIONS** · Display confident, calm manner. · Encourage ventilation of feelings and concerns. · Reduce distracting stimuli *to maintain quiet environment.* · See Anxiety, p. 4.	Anxiety will be managed.
Knowledge deficit *Related to:* New injury New treatment **DEFINING CHARACTERISTICS** Multiple questions Noncommunication Staring Change in behavior Guarding	**ONGOING ASSESSMENT** · Assess readiness to learn. · Assess baseline knowledge of injury and treatment. **THERAPEUTIC INTERVENTIONS** · Explain all procedures and tests. · Explain need for sterile techniques with dressing changes *to prevent infection.* · Explain reason for frequent assessment/orientation to environment. · Explain reason for frequent turning and repositioning *to gain patient's cooperation.* · *To alleviate fears,* explain reason for gloves and masks during sterile procedures.	Patient will verbalize knowledge and understanding of injury and treatment.

Originated by: Linda Marie St. Julien, RN, MS

Visual and Auditory Care Plans

DISORDERS
Otitis media
Visual impairment

THERAPEUTIC INTERVENTIONS
Cataract extraction: with and without
  intraocular lens implant

Otitis media

Infection and inflammation of the usually sterile middle ear caused by the introduction of bacteria. Otitis media is often seen in children under 3 years of age secondary to an upper respiratory infection. In this age group, the eustachian tube is horizontal in position between the middle ear and the nasopharynx. Upper airway secretions easily flow into the middle ear. After 3 years of age the eustachian tube slants downward to the nasopharynx. If untreated or partially treated, otitis media can lead to chronic otitis, mastoiditis, central nervous system damage, and permanent hearing loss.

NURSING DIAGNOSES / DEFINING CHARACTERISTICS	NURSING INTERVENTIONS / *RATIONALES*	EXPECTED OUTCOMES
Hyperthermia *Related to:* Bacterial infection Haemophilus influenzae β-hemolytic streptococci Pneumococci **DEFINING CHARACTERISTICS** Skin warm and flushed Persistent rise in body temperature Irritability Drowsy Presence of drainage from middle ear(s)	**ONGOING ASSESSMENT** • Monitor vital signs, especially temperature, q4h. If >38.5 °C, monitor q2h. • Observe for chilling. • Assess previous history and physical factors, including: 　Age 　Pattern of fever 　Previous ear infections **THERAPEUTIC INTERVENTIONS** • Plot temperature curve; observe for trends q4h. • Encourage oral fluids. • Use hypothermia blanket for elevated temperature as ordered. • Administer antipyretics as ordered. • Remove excessive clothing; use light blankets only if needed. • Maintain bedside humidifier. • Notify physician of temperature >38.5 °C. *Uncontrolled fever can lead to febrile seizures.*	Normal body temperature will be maintained.
Ineffective airway clearance *Related to:* Upper respiratory infection **DEFINING CHARACTERISTICS** Coarse breath sounds Rales and/or rhonchi Upper airway congestion Congested cough (productive and nonproductive) Nasal drainage	**ONGOING ASSESSMENT** • Assess respiratory status q4h and as needed for 　Respiratory rate 　Quality of respirations 　Breath sounds 　Retractions or nasal flaring 　Cough (quality and frequency) 　Rales and rhonchi • Assess vital signs q4h. • Monitor effectiveness of respiratory treatment: 　Chest percussion and drainage 　Suctioning 　Hand-held nebulizer **THERAPEUTIC INTERVENTIONS** • Maintain O_2 and humidity therapy as ordered by physician. • Position for optimal breathing. • Encourage deep breathing and position change q2h. • Provide mouth care q4h and as needed. • Refer to Airway clearance, ineffective, p. 3.	An open airway will be maintained.
Pain *Related to:* Inflammation and pressure in middle ear	**ONGOING ASSESSMENT** • Assess level of comfort by observing both verbal and nonverbal behaviors (see Defining Characteristics). **THERAPEUTIC INTERVENTIONS** • Instill eardrops as ordered. • Raise head of bed (HOB) *to decrease pressure in ears.*	Pain will be reduced.

Continued.

■ **Otitis media—cont'd**

NURSING DIAGNOSES / DEFINING CHARACTERISTICS	NURSING INTERVENTIONS / *RATIONALES*	EXPECTED OUTCOMES
DEFINING CHARACTERISTICS Irritability Restlessness Altered sleeping patterns Verbalized ear pain	· Use warm, moist compresses to affected ear(s). · Administer analgesics as ordered.	
Knowledge deficit *Related to:* Illness and hospitalization Lack of experience **DEFINING CHARACTERISTICS** Confusion Repetitive questions Lack of questions Disbelief	**ONGOING ASSESSMENT** · Assess knowledge of illness. · Assess level of understanding. · Evaluate ability to learn. **THERAPEUTIC INTERVENTIONS** · Provide information about cause of otitis media. · Provide instruction on signs/symptoms of otitis media. · Teach proper instillation of eardrops. · Discuss prevention and treatment of URIs. · Discuss administration and possible side effects of antibiotic therapy. *Full course of antibiotics must be taken to prevent recurrence and possible hearing impairment.*	Signs/symptoms, prevention, and treatment will be understood.

Originated by: Andrea So, RN, BSN

Visual impairment

(CATARACT; BLINDNESS; GLAUCOMA)

State in which an individual experiences a change in amount or patterning of incoming stimuli, accompanied by a diminished, exaggerated, distorted, or impaired response to such stimuli.

NURSING DIAGNOSES / DEFINING CHARACTERISTICS	NURSING INTERVENTIONS / *RATIONALES*	EXPECTED OUTCOMES
Sensory/perceptual alteration: visual *Related to:* Disease/trauma to visual pathways/cranial nerves II, III, IV, and VI secondary to: Stroke Intracranial aneurysms Brain tumor Trauma Myasthenia gravis Multiple sclerosis Glaucoma Cataract	**ONGOING ASSESSMENT** · Assess peripheral field of vision, corneal reflex, pupillary response, visual acuity, extraocular movements. · Assess central vision with each eye individually and together. · Determine nature of visual symptoms, onset, and degree of visual loss. · Inquire about previous visual complaints, eye injury, or ocular pain. · Assess eye and lid for inflammation, edema, positional defects, and deviation. · Inquire about patient/family history of systemic or CNS disease. · Evaluate patient's ability to function within limits of visual impairment. · Assess factors/aids that improve vision, such as glasses, contact lenses, bright lights.	Optimal functioning within limits of visual impairment will be achieved.

NURSING DIAGNOSES / DEFINING CHARACTERISTICS	NURSING INTERVENTIONS / *RATIONALES*	EXPECTED OUTCOMES

DEFINING CHARACTERISTICS
 	
Lack of eye-to-eye contact
Abnormal eye movement
Failure to locate distant objects
Squinting, frequent blinking
Bumping into things
Clumsy behavior
Closing of one eye to see
Frequent rubbing of eye
Deviation of eye
Gray opacities in eyes
Head tilting
	THERAPEUTIC INTERVENTIONS
	• Identify self to patient.
	• Orient patient to environment *to reduce fear related to unfamiliar environment.*
	• Provide adequate lighting:
	    Bright for patients with dimmed vision
	    Subdued for patients with photophobia
	• Place meal tray, tissues, water, and call light within patient's range of vision *to ensure safety.*
	• Place sign over bed indicating type and degree of impairment, contraindicated activities.
	• If patient has right-field cut, indicate in sign over bed to approach the patient from left.
	• Provide eye patch for affected eye for patient with diplopia.
	• Instruct patient with hemianopsia to scan environment visually *to optimize vision.*
	• Use visual aids (e.g., magnifying glass, large-type printed books and magazines), when appropriate.
	• If patient is blind:
	    Place sign in front of chart.
	    Inform him/her of date and time.
	    Explain arrangement of food on tray and plate, using clockwise sequence.
	    Place food on tray and plate in same place each meal.
	    Encourage use of sense of touch to become familiar with new objects.
	    Explain sounds.
	• Encourage use of radios, tapes. *Time passes slowly when one is inactive. Diversional activities should be encouraged. Radio, television increase awareness of day and time.*
	• Inform of availability of "talking books" through Library of Congress.	

Potential for injury *Related to:* Visual impairment Lack of awareness of environmental hazards **DEFINING CHARACTERISTICS** Stumbling into furniture Bruised legs Falls	**ONGOING ASSESSMENT** • Assess need for assistive devices. • Inquire about previous fall history related to visual impairment. • Evaluate ability to mobilize within environment. • Assess patient's fall-risk level. **THERAPEUTIC INTERVENTIONS** • Place sticker in front of patient's chart and over HOB indicating type and degree of visual impairment. • Remove environmental barriers *to ensure safety.* If furniture or waste baskets moved, notify patient of changes. • Encourage patient's roommate and other patients to avoid leaving doors partially open; should be fully open or closed. • Maintain bed in low position with side rails up, if appropriate. *Side rails help remind patient not to get up without help.* Keep bed in locked position. • Guide patient when ambulating, if appropriate. Walk ahead, with patient's arm around your elbow. Describe where you are walking; identify obstacles. • Instruct patient to hold both arms of chair before sitting. • Consult OT personnel for assistive devices and training in their use. • Supervise patient when smoking *to prevent accidental fires.*	Risk of fall and injury will be decreased.
Anxiety/fear *Related to:* Change in health status Visual impairment Change in role functioning	**ONGOING ASSESSMENT** • Recognize level of anxiety (mild, severe). • Assess normal coping patterns (by interview with patient/family/significant others/physician). **THERAPEUTIC INTERVENTIONS** • Display confident, calm manner and tolerant, understanding attitude.	Anxiety/fear will be reduced.

Continued.

NURSING DIAGNOSES / DEFINING CHARACTERISTICS	NURSING INTERVENTIONS / *RATIONALES*	EXPECTED OUTCOMES
Change in interaction patterns **DEFINING CHARACTERISTICS** Withdrawal Indifference Constant demands Uncooperative behavior Avoidance Crying Sleepless nights	• Encourage ventilation of feelings/concerns/dependence; listen carefully. Give unhurried, attentive response. • See Anxiety, p. 4 and Fear, p. 18.	
Self-concept disturbance *Related to:* Visual impairment **DEFINING CHARACTERISTICS** Patient's/significant others' report of changes in self-esteem/personal identity Withdrawal Irritability Tearfulness Anxiety Denial of problem Insomnia Refusal to participate in teaching/learning experiences Self-maligning statements	**ONGOING ASSESSMENT** • Assess patient for: 　Perception of self 　Level of anxiety 　Verbalization of changed self-concept 　Affect, behavior 　Ability to care for self 　Previous methods of coping **THERAPEUTIC INTERVENTIONS** • Encourage patient to verbalize fears and concerns. • Include significant others in discussions when possible. • Support by positive reinforcement patient's effort to adapt to constructive changes. • Provide patient/significant others opportunities to ask questions and verbalize feelings. • Use referral groups (other professional or lay persons) when appropriate *to facilitate patient's attempts at coping.*	Positive expression of self-worth will be verbalized.
Knowledge deficit *Related to:* Change in health status **DEFINING CHARACTERISTICS** Questioning Misconceptions Frequent use of call light	**ONGOING ASSESSMENT** • Assess patient's/significant others' knowledge of visual impairment. • Assess effects of visual impairment on ADL. **THERAPEUTIC INTERVENTIONS** • Involve significant others in patient's care and instructions. • Help them understand nature and limitations of disease. *Patient/family need information to plan strategies for coping with impairment.* • Reinforce physician's explanation of medical management and surgical procedures, if any. • Teach general eye care. • Demonstrate proper administration of eye drops or ointments. • Help family/significant others identify and make arrangements at home to provide for patient's safety, if indicated. • Make appropriate referrals to home health agency for nursing and social service follow-up. • Reinforce need to use community agencies, if indicated (e.g., American Foundation for the Blind, 15 West 16th St., New York, NY 10011).	Patient/significant others will demonstrate or verbalize knowledge of disease and care needed after discharge.

Originated by: Maria Dacanay, RN

Cataract extraction: with and without intraocular lens implant

A cataract is an opacity of the lens or lens capsule of the eye. It may be congenital, senile or degenerative, metabolic (diabetes), traumatic, or toxic in origin. Treatment consists of surgical extraction of the defective lens, either with or without intraocular lens implant.

NURSING DIAGNOSES / DEFINING CHARACTERISTICS	NURSING INTERVENTIONS / *RATIONALES*	EXPECTED OUTCOMES

Sensory/perceptual alteration: visual
Related to:
Opacity of crystalline lens of eye
 	
DEFINING CHARACTERISTICS
Gradual dimming, blurring of vision
Double vision
Progressive nearsightedness
Frequent need for new glasses
Glare haloes noted in bright light
Inability to find lighting bright enough for reading
Poor reading vision
	ONGOING ASSESSMENT
	· Observe gross appearance of affected eye, particularly pupil.
	· Assess patient's level of daily functioning, need for assistance, etc.
	
	THERAPEUTIC INTERVENTIONS
	· Orient patient to hospital environment:
	    Walk patient around room and unit.
	    Place objects (especially call light) with reach on unaffected side.
	· Provide assistance with ADL as needed.
	· Encourage patient to communicate concerns.
	· See Visual impairment, p. 492.
		Optimal functioning within limits of visual impairment will be achieved.

Knowledge deficit
Related to:
Unfamiliarity with preoperative routines
 	
DEFINING CHARACTERISTICS
Questions
Misconceptions
	ONGOING ASSESSMENT
	· Assess knowledge of preoperative routines/eye care.
	
	THERAPEUTIC INTERVENTIONS
	· Instruct patient about preparation of operative eye:
	    Place mydriatic solution in eye.
	    Press inner canthus for about 30-60 sec *to speed dilation, prevent systemic absorption, and prevent drops from running into nose.*
	    If more than one eye medication given at one time, wait at least 3-5 min between dosages *to allow absorption of each successive medication.*
	· Document appropriate pupil dilation after instillation of mydriatic solution.
	· Darken room; avoid bright lights.
	· Instruct about general postoperative procedures/care:
	    Eye patch and shield will cover eye postoperatively
	    Do not touch, squeeze, or rub eye postoperatively
	· Reassure patient of assistance by nurses to meet physical needs after surgery.
		Patient verbalizes required preoperative eye care and general postoperative precautions.

Potential for injury to operative eye *Related to:* Increased intraocular pressure resulting from bleeding, edema, hematoma **DEFINING CHARACTERISTICS** Severe eye pain Eye hemorrhage Symptoms of damage to optic nerve (blindness)	**ONGOING ASSESSMENT** · Observe/document/report amount of drainage on eye patch and shield. Notify physician immediately if drainage bright red and excessive. · Report complaints of eye pain *(may indicate hemorrhage/infection).* · If intraocular lens implanted, observe/document/report. presence of intraoclar lens implant, signs/symptoms of eye inflammation, irritation, increased tearing, soreness, pain. *Intraocular lens implant used for patients who cannot wear contact lenses or cataract glasses.* · Observe for and attempt to allay restlessness. **THERAPEUTIC INTERVENTIONS** · Maintain quiet, relaxed atmosphere. Avoid jarring bed. · Elevate HOB 30-45 degrees. Do not place patient flat in bed. · Position patient on nonoperative side or back, never on operative side.	Physical injury caused by increased intraocular pressure will be reduced.

Continued.

Visual and Auditory Care Plans

NURSING DIAGNOSES / DEFINING CHARACTERISTICS	NURSING INTERVENTIONS / *RATIONALES*	EXPECTED OUTCOMES

	• Maintain bed rest with bathroom privileges; provide assistance.
	• Instruct patient to change position *gradually*.
	• Instruct patient to:
	    Avoid rubbing, squeezing, scratching, or touching operative eye.
	    Avoid nose blowing and coughing first day after surgery *to prevent pressure buildup in eye*.
	    Avoid stooping and lowering head *to prevent increase in intraocular pressure*. Use step-in slippers and shoes.
	    Avoid turning head rapidly.
	    Avoid shaving, brushing teeth, combing hair, showering first day after surgery.
	• Instruct patient to notify nurse of nausea/vomiting *(increases intraocular pressure)*. Administer antiemetic as ordered.
	• Place personal items (i.e., call light, urinal, bedpan) within reach on unaffected side *to increase independence*.
	• Administer mydriatic drops as ordered *to dilate pupil*.
	• Medicate for discomfort as needed.	

Knowledge deficit
Related to:
Unfamiliarity with postdischarge eye care and self-care at home
 	
DEFINING CHARACTERISTICS
Many questions
Misconceptions
	ONGOING ASSESSMENT
	• Assess patient's/significant other's knowledge of and readiness for learning.
	
	THERAPEUTIC INTERVENTIONS
	• Teach specifics on eye care:
	    Wear eye shield at night *to prevent injury* for approximately 6 wk.
	    Wear glasses during day. Wear old glasses for unoperated eye.
	    Avoid heavy lifting, stooping, straining, bending 4-6 wk.
	    Reading and light activity permitted.
	    Avoid falls and bumping or jarring head. Take care entering and leaving car.
	    Avoid squeezing, scratching, or rubbing operative eye and lids.
	    Use proper eyedrop instillation technique.
	    Call physician if patient experiences severe pain, sudden loss of vision, or signs of infection.
	    Avoid constipation.
	• Reassure patient that vision will gradually improve in few weeks.
	• Inform that he/she will be fitted for contact lenses or glasses if lens implant not performed.
	• Instruct that several weeks needed to adjust to distortion from glasses and special contact lenses. Peripheral vision diminished with cataract glasses.
	• Encourage patient to carry intraocular lens implant ID card as appropriate.
		Patient/significant others will have adequate knowledge to care for eye on discharge.

Originated by: Laura Vieceli-Brooks, RN, BSN

Hematolymphatic and Oncologic Care Plans

DISORDERS

Anemia
Cellulitis
Disseminated intravascular coagulation
Granulocytopenia
Hemophilia
Leukemia, acute

Multiple myeloma
Sickle cell pain crisis
Stomatitis
Tumor lysis syndrome

THERAPEUTIC INTERVENTIONS

Autologous bone marrow transplantation
Blood and blood product transfusion
  therapy
Bone marrow harvest: care of the bone
  marrow donor
Cancer chemotherapy
Hickman right atrial catheter

Anemia

(APLASTIC ANEMIA; IRON DEFICIENCY ANEMIA; PERNICIOUS ANEMIA; HEMOLYTIC ANEMIA; VITAMIN B$_{12}$ DEFICIENCY)

Anemia implies low red cell count and below-normal hemoglobin or hematocrit level that reduces the oxygen-carrying capacity of the blood. It can occur secondary to decreased production of red cells (e.g., nutritional deficiency, malignancy, toxic exposure), loss of red cells through hemorrhage, or red cell lysis. Specific types of anemia include aplastic, iron deficiency, pernicious, and hemolytic.

NURSING DIAGNOSES / DEFINING CHARACTERISTICS	NURSING INTERVENTIONS / *RATIONALES*	EXPECTED OUTCOMES

Activity intolerance
Related to:
Decreased O$_2$ supply to cells
Decreased cellular ability to meet energy requirements
 	
Defining Characteristics
Weakness
Fatigue
Dyspnea on exertion
Abnormal respiratory response to activity
Abnormal cardiac response to activity
	Ongoing Assessment
	· Assess respiratory status before activity:
	  Respiratory rate
	  Use of accessory muscles
	  Need for supplemental O$_2$
	· Assess cardiac status before activity:
	  Pulse rate
	  Cardiac rhythm
	  BP
	  Skin color and perfusion
	· Assess patient's ability to perform ADL.
	· Assess potential for injury with activity.
	· Assess understanding of change in activity level and tolerance by patient/significant others.
	· Monitor patient for cardiac or respiratory complications.
	
	Therapeutic Interventions
	· Plan nursing activities *to provide adequate rest periods.*
	· Provide quiet atmosphere *to allow rest and decrease oxygen consumption.*
	· Provide assistance for activities patient cannot perform independently.
	· Increase activity levels as tolerated by patient.
	· Reassure patient that state is temporary (if accurate).
		Activity level will be maintained within limits of patient's capability.

Potential ineffective breathing pattern
Related to:
Decreased Hb level resulting in decreased blood O$_2$ content and O$_2$-carrying capacity
 	
Defining Characteristics
Dyspnea
Shortness of breath
Orthopnea
Tachypnea
Cyanosis
Tachycardia
Use of accessory muscles
Nasal flaring
Retractions
	Ongoing Assessment
	· Assess respiratory status:
	  Respiratory rate
	  Depth of respiration
	  Use of accessory muscles
	  Presence of flaring nostrils, retractions
	  Dyspnea, shortness of breath
	  Position for optimal breathing
	· Monitor vital signs.
	· Observe for changes in breathing patterns.
	· Monitor ABGs.
	
	Therapeutic Interventions
	· Pace activities to patient's tolerance.
	· Administer supplemental O$_2$ as ordered *to increase oxygen supply, improve lung expansion, and improve ventilation.*
	· Elevate HOB as needed.
	· See Breathing pattern, ineffective p. 8.
		Optimal breathing pattern will be maintained.

NURSING DIAGNOSES / DEFINING CHARACTERISTICS	NURSING INTERVENTIONS / *RATIONALES*	EXPECTED OUTCOMES
Potential for injury: cardiac complications of anemia (angina, myocardial infarction, congestive heart failure) *Related to:* High output state Tachycardia Tachypnea Increased metabolic needs Significantly decreased Hb levels **DEFINING CHARACTERISTICS** Shortness of breath Orthopnea Edema Palpitations Angina, chest pain Cold, clammy skin Changes in color of skin, mucous membranes Arrhythmias	**ONGOING ASSESSMENT** • Assess factors affecting anemia symptoms. 　Speed with which anemia developed 　Metabolic needs of patient 　Other physical disorders • Observe for changes in cardiac status *(so appropriate treatment can be initiated early)*: 　Pulse rate 　Cardiac rhythm 　BP 　Skin color and perfusion 　Complaints of angina, chest pain • Observe for angina and chest pain (see Angina pectoris, unstable, p. 69). • Observe for conditions increasing metabolic needs *that might precipitate complications.* **THERAPEUTIC INTERVENTIONS** • Pace activities to patient's tolerance *to reduce development of complications.*	Optimal cardiac status will be maintained.
Potential impaired skin integrity *Related to:* Decreased blood and O_2 supply to skin **DEFINING CHARACTERISTICS** Skin cool to touch Altered circulation Altered sensation Altered nutrition	**ONGOING ASSESSMENT** • Assess skin integrity: color, moisture, temperature, texture, presence of existing lesions. • Assess nutritional status: diet, laboratory data, weight. • Assess physical impairments that may contribute to breakdown: altered circulation, altered sensation. **THERAPEUTIC INTERVENTIONS** • Reposition patient frequently (at least q2h) *to improve circulation to skin and tissues.* • Use pressure-relieving devices as necessary. • Provide extra blankets and clothing for warmth. • Teach patient to avoid heating pads *to reduce risk of skin injury.* • Provide adequate nutritional support.	Optimal skin integrity will be maintained.
Altered nutrition: less than body requirements *Related to:* Decreased intake of iron, protein Disease of GI tract, liver Deficiency in nutrient metabolism Increased need for nutrients above normal intake Blood loss	**ONGOING ASSESSMENT** • Document patient's weight. • Obtain nutritional history. • Determine presence of underlying disease process (iron, vitamin deficiency, etc.). • Obtain baseline laboratory values: 　Serum iron *to identify amount of iron available* 　Total iron-binding capacity 　RBC 　Hb; Hb electrophoresis *to determine whether adequate amount hemoglobin present* 　Reticulocyte count *to identify increased number of immature RBCs* 　Red cell shape and size *(may not carry adequate amounts of oxygen)* 　Bilirubin *to identify increased breakdown of RBCs*	Optimal nutrition will be achieved.

Continued.

NURSING DIAGNOSES / DEFINING CHARACTERISTICS	NURSING INTERVENTIONS / *RATIONALES*	EXPECTED OUTCOMES
DEFINING CHARACTERISTICS Loss of weight Nausea/vomiting Anorexia	Bone marrow examination *to determine whether adequate precursors present* Bleeding/coagulation studies *to identify bleeding/loss of RBCs* Occult blood in urine/stool *to identify bleeding/loss of RBCs* **THERAPEUTIC INTERVENTIONS** • Assist patient in selecting meals. • Provide high-protein, high-carbohydrate, iron-containing foods *to improve nutrients (to meet energy needs)*. • Encourage good oral hygiene. • Provide small, frequent meals. • Administer vitamin and mineral supplements as ordered. • Administer nutritional supplements as ordered.	
Constipation and/or diarrhea *Related to:* Decreased dietary intake Decreased digestive processes Decreased activity level Drug therapy **DEFINING CHARACTERISTICS** *Constipation:* Frequency less than usual pattern Straining at stool Hard-formed stool Passage of liquid feces around impaction Abdominal distention Nausea/vomiting Fecal incontinence Decreased bowel sounds *Diarrhea:* Increased frequency of stool Loose/liquid stool Urgency Cramping Abdominal pain Hyperactive bowel sounds	**ONGOING ASSESSMENT** • Establish history of elimination. • Determine if medications used for regular elimination. • Observe stool for color, consistency, frequency, amount. **THERAPEUTIC INTERVENTIONS** • Provide adequate food/fluid intake *to decrease risk of constipation or diarrhea*. • Administer medications for diarrhea or constipation as ordered. • See Constipation, p. 12; Diarrhea, p. 16.	Normal bowel function will be maintained.
Potential altered levels of consciousness *Related to:* Decreased blood and O$_2$ supply to vital organs **DEFINING CHARACTERISTICS** Visual changes Dizziness Fainting	**ONGOING ASSESSMENT** • Assess ability to carry out ADL. • Assess potential for injury. • Observe for changes in orientation, neurologic function, vision *to identify development of complications*. **THERAPEUTIC INTERVENTIONS** • Provide patient with assistance in completing ADL. • Teach patient to avoid sudden movements (e.g., sitting up too quickly or getting out of bed rapidly) *to reduce risk of injury*. • Place objects within patient's reach. • If signs of altered LOC noted, see Consciousness, alteration in level of, p. 234	Optimal state of consciousness will be maintained.

Anemia—cont'd

NURSING DIAGNOSES / DEFINING CHARACTERISTICS	NURSING INTERVENTIONS / *RATIONALES*	EXPECTED OUTCOMES
Postural hypotension Change in alertness Memory impairment Impaired judgment		

Knowledge deficit
Related to:
Unfamiliarity with disease process, treatment plan, and complications
 	
Defining Characteristics
Multiple questions by patient/significant others
Lack of questions
Confusion about treatment
Inability to comply with treatment regimen
Development of complications
	Ongoing Assessment
	• Determine patient's/significant others' understanding of disease process, treatment, and complications.
	• Evaluate understanding of information after teaching sessions *to identify areas for further teaching and reinforcement.*
	• Observe compliance with treatment program:
	    Improved activity tolerance
	    Ability to manage ADL more effectively
	    Increased Hct and Hb
	    Selection of well-balance diet
	    Compliance with medication regimen (e.g., vitamin, iron, mineral, and nutritional supplements)
	• Observe for development of complications *to allow early treatment and reduce risk of injury*:
	    Dyspnea
	    Angina, myocardial infarction
	    Skin breakdown
	    Constipation, diarrhea
	    Altered LOC
	
	Therapeutic Interventions
	• Encourage patient/significant others to ask questions.
	• Provide patient/significant others information about disease process, treatment, and complications.
		Patient will demonstrate understanding of and compliance with treatment regimen.

Originated by: Martha Dickerson, RN, MS, CCRN

Cellulitis

(TISSUE TRAUMA)

An infection of the skin at the cellular level. Cellulitis usually results from an initial minor injury (i.e., small cut, insect bite) that does not produce an adequate immune response in the host.

NURSING DIAGNOSES / DEFINING CHARACTERISTICS	NURSING INTERVENTIONS / *RATIONALES*	EXPECTED OUTCOMES

Impaired skin integrity
Related to:
Trauma infection
 	
Defining Characteristics
Affected area hot and tender to touch
Skin purplish red
Swelling around initial injury
	Ongoing Assessment
	• Elicit details of initial injury and treatment.
	• Assess current skin condition:
	    Swelling/size
	    Itching
	    Burning
	    Pain
	    Scaling
	    Oozing
	    Open lesions
	• Refer to Skin integrity, impaired, p. 48.
		Skin damage is reduced.

Continued.

Hematolymphatic and Oncologic Care Plans

NURSING DIAGNOSES / DEFINING CHARACTERISTICS	NURSING INTERVENTIONS / *RATIONALES*	EXPECTED OUTCOMES

	THERAPEUTIC INTERVENTIONS
	· Apply continuous or intermittent wet dressings *to reduce intensity of inflammation.*
	· Protect healthy skin from maceration when wet dressings applied:
	  Remove moisture by blotting gently; avoid friction.
	  Consider use of liquid skin barriers.
	· Advise patient to avoid rubbing and scratching *(can cause further injury and delay healing).* Provide gloves or clip nails if necessary.
	· Provide medicated soaks for open wounds, as ordered.
	· Administer IV antibiotics as ordered.	

Hyperthermia
Related to:
Tissue trauma
Infectious process
 	
DEFINING CHARACTERISTICS
Temperature
  >38.5 °C
	ONGOING ASSESSMENT
	· Monitor temperature q2h:
	  Use same instrument each time.
	  Document change in methods (axillary versus rectal) *so temperature change can be accounted for accurately*
	· Assess for temperature fluctuations/patterns *to evaluate treatment effectiveness.*
	· Monitor lab results.
	· Monitor I & O.
	
	THERAPEUTIC INTERVENTIONS
	· Administer antipyretics and antibiotics as ordered.
	· Encourage fluid intake.
	· See Hyperthermia, p. 31.
		Normal body temperature will be maintained.

Pain
Related to:
Skin trauma
Swelling
 	
DEFINING CHARACTERISTICS
Verbal complaint of
  pain
Grimacing
Crying
Protectiveness toward
  site
	ONGOING ASSESSMENT
	· Assess for type and level of pain.
	· Assess effectiveness of treatments.
	
	THERAPEUTIC INTERVENTIONS
	· Provide warm or cool soaks as desired *to alter pain perception.*
	· Provide pain medications.
	· See Pain, p. 39.
		Discomfort will be relieved.

Potential knowledge deficit *Related to:* New diagnosis Treatment regimen **DEFINING CHARACTERISTICS** Questioning Confusion	**ONGOING ASSESSMENT** · Assess current level of understanding. · Assess ability to learn. **THERAPEUTIC INTERVENTIONS** · Provide information about disease process and treatments. · Explain necessity for antibiotics. · Explain follow-up care and preventive health maintenance measures. *Good general health and appropriate treatment of injury often prevent cellulitis.*	Patient will understand diagnosis, treatment, and preventive measures.

Originated by: Sherry Adams, RN, ADN

Disseminated intravascular coagulation (DIC)

(COAGULOPATHY; DEFIBRINATION SYNDROME)

Inappropriate, accelerated consumption of coagulation factors resulting in hemorrhage. Disseminated intravascular coagulation always occurs secondary to some other pathology and is associated with infection, neoplastic disorders, obstetric complications, tissue trauma, and burns.

NURSING DIAGNOSES / DEFINING CHARACTERISTICS	NURSING INTERVENTIONS / *RATIONALES*	EXPECTED OUTCOMES

Fluid volume deficit
Related to:
Blood loss
Depleted coagulation factors
 	
DEFINING CHARACTERISTICS
Prothrombin time (PT) >15 sec
Partial thromboplastin time (PTT) >60-90 sec
Hypofibrinogenemia
Thrombocytopenia
Elevated fibrin split products
Prolonged bleeding time
Oozing of blood from IV sites, drains, or wounds
Petechiae, purpura, hematomas
Bleeding from mucous membranes
Hematuria, hemoptysis, blood in stools
Cardiovascular changes (hypotension, arrhythmias)
CNS changes (decreased mental status, possible cerebral hemorrhage)
	ONGOING ASSESSMENT
	· Examine skin surface for signs of bleeding. Note:
	  Petechiae, purpura, hematomas
	  Oozing of blood from IV sites, drains, and wounds
	  Bleeding from mucous membranes
	· Observe for signs of bleeding from GI/GU tracts.
	· Note any hemoptysis or blood obtained during suctioning.
	· Observe for changes in mental status; institute neurologic checklist.
	· Monitor vital signs.
	· Monitor coagulation profile.
	· Monitor Hct and Hb.
	· Document amount and character of drainage on dressings; note frequency of dressing changes.
	· Observe for any increase in bleeding after initiating heparin therapy. If bleeding increased, notify physician of possible need to decrease drip.
	
	THERAPEUTIC INTERVENTIONS
	· Protect patient from bleeding:
	  Eliminate pressure by turning patient.
	  If patient confused/agitated, pad side rails *to prevent bruising*.
	  Minimize IM/SC injections; apply pressure to injection site if puncture unavoidable.
	  Prevent stable clots from dislodging; if clot dislodges, apply pressure and cold compress.
	  Apply pressure to any oozing site.
	  Prevent trauma to catheters/tubes by proper taping; minimize pulling.
	  Minimize number of cuff BPs; maintain arterial line.
	  Use gentle suctioning *to prevent trauma to respiratory mucosa*.
	· Administer fluids as ordered.
	· Administer blood products as ordered; monitor patient response. (Observe for transfusion reaction.)
	· Administer heparin therapy as ordered to interrupt abnormal accelerated coagulation. *Heparin interferes with production of thrombin, which is necessary for clot formation.*
	  Infuse continuous heparin drip on infusion device (usually 1000-1500 U/hr).
	  Maintain PTT at 2 times normal.
	  Consider dosage alteration in patients with hepatic or renal failure.
	· See Fluid volume deficit, p. 20.
		Optimal fluid balance will be maintained.

Anxiety *Related to:* Presenting symptoms of DIC and/or staff reaction to disease process **DEFINING CHARACTERISTICS** Restlessness Increased awareness Increased questioning	**ONGOING ASSESSMENT** · Assess anxiety level. · Assess normal coping patterns. **THERAPEUTIC INTERVENTIONS** · Inform significant others of patient's prognosis; prepare them for patient's appearance. *Bleeding site/clots must be left undisturbed, result in sometimes shocking appearance.* · Minimize staff conversations at bedside. · Use calm approach with patient. · See Anxiety, p. 4.	Anxiety will be reduced.

Continued.

NURSING DIAGNOSES / DEFINING CHARACTERISTICS	NURSING INTERVENTIONS / *RATIONALES*	EXPECTED OUTCOMES
Potential for injury *Related to:* Excess heparin Insufficient heparin *Note that heparin aborts clotting process by blocking thrombin production* **DEFINING CHARACTERISTICS** *Excess heparin:* Bleeding from IV sites, drains, wounds Petechiae, purpura, hematomas Bleeding from mucous membranes GI, GU bleeding Bleeding from respiratory tract PTT >2 times normal *Insufficient heparin:* Continued evidence of further clot formation (e.g., newly developed signs of pulmonary emboli or peripheral thromboemboli) Continued evidence of bleeding from DIC (abnormal clotting) PTT < twice normal	**ONGOING ASSESSMENT** · Note adverse effects of heparin therapy: Any increase in bleeding from IV sites, GI/GU tracts, respiratory tract, wounds Development of new purpura, petechiae, or hematomas **THERAPEUTIC INTERVENTIONS** · Maintain constant, uninterrupted infusion of heparin titrated to lab values and clinical situation. *As clinical situation improves, heparin need decreases. Challenge lies in differentiating blood loss as untoward effect of heparin therapy from worsening of DIC.*	Side effects of heparin therapy will be reduced.
Impaired gas exchange *Related to:* Inappropriate coagulation Possible blood loss Decreased Hct and Hb Acidosis Decreased circulation Poor O_2 exchange at cellular level Generalized systemic microvascular clot formation **DEFINING CHARACTERISTICS** Dyspnea Poor capillary refill Acral cyanosis Changes in mental status (confusion) Decreased Po_2 or decreased O_2 saturation Decreased Hb	**ONGOING ASSESSMENT** · Observe for signs of dyspnea, respiratory distress, poor capillary refill, acral cyanosis. · Assess for confusion. · Monitor vital signs. · Monitor ABGs. **THERAPEUTIC INTERVENTIONS** · Maintain airway: Encourage coughing. Use suction as needed. Elevate HOB >45 degrees *for dyspnea.* · Administer O_2 as ordered. · Correct acid-base imbalances. · See Mechanical ventilation, p. 213, if appropriate.	Gas exchange will be adequate.

Disseminated intravascular coagulation—cont'd

NURSING DIAGNOSES / DEFINING CHARACTERISTICS	NURSING INTERVENTIONS / *RATIONALES*	EXPECTED OUTCOMES
Increased P_{CO_2} Blood pH >7.3 Bicarbonate <22 mEq/L Acidic urine pH 4.6-5.02		
Knowledge deficit *Related to:* Lack of familiarity with procedures Unfamiliar environment **DEFINING CHARACTERISTICS** Increased questioning Lack of questions	**ONGOING ASSESSMENT** ▪ Assess knowledge and readiness to learn. **THERAPEUTIC INTERVENTIONS** ▪ Instruct patient to notify nurse of bleeding from wounds, IV sites, etc. ▪ Instruct patient to inform nurse of fatigue or dizziness. ▪ Instruct patient to try to avoid trauma *(may precipitate further bleeding)*. ▪ Explain purpose of drug/transfusion therapy. ▪ Explain rationale for therapy to significant others; encourage them and other visitors to remain calm while visiting.	Patient/significant others verbalize basic understanding of DIC and its management.

Originated by: Gail L. Dykstra, RN
                  Audrey Klopp, RN, PhD, ET

Granulocytopenia: risk for infection

(DISORDER OF NEUTROPHILS)

There are three types of granulocytes: basophils, eosinophils, and neutrophils. Granulocytopenia and its complications actually center around the neutrophilic granulocyte. A substantial decrease in the number of circulating neutrophils may result in overwhelming, potentially life-threatening infection. Neutrophils constitute 60-70 percent of all white blood cells. Their primary function is phagocytosis, the digestion and subsequent destruction of microorganisms, and as such, they form one of the body's most powerful defenses against infection.

NURSING DIAGNOSES / DEFINING CHARACTERISTICS	NURSING INTERVENTIONS / *RATIONALES*	EXPECTED OUTCOMES

Potential for infection
Related to:
Granulocytopenia, secondary to:
  Radiation therapy
  Chemotherapy
  Hypersplenism
  Bone marrow depression/failure
  Autoimmune responses
	ONGOING ASSESSMENT
	▪ Monitor WBC (especially neutrophils/bands).
	▪ Identify source(s) of low WBC.
	▪ Identify sites posing risk of infection (e.g., orifices, wounds, catheter sites).
	▪ Note abnormalities in color/character of sputum/urine/stool.
	▪ Monitor vital signs q4h around the clock.
	▪ Observe closely for fever/chills *(may be initial presentation of infection since in absence of granulocytes locus of infection may develop without characteristic inflammation/pus formation at site)*.
	▪ Assess for local/systemic infection signs/symptoms (e.g., fever, chills, diaphoresis, local redness, heat, pain, excessive malaise, sore throat, dysphagia, or cellulitis). Note that inflammation and exudate may be absent because of decrease or lack of neutrophils.
	▪ Identify medication patient may have taken that would mask infection signs/symptoms (e.g., steroids, antipyretics).
		The risk of infection will be reduced.

Continued.

Hematolymphatic and Oncologic Care Plans

NURSING DIAGNOSES / DEFINING CHARACTERISTICS	NURSING INTERVENTIONS / *RATIONALES*	EXPECTED OUTCOMES
DEFINING CHARACTERISTICS Decrease in circulating granulocytes Total neutrophil level <1000/mm³	• Send cultures as ordered for temperature >38.5 °C. • Identify nosocomial pathogens in patient care area (e.g., respiratory or urine bacteria). **THERAPEUTIC INTERVENTIONS** • Wash hands thoroughly before physical contact with patient *(removes transient and residual bacteria from hands and prevents transmission to patient). Because microorganisms can also be transmitted from one site of infection to other portals of entry, thorough handwashing also important between patient care activities (central line dressing change, mouth care, perineal care, etc.).* • Use sterile technique with dressing changes and catheter care. • Use isolation procedures as ordered or appropriate *to protect patient from exposure to environmental contagions.* • Limit visitors. Discourage anyone with current or recent infection from visiting. • Encourage daily shower and perineal care (with soap and water) after urination and defecation *(perineal area is source of many pathogens, frequent portal of entry for microorganisms).* • Encourage meticulous oral hygiene before and after each meal and at bedtime *(important in prevention of periodontal disease as locus of infection).* • Encourage oral fluids. • Assist patient selection of high-protein, high-vitamin, high-calorie diet (refer to dietitian as needed). • Avoid unnecessary invasive procedures. • Notify physician immediately of temperature >38.5 °C, chills, hypotension, other signs/symptoms of acute systemic infection. • Initiate measures for fever control (e.g., cool sponge bath, blanket, light covers). • Initiate anibiotic therapy promptly as ordered *to prevent early dissemination of suspected infection.* • Administer medications as ordered to prevent mucosal damage (stool softeners) and allay signs/symptoms of infections (antipyretics).	

Knowledge deficit
Related to:
Unfamiliarity with nature, treatment of condition
 	
DEFINING CHARACTERISTICS
Multiple questions
Lack of questions
Misconceptions
Request for information
	ONGOING ASSESSMENT
	• Assess patient's/significant others' readiness for teaching.
	• Assess knowledge base about infection (recognition of, plan of care for, evaluation of care).
	
	THERAPEUTIC INTERVENTIONS
	• Explain to patient/significant others that low WBC and neurophil counts produce high susceptibility to infection.
	• Explain factors that contributed to low WBC (e.g., chemotherapy, drug sensitivity, etc.).
	• Explain signs/symptoms of infection to patient/significant others; instruct them to contact appropriate health team member immediately if any occurs or is suspected.
	• Explain plan of care to patient/significant others (e.g., need for private room, isolation, etc.) *to decrease fear/anxiety about therapeutic regime.*
	• Instruct patient/significant others about:
	    Use of prescribed medications (indications, dosages, side effects)
	    Avoidance of activities that may result in bodily injury. Suggest alternatives where appropriate (e.g., oral/axillary temperatures instead of rectal, electric razor instead of razor blades, sanitary napkins instead of tampons, tooth sponge instead of toothbrush).
	    Avoidance of crowds and persons with current or recent infection
	    Avoidance of shared drinking and eating utensils
	    Avoidance of animal excreta
	• Instruct patient to make routine dental visits.
		Patient/significant others will demonstrate understanding of medical diagnosis, treatment plan, safety measures, and follow-up care.

Originated by: Vanessa Randle, RN

Hemophilia

(CHRISTMAS DISEASE; COAGULATION
DISORDERS; BLEEDING DISORDER)

An inherited disorder of the clotting mechanism caused by diminished or absent factors necessary to the formation of prothrombin activator (the catalyst to clot formation). Classic hemophilia (type A) is caused by lack of factor VIII; it is the most common and usually most severe type of hemophilia. Type B (Christmas disease) and type C hemophilia are caused by the lack of factors IX and XI, respectively. Symptom severity is directly proportional to plasma levels of available clotting factors; depending on these levels, the disease is classified as mild, moderate, or severe. Patients with close to normal factor levels may only experience frequent bruising and slightly prolonged bleeding times. This care plan addresses the more severe symptoms of hemophilia.

NURSING DIAGNOSES / DEFINING CHARACTERISTICS	NURSING INTERVENTIONS / *RATIONALES*	EXPECTED OUTCOMES

Potential for injury: hemorrhage
Related to:
Decreased concentration of clotting factors circulating in blood: identified as factor VIII, factor IX, or factor XI
 	
DEFINING CHARACTERISTICS
Frequent bruising
Prolonged bleeding
Petechiae
Joint pain, swelling
GI bleed
Hematuria
	ONGOING ASSESSMENT
	• Assess for history of bruising/bleeding.
	• Assess for type and severity of disease.
	• Perform physical assessment to determine bruising and bleeding sites.
	• Assess for pain and swelling *(may indicate internal bleeding)*.
	• Monitor vital signs, Hb, and Hct.
	• Observe for reaction to blood product transfusion.
	
	THERAPEUTIC INTERVENTIONS
	• Provide safe environment:
	    Minimize trauma from temperature and BP measurements. Perform care gently.
	    Provide medications in oral form if possible; otherwise rotate injection/IV sites; apply pressure as needed.
	• Apply sterile dressings to wounds. *Counting soaked dressings may help determine blood loss.* Apply pressure to bleeding site.
	• Anticipate need for blood replacement. *Excessive blood loss may indicate need for IV fluid replacement and whole or packed cell blood transfusion-Note: Maintain universal precautions: hemophiliacs who have received factor or other blood products are at high risk for development of AIDS.*
	• If bleeding in joint (hemarthrosis), elevate and immobilize affected limb. Apply ice packs.
	• Control hemorrhage by administering cryoprecipitate or concentrated factor.
	• Document blood product transfusion per hospital policy. See Blood and blood product transfusion, p. 538.
		Risk of injury caused by hemorrhage will be reduced.

Pain
Related to:
Hemarthrosis
Open wound
Nerve compression caused by bleeding and swelling
 	
DEFINING CHARACTERISTICS
Verbalized pain
Crying
Irritability
	ONGOING ASSESSMENT
	• Assess pain and monitor for changes:
	    Headache *may indicate intracranial bleed.*
	    Joint pain *may indicate hemarthrosis.*
	    Abdominal pain *may indicate trauma and bleeding of major organ.*
	• Assess for permanent damage to limb.
	    Paresthesia
	    Joint changes, contractures
	
	THERAPEUTIC INTERVENTIONS
	• Provide analgesia or sedation if needed *(may not be allowed if head trauma suspected)*.
	• Immobilize affected limbs/joints.
	• Apply ice packs to painful joints.
	• Provide care gently, carefully.
		Pain will be relieved.

Continued.

507

NURSING DIAGNOSES / DEFINING CHARACTERISTICS	NURSING INTERVENTIONS / *RATIONALES*	EXPECTED OUTCOMES
Potential ineffective airway clearance *Related to:* Bleeding in or around airway, neck, nose, pharynx, esophagus Blood seen/not seen, depending on site Obstruction caused by tissue swelling **DEFINING CHARACTERISTICS** Dyspnea Abnormal breath sounds Verbalized difficultty in breathing	**ONGOING ASSESSMENT** · Assess for known trauma sites. · Observe for bleeding in or around airway. · Monitor vital signs, especially respiratory rate and breath sounds. **THERAPEUTIC INTERVENTIONS** · If neck or pharyngeal injury suspected: Keep an oral airway and suction nearby. Keep tracheostomy setup available. Prepare for intubation. Administer required clotting factors *to stop bleeding in or around airway.*	Risk of ineffective airway clearance is reduced.
Potential altered level of consciousness *Related to:* Intracranial bleed **DEFINING CHARACTERISTICS** Headache Nausea, vomiting Inappropriate affect Impaired judgment or thought processes Impaired memory Dizziness Pupil changes Lethargy Coma	**ONGOING ASSESSMENT** · Assess for known trauma sites. *Patient may not remember head trauma; bruising may be hidden by hair.* · Perform neurologic assessment, maintain neurologic flow sheet for serial documentation and reference. **THERAPEUTIC INTERVENTIONS** · Notify physician immediately of signs of neurologic compromise (see Defining Characteristics). · Administer clotting factors as ordered. · Prepare for surgical intervention. *Intracranial bleeding is life-threatening complication.*	Risk of neurologic injury will be reduced.
Potential impaired physical mobility *Related to:* Hemarthrosis Joint degeneration **DEFINING CHARACTERISTICS** Joint pain, swelling, discoloration Limited ROM	**ONGOING ASSESSMENT** · Assess current limitations. *Actively bleeding patients should have restricted mobility.* · When bleeding controlled, assess for limited ROM, contractures, and bony changes in the joints. *Repeated joint bleeds cause bone destruction, permanent deformities, and crippling.* **THERAPEUTIC INTERVENTIONS** · Provide gentle, passive ROM exercise when stable. · Encourage progression to active exercise as tolerated. · Provide assistive devices when needed. · Refer for PT/OT and orthopedic consultation as required. · Instruct patient on preventive measures (e.g., administration of factor products and application of protective gear). *Prevention of injury and hemarthrosis best method of maintaining joint/limb mobility and use.*	Risk of impaired physical mobility will be reduced.
Body image disturbance *Related to:* Limited activity Deformities	**ONGOING ASSESSMENT** · Assess current perceptions of self-concept and body image. *Self-perceptions differ, depending on age and severity of illness.* · Assess attitude toward assistive/protective devices, limitations, and required medications.	Self-concept/body image disturbance will be reduced.

NURSING DIAGNOSES / DEFINING CHARACTERISTICS	NURSING INTERVENTIONS / *RATIONALES*	EXPECTED OUTCOMES
Scarring Presence of ambulatory aids or protective devices Medication administration Hospitalization Bruising Bleeding **DEFINING CHARACTERISTICS** Withdrawn or flat affect Self-deprecating remarks	**THERAPEUTIC INTERVENTIONS** • Allow verbalization of feelings. • Correct misconceptions. • Provide alternatives to current protective devices (*may require creativity of nurse and patient*). • Encourage participation in safe activities (i.e., *swimming may be acceptable, as opposed to football or wrestling*). • Provide positive feedback.	
Ineffective individual coping: parent/ mother *Related to:* Hereditary cause of illness **DEFINING CHARACTERISTICS** Tearfulness Anxiousness Withdrawal Demandingness Overcautiousness Agitation	**ONGOING ASSESSMENT** • Assess patient's mother for signs of ineffective coping. *Hemophilia is genetic disorder transmitted by female carrier to children, primarily males. Associated guilt feelings may interfere with usual coping behaviors.* • Assess available family structure and support systems. **THERAPEUTIC INTERVENTIONS** • Acknowledge mother's feelings and their normalcy. • Correct psychological or social work referrals if needed. • Provide psychological or social work referrals if needed. • Initiate contact with other hemophiliac families. Contact National Hemophilia Foundation for information about parent groups.	Effective coping behaviors will be observed.
Anxiety *Related to:* Potential trauma Death AIDS **DEFINING CHARACTERISTICS** Agitation Tearfulness Unexplained fears Verbalized fear of death, hemorrhage, AIDS	**ONGOING ASSESSMENT** • Assess level of anxiety. • Identify fears if possible; assess odds of occurrence. • Assess available supportive relationships. **THERAPEUTIC INTERVENTIONS** • Allow expression of fears, anger, and other feelings. • Discuss actual fears, likelihood of occurrence, and preventive measures if available. • Provide psychiatric referral if necessary. *Hemophiliac may need help controlling fears and anxiety. Fear of AIDS especially destructive; assistance may be needed to prevent fear from controlling life.*	Anxiety/fears will be reduced.

Knowledge deficit
Related to:
New diagnosis
Emergency situation
Surgical/dental needs
 	
DEFINING CHARACTERISTICS
Questioning
Verbalized lack of understanding
	ONGOING ASSESSMENT
	• Assess current knowledge and physical abilities.
	• Assess cognitive abilities and readiness to learn.
	
	THERAPEUTIC INTERVENTIONS
	• Provide information about disease type, treatment, and progression.
	• Explain genetic transference to those of childbearing age. Refer for genetic counseling if needed.
	• Discuss safety and prevention:
	    Safe physical activities
	    Avoidance of aspirin products
	    Emergency care
		Patient/parent will understand hemophilia, its treatment, and home care.

Continued.

509

■ **Hemophilia—cont'd**

NURSING DIAGNOSES/ DEFINING CHARACTERISTICS	NURSING INTERVENTIONS/*RATIONALES*	EXPECTED OUTCOMES
	· Provide instruction on self-administration of IV factors, if applicable. · Discuss prophylactic treatment with factors or cryoprecipitate *to prevent bleeding during dental or surgical procedures*. · Provide follow-up appointments and emergency numbers.	

Originated by: Michele Knoll Puzas, RN,C, MHPE

Leukemia, acute

Abnormal proliferation of immature leukocytes, or blasts.

(ACUTE LYMPHOCYTIC LEUKEMIA [ALL])

NURSING DIAGNOSES / DEFINING CHARACTERISTICS	NURSING INTERVENTIONS / *RATIONALES*	EXPECTED OUTCOMES

Potential ineffective coping
Related to:
Situational crisis
Inadequate support system
Inadequate coping methods
 	
DEFINING CHARACTERISTICS
Verbalization of fear, anxiety, and feelings of hopelessness/ meaninglessness
Questions about illness, procedures, and therapy
Noncompliance with diet, medications, precautionary measures
	ONGOING ASSESSMENT
	· Assess patient's concept and knowledge of disease.
	· Assess for:
	  Events/illnesses preceding hospitalization
	  Awareness and comprehension of illness, importance of procedures, importance of hospitalization
	  Coping mechanisms used in previous illnesses and hospitalization experiences
	  Level of understanding, modes of communication, and readiness to learn
	  Dynamics of relationship with significant others
	· Assess patient's readiness and need for information.
	
	THERAPEUTIC INTERVENTIONS
	· Establish open lines of communication:
	  Initiate brief visits to patient.
	  Define your role as patient informant and advocate.
	  Understand grieving process, respect patient's feelings as they ensue.
	    Request break when you have approached your emotional limit.
	    Introduce patient to unit's physical environment and staff.
	· Meet with medical team to discuss plan of care *(facilitates/maintains consistency)*.
	· Assist patient/significant others in redefining hopes, components of individuality (e.g., roles, values, and attitudes).
	· Provide reading materials and resource persons as needed.
	· Introduce new information about disease treatment:
	  Use simple terms.
	  Add to current knowledge.
	  Reinforce instructions/repeat information as necessary.
	· Use calm approach with patient/significant others.
	· See Grief over long-term illness/disability, p. 618.
		Coping mechanisms will be maximized.

510

NURSING DIAGNOSES / DEFINING CHARACTERISTICS	NURSING INTERVENTIONS / *RATIONALES*	EXPECTED OUTCOMES

Potential for infection
Related to:
Altered immunologic responses related to disease process
Immunosuppression secondary to chemotherapy
 	
DEFINING CHARACTERISTICS
Rales
Cyanosis
Decreased breath sounds
Rhonchi
Cough
Tachypnea
Changes in color or character of sputum, urine, stool; urinary frequency, burning; vaginal discharge
Redness/tenderness in perineal/rectal area
Redness/tenderness over peripheral (IV) or central catheter site(s)
Fever
Shaking chills
Decreased BP
Increased pulse
	ONGOING ASSESSMENT
	• Auscultate lung fields every day or as necessary.
	• Observe patient for coughing spells, sputum nature, character.
	• Observe for changes in color, character, frequency of urine and stool.
	• Inspect body sites with high infection potential (mouth, throat, axilla, perineum, rectum) daily.
	• Inspect IV/central catheter sites daily.
	• Monitor vital signs q4h or as needed.
	
	THERAPEUTIC INTERVENTIONS
	• Report findings to physician; initiate treatment as follows.
	• Place patient in protective isolation if lab results indicate neutropenia:
	  Inform patient/significant others.
	  Screen visitors to minimize room traffic.
	  Implement thorough staff/visitors handwashing before physical contact with patient *to remove transient and resident bacteria from hands, thus minimizing/preventing transmission to patient.*
	  Administer antibiotic/antifungal/antiviral drugs as ordered on time *to maintain therapeutic drug level(s).*
	• Initiate meticulous oral hygiene. Instruct patient:
	  To brush teeth with soft toothbrush qid and as necessary
	  To remove dentures at night.
	  To rinse mouth after each emesis or when expectorating phlegm
	  Refer to Stomatitits, p. 521.
	• Instruct patient to maintain personal hygiene:
	  To wash hands well before eating and after using bathroom
	  To wipe perineal area from front to back
	  Bathe with chlorhexidine (Hibiclens) before initially entering room and every day thereafter.
	• Observe aseptic technique for all invasive procedures.
	• Minimize risk of infection from central lines and arteriovenous punctures:
	  Observe patient closely for evidence of infection (*in absence of granulocytes, site of infection may develop without characteristic pus formation*).
	  Obtain cultures as ordered; send to lab for antibiotic sensitivity determination and fungi.
	• Observe strict aseptic technique when changing dressings.
	• Avoid wetting central catheter dressings.
	• Apply lotion to intact skin every morning and as needed.
	• Explain definition, etiology, and effects of leukopenia:
	  Normal range of blood count
	  Function of leukocytes and neutrophils
	• Instruct patient to observe for fever spikes, flulike symptoms (malaise, weakness, and myalgia); notify nurse/physician if they occur.
	• Instruct patient to avoid crowds or contact with contagious persons.
	• Teach patient to take oral and axillary temperature.
	• Encourage patient to observe good handwashing technique.
	• Teach patient to monitor blood counts and report those not within normal limits.
	• Refer patient to dietitian for instructions on maintenance of well-balanced diet.
	• Explain to patient importance of regular medical and dental checkups.
	• Teach patient to inspect oropharyngeal area daily for:
	  White patches in mouth
	  Coated/encrusted oral ulcerations
	  Swollen and erythematous tongue with white/brown coating
	  Infected throat and pain on swallowing
	  Texture, color, and character of oropharynx
	  Debris on teeth
	  Ill-fitting dentures
		Risk of local/systemic infection will be reduced.

Continued.

NURSING DIAGNOSES / DEFINING CHARACTERISTICS	NURSING INTERVENTIONS / *RATIONALES*	EXPECTED OUTCOMES

	Amount and viscosity of saliva
	Changes in vocal tone
	• Teach patient to:
	    Avoid mouthwashes that contain alcohol *(drying effect on mucous membranes)*
	    Avoid irritating foods/acidic drinks
	• Teach patient to use prescribed topical medications (e.g., nystatin [Nilstat] and lidocaine [Xylocaine]).
	• See Stomatitis, p. 521.	

Potential for injury: bleeding
Related to:
Bone marrow depression secondary to chemotherapy
Proliferation of leukemic cells
 	
DEFINING CHARACTERISTICS
 	
Decrease in total circulating platelet <50,000/mm^3
Petechiae and bruising, especially venipuncture sites
Headaches and changes in mental and visual acuity
Hemoptysis
Hematemesis
Hematochezia
Melena
Vaginal bleeding
Dizziness
Orthostatic changes
Decreased BP
Increased pulse rate
	ONGOING ASSESSMENT
	• Monitor platelet count daily.
	• Observe for changes in neurologic status q4h.
	• Monitor vital signs q4h and as needed.
	• Note change in color of emesis, urine, and stool.
	• Note bleeding at puncture sites (e.g., venipuncture, bone marrow aspiration site).
	
	THERAPEUTIC INTERVENTIONS
	• Institute bleeding precautions for platelet count <50,000/mm^3:
	    Avoid use of toothpicks and dental floss *to prevent gum trauma.*
	    Avoid rectal suppositories, thermometers, enemas, constipation, vaginal douches, and tampons.
	    Avoid IM/SC injections. If necessary, use small-bore needles for injections; apply pressure to site for 10 min. Observe for oozing from site.
	    Avoid straight-edged razors.
	    Avoid aspirin, alcohol, anticoagulants, or products containing them.
	    Avoid coarse foods/snacks.
	    Administer antacids as ordered for patients taking steroids.
	    Avoid straining with stool, forceful nose blowing, coughing *(increase risk for bleeding).*
	    Inspect gums for oozing.
	    Count used sanitary pads during menstruation.
	    Place sign over patient's bed as reminder to apply pressure after venipunctures.
	    Use fingerstick if possible. Coordinate lab work so all tests done at one time.
	    Apply pressure/dressing/sandbag to bone marrow aspiration site.
	    Inflate BP cuff as little as possible to get accurate reading.
	    Check urine, emesis, and stool for blood.
	• Maintain safe environment for patient, especially during episodes of chills, fever, confusion, and weakness. Assist patient during ambulation and shower/tub bath.
	• Encourage rest to decrease pulse rate, *thus assisting clot formation.*
	• Apply ice or topical thrombin promptly as ordered for bleeding mucous membranes.
	• Ensure availability and readiness of blood products.
	• Assess vital signs during and after blood transfusion(s).
	• Explain to patient/significant others definition, etiology, and symptoms of thrombocytopenia and functions of platelets:
	    Normal range of platelet count
	    Effects of thrombocytopenia
	    Rationale of bleeding precautions
	• Instruct patient to:
	    Use electric razor *to prevent accidental break in skin.*
	    Avoid sharp objects such as scissors.
	    Use emery boards.
	    Avoid wearing tight/constrictive clothing.
	    Lubricate nostrils with saline drops as necessary.
		Potential for bleeding related to low platelet count will be reduced.

NURSING DIAGNOSES / DEFINING CHARACTERISTICS	NURSING INTERVENTIONS/ *RATIONALES*	EXPECTED OUTCOMES
	Protect self from injury/trauma (e.g., falls, bumps, strenuous exercises). Report menstrual cycle changes to physician. ▪ Advise patient to be gentle during intercourse, use lubrication, and avoid trauma.	
Potential fluid volume deficit *Related to:* Side effects of chemotherapy **DEFINING CHARACTERISTICS** Parched tongue Poor skin turgor Weight loss with output exceeding intake Thirst Weakness Lethargy Change in pulse Change in BP Increased serum BUN and creatinine levels	**ONGOING ASSESSMENT** ▪ Assess for presence of Defining Characteristics. **THERAPEUTIC INTERVENTIONS** ▪ Refer to Fluid volume deficit, p. 20; Cancer chemotherapy, p. 543.	Optimal fluid status will be maintained.
Altered nutrition: less than body requirements *Related to:* Disease process Side effects of chemotherapy (e.g., nausea, vomiting, stomatitis) **DEFINING CHARACTERISTICS** Parched tongue Poor skin turgor Weight loss with output exceeding intake Thirst Weakness Lethargy Change in pulse Change in BP Increased serum BUN and creatinine levels	**ONGOING ASSESSMENT** ▪ Assess for presence of Defining Characteristics. **THERAPEUTIC INTERVENTIONS** ▪ See Nutrition, altered: less than body requirements, p. 37.	Present weight will be maintained or patient will not lose more than 10% of original body weight.
Impaired physical mobility *Related to:* Fluid volume deficit secondary to chemotherapy side effects Pain and discomfort Depression/severe anxiety	**ONGOING ASSESSMENT** ▪ Assess for presence of Defining Characteristics. **THERAPEUTIC INTERVENTIONS** ▪ See Mobility, impaired physical, p. 35.	Optimal state of mobility will be maintained.

Continued.

NURSING DIAGNOSES / DEFINING CHARACTERISTICS	NURSING INTERVENTIONS/ *RATIONALES*	EXPECTED OUTCOMES
DEFINING CHARACTERISTICS Weakness Lethargy Decreased attempt to move Physical restrictions on movements (e.g., protective isolation) Need for help during meals/ambulation Verbalized inability to move freely without fear of falling Remaining in bed most of time		

Potential social isolation
Related to:
Protective isolation
Impaired mobility secondary to disease entity
 	
DEFINING CHARACTERISTICS
Verbalization of isolation ("I want to get out of here")
Reduced social acceptance and interactions
Unrealistic self-expectations
Outbursts
Withdrawal
Impaired ability to ambulate
	ONGOING ASSESSMENT
	• Recognize early verbal/nonverbal communication cues reflecting need to socialize.
	• Monitor blood counts to determine duration of isolation.
	• Observe patient closely for behavioral changes.
	• Assess anxiety level.
	
	THERAPEUTIC INTERVENTIONS
	• Allow patient to exert some control over environment:
	    Remove unnecessary equipment *to provide space.*
	    Open blinds during daytime.
	    Dim lights at night.
	    Ask significant others to bring in familiar objects (e.g., pictures and pillows).
	    Muffle noises.
	• Visit and talk with patient frequently *to minimize social isolation.*
	• Avoid using intercom when responding to patient's call.
	• Provide normal aids for interaction (e.g., eyeglasses, hearing aids, writing materials).
	• Encourage participation of significant others through visits and telephone calls.
	• Provide diversional therapy/activities (e.g., radio, television, magazines, occupational therapy).
	• Assist patient in grooming when entertaining visitors:
	    Encourage use of makeup.
	    Encourage use of wig during daytime.
	• Encourage patient to ambulate during course of protective isolation as permitted by physician and physical limitations.
	• Leave patient's door open.
	• Acknowledge patient's efforts in maintaining sense of well-being.
		Optimal state of socialization will be maintained.

Originated by: Marlene T. de la Cruz, RN, BSN
Christa M. Schroeder, RN, MSN

Multiple myeloma

(PLASMACYTOMA; MYELOMATOSIS; PLASMA CELL MYELOMA)

Seen in the elderly, this terminal disease is characterized by infiltration of bone and marrow by malignant plasma cells. This infiltration causes demineralization, fractures, and pain. Late stages of the disease involve kidney, liver, spleen, and lymph node infiltration. Occasionally this disease converts to acute leukemia. Etiology is unknown.

NURSING DIAGNOSES / DEFINING CHARACTERISTICS	NURSING INTERVENTIONS / *RATIONALES*	EXPECTED OUTCOMES

Pain
Related to:
Invasion of marrow and bone by plasma cells
Pathological fractures
 	
DEFINING CHARACTERISTICS
Constant, severe bone pain on movement
Low back pain
Abdominal pain
Swelling, tenderness
Guarding behavior
Decreased physical activity
Moaning, crying
Pacing, restlessness, irritability, altered sleep pattern
	ONGOING ASSESSMENT
	• Assess pain characteristics:
	  Quality (sharp, dull, aching, shooting, stabbing, or burning)
	  Severity of pain (scale of 1 to 10, 10 most severe)
	  Location
	  Precipitating factors
	  Duration of pain (intermittent or continuous)
	• Assess effectiveness of relief measures and adjust dosage, drug, or route as needed. *Accurate assessment essential to define cause and determine interventions that will not cause further suffering. Early in disease, pain most often bone-originated: ribs, vertebrae, hips. In late stages abdominal pain may be present caused by spleen, liver and kidney involvement.*
	
	THERAPEUTIC INTERVENTIONS
	• Anticipate need for pain medication.
	• Provide analgesics in dosage, route, and frequency best suited to individual patient.
	• Consider around-the-clock injections, continuous infusion, or PCA *to control pain.*
	• Consider combination analgesics *to arrest pain cycle at varied levels.*
	• Notify physician if pain medications ineffective *so other methods may be implemented; braces and splints may be used for support and/or radiation therapy may be required to decrease size of lesions causing pain.*
	• Use additional measures for comfort.
	  Decreased noise and activity
	  Relaxation techniques
	  Good body alignment
	  Clean, comfortable bed
	  Additional rest and sleep periods
	  Ambulation unless contraindicated (i.e., spinal lesions)
		Pain will be reduced.

Impaired physical mobility *Related to:* Bone weakness Pain Generalized weakness caused by chemotherapy **DEFINING CHARACTERISTICS** Inability to move purposefully within physical environment Decrease in ADL Reluctance to attempt movement Limited ROM Decreased muscle strength or control Restricted movement and impaired coordination	**ONGOING ASSESSMENT** • Assess ability to carry out ADL. • Assess ROM and muscle strength. **THERAPEUTIC INTERVENTIONS** • Assist patient with ADL. • Provide supportive aids (e.g., walker, cane, back brace) as needed. • Encourage ambulation *to prevent further bony demineralization.* • Prevent contractions of upper and lower extremities by passive ROM. • Allow rest periods after ambulation. • Maintain uncluttered environment *to prevent unnecessary trauma to extremities.*	Optimal state of mobility will be maintained.

Continued.

NURSING DIAGNOSES / DEFINING CHARACTERISTICS	NURSING INTERVENTIONS / *RATIONALES*	EXPECTED OUTCOMES
Potential for injury: anemia *Related to:* Bone marrow depression or failure Replacement or invasion of bone marrow by neoplastic plasma cells Abnormal hepatic or renal function Bleeding **DEFINING CHARACTERISTICS** Petechiae Purpura Hematomas Unexplained bruises or areas of ecchymoses Bleeding from any body orifice Prolonged oozing of blood from IM, IV, venipuncture, or bone marrow sites	**ONGOING ASSESSMENT** · Monitor vital signs. · Monitor lab values: Hb, Hct, platelet count. · Identify factors that lower platelet count or predispose patient to bleeding. · Check current chemotherapy regimens for potential myelosuppression. · Identify drugs interfering with platelet function. · Observe and report signs/symptoms of spontaneous or excessive bleeding. **THERAPEUTIC INTERVENTIONS** · Avoid unnecessary trauma: Draw all blood for lab work with one daily venipuncture (fingerstick when possible). Avoid IM injection; if necessary, use smallest needle possible. Apply direct pressure for 3-5 min after IM injection, venipuncture, and bone marrow aspiration. Avoid rectal temperatures and enemas. *Axillary route may be least harmful.* Prevent constipation by increased oral fluid intake/stool softeners as ordered per physician. *Straining causes breakage of small blood vessels around anus.* Use soft toothbrushes. Use electric razor, not blades. · Avoid aspirin, aspirin compounds, and other drugs interfering with hemostatic platelet function. · Place sign near patient, informing other health team members of bleeding precautions. · Transfuse platelet/packed red cells as ordered. · Administer chemotherapy and hormones (steroids/androgens) *to stimulate red cell production.*	Risk of injury will be reduced.
Potential for infection *Related to:* Decrease in synthesis of immunoglobulin by plasma cells secondary to: Bone marrow depression/failure Decrease in normal circulating antibodies Decreased autoimmune response Chemotherapy **DEFINING CHARACTERISTICS** Temperature >37.7 °C (100 °F)) Chills Fever Localized swelling Soreness Redness Pain	**ONGOING ASSESSMENT** · Check body for general skin appearance: Open wounds Skin breakdown Swelling Redness · Monitor temperature q4h. · Monitor urine output, color, and odor; pain or burning on urination. · Watch for signs/symptoms of bronchopneumonia, coughing (productive and nonproductive), and color and odor of sputum. · Obtain urine, sputum, and blood for culture and sensitivity if temperature >37.7 °C. · Check medications. *Patient taking steroids may not have overt infection symptoms.* **THERAPEUTIC INTERVENTIONS** · Use good handwashing technique before and after each patient contact. · Use sterile technique for dressing change and catheter care. · Maintain reverse isolation as ordered. · Discourage visitors with current or recent infection (e.g., family member who has upper respiratory infection but must visit, wears mask and limits stay to 10 min). · Avoid unnecessary invasive procedures. · Maintain normal or near-normal body temperature: Medications as ordered per physician Tepid bath Cooling blanket · Notify physician of untoward signs *so appropriate treatment can be initiated.* · See Cancer chemotherapy, p. 543.	Risk of infection will be decreased.

Multiple myeloma—cont'd

NURSING DIAGNOSES / DEFINING CHARACTERISTICS	NURSING INTERVENTIONS / *RATIONALES*	EXPECTED OUTCOMES
Potential altered urinary elimination *Related to:* Immunoglobulin precipitates Hypercalcemia/ hypercalcuria Hyperuricemia Pyelonephritis Myeloma kidney Renal vein thrombosis Spinal cord compression **DEFINING CHARACTERISTICS** Decreased urine output Increased BUN, creatinine, Ca, and uric acid levels Repeated urinary tract infection (UTI) Hypertension Increase in weight Pedal edema Puffy eyes Oliguria Anuria	**ONGOING ASSESSMENT** - Monitor serum laboratory values (BUN, creatinine, Ca, K^+, and uric acid). - Monitor I & O. - Monitor urine for specific gravity, color, odor, and blood. - Observe for dyspnea, tachycardia, pneumonia, pulmonary edema, distended neck veins, peripheral edema; monitor weight daily *to evaluate for fluid retention.* - Assess for bladder distention *(may indicate spinal cord compression).* **THERAPEUTIC INTERVENTIONS** - If hypercalcemia present, push fluids 2500-3000 ml/day as ordered. - Provide IV fluids if necessary *to prevent dehydration, which may precede acute renal failure.* - Notify physician of decrease in urine output or increase in K^+, BUN, or creatinine. - Provide renal diet if ordered; restrict sodium and protein. - Administer medications; *prednisone may be used for hypercalcemia, allopurinol for hyperuricemia.* - Place indwelling catheter *to determine I & O and decrease bladder distention. Patient with spinal compression will require further intervention (e.g., laminectomy or radiation therapy).* - Prepare for dialysis if renal failure impending. - See Renal failure, acute, p. 343; Hypercalcemia, p. 388.	Optimal renal function will be maintained.
Potential altered nutrition: less than body requirements *Related to:* Chemotherapy side effects Limited menu Pain Immobility Lethargy **DEFINING CHARACTERISTICS** Nausea Vomiting Anorexia Diarrhea Weight loss	**ONGOING ASSESSMENT** - Monitor food intake; obtain diet list. - Assess food preferences. - Assess for signs of nausea, vomiting, anorexia, diarrhea, weight loss. - Check food for protein, carbohydrate, and fat content. Consult dietitian as appropriate. **THERAPEUTIC INTERVENTIONS** - Increase diet when patient able to tolerate. - Obtain food patient likes; supplement (e.g., Ensure shakes). - Provide antiemetic as needed. - Encourage family/friends to dine with patient; *mealtime social occasion; appetite may improve.* - Provide hyperalimentation if necessary. See Total parenteral nutrition, p. 324.	Patient's nutritional status will be improved.

Acute grieving *Related to:* Terminal illness **DEFINING CHARACTERISTICS** Fear Denial Regression Depression Anger	**ONGOING ASSESSMENT**
	- Assess awareness of disease.
	- Monitor mental state:
	  Withdrawal
	  Anger
	  Crying
	  Disbelief
	
	THERAPEUTIC INTERVENTIONS
	- Work with patient during grieving stage.
	  Give time to adjust to diagnosis.
		Grieving will be initiated.

Continued.

NURSING DIAGONOSES/ DEFINING CHARACTERISTICS	NURSING INTERVENTIONS/*RATIONALES*	EXPECTED OUTCOMES
Shame Guilt Grief "Why me?" attitude	Have patient express feelings. Listen to complaints. Channel some of patient's anger. *Each person will deal with grief in a personal, individual manner.* · Include family/significant other if desired. · Answer questions as honestly as possible. · Provide consultants (social work, psychologist, clergy) as needed. Contact local chapter of multiple myeloma support groups (if available in area). · Refer to Grieving, anticipatory, p. 22.	

Knowledge deficit
Related to:
New diagnosis
Unfamiliarity with disease process and treatment
 	
DEFINING CHARACTERISTICS
Questions
Lack of questions
Confusion over disease and outcome
	ONGOING ASSESSMENT
	· Assess physical and mental status for ability to learn and perform self-care.
	· Assess patient's/significant others' knowledge of:
	    Pain and medications
	    Possible infection
	    Bleeding disorders
	    Mobility
	    Dietary and fluid restriction
	
	THERAPEUTIC INTERVENTIONS
	· Provide instruction on pain control, infection signs and prevention, diet and fluid therapy, bleeding tendencies, and need for continued mobility.
	· Explain all medications, tests, and procedures.
	· Obtain literature for patient:
	    Contact U.S. Department of Health and Human Services for information on multiple myeloma.
	    Contact American Cancer Society.
		Patient/significant others will be aware of various components of disease entity and treatments.

Originated by: Geraldine Rowden, RN
             Michele Knoll Puzas, RN, C, MHPE

Sickle cell pain crisis

(VASO-OCCLUSIVE CRISIS; SICKLE CELL ANEMIA)

Severe pain, usually in the extremities, caused by the occlusion of small blood vessels by the sickle shaped red cells seen in sickle cell anemia. Abdominal pain, back pain, and central nervous system changes indicate occlusion, ischemia, and possibly infarction in the spleen, liver, and brain. This chronic disease causes impaired kidney, liver, and spleen functions; strokes; blindness; increased susceptibility to infection; and ultimately decreased life span.

NURSING DIAGNOSES / DEFINING CHARACTERISTICS	NURSING INTERVENTIONS / *RATIONALES*	EXPECTED OUTCOMES

Pain
Related to:
Vaso-occlusive crisis
Hypoxia, which causes cells to become rigid and elongated, forming crescent shape
Stasis of RBCs
	ONGOING ASSESSMENT
	· Assess pain q2-4h:
	    Precipitation
	    Quality
	    Radiation
	    Severity
	    Timing
	· Check lab values (e.g., Hb electrophoresis for amount of sickling and RBC count). *Severe decrease in functioning RBCs may indicate need for transfusion.*
		Pain will be reduced or relieved.

Sickle cell pain crisis—cont'd

NURSING DIAGNOSES / DEFINING CHARACTERISTICS	NURSING INTERVENTIONS / *RATIONALES*	EXPECTED OUTCOMES

DEFINING CHARACTERISTICS
Complaint of generalized or localized pain
Tenderness on palpation
Inability to move affected joint
Swelling of area
Deformity of joint
Warmth, discoloration
	THERAPEUTIC INTERVENTIONS
	• Administer medications according to sickle cell pain protocol:
	  Administer IM injections (meperidine [Demerol] or MSO_4) q3h for first 48 hr.
	  Use anti-inflammatory agent simultaneously with IM injections q3h aspirin [Ascriptin] 2 tablets).
	  Start oral analgesic 48 hr after admission (Tylenol No. 3, Empirin, Percodan, Darvocet-N, or Darvon).
	• Apply warm compresses to swollen and painful areas.
	• Position to promote comfort.
	• Initiate use of PCA pump, *which allows some control over amount and frequency of IV pain medication received in 1-hr period.*
	• Use additional comfort measures:
	  Alteration in environment
	  Distractional devices
	  Relaxation techniques
	• Provide rest periods *to facilitate comfort, sleep, and relaxation.*	

Potential altered nutrition: less than body requirements *Related to:* Nutrient resources expended in response to illness Poor appetite **DEFINING CHARACTERISTICS** Loss of weight with/ without adequate caloric intake Current weight 10 percent or more below ideal Caloric intake inadequate to keep pace with disease/ metabolic state	**ONGOING ASSESSMENT** • Document patient's actual weight on admission. • Obtain nutritional history as appropriate. • Document appetite and I & O: • Encourage patient participation (daily log). **THERAPEUTIC INTERVENTIONS** • Assist patient with meals as needed. • Consult dietitian when appropriate *to determine ideal weight, implement steps to ensure intake required to meet demands on body during illness.* • If inadequate nutrition noted, see Nutrition, altered: less than body requirements, p. 37.	Adequate nutrition will be maintained.

Potential fluid volume deficit
Related to:
Inability to take fluids by mouth
Pain
 	
DEFINING CHARACTERISTICS
Decreased urine output
Concentrated urine
Output greater than intake
Sudden weight loss
Decreased skin turgor
Increased thirst
	ONGOING ASSESSMENT
	• Assess hydrational status:
	  Skin turgor
	  Mucous membranes
	  Daily weight
	• Monitor strict I & O q4-8h.
	• Report urine output <30 ml/hr for consecutive 2 hr.
	• Monitor serum/urine electrolytes and specific gravity.
	• Monitor and document vital signs. Report any abnormal findings.
	
	THERAPEUTIC INTERVENTIONS
	• Administer parenteral fluids as ordered:
	  Administer $D_5W.2NS$ at 1½ times maintenance.
	  Maintain patent IV flow rate.
	  Continue IV fluids 24-48 hr after oral pain management begins *to prevent dehydration and recurrence of pain crisis.*
	• Push oral fluids as soon as possible.
	• Provide desired fluids (e.g., ice, tea, popsicles, milk).
		Fluid and electrolyte balance will be maintained.

NURSING DIAGNOSES / DEFINING CHARACTERISTICS	NURSING INTERVENTIONS / *RATIONALES*	EXPECTED OUTCOMES
Dry mucous membranes Hypokalemia Hyponatremia		
Hyperthermia *Related to:* Infections of bone/organ infarcts Splenic infarction causing spleen to lose ability to filter bacteria Decreased splenic production of phagocyte **DEFINING CHARACTERISTICS** Persistent rise in body temperature to >38.3 °C (101 °F) 24-48 hr Positive blood, urine, or sputum cultures Positive x-rays for bony infarcts	**ONGOING ASSESSMENT** • Monitor vital signs q2-4h. • Observe for excessive chills resulting from body's attempt to fight off fever. • Observe for profuse diaphoresis. • Assess joints for redness, warmth, and swelling. • Observe skin for wounds with drainage. • Review x-ray films and lab results with physician. **THERAPEUTIC INTERVENTIONS** • Administer antipyretics as ordered *to control fever*. • Provide cool sponge baths. • Keep patient's body and linen clean and dry. • Administer antibiotics as ordered *to destroy invading bacteria*. • Push fluids as appropriate.	Normal temperature will be maintained.

Potential ineffective individual/family coping
Related to:
Repeated hospitalizations; chronic status of disease
 	
DEFINING CHARACTERISTICS
Frequent hospitalization
Poor attendance at work/school
Poor performance
Withdrawal
Poor self-image
	ONGOING ASSESSMENT
	• Assess patient's ability to express feelings about disease openly.
	• Assess family involvement with patient care.
	
	THERAPEUTIC INTERVENTIONS
	• Provide primary nurse relationship.
	• Set aside talk times when pain controlled; *patient in pain unable to communicate concerns effectively*.
	• Identify needs/provide information on coping mechanisms for patient and family:
	    Outside activities
	    Exercise programs (YMCA, health clubs)
	    Support systems available (e.g., National Association of Sickle Cell Anemia, in-house support group if available).
	• Use other resource persons:
	    Pediatric nurse clinicians
	    Clinical specialist
	    Psychiatric liaison personnel
	    Social workers
		Coping strategies will be maximized.

Knowledge deficit
Related to:
Unfamiliarity with disease process, treatment, complications
 	
DEFINING CHARACTERISTICS
Inability to define sickle cell disease
	ONGOING ASSESSMENT
	• Assess level of understanding, developmental stage, and ability to learn.
	• Assess family involvement and readiness to learn.
	
	THERAPEUTIC INTERVENTIONS
	• Explain cause of sickle cell disease.
	• Instruct patient/family on signs of impending crisis:
	    Verbal complaint of pain
	    Persistent low-grade temperature
	    Decreased appetite
	    Decreased fluid intake
	    Increased sleeping time
		Patient/family will verbalize understanding of sickle cell disease, prevention of crisis, and appropriate treatment.

Sickle cell pain crisis—cont'd

Stomatitis

NURSING DIAGNOSES / DEFINING CHARACTERISTICS	NURSING INTERVENTIONS / *RATIONALES*	EXPECTED OUTCOMES
Inability to list signs/ symptoms of crisis/ infection Lack of understanding of self-care/ preventive measures	Swollen joints • Instruct on necessity of informing physician of signs of infection *that may lead to crisis.* • Inform of importance of: Fluids, water, and juice Food high in carbohydrates and protein; three balanced meals per day Dressing appropriately for weather conditions. *(Added stress, such as severe cold weather, increases likelihood of crisis.)* • Provide information about medications as ordered: Pain medications Anti-inflammatory agents Antibiotics • Stress importance of keeping clinic appointments and wearing Medic-Alert tag. • Inform patient/family of support groups and importance of genetic counsel in family planning.	

Originated by: Carol Boyd, RN

Stomatitis

(ORAL MUCOSITIS; MOUTH CARE)

Inflammatory response and ulcerative lesions of the mouth and oropharynx which develop as a reaction to the stress of chemotherapy and radiation therapy.

NURSING DIAGNOSIS/DEFINING CHARACTERISTICS	NURSING INTERVENTIONS/*RATIONALES*	EXPECTED OUTCOMES
Alteration in integrity of oral/ oropharyngeal mucosa *Related to:* Inadequate replacement of damaged and destroyed epithelial cells Immunosuppression and myelosuppression resulting from cancer and chemotherapy Dehydration Protein malnutrition Poor oral hygiene **DEFINING CHARACTERISTICS** Oral dryness Reddened mucosa Hemorrhage Secondary infection	**ONGOING ASSESSMENT** • Assess status of oral mucosa: Use adequate source of light. Remove dental appliances. Use an oral assessment guide *as a baseline comparison.* Use a moist padded tongue blade to gently pull back the cheeks and tongue *in order to expose all areas of oral cavity for inspection.* • Assess status of oral tissue twice daily and report changes in appearance, taste and sensation. **THERAPEUTIC INTERVENTIONS** • Implement meticulous mouth care regime after each meal and q 4h while awake *to prevent buildup of oral plaque and bacteria.* • Instruct patient to: Gently brush all surfaces of teeth, gums, and tongue with a soft nylon brush q.i.d. and as needed. Brush with a non-irritating dentifrice such as baking soda. Remove and brush dentures thoroughly after meals and as needed. Rinse the mouth thoroughly during and after brushing. Avoid alcohol containing mouthwashes *as these may dry oral mucous membranes.* Recommended mouth rinses include: Hydrogen peroxide and saline or water (1:2 or 1:4). Peroxide solutions should be mixed immediately before use *to maintain oxydizing property* and held in mouth for 1-1½ minutes. Follow with a rinse of water or saline.	Development of stomatitis related to cancer therapy is prevented or reduced.

Continued.

521

Hematolymphatic and Oncologic Care Plans

NURSING DIAGNOSIS/DEFINING CHARACTERISTICS	NURSING INTERVENTIONS / *RATIONALES*	EXPECTED OUTCOMES

	Baking soda and water (1 tsp in 500 ml).
	Salt (½ tsp), baking soda (1 tsp), and water (100 ml).
	Keep lips moist *to prevent drying and cracking.* Use a water soluble lubricant (K-Y jelly, Aquaphor Cream) *to minimize risk of aspirating non–water-soluble agent.*
	Include food items with each meal that require chewing *as this stimulates gingival tissue and promotes circulation.*
	Minimize trauma to mucous membranes. Avoid use of tobacco and alcohol *as these are irritating and drying to the mucosa.* Avoid extremely hot or cold foods. Avoid acidic or highly spiced foods. Note and remove any loose-fitting dentures.
	If signs of mild stomatitis occur (sensation of dryness and burning; mild erythema and edema along the mucocutaneous junction):
	  Increase frequency of oral hygiene by rinsing with one of the suggested solutions between brushings and once during the night.
	  Discontinue flossing if it causes pain.
	  Use systemic or topical analgesics as ordered by physician.	

Pain
Related to:
Sloughing of mucosal membrane that progresses to ulceration
Increased sensitivity/pain due to thinning of oral mucosal lining
 	
Defining Characteristics
Complaints of burning/tightness in mouth
Complaints of mouth pain when drinking, chewing, and/or swallowing
	Ongoing Assessment
	• Assess for extensiveness of ulcerations involving the intraoral soft tissues, including palate, tongue, gums, and lips.
	
	Therapeutic Interventions
	• Administer systemic and/or topical analgesics, particularly if the amount of pain is severe.
	• Instruct patient that topical analgesics can be administered as "swished and swallow" or "swish and spit" 15 to 20 minutes before meals, or painted on each lesion immediately prior to mealtime.
	  Topical analgesics include:
	  Dyclone 1%
	  Viscous lidocaine (10 ml per dose up to 120 ml in 24 hours)
	  Xylocaine (viscous 2%), Benadryl elixir (12.5 mg per 5 ml) and an antacid mixed in equal proportions.
	• Instruct patient to hold solution for several minutes before expectorating, and not to use solution if mucosa is severely ulcerated and if drug sensitivity exists.
	• Caution client to chew or swallow after each dose *as numbness of throat may be experienced.*
	• Explain use of topical protective agent *to promote healing* as prescribed:
	  Kaolin preparations
	  Substrate of an antacid. This substance is prepared by allowing antacid to settle. The pasty residue is swabbed onto the inflamed areas and, after 15-20 min, rinsed with saline or water.
		Discomfort will be reduced or relieved.

Altered nutrition: less than body requirements *Related to:* Inability to chew and swallow secondary to pain of inflamed/ulcerated oral and/or oropharyngeal mucous membranes **Defining Characteristics** Poor skin turgor Parched tongue	**Ongoing Assessment** • Assess for Defining Characteristics. **Therapeutic Interventions** • Maintain optimum oral intake. • Encourage diet high in protein and vitamins *to promote healing and new tissue growth.* • Serve foods and fluids lukewarm or cold *as this may feel soothing to the oral mucosa.* • Serve frequent small meals/snacks spaced throughout the day. • Encourage soft foods (mashed potatoes, puddings, custards, creamy cereals) *to avoid tissue trauma and pain.* • Refer patient to dietitian for instructions on maintenance of a well-balanced diet. • See Nutrition, altered: less than body requirements, p. 37	Optimal nutritional intake will be maintained.

NURSING DIAGNOSIS/DEFINING CHARACTERISTICS	NURSING INTERVENTIONS / *RATIONALES*	EXPECTED OUTCOMES
Weight loss Weakness/lethargy Increased serum BUN and creatinine levels		
Fluid volume deficit: potential *Related to:* Inability to take fluids by mouth **DEFINING CHARACTERISTICS** Poor skin turgor Dry skin Thirst Weakness/lethargy Change in BP Changes in pulse Increased serum BUN and creatinine levels Decrease in Hgb/Hct	**ONGOING ASSESSMENT** • Assess for Defining Characteristics. **THERAPEUTIC INTERVENTIONS** • Encourage use of a straw *to make swallowing easier.* • Encourage peach, pear, or apricot nectars and fruit drinks instead of fruit juices *as these are not irritating and are easier to swallow.* • See Fluid volume deficit, p. 20	Optimal fluids status will be maintained.

Potential for systemic infection
Related to:
Severe mucositis
 	
DEFINING CHARACTERISTICS
Candidiasis:
  Cottage cheese-like white or pale yellowish patches on tongue, buccal mucosa and palate
Herpes simplex:
  Painful itching vesicle (typically on upper lips) that ruptures within 12 hours and becomes encrusted with a dried exudate
Gram positive bacterial infection, specifically staphylococcal and streptococcal infections:
  Dry, raised wart-like yellowish-brown, round plaques on buccal mucosa
Gram negative bacterial infections:
  Creamy to yellow-white shiny, non-purulent patches often seated on painful, red, superficial, mucosal ulcers, and erosions.
Fever, chills, rigors
	ONGOING ASSESSMENT
	• Assess for Defining Characteristics.
	• Monitor vital signs q4h or more frequently as indicated.
	• Observe for evidence of infection and report to physician.
	
	THERAPEUTIC INTERVENTIONS
	• Increase frequency of oral hygiene to q2h while awake and once during the night.
	• Administer local antibiotics and/or antifungal agents as ordered by physician.
	• Discontinue use of toothbrush and flossing *as this will increase damage to ulcerated tissues. A disposable foamstick ("Toothette") or sterile cotton swab are gentle ways to apply cleansing solutions.*
	• Continue use of lubricating ointment on the lips.
		Risk of local/systemic infection will be reduced.

Continued.

NURSING DIAGNOSIS/DEFINING CHARACTERISTICS	NURSING INTERVENTIONS / *RATIONALES*	EXPECTED OUTCOMES
Knowledge deficit *Related to:* Unfamiliarity with potential side effects of chemo/radiation therapy **DEFINING CHARACTERISTICS** Lack of questions Multiple questions Misconceptions Verbalized knowledge deficit	**ONGOING ASSESSMENT** • Assess patient's understanding of potential side effects of chemo/radiation therapy. **THERAPEUTIC INTERVENTIONS** • Provide available patient teaching booklets. • Discuss booklets with patient/significant others and answer questions. • See mouth care instructions on p. 521.	Patient will verbalize knowledge about mucositis and the importance of practicing meticulous oral hygiene.

Originated by: Marina Bautista, RN, BSN

Tumor lysis syndrome

Rapid necrosis of malignant tumor cells induced by chemotherapy/radiation resulting in hyperkalemia, hyperphosphatemia with hypocalcemia, azotemia, and hyperuricemia.

NURSING DIAGNOSES / DEFINING CHARACTERISTICS	NURSING INTERVENTIONS / *RATIONALES*	EXPECTED OUTCOMES

Altered body fluid composition
Related to:
Renal impairment
Chemotherapy
Radiation
 	
DEFINING CHARACTERISTICS
Potassium level >5.1 mEq/L
Calcium level <8.6 mg/dl
Bradycardia
Ventricular tachycardia
Ventricular arrhythmias
Changes in ECG
Prolonged PR and QT intervals
Depressed ST segments
Tall, peaked T waves
Widened QRS complex
	ONGOING ASSESSMENT
	• Assess cardiac status:
	    Monitor apical pulse q4h.
	    Assess rate and rhythm.
	    Assess for arrhythmias.
	• If ECG monitoring available:
	    Monitor ECG tracing for tall peaked T waves, depressed ST segment, widened QRS complex, presence of ventricular arrhythmias.
	• Notify physician of changes in cardiac status.
	• Assess serum potassium and calcium levels daily.
	
	THERAPEUTIC INTERVENTIONS
	• Restrict K^+ containing foods *to decrease K^+ intake* (e.g., restrict bananas, grapes, dried fruits, chocolate, meats).
	• Encourage Na intake *(promotes K^+ loss if not restricted)*.
	• Administer diuretics as ordered; monitor intake/output q8h.
	• Administer cation-exchange resins (Kayexelate) *(exchanges Na^+ ions for K^+ ions through GI mucosa, then excreted K^+)*.
	• Administer calcium gluconate IV as ordered by physician.
	• Administer $NaHCO_3$/IV glucose with insulin *(moves K^+ back into cell)* as ordered.
	• Prepare patient for dialysis if other measures unsuccessful.
		Body fluid composition will be maximized.

Tumor lysis syndrome—cont'd

NURSING DIAGNOSES / DEFINING CHARACTERISTICS	NURSING INTERVENTIONS / *RATIONALES*	EXPECTED OUTCOMES
Potential for injury: neuromuscular system *Related to:* Hyperphosphatemia Chemotherapy Radiation Hypocalcemia **DEFINING CHARACTERISTICS** Serum calcium less than 8.6 mg/dl Muscle cramps Carpopedal spasms and laryngospasm Tetany Seizures Confusion Positive Chvostek's and Trousseau's signs Phosphate level >5.0 mEq/L	**ONGOING ASSESSMENT** • Assess patient for neuromuscular changes q4h; observe for: Tetany Carpopedal spasms Chvostek's sign *(Tap face over facial nerve in front of temple; face will twitch.)* Trousseau's sign *(Inflate BP cuff above systolic pressure for 3 min; contraction of hand will occur.)* • Assess for changes in mental status (confusion). • Monitor for seizure activity. • Monitor serum calcium and phosphate levels daily. **THERAPEUTIC INTERVENTIONS** • Teach patient signs/symptoms of hypocalcemia (muscle cramps, paresthesias). Instruct patient to notify physician if they occur. • Teach patient to avoid putting direct pressure on motor nerves (e.g., by crossing legs), *which exacerbates tetany.* • Teach patient importance of relaxation. *Tetany can be potentiated by stress.* • If confusion present: Reorient as needed. Assist with ADLs. Maintain safety precautions *to prevent injury.* • Maintain seizure precautions: Airway at bedside Padded side rails • Increase calcium in diet. • Administer phosphate binders (e.g., aluminum hydroxide gels): Monitor for constipation. Provide stool softeners. • Administer calcium gluconate IV *to treat acute Ca^{++} deficit.*	Potential for injury will be reduced.
Potential for injury: renal damage *Related to:* Uric acid Nephropathy resulting from: Increased uric acid precipitation in renal tubules Release of nucleic acids from tumor cell lysis **DEFINING CHARACTERISTICS** Increased serum uric acid (normal: 2.0-7.5 mg/dl) Elevated blood urea nitrogen (normal: 8-25 mg/dl) Elevated serum creatinine (normal: 0.5-1.3 mg/dl) Decreased urine output Acidic urine	**ONGOING ASSESSMENT** • Monitor accurate intake/output: Maintain strict I & O q6h. Note decreasing output. • Monitor urine pH q6h: Maintain alkalized urine pH >7.0. • Monitor serum lab values: Uric acid BUN Creatinine • Monitor for allopurinol side effects: Rash Fever Abnormal liver function tests Acute renal failure • See Renal failure, acute, p. 343, as needed. **THERAPEUTIC INTERVENTIONS** • Administer fluids as ordered. IV hydration should begin 1-2 days before chemotherapy, continue 2-3 days after chemotherapy completed *to prevent uric acid precipitation in urine.* • Administer $NaHCO_3$ or Diamox as ordered *to maintain alkalized urine.* • Notify physician of abnormal lab value. • Administer allopurinol as ordered *to reduce chance of nephropathy.*	Potential for renal damage will be reduced.

Continued.

NURSING DIAGNOSES / DEFINING CHARACTERISTICS	NURSING INTERVENTIONS / *RATIONALES*	EXPECTED OUTCOMES

Potential fluid volume overload
Related to:
IV hydration
Chemotherapy
 	
DEFINING CHARACTERISTICS
Weight gain
Edema
Effusion (pleural/pericardial)
Changes in respiratory pattern
Intake > output
Shortness of breath
Pulmonary congestion
Abnormal breath sounds: crackles/rales
Changes in vital signs
Jugular vein distention
Electrolyte imbalance
	ONGOING ASSESSMENT
	· Monitor vital signs q4h.
	· Monitor daily weight after breakfast.
	· Weigh patient on same scale every day. *Monitoring vital signs, weight, and urinary output helps assess changes in fluid shifts and effectiveness of therapy.*
	· Observe for edema: pedal, sacral, generalized.
	· Monitor accurate I & O.
	· Observe for jugular vein distention.
	· Auscultate lung fields q4h:
	   Observe respiration quality and rate q8h.
	   Note presence of rales.
	   Observe for shortness of breath at rest/with exertion.
	· Auscultate apical heart rate q8h:
	   Note tachycardia.
	   Note third heart sound.
	· Monitor daily lab data:
	   Electrolytes
	   Uric acid levels
	   Lactic dehydrogenase (LDH) levels
	   BUN, creatinine
	
	THERAPEUTIC INTERVENTIONS
	· Notify physician of deviation from baseline vital signs.
	· Elevate feet while sitting.
	· Apply elastic stockings (TED hose).
	· Notify physician of all findings.
	· Restrict fluids as necessary: set up 24-hr schedule for fluid intake. Restrict Na$^+$ intake.
	· Notify physician if intake > output by 1 L/24 hrs.
	· Place patient in semi- to high Fowler's position; encourage ambulation *(improves lung expansion)*.
	· Encourage frequent rest periods.
	· Notify physician of abnormal lab data.
	· Administer electrolyte supplements as necessary, as ordered.
	· Administer diuretics as ordered *to decrease fluid liquid*.
		Fluid overload will be prevented/corrected.

Potential knowledge deficit
Related to:
Change in body function
Unfamiliarity with disease process
Misintepretation of disease process
 	
DEFINING CHARACTERISTICS
Multiple questions
Patient's/significant others' questions and concerns about patient's condition, procedures, and treatments
Noncompliance with medications and diet
	ONGOING ASSESSMENT
	· Assess patient's/significant others' understanding of condition, procedures, and treatments.
	
	THERAPEUTIC INTERVENTIONS
	· Inform patient of severity of condition and necessary treatments.
	· Prepare patient and family members for possible dialysis, if necessary:
	   Teach about venous access: peripheral/vascular.
	   Teach about rationale for dialysis.
	· See Renal failure, acute, p. 343.
		Patient/family verbalize understanding of treatment, procedures, and condition.

Originated by: Sharon Flucus, RN, BSN
Carol Nawrocki, RN, BSN

Autologous bone marrow transplantation

An autologous bone marrow transplant uses the patient's own bone marrow to prevent potentially lethal marrow toxicities resulting from treatment with high-dose chemotherapy alone or in combination with radiation therapy.

NURSING DIAGNOSES / DEFINING CHARACTERISTICS	NURSING INTERVENTIONS / *RATIONALES*	EXPECTED OUTCOMES

Knowledge deficit
Related to:
Unfamiliarity with procedures and treatments in bone marrow transplantation
Unfamiliarity with overall schedule of events
Unfamiliarity with discharge/follow-up care
 	
Defining Characteristics
Verbalized lack of knowledge
Expressed need for information
Multiple questions
Lack of questions
Verbalized misconceptions
	Ongoing Assessment
	• Solicit patient's/significant others' understanding of:
	   Procedure(s)
	   Treatment protocol
	   Potential side effects/complications
	   Schedule of overall treatment plan
	   Anticipated length of hospitalization
	   Follow-up care after discharge
	• Assess patient's/significant other's learning capabilities.
	• Assess patient's/significant other's willingness to learn.
	• See Knowledge deficit, p. 33.
	
	Therapeutic Interventions
	• Provide patient teaching materials (booklets, videotape, slide presentation, etc.).
	• Discuss teaching materials with patient/significant other.
	• Reinforce and restate information *to clarify misconceptions and promote better understanding of bone marrow transplant process.*
	• Share with patient written calendar/schedule of overall treatment plan.
	• Instruct patient (significant other as needed) about Hickman catheter insertion (if central venous catheter not already in place):
	   Preoperative care
	   Postoperative care
	   Potential complications (See also Hickman right atrial catheter, p. 553.)
	• Explain bone marrow harvest (if bone marrow not already collected):
	   Preoperative care
	   Collection/storage of bone marrow
	   Postoperative care
	   Potential complications (See also Bone marrow harvest, p. 540.)
	• Discuss high-dose chemotherapy/radiation therapy administration:
	   Potential short- and long-term side effects/toxicities
	   Preventive measures to minimize/alleviate toxicities (antiemetic, oral/skin care regimens, pain control, etc.)
	• Discuss bone marrow transplantation:
	   Procedure for bone marrow reinfusion
	   Potential complications
	   Preventive measures to minimize/alleviate potential complications
	   Time frame for marrow engraftment
	• Determine anticipated supportive care:
	   Protective environment (private room, laminar air flow room, etc.) *to protect patient from environmental contagions during myelosuppression period*
	• Provide information about isolation techniques/procedures.
	• Discuss blood component transfusions (i.e., packed red cells, white cells, and platelets) *which constitute adjunct management of anemia, infections, and thrombocytopenia.* Encourage patient/significant other to participate in blood component donor accrual to fulfill frequent, often prolonged transfusion requirements.
		Patient/significant other verbalize basic understanding of procedures, treatments, possible complications, and follow-up care and properly performs care as appropriate.

Continued.

Autologous bone marrow transplantation—cont'd

NURSING DIAGNOSES / DEFINING CHARACTERISTICS	NURSING INTERVENTIONS / *RATIONALES*	EXPECTED OUTCOMES

	• Discuss antibacterial, antiprotozoal, antifungal, and antiviral therapy *to prevent/treat infections. Oral nonabsorbable antibiotics (Gentamicin/Vancomycin/Nystatin/Polymyxin) may be administered prophylactically to suppress patient's own GI flora, which, during myelosuppression, potentially become pathogenic and eventually are source of infection/sepsis. Efficacy of oral nonabsorbable antibiotics controversial; patient compliance/tolerance generally poor.*
	• Discuss dietary modifications that may include low-bacterial diet (no fresh fruits/vegetables, "well cooked" food items) *to decrease bacterial contamination of alimentary tract. Total parenteral nutrition (TPN) initiated when patient's oral intake no longer meet daily nutritional requirements.*
	• Explain need for frequent blood sampling *to assess for electrolyte and metabolic changes, cardiac/pulmonary/renal alterations, bone marrow function, need for blood component transfusion(s), and presence of infection.*
	• Explain need for frequent inspection/culturing of all orifices/potential infection sites *for surveillance of opportunitistic microorganisms, early detection, and prompt treatment of infection.*
	• Discuss discharge planning/teaching. *(Depends on course of postengraftment period, but usually begins about 2 wk after transplantation. Discharge criteria include absolute granulocyte count of >1000/mm³, oral intake 1000 cal/day, and no evidence of infection):*
	    ADLs
	    Sexual relations/contraception
	    Return to work or school
	    Hickman catheter care
	    Recognition/report of signs/symptoms of bleeding, low red blood cell count, and infection
	    Measures to prevent infection *(patient's immune function not fully restored until about 6-9 months after transplantation)*
	    Medications after discharge
	    Importance of balanced diet and adequate fluid intake
	    Outpatient follow-up care after discharge	

Anxiety/fear *Related to:* Fear of unknown Fear of prognosis Fear of treatment Threat of death Experience with chemotherapy/radiation therapy Diagnosis of cancer Hospitalization Fear of infection at time of discharge (i.e., leaving "protective isolation" environment) **DEFINING CHARACTERISTICS** Increased questioning Lack of questioning Tense appearance Restlessness Tearfulness Irritability Demandingness	**ONGOING ASSESSMENT** • Assess patient's/significant other's level of anxiety/fear. • Solicit how patient/significant other coped with stress in past. • Identify patient's support system. **THERAPEUTIC INTERVENTIONS** • Reassure patient/significant other that anxiety is normal. • Encourage patient to identify and verbalize feelings, fears, and concerns. • Approach patient with receptiveness, warmth, and consistency. • Encourage patient to identify previously effective coping mechanisms *(may be helpful in minimizing or alleviating fear/anxiety).* • Involve other departments (social worker, psychiatric liaison, clergy) *in counseling as needed.* • See Anxiety, p. 4 and Fear, p. 18.	Anxiety/fear will be reduced.

Autologous bone marrow transplantation—cont'd

NURSING DIAGNOSES / DEFINING CHARACTERISTICS	NURSING INTERVENTIONS / *RATIONALES*	EXPECTED OUTCOMES
Impaired physical mobility *Related to:* Treatment-related side effects Disease process Pain and discomfort Depression/severe anxiety Generalized weakness/ deconditioning Physical restrictions on movement (i.e., protective isolation) **DEFINING CHARACTERISTICS** Pain/discomfort on movement Weakness/lethargy Decreased attempt to move In bed most of time	**ONGOING ASSESSMENT** · Assess for presence of Defining Characteristics. **THERAPEUTIC INTERVENTIONS** · Teach importance of activity and possible hazards of immobility. *(Thorough explanation of purpose, goal, and importance of activity often increases patient compliance.)* · Notify PT of patient's admission *for assessment and formalization of individualized activity regimen* (after clearance with physician). · Facilitate procurement of stationary bicycle *to assist patient in maintaining muscle strength.* · Encourage daily use of exercise bicycle as appropriate. · Encourage patient involvement/participation in patient care activities. · See Mobility, impaired physical, p. 35.	Optimal level of physical mobility and independence will be achieved.
Nausea/vomiting *Related to:* Side effects of chemotherapy/ radiation therapy Antibiotic therapy Infection **DEFINING CHARACTERISTICS** Complaints of nausea/ vomiting Retching Straining Expulsion of gastric contents Queasy stomach Inability to look at or smell food	**ONGOING ASSESSMENT** · Assess for presence of Defining Characteristics. · Obtain history of side effects of previous chemotherapy/radiation therapy and treatment measures effective in past. · Solicit patient's description, including: Onset Severity Duration Precipitating factors · Monitor daily calorie counts *to determine whether patient's oral intake meets daily nutritional requirements.* · Evaluate effectiveness of antiemetic regimen. **THERAPEUTIC INTERVENTIONS** · Administer chemotherapy at night or in late afternoon if possible. · Administer antiemetic on timed rather than "prn" schedule before, during, and after chemotherapy/radiation therapy *to maintain adequate blood levels.* · Teach methods to minimize/prevent nausea/vomiting: Small dietary intake before treatments Foods with low potential for nausea (e.g., dry toast, crackers, ginger ale, cola, popsicles, gelatin, baked/boiled potatoes) Avoidance of spices, gravy, greasy foods Modification of food consistency/type as needed Small, frequent nutritious meals Attractive servings Sufficient time for meals Rest periods before and after meals Quiet, restful environment Comfortable position Oral hygiene measures Avoidance of coaxing, bribing, or threatening in relation to intake Antiemetic half-hour before meals as ordered · Identify and provide favorite foods; avoid serving them during periods of nausea/vomiting *as patient may develop aversion.*	Nausea/vomiting and related discomforts will be diminished.

Continued.

NURSING DIAGNOSES / DEFINING CHARACTERISTICS	NURSING INTERVENTIONS / *RATIONALES*	EXPECTED OUTCOMES
	· Administer supplemental feedings and fluids as ordered. · Keep clean emesis basin, tissue, mouthwash within reach; remove emesis promptly. · See Cancer chemotherapy, p. 543.	
Diarrhea *Related to:* Side effects of chemotherapy/ radiation therapy Antibiotic therapy Infection **Defining Characteristics** Abdominal pain Cramping Frequency of stools Loose/liquid stools Urgency Hyperactive bowel sounds/sensations	**Ongoing Assessment** · Assess for presence of Defining Characteristics. · Check bowel sounds q4h; observe for abdominal distention/rigidity. · Observe stool pattern; record frequency, character, and volume. · Obtain stool specimen for culture and sensitivity as ordered. **Therapeutic Interventions** · Administer antidiarrheal, antispasmodic as ordered; document effectiveness. · Administer IV analgesics *to relieve abdominal pain/cramping.* · Implement meticulous perianal care regimen *to prevent mucosal irritation/ breakdown.* · Administer parenteral nutrition as ordered *to maintain optimal nutritional support in view of inadequate PO intake/decreased absorption secondary to diarrhea.* · See Diarrhea, p. 16.	Normal elimination pattern will be achieved.
Potential for injury: bleeding *Related to:* Invasion of bone marrow by malignant cells Bone marrow suppression secondary to chemotherapy/ radiation therapy Prolonged bone marrow regeneration Failure of bone marrow graft Infection/sepsis Bacteremia DIC Tumor erosion ulcerations (i.e. stress ulcer, gastrointestinal mucosal sloughing secondary to chemotherapy/ radiation therapy) Hemorrhagic cystitis secondary to high-dose Cytoxan therapy **Defining Characteristics** Decrease in total circulating platelets <50,000/mm³ Petechiae, bruises, areas of ecchymoses	**Ongoing Assessment** · Assess for presence of Defining Characteristics. · Monitor vital signs q4h and as needed. · Monitor platelets, Hb/Hct daily *to detect changes early.* **Therapeutic Interventions** · Implement bleeding precautions for platelet count <50,000/mm³ *(level at which spontaneous bleeding occurs).* · Communicate anticipated need for platelet support to transfusion center *to assure availability and readiness of platelets.* · Transfuse single or random donor platelet as ordered. *Note: Orders to irradiate all blood products before administration (except bone marrow reinfusion) may be written to prevent mild form of graft-versus-host disease (GVHD), which, in autologus bone marrow transplant patient, may be caused by imbalance in T_4/T_8 ratio, as well as presence of component donor's white blood cells. Irradiation of blood components continues about 6-12 months after patient discharge.* · Maintain a current blood sample for "type and screen" in transfusion center *to ensure availability and readiness of packed red blood cells.* · If significant drop in Hb and Hct noted, transfuse packed red cells as ordered *to restore Hb/Hct to levels where patient experiences minimal symptoms.* (Check whether blood components irradiated before transfusion.) · See Anemia, p. 498; Leukemia, acute, p. 510.	Risks for and complications of bleeding will be reduced.

NURSING DIAGNOSES / DEFINING CHARACTERISTICS	NURSING INTERVENTIONS / *RATIONALES*	EXPECTED OUTCOMES
Epistaxis Bleeding gums Hematemesis Hemoptysis Retinal hemorrhages Melena Hematuria Vaginal bleeding Headaches and changes in mental and visual acuity Dizziness Orthostatic changes Increased pulse rate Decreased Hb/Hct Fever Positive blood culture		
Potential for injury: liver dysfunction *Related to:* Veno-occlusive disease (VOD) Hepatitis Infection Fatty liver (from parenteral nutrition) Drug injury (chemotherapy/ antibiotic therapy) Hepatic malignancy Liver failure **DEFINING CHARACTERISTICS** *Typically, symptoms develop 1-3 wk after transplant. Patients usually present with some, but not all symptoms:* Sudden weight gain Enlarged liver Right upper quadrant pain Increased abdominal girth Jaundice Tea-colored urine Labored, shallow respirations Dyspnea Confusion Drowsiness Lethargy Increased alkaline phosphatase Increased bilirubin	**ONGOING ASSESSMENT** - Assess for presence of Defining Characteristics. - Monitor appropriate lab values daily. - Monitor daily weight. - Measure abdominal girth; document changes. - Monitor I & O. **THERAPEUTIC INTERVENTIONS** - Maintain sodium restriction as indicated. - Restrict fluids (as ordered). - Administer IV medications with minimal amount of solution. - Apply heparin lock to unused ports on central venous catheter(s). - Administer 25% normal serum albumin (human) as ordered *to keep serum levels within normal range and maintain plasma oncotic pressure.* - Administer diuretics as ordered *to decrease amount of ascites by promoting water and sodium excretion.* Monitor for side effects; document appropriately.	Physical and physiologic complications will be reduced.

Continued.

NURSING DIAGNOSES / DEFINING CHARACTERISTICS	NURSING INTERVENTIONS / *RATIONALES*	EXPECTED OUTCOMES
Increased serum glutamic oxaloacetic transaminase (SGOT)/serum glutamic pyruvic transaminase(SGPT)/ Lactic dehydrogenase (LDH) Decreased serum albumin Electrolyte imbalance Abnormal coagulation profile Increased serum ammonia		

Potential for infection
Related to:
Altered immunologic responses related to immunosuppression secondary to high-dose chemotherapy/ radiation therapy
Bone marrow suppression
Antibiotic therapy (i.e., superimposed infection)
Prolonged bone marrow regeneration
Failure of bone marrow graft
 	
DEFINING CHARACTERISTICS
Fever
Flushed appearance
Diaphoresis
Increased pulse and respirations
Decreased BP
Rigors
Shaking chills
Sore throat
Rales
Decreased breath sounds
Pleuritic pain
Abnormal sputum
Conjunctivitis
Urinary frequency/ burning
Vaginal discharge
	ONGOING ASSESSMENT
	· Assess for presence of Defining Characteristics
	· Monitor WBC/differential daily *for evidence of rising/falling counts. Gradually rising blood counts signal successful bone marrow engraftment/ function (generally occurs 14-20 days after transplantation).*
	· Monitor vital signs q4h and as needed.
	· Auscultate lung field every shift and as needed.
	· Note presence/type of cough.
	· Observe for changes in color/character of sputum, urine, stool.
	· Inspect body sites with high potential for infection (mouth, throat, axilla, perineum, rectum) daily.
	· Inspect peripheral IV/central catheter site(s) daily.
	
	THERAPEUTIC INTERVENTIONS
	· Place patient in protective isolation per transplant protocol.
	· Ensure thorough handwashing (using vigorous friction) by staff/visitors before physical contact with patient *to remove transient/resident bacteria from hands, thus minimizing/preventing transmission to patient.*
	· Provide care for neutropenic patients before other patients, taking strict precautions to prevent transferring infectious agent(s) to neutropenic patients.
	· Teach/provide meticulous total body hygiene with special attention to high-risk area *(often sites of infection).*
	· Use aseptic/sterile technique in patient care/treatments per isolation protocol/procedure.
	· Use separate towel/washcloth for area of infection *to prevent cross contamination.*
	· See Leukemia, acute, p. 510.
	· See Granulocytopenia, p. 505.
	· See Hickman right atrial catheter, p. 553.
	· Implement meticulous oral hygiene regimen.
	· See Stomatitis, p. 521.
	· Administer antibacterial/antifungal/antiviral/antiprotozoal drugs as ordered on time *to maintain therapeutic drug levels.*
	· Describe to patient/significant other WBC role in infection prevention:
	    Normal range of WBC
	    Function of leukocytes and neutrophils
	    Meaning/importance of "absolute" neutrophil count
	    Risk of bacterial infection associated with "absolute" neutrophil count
		Risk of local/systemic infection will be reduced.

Autologous bone marrow transplantation—cont'd

NURSING DIAGNOSES / DEFINING CHARACTERISTICS	NURSING INTERVENTIONS / *RATIONALES*	EXPECTED OUTCOMES

Redness/tenderness over peripheral IV puncture or indwelling venous catheter sites
 	
Decrease in circulating white blood cells characterized by profound decrease/absence of neutrophils
	$<500/mm^3$: severe risk
	$500/mm^3$: moderate risk
	$>1000/mm^3$: minimal risk
	$1500\text{-}2000/mm^3$: no significant risk
	• Explain effects of chemotherapy/radiation therapy on immune system.
	• Teach patient/significant other measures *to prevent infection after discharge until immune function fully restored* (about 6-9 mon after transplantation):
	  Avoid crowds or contact with persons with known infections.
	  Avoid cleaning cat-litter boxes, fish tanks, or bird cages.
	  Avoid contact with dog/human excreta.
	  Avoid contact with barnyard animals.
	  Avoid swimming in private/public pools.
	  Practice meticulous oral/body hygiene, including frequent handwashing.
	  Use aseptic technique when caring for central venous catheter.
	  Maintain balanced diet with sufficient protein, calories, vitamins, minerals, and fluids.
	  Limit number of sexual partners; practice "gentle" sex; use adequate lubrication; avoid rectal intercourse/douching; use contraceptive method(s) approved by physician.	

Potential fluid volume overload *Related to:* Aggressive IV hydration with high-dose Cytoxan-based preparatory regimen Antidiuretic effect of Cytoxan Bone marrow reinfusion Multiple IV drug therapy (oral route unsuitable secondary to nausea, vomiting, mucositis, etc.) Parenteral nutrition Blood component transfusions **Defining Characteristics** Weight gain Fluid intake > urine output Shortness of breath Dyspnea Rales Rhonchi Edema Distended neck veins Changes in vital signs (BP, heart rate, respiratory rate) Anxiety Restlessness	**Ongoing Assessment** • Monitor vital signs q4h. • Auscultate chest q4h and as needed. • Weigh patient daily at same time with same scale *to assure accuracy.* • Record accurate I & O. **Therapeutic Interventions** • Administer diuretics as ordered; monitor for effectiveness and side effects; document. • Administer IV medications with minimal amount of solution. • Infuse IV solutions as ordered via infusion control device *to assure accurate flow rate and prevent unintentional fluid overload.* • Provide measures to decrease anxiety/stress. • Plan activities *to allow minimum energy expenditure with adequate rest periods.* • Administer O_2 as ordered. • See Breathing pattern, ineffective, p. 8.	Optimal fluid balance will be maintained.

Continued.

Hematolymphatic and Oncologic Care Plans

NURSING DIAGNOSES / DEFINING CHARACTERISTICS	NURSING INTERVENTIONS / *RATIONALES*	EXPECTED OUTCOMES
Potential fluid volume deficit *Related to:* Side effects of chemotherapy/ radiation therapy Muscositis Dysphagia Nausea Vomiting Diarrhea Diuretic therapy **Defining Characteristics** Decreased urine ouput Output > intake Dilute urine Decreased skin turgor Dry mucous membranes Thirst Possible weight gain Edema Increased pulse rate Decreased pulse volume/pressure Weakness Decreased serum potassium Increased serum sodium Increased serum BUN/ creatinine Hemoconcentration	**Ongoing Assessment** · Assess for presence of Defining Characteristics. **Therapeutic Interventions** · See Fluid volume deficit, p. 20. · See Cancer chemotherapy, p. 543.	Optimal fluid status and electrolyte balance will be maintained.
Altered nutrition: less than body requirements *Related to:* Side effects of chemotherapy (inability to taste and smell foods, loss of appetite, nausea, vomiting, mucositis, abdominal cramping, diarrhea, indifference to food) Mouth lesions Pain on chewing, swallowing Increased metabolic rate secondary to fever/infection **Defining Characteristics** Weight loss Documented inadequate caloric intake	**Ongoing Assessment** · Assess for presence of Defining Characteristics. **Therapeutic Interventions** · See Nutrition, altered: less than body requirements, p. 37.	Optimal nutritional status will be maintained.

NURSING DIAGNOSES / DEFINING CHARACTERISTICS	NURSING INTERVENTIONS / *RATIONALES*	EXPECTED OUTCOMES
Potential decreased cardiac output *Related to:* Cardiomyopathy secondary to high-dose Cytoxan therapy **DEFINING CHARACTERISTICS** Variations in hemodynamic parameters (BP, heart rate, neck veins, etc.) Abnormal heart sounds. Decreased peripheral pulses Shortness of breath Cold, clammy skin Arrhythmias ECG changes Abnormal lung sounds	**ONGOING ASSESSMENT** • Assess for significant alterations in: Radial/apical/peripheral pulses, cardiac rhythm, respiration BP, pulsus paradoxus Heart sounds Lung sounds Jugular venous distention Skin color, moisture, temperature Fluid balance: I & O, weight, presence of peripheral edema ABGs, chest x-ray • Monitor ECG rate, rhythm, and change in PR, QRS, and QT intervals daily during high-dose Cytoxan therapy. *Note that nonspecific ST changes not uncommon with high-dose Cytoxan therapy.* Continue to monitor 48 hr after administration of last Cytoxan dose *to assess for potential myocardial damage.* **THERAPEUTIC INTERVENTIONS** • Administer O_2 as indicated. • Administer medications as ordered. • See Cardiac output, decreased, p. 9.	Optimal hemodynamic function will be maintained.
Potential for injury *Related to:* Chemotherapy Radiation therapy Antiemetic drugs Antifungal drugs Bone marrow reinfusion Blood component transfusion(s) **DEFINING CHARACTERISTICS** *Chemotherapeutic drugs:* Restlessness Facial edema/flushing Wheezing Skin rash Tachycardia Hypotension Hematuria (Cytoxan) Increased uric acid levels *Radiation therapy:* Nausea/vomiting Fever Diarrhea Flushing Swelling of parotid glands Pancreatitis *Antiemetic drugs:* Agitation Hypotension Irritability	**ONGOING ASSESSMENT** • Assess for presence of Defining Characteristics. • Check for history of drug allergies. • Monitor vital signs q4h. • Monitor serum electrolyte levels. *(Diuretic therapy may produce electrolyte depletion, i.e., hypokalemia.)* • Check urine pH as ordered until 48 hr after administration of last Cytoxan dose. • Test urine for blood *to check for hematuria caused by irritation of bladder lining secondary to metabolites from Cytoxan therapy. High urine flow, alkalinization of urine, and frequent voiding help prevent concentration of Cytoxan metabolites in bladder, thus reducing risk of hemorrhagic cystitis.* • Perform pretransplant assessment before bone marrow infusion: Take baseline vital signs. Auscultate chest and heart. Check patency of central venous catheter; *24-72 hr after completion of chemotherapy (depending on biologic clearance rates of drugs given), frozen marrow is taken to patient's bedside, thawed in water bath, and administered to patient intravenously via Hickman catheter.* • Monitor vital signs throughout, after transplant procedure. **THERAPEUTIC INTERVENTIONS** • Perform the following when drug/transfusion reaction suspected: Stop infusion. Notify physician. Administer emergency drugs as ordered. Reassure patient. See also Blood and blood product transfusion therapy, p. 538. • Administer premedications as ordered; monitor for effectiveness; document. • Keep emergency drugs (IV Benadryl, hydrocortisone, Epinephrine 1:1000) readily available. • Administer IV fluids and diuretics before, during, and after Cytoxan therapy as ordered *to maintain good urine output and counteract antidiuretic effect of Cytoxan. As chemotherapy destroys tumor cells, uric acid is liberated and accumulates in blood. High urine flow prevents uric acid deposits in kidneys.* See also Tumor lysis syndrome, p. 524.	Injury from drug/radiation/blood therapy will be reduced.

Continued.

NURSING DIAGNOSES / DEFINING CHARACTERISTICS	NURSING INTERVENTIONS / *RATIONALES*	EXPECTED OUTCOMES
Spasm of neck muscles Dystonias *Antifungal drugs:* Fever Chills Rigors Hypotension Headache Nausea/vomiting Hypokalemia *Bone marrow reinfusion:* Chills Rigors Fever Nausea/vomiting Dyspnea Shortness of breath Chest pain Sensation of tightness, fullness in throat *Packed red cell/ platelet transfusion:* Fever Chills Rigors Hives	• Administer supplemental sodium bicarbonate as ordered to maintain urine pH above 7, *thus increasing solubility of uric acid in urine and diminishing changes of crystalline deposits in kidneys, which could potentially cause uric acid nephropathy. Allopurinol may be added.* • Instruct patient to void q1-2 h until 24 hr after completion of last Cytoxan dose. • Administer analgesics as needed; apply topical ice packs to swollen parotid gland(s) *(helps reduce pain of parotitis). Symptomatic parotitis may occur 4-24 hr after single-dose 1000-rad total body irradiation (TBI); generally resolves in 1-4 days. Side effect less frequent when TBI administered in divided (fractionated) doses.* • Have patient void before bone marrow reinfusion and assist in assuming position of optimal comfort *(prevents/minimizes interruptions to transplant procedure).* • Premedicate patient with antiemetic and antihistamine as ordered before to bone marrow reinfusion *to reduce incidence of nausea/vomiting and allergic reactions. Nausea/vomiting caused by garlic-like odor of dimethyl sulfoxide (DMSO) chemical used to preserve bone marrow. Allergic reactions, including shortness of breath (SOB), possible results of liberation of histamines from broken marrow cells.* • Provide warm blankets if chills occur during bone marrow reinfusion. *Chills usually secondary to cool temperature of thawed marrow.* • See Pulmonary thromboembolism, p. 200 for cardiopulmonary problems. • See Anaphylactic shock, p. 64, if allergic reactions during or after transplant procedure. • Inform patient that urine will be pink or red for several hours after transplant procedure *because of red color of tissue culture medium contained in reinfused marrow.*	

Potential impaired skin integrity
Related to:
Side effects of chemotherapy/ radiation therapy
Malignant skin lesions
Impaired physical mobility secondary to treatment-related side effects
Allergic reaction secondary to drug/blood component therapy
Infection
 	
DEFINING CHARACTERISTICS
Redness
Tenderness
Pain
Dryness
Scaling
Peeling
Itching
Erythematous patches
Maculas
Papules
Vesicles
	ONGOING ASSESSMENT
	• Assess for presence of Defining Characteristics.
	• Assess skin integrity daily; note color, moisture, texture, and temperature.
	• Inspect "high risk" areas daily for skin breakdown:
	  Bony prominences
	  Skin folds (e.g., axillae, breast folds, buttocks, perineum, groin)
	  Radiation port and exit site(s)
	• Assess movement/positioning ability.
	
	THERAPEUTIC INTERVENTIONS
	• See Skin integrity, impaired, p. 48.
	• See Shingles, p. 484.
	• Promote comfort:
	  Bed cradle to keep linen off body
	  Egg crate, alternating-pressure mattress
	  Nonadherent disposable sheets
	  Body positioning and supports
	  Systemic analgesics
	• Maintain dressing placement with Kerlix wrap or Surgiflex *to avoid use of tape on sensitive skin.*
	• Implement measures to prevent dryness of nonirradiated skin:
	  Include Alpha Keri Oil in bath water.
	  Apply Eucerin lotion liberally.
	• Implement measures *to prevent irritation to irradiated skin:*
	  Avoid constricting clothing.
	  Avoid irritating substances (e.g., perfumed soap, perfume, ointments, lotions, cosmetics, talcum).
		Impaired skin integrity will be reduced/ controlled.

NURSING DIAGNOSES / DEFINING CHARACTERISTICS	NURSING INTERVENTIONS / *RATIONALES*	EXPECTED OUTCOMES
Hypothermia/ hyperthermia Hyperpigmentation	Avoid use of oil-based creams, ointments, and lotions during treatment *(may contain heavy metals and leave coating on skin that may interfere with radiation therapy).* Use only topical ointments, creams, powders, etc., as prescribed by radiologist *for skin tenderness, dryness, and itching.* Avoid hot or cold applications (e.g., heating pad, ice compress) as well as sun exposure *(may increase irritation).* Avoid vigorous scrubbing of skin. Avoid scratching/peeling skin. Wear soft cotton clothing. Inform patient that discoloration temporary; skin will return to normal color though texture may continue to be dry.	
Body image disturbance *Related to* Loss of hair Central venous catheter(s) protruding from chest Local/generalized edema Generalized "wasting" Changes in skin color/ texture Breakage/loss of fingernails secondary to high-dose chemotherapy **DEFINING CHARACTERISTICS** Self-deprecating remarks Refusal to look at self in mirror Crying Anger Decreased attention to grooming Verbalization of ambivalence Compensatory use of concealing clothing, devices	**ONGOING ASSESSMENT** • Assess for presence of Defining Characteristics. • Observe for verbal/nonverbal cues *to note body image alteration.* **THERAPEUTIC INTERVENTIONS** • Refer to Body image disturbance, p. 6. • Acknowledge normalcy of emotional response to actual or perceived changes in physical appearance. • Encourage verbalization of feelings, listen to concerns *to alleviate anxiety.* • Convey feelings of acceptance and understanding. • Offer realistic reassurance of temporary nature of some changes of physical appearance (i.e., hair/nails will regrow; catheter(s) will eventually be removed, etc.). • Involve other staff (social worker, psychiatric liaison) as indicated *for counseling as needed.*	Feelings about changes in body image will be acknowledged.
Potential ineffective coping *Related to:* Situational crisis Disturbances in self-concept/self-esteem/ body image Disturbances in lifestyle/role Inadequate coping methods Prolonged hospitalization	**ONGOING ASSESSMENT** • Assess for presence of Defining Characteristics. • Assess patient's specific stressors. • Determine patient's perception of stressors and events, beliefs about their causes. • Evaluate patient's available resources/support systems. • Determine patient's available/useful past and present coping strategies. • Ascertain patient's ability to solve problems. **THERAPEUTIC INTERVENTIONS** • Establish open lines of communication. • Provide atmosphere of acceptance by listening attentively to patients, *thereby promoting expression of feelings.*	Positive coping strategies will be enhanced.

Continued.

NURSING DIAGNOSES / DEFINING CHARACTERISTICS	NURSING INTERVENTIONS / *RATIONALES*	EXPECTED OUTCOMES
Perceived personal stress resulting from disease/treatment Lack of support system(s) **DEFINING CHARACTERISTICS** Verbalized fear, anxiety, and feeling of meaninglessness Crying Noncompliance with diet, medications, precautionary measures Difficulty in expressing feelings, especially anger, guilt, fear Nonperformance of ADLs Questions about illness, procedures, and therapy Sense of helplessness/hopelessness Unrealistic expectations of treatments	• Encourage and support patient's search for information. • Answer questions with pertinent, useful information; clarify misconceptions. • Encourage, reinforce, and reward emotional release of energy with regard to stressor events, situations, or changes imposed by disease, treatment, and adaptation. • Encourage patient to identify/use previously effective coping mechanisms. • Implement strategies to foster/enhance self-esteem (e.g., participating in plan of care, caring for self, improving physical appearance, offering realistic reassurance about returning to home and work). • Involve other staff (social workers, psychiatric liaisons, clergy) as indicated *for counseling as needed.* • See Grief over long-term illness/disability, p. 618.	

Originated by: Victoria Frazier-Jones, RN, BSN
                 Christa M. Schroeder, RN, MSN

Blood and blood product transfusion therapy

Homologous donated blood or autologous blood or blood components infused to achieve hemodynamic equilibrium.

(WHOLE BLOOD; PACKED RBCS; PLATELETS; GRANULOCYTES; FRESH FROZEN PLASMA; ALBUMIN; FACTOR VII CRYOPRECIPITATION)

NURSING DIAGNOSES / DEFINING CHARACTERISTICS	NURSING INTEVENTIONS / *RATIONALES*	EXPECTED OUTCOMES
Potential for injury: anaphylactic shock, pulmonary congestion, circulatory overload, hyperkalemia, hematoma *Related to:* Hemolytic/allergic reaction to blood	**ONGOING ASSESSMENT** • Assess for previous transfusions or reactions. • Assess adequacy of venous access. • Check that component order appropriate, that volume order within safe range, and that rate of transfusion appropriate. • Check for signed consent for blood transfusion. *Infusion of blood product should begin within 30 min of receipt of blood on unit.* • Check blood product and patient ID along with blood type and expiration date. Discrepancies must be resolved before product administered.	Risk of transfusion reaction will be reduced.

Blood and blood product transfusion therapy—cont'd

NURSING DIAGNOSES / DEFINING CHARACTERISTICS	NURSING INTERVENTIONS / *RATIONALES*	EXPECTED OUTCOMES

Volume overload
Aged blood
Inadequate IV access
 	
DEFINING CHARACTERISTICS
Chills/fever
Headache/nausea/
vomiting
Urticaria/flushing
Chest pain
Flank pain
Change in vital signs
Change in mentation
	• Obtain baseline vital signs (temperature, pulse, respiratory rate, BP).
	• Take vital signs before therapy begins, then q15min for next hour; then q4h thereafter.
	• Assess patient's cardiorespiratory status to determine amount and rate of infusion.
	• Assess patient for signs/symptoms of reaction to blood product.
	
	THERAPEUTIC INTERVENTIONS
	• Follow hospital policy for obtaining blood product from blood bank.
	• Prime blood tubing with normal saline, IV blood; connect to patient access. *Where fluid volume strictly controlled, only 1 cc normal saline necessary as barrier between IV maintenance solution and blood product to prevent hemolysis.*
	• If a reaction occurs:
	  Stop transfusion; infuse normal saline.
	  Call physician.
	  Administer oxygen as ordered; monitor effectiveness.
	  Treat life-threatening reaction with Benadryl, Epinephrine, as ordered by physician. *Epinephrine: adrenergic agent used to control allergic reactions and acute anaphylactic reactions. Benadryl: antihistamine used to prevent vasodilator effects of histamine, thus preventing edema, itching, bronchospasm if reaction occurs.*
	  Continue to monitor vital signs.
	  Record I & O; obtain blood and urine specimen according to hospital policy for presence of hemoglobin *(which indicates intravascular hemolysis).*
	  Observe for signs of hemorrhage resulting from intravascular coagulation.
	• If no reaction occurs:
	  Infuse total IV ordered blood; flush catheter with normal saline; and reconnect maintenance solution.
	  Obtain post-transfusion vital signs.
	  Complete documentation of transfusion per hospital policy.	

Knowledge deficit *Related to:* Unfamiliarity with transfusion process Misinformation about risks of transfusion **DEFINING CHARACTERISTICS** Questioning Verbalized misconceptions Refusal to permit transfusion	**ONGOING ASSESSMENT** • Assess patient's/family's knowledge of the transfusion process. **THERAPEUTIC INTERVENTIONS** • Reinforce physician explanations; allow time for patient/family to express concerns. • Offer explanations of precautionary measures employed by blood bank; *blood tested for hepatitis B, non-A, non-B, and syphilis; also tested for HIV antibody.* • Acknowledge concerns. • Explain procedure for administering blood so patient not concerned when vital signs taken frequently, etc. Help decrease fear of unknown.	Patient/family will verbalize understanding of need for transfusion and screening process performed before transfusion.

Originated by: Nedra Skale, RN, MS, CNA

Bone marrow harvest: care of the bone marrow donor

The collection of bone marrow via multiple needle aspirations from the posterior iliac crest under general or spinal anesthesia. The anterior iliac crest and sternum may also be used. Bone marrow needles are placed through the skin into the inner cavity of the bone, marrow, along with some blood, is withdrawn. Approximately 200 aspirations are required to collect the desired amount of bone marrow, which is usually 1 to 1½ quarts or about 10% of the patient's total marrow volume.

NURSING DIAGNOSES / DEFINING CHARACTERISTICS	NURSING INTERVENTIONS / *RATIONALES*	EXPECTED OUTCOMES

Knowledge deficit
Related to:
Unfamiliarity with procedure, postoperative care, recovery
Unfamiliarity with discharge activity
 	
Defining Characteristics
Verbalized lack of knowledge or misconceptions
Expressed need for information
Multiple questions
Increased anxiety
	Ongoing Assessment
	• Solicit patient's description and understanding of:
	  Procedure
	  Postoperative care
	  Self-care of bone marrow aspiration sites
	  Potential complications
	  Marrow recovery
	• Assess patient's/significant others' learning capabilities.
	• See Knowledge deficit, p. 33.
	
	Therapeutic Interventions
	• Provide available patient teaching booklets.
	• Discuss pamphlets with patient/significant others; answer questions.
	• Provide private, quite environment for patient teaching.
	• Instruct patient on the following:
	Procedure:
	  Preoperative care
	  Bone marrow aspirations
	  Postoperative care
	  Potential complications
	Site care:
	  Importance of keeping puncture sites clean and dressed for 3 days
	  Importance of keeping sites dry
	  Choice of sponge bath rather than shower or tub bath for 3 days after harvest *to keep puncture sites dry and thus minimize potential risk of infection*
	Pain management:
	  Use of analgesics before pain becomes severe
	  Avoidance of pressure against iliac crest; wearing of loose, nonrestrictive clothing
	  Use of shoes with low heels (sandals, tennis shoes)
	Activity:
	  Return to all activities as tolerated. Inform physician of signs of infection
		Patient/significant others verbalize a basic understanding of bone marrow harvest procedure and recovery and demonstrate knowledge of aspiration site care and potential complications.

Anxiety/fear *Related to:* Impending surgery Fear of anesthesia Fear of pain Threat to or change in health status Threat of death Feelings about bone marrow recipient Responsibility of being donor Fear of unknown	**Ongoing Assessment** • Assess patient's level of anxiety/fear and normal coping patterns. • Assess patient's relationship with bone marrow recipient if appropriate. **Therapeutic Interventions** • Reassure patient that anxiety normal. • Encourage verbalization of feeings, especially about donor role, if appropriate. • Explain patient's relationship with bone marrow recipient *as patient may feel "obligated" or "pressured" to donate marrow especially when only tissue "match" suitable for transplantation.* • Explore potential economic hardships (e.g., loss of work time, cost of travel and hospitalization).	Anxiety/fear will be reduced.

NURSING DIAGNOSES / DEFINING CHARACTERISTICS	NURSING INTERVENTIONS / *RATIONALES*	EXPECTED OUTCOMES
DEFINING CHARACTERISTICS Increased questioning Lack of questioning Restlessness Tense appearance Crying	• Involve other staff (social work, psychiatric liaison, etc.) as indicated. • Assist patient in use of previously successful coping measures. • Provide environment of confidence and reassurance. • See Anxiety, p. 4; and Fear, p. 18.	
Potential fluid volume deficit *Related to:* Restricted intake before procedure Bone marrow volume loss Peripheral blood volume loss Bleeding from bone marrow aspiration sites Postanesthesia vomiting **DEFINING CHARACTERISTICS** Dizziness, lightheadedness Pale, cool, clammy skin Tachycardia Hypotension Weakness Decreased skin turgor Hemoconcentration Decreased urine output	**ONGOING ASSESSMENT** • Assess for Defining Characteristics. • Monitor postoperative vital signs as ordered and more frequently if indicated. • Review OR records to determine total volume of bone marrow collected. • Assess I & O from IV infusions, packed RBC transfusions (intra- and postoperative), vomitus, urine as appropriate. • Maintain accurate I & O recordings. • Monitor lab (e.g., serum electrolytes, Hct) as ordered. • Inspect pressure dressings over bone marrow aspiration site(s) frequently *to detect signs of undue oozing or hemorrhage. Dressings may have small areas of blood (normal).* • Obtain blood sample for PT/PTT as ordered. **THERAPEUTIC INTERVENTIONS** • Initiate IV therapy with lactated Ringer's solution or normal saline as ordered. • Reinfuse patient's own red cells as soon as available (if patient is own donor, i.e., autologous marrow). • Give patient clear liquid diet and advance as tolerated. • Administer antiemetics as ordered. • Document and report to physician bleeding from bone marrow aspiration sites *(may be caused by residual effects of preoperative heparin bolus administered to facilitate easier marrow aspiration).* • Reinforce pressure dressings as needed. • Prepare protamine sulfate if ordered for physician to administer *(drug neutralizes heparin).* • Instruct patient to move slowly and dangle at bedside before getting out of bed *to prevent dizziness/hypotension.* • See Fluid volume deficit, p. 20	Alteration in fluid/electrolyte balance will be reduced.
Potential ineffective breathing pattern *Related to:* Anesthesia Inability to cough and deep breathe adequately **DEFINING CHARACTERISTICS** Auscultation of wheezes, rhonchi, congestion Decreased breath sounds Increased respirations >24/min Decreased respirations <10/min Complaints of shortness of breath or dyspnea	**ONGOING ASSESSMENT** • Assess for Defining Characteristics. • Auscultate lungs q4h and as needed for presence of/change in breath sounds. **THERAPEUTIC INTERVENTIONS** • Encourage patient to turn, cough, and deep breathe q2h *(expands lungs and helps prevent possible infection).* • Encourage patient to use incentive spirometer as indicated.	Optimal respiratory status will be maintained.

Continued.

NURSING DIAGNOSES / DEFINING CHARACTERISTICS	NURSING INTERVENTIONS / *RATIONALES*	EXPECTED OUTCOMES
Pain *Related to:* Multiple puncture wounds in skin and bone Endotracheal intubation (if procedure performed under general anesthesia) Injection site of local anesthetic (if procedure performed under spinal anesthesia) **DEFINING CHARACTERISTICS** Facial grimacing Moaning Verbal complaints of discomfort and pain Restlessness Autonomic responses seen in acute pain (diaphoresis, changes in BP, pulse rate, increased or decreased respiratory rate) Sore throat Headache	**ONGOING ASSESSMENT** - Assess patient for signs/symptoms of discomfort (see Defining Characteristics). - Evaluate effectiveness of pain medication and nonmedication measures to relieve pain. - See Pain, p. 39. **THERAPEUTIC INTERVENTIONS** - Encourage patient to describe discomfort: location, character, intensity, radiation, precipitating factor(s). - Encourage patient to request analgesic at early sign of discomfort *to prevent severe pain.* - Administer analgesics as ordered; evaluate effectiveness, observe for any signs/symptoms of adverse effects. - Provide throat lozenges as needed. - Offer popsicles/cold beverages *(soothing to irritated throat mucous membrane).* - Reposition as needed; use pillows for support. - Handle patient gently and carefully. - Avoid use of rolling board *to prevent exacerbation of discomfort/pain.* - Maintain therapeutic environment (temperature, ventilation, noise control, diversional activities, etc.).	Pain will be reduced or relieved.
Impaired physical mobility *Related to:* Pain **DEFINING CHARACTERISTICS** Reluctance to move Complaints of pain with movement and position changes	**ONGOING ASSESSMENT** - Assess for impaired mobility. - See Mobility, impaired physical, p. 35. **THERAPEUTIC INTERVENTIONS** - Encourage early ADL when possible *to prevent postoperative complications related to prolonged bed rest.* - Instruct patient to change position gradually. - Instruct patient to ambulate slowly and ask for assistance as needed. - Anticipate need for analgesics, especially before activities.	Optimal physical mobility will be maintained.

Potential for infection
Related to:
Interruption of skin and bone integrity secondary to bone marrow aspirations
 	
DEFINING CHARACTERISTICS
Presence of drainage, redness, or swelling at puncture sites
Elevated temperature, pulse, and respiratory rate
Changes in local temperature
	ONGOING ASSESSMENT
	- Assess for Defining Characteristics.
	- Observe puncture sites at time of dressing change for evidence of infection:
	  Skin puncture sites red, tender, warm, swollen
	  Drainage from skin puncture sites
	  Persisting or increasing pain at operative site or near surrounding area
	  Elevated body temperature
	- Obtain culture if ordered before wound cleansed *to obtain true sample of microorganisms present.*
	- Report abnormalities in assessment to physician.
	
	THERAPEUTIC INTERVENTION
	- Change postoperative pressure dressing day after harvest.
	- Use aseptic technique when performing daily dressing changes for 3 days:
	  Wipe over *each* skin puncture site with *new* Betadine wipe; let dry.
	  Apply small amount of Betadine ointment to each puncture site.
	  Cover with sterile adhesive bandage; keep dressings dry and intact.
	- Report signs of infection.
		Risk of infection will be reduced.

Originated by: Victoria Frazier-Jones, RN, BSN

Cancer chemotherapy

Cancer chemotherapy is the administration of cytotoxic drugs by various routes (topical, oral, intramuscular, subcutaneous (SQ), intravenous, intra-arterial, intracavitary, intrathecal, and intravesicular), for the purpose of destroying malignant cells. The goal of chemotherapy may be cure, palliation, or symptom relief.

NURSING DIAGNOSES / DEFINING CHARACTERISTICS	NURSING INTERVENTIONS / *RATIONALES*	EXPECTED OUTCOMES
Knowledge deficit *Related to:* Unfamiliarity with proposed treatment plan/procedures Misinterpretations of information Unfamiliarity with discharge/follow-up care **DEFINING CHARACTERISTICS** Verbalized lack of knowledge Expressed need for information Multiple questions Lack of questions Verbalized misconceptions Verbalized confusion over events	**ONGOING ASSESSMENT** • Solicit patient's/significant others' understanding of: Diagnosis Rationale for chemotherapy Goal of treatment Chemotherapeutic agents to be used Rationale for occurrence of side effects Strategies (including interventions for self-management) aimed at prevent/control of adverse side effects Method of chemotherapy administration Potential problems experienced during chemotherapy administration Schedule of overall treatment plan Anticipated length and number of hospitalizations, clinic/office visits Follow-up care • Assess patient's/significant other's learning capabilities. • Assess patient's/significant other's readiness/willingness to learn. • Assess resources available to ensure compliance with treatment plan. • See Knowledge deficit, p. 33. **THERAPEUTIC INTERVENTIONS** • Provide patient teaching materials (booklets, drug cards, videotape, slide presentation, etc.) as adjunct to individualized education. • Contact National Cancer Institute in Bethesda, Maryland, (1-800-4-CANCER) or oncology clinical nurse specialist for additional patient teaching materials related to chemotherapy. • Discuss teaching materials with patient/significant other. • Restate and reinforce information *to clarify misconceptions and promote better understanding of treatment plan.* • Instruct patient/significant others as needed about: *Treatment plan:* Schedule and need for laboratory tests before and during treatment *to assess for electrolyte and metabolic changes, cardiac/pulmonary/renal alterations, bone marrow function, need for blood component transfusion(s), and presence of infection* Chemotherapy agents to be used Method of administration Schedule of administration *Chemotherapy:* Potential short- and long-term side effects/toxicities Period of anticipated side effects/toxicities Preventive measures to minimize/alleviate potential side effects/toxicities *Discharge planning/teaching:* ADLs Return to work or school Sexual relations/contraception Catheter care (central venous, arterial, intraperitoneal catheters/devices) Signs/symptoms to report to health care professionals (e.g., bleeding, fever, shortness of breath, intractable nausea/vomiting, inability to eat/drink, diarrhea) Measures to prevent infection (*patient's immune function impaired by chemotherapy-induced bone marrow suppression*) Importance of balanced diet and adequate fluid intake Dietary/medications restrictions if indicated	Patient/significant other will verbalize basic understanding of chemotherapy treatment.

Continued.

NURSING DIAGNOSES / DEFINING CHARACTERISTICS	NURSING INTERVENTIONS / *RATIONALES*	EXPECTED OUTCOMES
	Medication(s) after discharge Outpatient follow-up care after discharge Community resources/support systems	
Anxiety/fear *Related to:* Diagnosis of cancer Fear of prognosis Threat of death Past experience with chemotherapy No previous experience with chemotherapy Fear of treatment ("may be worse than disease itself") Fear of pain Fear of unknown Socioeconomic factors (treatment cost, loss of ability to work, etc.) **DEFINING CHARACTERISTICS** Increased questioning Lack of questioning Restlessness Irritability Tearfulness Tense appearance Apprehension Demandingness Anger Withdrawal	**ONGOING ASSESSMENT** · Assess patient's/significant other's anxiety and fear; note verbal and nonverbal cues. · Solicit how patient/significant others coped with stress in past. · Assess patient's/significant other's experience(s) with chemotherapy, perceived degree of treatment success/failure. · Identify patient's support system. **THERAPEUTIC INTERVENTIONS** · Reassure patient/significant other that anxiety normal. · Approach patient with warmth, receptiveness, and consistency. · Encourage patient to identify and verbalize feelings, fears, and concerns. · Correct misconceptions; fill in knowledge gaps. · Encourage patient to identify previously effective coping mechanisms *(may help minimize/alleviate fear/anxiety)*. · Involve other staff (social worker, psychiatric liaison, clergy) *for counseling as needed*. · See Anxiety, p. 4; and Fear, p. 18.	Anxiety/fear will be reduced.
Body image disturbance *Related to:* Loss of hair (scalp, eyebrows, eyelashes, pubic/body hair) Discoloration of fingernails, veins Breakage/loss of fingernails Changes in skin color/texture Generalized "wasting" **DEFINING CHARACTERISTICS** Self-deprecating remarks Refusal to look at self in mirror Crying Anger	**ONGOING ASSESSMENT** · Assess for presence of Defining Characteristics. · Observe for verbal/nonverbal cues to note image alteration. **THERAPEUTIC INTERVENTIONS** · See Body image disturbance, p. 6. · Acknowledge normalcy of emotional response to actual/perceived changes in physical appearance. · Encourage verbalization of feelings, listen to concerns *to alleviate anxiety*. · Convey feelings of acceptance and understanding. · Provide anticipatory guidance on hair alternatives, makeup, skin care, and clothing by supplying/recommending appropriate teaching materials. · Offer realistic assurance of temporary nature of some physical changes (i.e., hair/nails will regrow; external/implanted access devices will eventually be removed, etc.). · Involve other staff (social worker, psychiatric liaison) as indicated *for counseling as needed*.	Feelings about changes in body image will be acknowledged.

NURSING DIAGNOSES / DEFINING CHARACTERISTICS	NURSING INTERVENTIONS / *RATIONALES*	EXPECTED OUTCOMES
Decreased attention to grooming Verbalized ambivalence Compensatory use of makeup, concealing makeup, clothing, devices Decreased social interaction		

NURSING DIAGNOSES / DEFINING CHARACTERISTICS	NURSING INTERVENTIONS / *RATIONALES*	EXPECTED OUTCOMES
Nausea/vomiting *Related to:* *Treatment effects:* Side effects of chemotherapy Side effects of radiation therapy (brain, esophagus, stomach, and/or intestines involved in treatment fields) Medications (e.g., narcotics, antibiotics, vitamins, iron, digitalis) *Disease effects:* Primary malignancy/metastasis to CNS Increased intracranial pressure resulting from tumor, intracranial bleeding Obstruction of GI tract by tumor Tumor waste products Renal dysfunction Electrolyte imbalances (e.g., hypercalcemia, hyponatremia) Pain *Psychogenic effects:* Conditioning to adversive stimuli (e.g., anticipatory nausea/vomiting; tension, anxiety, stress) **DEFINING CHARACTERISTICS** Nausea "Greasy" stomach Retching Straining Expulsion of gastric contents through mouth Inability to look at/smell food	**ONGOING ASSESSMENT** - Assess for presence of Defining Characteristics. - Obtain history of previous patterns of nausea/vomiting, treatment measures effective in past. - Solicit patient's description of nausea/vomiting pattern: Onset Severity Duration Precipitating factors - Evaluate effectiveness of antiemetic/comfort measure regimens. - Observe patient for potential complications of prolonged nausea/vomiting: Fluid/electrolyte imbalance (e.g., dehydration, hypokalemia, decreased H and Cl) Weight loss Decreased activity level Weakness, lethargy, apathy, anxiety Aspiration pneumonia Esophageal trauma Tenderness/pain in abdomen and chest **THERAPEUTIC INTERVENTIONS** - Administer chemotherapy in late afternoon, at night if possible. - Administer antiemetics around the clock rather than "prn" during periods of high incidence of nausea/vomiting. *(Maintain adequate plasma levels and thus increase effectiveness of antiemetic therapy.)* - Adjust antiemetic regimen as appropriate in consultation with physician. - Institute/teach measures to minimize/prevent nausea/vomiting: Small dietary intake before treatment(s) Foods with low potential to cause nausea/vomiting (e.g., dry toast, crackers, ginger ale, cola, popsicles, gelatin, baked/boiled potatoes, fresh/canned fruit) Avoidance of spices, gravy, or greasy foods Modifications in diet (e.g., choice of bland foods) Small, frequent nutritious meals Attractive servings Avoidance of coaxing, bribing, or threatening in relation to intake. (Help family to avoid being "food pushers.") Sufficient time for meals Rest periods before and after meals Sucking on hard candy while receiving chemotherapeutic drugs with "metallic taste" (e.g., Cytoxan, Dacarbazine (DTIC), Cisplatinum, Actinomycin D, Mustargen, Methotrexate) Minimal physical activity and no sudden rapid movement during times of increased nausea *(may actually potentiate nausea/vomiting)* Quiet, restful, cool, well-ventilated environment Comfortable position Diversional activities Relaxation/distraction techniques Antiemetic half hour before meals as ordered	Occurrence of nausea/vomiting will be reduced, controlled, or absent.

Continued.

NURSING DIAGNOSES / DEFINING CHARACTERISTICS	NURSING INTERVENTIONS / *RATIONALES*	EXPECTED OUTCOMES
Nausea/vomiting before therapy or contact with health care personnel/system	• Identify and provide favorite foods; avoid serving during nausea/vomiting. *(Patient may develop aversion.)* • Keep clean emesis basin/tissue/mouthwash within reach; remove emesis promptly. • Provide/encourage mouth care after vomiting; wash face with cool cloth. • Position patient during vomiting episode *to decrease aspiration risk.*	
Altered integrity of oral/oropharyngeal mucosa *Related to:* Side effect of chemotherapy (damaged and destroyed epithelial cells; immunosuppression/ myelosupression Dehydration Protein malnutrition Poor oral hygiene **DEFINING CHARACTERISTICS** Reddened mucosa Dry, shiny oral mucosa Burning/tightness in mouth Pain when drinking, chewing, and/or swallowing Mucosal ulceration Mucosal sloughing Bleeding	**ONGOING ASSESSMENT** • Assess for Defining Characteristics. • Assess status of oral tissue twice daily; report changes in appearance, taste, and sensation *to identify changes in mucosal integrity.* **THERAPEUTIC INTERVENTIONS** See Stomatitis, p. 521.	Development of stomatitis related to cancer chemotherapy will be reduced or prevented.

Diarrhea
Related to:
Side effect of chemotherapy
Side effect of radiation therapy with bowel involved in treatment field
Side effect of antiemetic therapy (e.g., metaclopramide)
Concentrated supplemental feedings
Laxatives/stool softeners
 	
DEFINING CHARACTERISTICS
Loose/liquid stools
Frequent stools
Urge to defecate
Cramping
Abdominal pain
Hyperactive bowel sounds/sensations
Flatus
	ONGOING ASSESSMENT
	• Assess for presence of Defining Characteristics.
	• Obtain history of patient's usual bowel pattern:
	  Frequency
	  Character of stool:
	    Color
	    Amount
	    Odor
	    Consistency
	  Type/frequency of laxative/stool softener used by patient *to prevent constipation secondary to medication(s) (e.g., narcotics)*
	• Observe stool pattern. Record frequency, character, and volume.
	• Monitor I & O.
	• Obtain stool specimen for culture and sensitivity as ordered.
	
	THERAPEUTIC INTERVENTIONS
	• Administer antidiarrheal antispasmodics as ordered; document effectiveness.
	• Implement meticulous perineal hygiene measures after bowel movements *to prevent mucosal irritation/breakdown.*
	• See Leukemia, acute, p. 510.
	• Modify diet *to decrease diarrhea risk/potentiation:*
	  Avoid concentrated supplemental feedings.
	  Serve foods at room temperature; avoid ice chips, popsicles until cramping/diarrhea subsides.
		Normal elimination pattern will be maintained/achieved.

NURSING DIAGNOSES / DEFINING CHARACTERISTICS	NURSING INTERVENTIONS / *RATIONALES*	EXPECTED OUTCOMES
	Provide clear, liquid diet during diarrhea episodes.	
	• Replace fluids lost via emesis with high caloric, electrolyte-rich liquids (e.g., Gatorade, soft drinks).	
	• See also Diarrhea, p. 16.	
Potential fluid volume deficit *Related to:* Side effects of chemotherapy: Nausea Vomiting Diarrhea Mucositis Diuretic therapy administered as adjunct to certain chemotherapy regimens (e.g., cisplatin, high-dose Cytoxan)	**ONGOING ASSESSMENT** • Assess for presence of Defining Characteristics. • Assess type and amount of fluid I & O; record accurately. • Monitor appropriate lab values (e.g., electrolytes, BUN, creatinine, serum osmolality). • Check daily weight. • Monitor vital signs for changes; *tachycardia can be an early sign of dehydration.* **THERAPEUTIC INTERVENTIONS** • See Fluid volume deficit, p. 20.	Optimal fluid status and electrolyte balance will be maintained.
DEFINING CHARACTERISTICS Decreased urine output Output > intake Thirst Decreased skin turgor Dry mucous membranes Increased pulse rate Decreased pulse volume/pressure Weakness Edema Possible weight gain Possible weight loss Decreased serum potassium Increased serum sodium Increased serum BUN/ creatinine Hemoconcentration		
Potential fluid volume overload *Related to:* Aggressive IV hydration (e.g., with cisplatin/ methotrexate/high dose Cytoxan-based treatment regimens) **DEFINING CHARACTERISTICS** Fluid intake > urine output Weight gain	**ONGOING ASSESSMENT** • Assess for Defining Characteristics. • Monitor vital signs q4h and as needed. • Weight patient at same time with same scale daily *to assure accuracy.* • Record accurate I & O. **THERAPEUTIC INTERVENTIONS** • Administer diuretics as ordered: observe for effectiveness and side effects; document. • Infuse IV solutions as ordered via infusion control device *to assure accurate flow rate and prevent unintentional fluid overload.* • Provide measures to decrease anxiety/stress. • Plan activities to allow minimum energy expenditure with adequate rest periods.	Fluid overload will be reduced or prevented.

Continued.

NURSING DIAGNOSES / DEFINING CHARACTERISTICS	NURSING INTERVENTIONS / *RATIONALES*	EXPECTED OUTCOMES
Shortness of breath Dyspnea Rales Rhonchi Edema Distended neck veins Changes in vital signs (BP, heart/respiratory rate) Anxiety Restlessness	- Position patient in semi-Fowler's or Fowler's position *to facilitate breathing.* - Administer O$_2$ as ordered. - See Breathing pattern, ineffective, p. 8.	

Altered nutrition: less than body requirements
Related to:
Side effects of chemotherapy (inability to taste and smell foods, loss of appetite, nausea, vomiting, mucositis, dry mouth, diarrhea)
Depression
Circulating tumor byproducts
Pain
 	
DEFINING CHARACTERISTICS
Weight loss
Documented inadequate caloric intake
Indifference to food
Irritability
Weakness
Fatigue
Poor skin turgor
Dry, shiny oral mucous membranes
Thick, scanty saliva
Muscle wasting
	ONGOING ASSESSMENT
	- Assess for presence of Defining Characteristics.
	- Weigh patient daily at same time with same scale *to assure accuracy.*
	- Monitor calorie counts daily *to determine whether oral intake meets daily nutritional requirement.*
	- Monitor appropriate lab values (e.g., CBC/differential, electrolytes, serum iron, TIBC, total protein, albumin).
	- Evaluate effectiveness of antiemetic/analgesic management.
	
	THERAPEUTIC INTERVENTIONS
	- See Nutrition, altered: less than body requirements, p. 37.
	- Explain rationale and measures to increase sensitivity of taste buds:
	  Perform mouth care before and after meals.
	  Change seasonings to compensate for altered sweet/sour threshold.
	  Increase use of sweeteners/flavorings in foods.
	  Warm foods to increase aroma.
	- Serve foods cold if odors cause aversions.
	- Offer meat dishes in morning. *(Aversions tend to increase during day: chicken, cheese, eggs, fish usually well-tolerated protein sources.)*
	- Serve supplements between meals; have patient sip slowly *to prevent bloating/nausea/vomiting/diarrhea.*
	- Explain rationale and measures to provide moisture in oral cavity if indicated:
	  Frequent intake of nonirritating fluids (e.g., grape or apple juice)
	  Sucking on smooth, flat substances (e.g., lozenges; tart, sugar-free candy; hot tea with lemon) *to increase saliva flow*
	  Use of artificial saliva
	  Liquids sipped with meals
	  Foods moistened with sauces/liquids
	  Strict oral hygiene before and after meals; avoidance of alcohol-containing commercial mouthwashes or lemon-glycerin swabs *(drying to oral mucosa)*
	  Lips moistened with balm, water-soluble lubricating jelly, lanolin, or coca butter
	  Humid environment air via vaporizer or pan of water near heat *(except when patient luekopenic because of risk of* Pseudomonas *infection).*
	- Titrate dosage/frequency of antiemetic(s)/analgesic(s) within prescribed parameters as needed until effective therapeutic levels achieved.
		Optimal nutritional status will be maintained.

NURSING DIAGNOSES / DEFINING CHARACTERISTICS	NURSING INTERVENTIONS / *RATIONALES*	EXPECTED OUTCOMES
Potential for infection *Related to:* *Treatment effects:* Granulocytopenia/ leukopenia secondary bone marrow toxicity of chemotherapy Side effect of radiation therapy with bone marrow producing sites in treatment field (e.g., skull, sternum, ribs, vertebrae, pelvis, ends of long bones) *Disease effects:* Invasion or "crowding" of bone marrow by malignant cells (especially secondary to hematologic malignancies, e.g., leukemia, lymphoma, multiple myeloma) Anergy (absence of immune response) **DEFINING CHARACTERISTICS** Fever Sore throat Flushed appearance Diaphoresis Rigors Shaking chill Abnormal sputum Rales Decreased breath sounds Pleuritic pain Increased pulse and respiratons Decreased BP Urinary frequency/ burning Vaginal discharge Redness/tenderness over peripheral IV puncture or indwelling venous catheter sites Decrease in circulating white blood cells characterized by profound decrease of neutrophils	**ONGOING ASSESSMENT** • Assess for Defining Characteristics. • Monitor WBC, differential, and absolute granulocyte count daily. *Absolute granulocyte count (AGC) calculated by multiplying WBC count by percentage of granulocytes in differential (e.g., AGC = WBC × % granulocytes).* **THERAPEUTIC INTERVENTIONS** • Determine anticipated nadir and recovery of bone marrow after chemotherapy administration *to plan for appropriate nursing care measures. Nadir: time of greatest bone marrow supression (e.g., when RBCs, WBCs, and platelets at lowest points). Each chemotherapeutic agent causes nadir at different time for each blood element; however, most drugs demonstrate nadir 7-14 days after start of chemotherapy with bone marrow recovery over another 5-10 days.* • See Granulocytopenia, p. 505. • See Leukemia, acute, p. 510. • See Autologous bone marrow transplantation, p. 527.	Risk of local/systemic infection will be decreased.

Continued.

Cancer chemotherapy—cont'd

NURSING DIAGNOSES / DEFINING CHARACTERISTICS	NURSING INTERVENTIONS / *RATIONALES*	EXPECTED OUTCOMES
Injury: potential for bleeding *Related to:* *Treatment effects:* 　Thrombocytopenia secondary to bone marrow toxicity of chemotherapy/ radiation therapy 　Mucosal soughing 　Anticoagulants *Disease effects:* 　Invasion of bone marrow by malignant cells 　Disease of bone marrow 　Genetically transmitted platelet deficiency 　coagulopathies (tumor-related or other) 　Abnormal hepatic/ renal function 　Fever 　Infection/sepsis 　DIC *Pharmacologic effects:* 　Aspirin use 　Thiazides, estrogens 　Alcohol **DEFINING CHARACTERISTICS** Decreased total circulating platelets and platelet percursors Prolonged oozing of blood from IM, IV, venipuncture, or bone marrow sites Oozing of blood from gums Epistaxis Spontaneous bruises, ecchymoses, hematomas, petachiae Hematemesis Hemoptysis Hematuria Vaginal bleeding Hypermenorrhea Black, tarry stools Neurologic status changes (i.e., headaches, blurred vision, disorientation, loss of coordination) Orthostatic changes	**ONGOING ASSESSMENT** • Assess for Defining Characteristics. • Monitor platelets/Hb/Hct daily *to detect changes early;* anticipate platelet count nadir. • Monitor coagulation parameters (fibrinogen, thrombin time, bleeding time, fibrin degradation products) if indicated. Changes in coagulation profile may be marked by: 　Ecchymoses 　Hematomas 　Petechia 　Blood in body excretions 　Bleeding from body orifices 　Change in neurologic status 　Changes in vital signs • Monitor vital signs q4h and as indicated. • Inspect patient at regularly (every shift) daily for evidence of: 　Spontaneous petechiae (all skin surfaces, including oral mucosa) 　Prolonged bleeding or new areas of ecchymoses or hematoma from invasive procedures (venipuncture, injection, and bone marrow sites) 　Oozing of blood from nose/gums **THERAPEUTIC INTERVENTIONS** • Determine nadir and anticipated recovery of bone marrow after administration. • Inform patient/significant other of relationship between platelets and bleeding: 　Platelet function 　Normal platelet count 　Effects of chemotherapy on bone marrow function, platelet count 　Risk of bleeding associated with decreased platelet count: 　　$<20,000/mm^3$: severe risk 　　$20,000\text{-}50,000/mm^3$: moderately severe risk 　　$50,000\text{-}100,000/mm^3$: mild risk 　　$>100,000/mm^3$: no significant risk • Implement bleeding precautions for platelet count $<50,000/mm^3$. *(At this level spontaneous bleeding can occur.)* • See Leukemia, acute, p. 510, for bleeding precautions/nursing interventions. • Emphasize to patient/significant other importance of consistent practice of measures to prevent bleeding and prompt reporting of all signs/symptoms of suspected or actual bleeding. • Communicate anticipated need for platelet support to transfusion center *to assure availability, readiness of platelets when needed.* • Transfuse single or random donor platelets as ordered. • Administer fresh frozen plasma or coagluation factors as ordered *to replace needed clotting factors.* • Transfuse packed red blood cells as ordered if significant drop in Hb/Hct noted.	Complications of bleeding will be reduced or prevented.

NURSING DIAGNOSES / DEFINING CHARACTERISTICS	NURSING INTERVENTIONS / *RATIONALES*	EXPECTED OUTCOMES
Increased pulse rate Decreased Hb/Hct Fever Weakness/lethargy		
Potential for injury: anemia *Related to:* *Treatment effects:* Anemia secondary to bone marrow toxicity of chemotherapy/ radiation therapy *Disease effects:* Primary disease bone marrow (e.g., leukemia, aplastic anemia) Infiltration of bone marrow by malig- nant cells Autoimmune disor- ders Renal disease Exposure to toxic substances (e.g., benzene, antibiot- ics) Nutritional deficien- cies (e.g., de- creased vitamin K, folic acid, B_{12}, iron intake absorption/use)	**ONGOING ASSESSMENT** • Assess for Defining Characteristics. • Monitor Hb/Hct daily *to detect changes early;* anticipate nadir. • Determine nadir, anticipated recovery of bone marrow after chemotherapy administration. **THERAPEUTIC INTERVENTIONS** • Estimate energy expenditures of ADLs; prioritize activities accordingly. • Plan/promote rest periods *to lower body's oxygen requirement and decrease cardiopulmonary strain.* • Provide warm clothing/blankets, comfortable environment; avoid drafts. • See Anemia, p. 498. • Maintain current blood sample for "type and screen" in transfusion center *to assure availability, readiness of packed red blood cells when needed.* • Transfuse packed red cells as ordered *to restore Hb/Hct to levels where patient experiences minimal symptoms.* • See Blood and blood product transfusion therapy, p. 538.	Potential complica-tions of anemia will be reduced/prevented.
DEFINING CHARACTERISTICS Decreased Hb/Hct Decreased red blood cell indices Tiredness Weakness Lethargy Fatigue Listlessness Pallor (skin, nailbeds, conjunctiva, circu- moral) Dyspnea on exertion Changes in vital signs: increased pulse respi- rations, and pulse pressure, decreased blood pressure Palpitations/chest pain on exertion Dizziness/syncope Hypersensitivity to cold		

Continued.

NURSING DIAGNOSES / DEFINING CHARACTERISTICS	NURSING INTERVENTIONS / *RATIONALES*	EXPECTED OUTCOMES

Potential for injury
Related to:
Hypersensitivity to drug(s)
Potential side effects/ toxicities of drug(s)
 	
Defining Characteristics
Chemotherapeutic drugs:
  Restlessness
  Facial edema/ flushing
  Wheezes
  Bronchospasms
  Tachycardia
  Hypotension
  Diaphoresis
  Fever
  Increased uric acid levels
  Runny nose
  Skin rash
Antiemetic drugs:
  Agitation
  Hypotension
  Irritability
  Facial flushing
  Extrapyramidal reactions
	Ongoing Assessment
	• Note allergy history.
	• Monitor relevant data (CBC, differential, platelets, other laboratory values, ECGs if indicated) on ongoing basis and before chemotherapy administration.
	• Monitor vital signs q4h and as needed.
	• Obtain, record vital signs before antiemetic/chemotherapy *to serve as baseline throughout and after administration.*
	• Observe closely for changes in patient's status and potential immediate/ delayed adverse side effects and toxicities.
	• See Tumor lysis syndrome, p. 524.
	
	Therapeutic Interventions
	• Verify physician's written order for specific drug name, dose, route, time, and frequency of administration.
	• Recalculate drug dosage if indicated.
	• Know immediate and delayed side effects of drug(s) to be administered.
	• Inform patient/significant other to report adverse effects. *Delineate which changes indicate emergencies that must be reported immediately (changes patient perceives as "minor" may be highly significant).*
	• Maintain/restore adequate fluid balance *to reduce potential drug toxicity as fluids help clear body of accumulated metabolic by-products.*
	• Keep emergency drugs (IV Benadryl, hydrocortisone, Epinephrine 1:1000) readily available when administering chemotherapeutic drugs with higher than usual risk for anaphylaxis (e.g., Bleomycin, Elspar, Cis-Platin, and Etoposide).
	• When adverse drug reaction suspected:
	  Stop infusion.
	  Administer emergency drugs as ordered.
	  Notify physician.
	  Take and record vital signs.
	  Maintain KVO IV with NS solution.
	  Reassure patient.
	• See Anaphylactic shock, p. 64.
		Risk of injury from drug therapy will be reduced.

Potential for injury
Related to:
Extravasation
Infiltration or leakage of chemotherapeutic drug from vein, defective or malpositioned indwelling central venous catheter/access device into local subcutaneous tissue surrounding administration site
 	
Defining Characteristics
Tenderness, pain, stinging, burning, and swelling at IV site and surrounding area
Pink or red "streaking" extending from IV site along source of affected vein and tissue
	Ongoing Assessment
	• Observe injection/infusion site closely during chemotherapy administration.
	• Assess at frequent intervals per established hospital policy/procedure:
	  Blood return
	  Patency of vein/catheter
	  Signs of infiltration outlined in Defining Characteristics
	• Instruct patient to report tenderness, stinging, burning, or other unusual sensation at IV site immediately.
	
	Therapeutic Interventions
	• Know local toxicity of chemotherapeutic agent(s) administered and hospital policy/procedure of intervention in event of extravasation.
	• Select veins most suitable for administration of chemotherapeutic agents (e.g., cephalic, median brachial, and basilic vein in midforearm area).
	• Avoid veins in anticubital fossa, near wrist, or dorsal surface of hand. *(Damage to underlying tendons/nerves may occur in event of drug extravasation.)*
	• Keep extravasation kit accessible; contents vary according to hospital policy.
	• Evaluate patient complaints of "painful infusion"; rule out source extravasation versus other causes of pain (may include chemical composition of drug, venous spasm, phlebitis, and/or psychogenic factors).
	• When drug extravasation suspected
	  Stop infusion.
	  Initiate extravasation management appropriate for chemotherapeutic drug infiltrated.
		Incidence/ complications of drug extravasation will be reduced or prevented.

Cancer chemotherapy—cont'd

NURSING DIAGNOSES / DEFINING CHARACTERISTICS	NURSING INTERVENTIONS / *RATIONALES*	EXPECTED OUTCOMES
Scanty or no blood return via peripheral IV or central venous catheter Edema, erythema, coldness, or warmth at infusion site extending to surrounding area	Notify physician. Reassure patient. Document incident per hospital policy/procedure. *Management of site after extravasation remains a controversial issue in chemotherapy administration. However, most hospitals/agencies have developed care standards in management of extravasation of drugs classified as "vesicants." These agents potentially cause cellular damage, ulceration, and tissue necrosis. Plastic surgeon may be consulted for consideration of débridement/skin grafting.*	

Originated by: Concordia Solita, RN, BSN
             Christa M. Schroeder, RN, MSN

Hickman right atrial catheter

(CENTRAL LINE)

Indwelling silicone rubber catheter placed in the right atrium for access to the venous system, used for long-term intravenous therapy.

NURSING DIAGNOSES / DEFINING CHARACTERISTICS	NURSING INTERVENTIONS / *RATIONALES*	EXPECTED OUTCOMES

Knowledge deficit
Related to:
Newness, complexity of procedure
 	
DEFINING CHARACTERISTICS
Several questions
Excessive anxiety
Inability to talk about procedure
Lack of questions
Inability to enumerate uses of Hickman catheter
Inability to identify potential catheter-related complications
	ONGOING ASSESSMENT
	• Assess current level of knowledge.
	• Assess patient's/significant other's learning capabilities.
	
	THERAPEUTIC INTERVENTIONS
	• Provide patient/significant others information about Hickman catheter:
	    Purpose
	    Procedure
	    Complications
	    Ongoing care
	    Duration
	• Provide printed teaching handouts as references.
	• Reinforce previous learning.
	• Encourage questions *(misunderstanding/lack of knowledge often basis for fear/anxiety)*.
	• Develop family rapport.
		Patient/significant others will state purpose, function, and care of Hickman catheter.

Potential for injury: hemorrhage *Related to:* Subclavian or carotid artery injury **DEFINING CHARACTERISTICS** Patient complaints of shortness of breath Hemoptysis Hypertension Swelling on affected side	**ONGOING ASSESSMENT** • Assess character of respiration. • Check for changes in vital signs, drop in blood pressure, increased respiratory rate. **THERAPEUTIC INTERVENTIONS** • Elevate HOB *to improve lung expansion.* • Notify physician of changes in vital signs and respiratory status. • Prepare/set up intervention (oxygen, thoracentesis, blood transfusion). • Alleviate patient's fear/anxiety *to promote ease of respiration.*	Effect of subclavian or carotid artery injury is reduced.

Continued.

NURSING DIAGNOSES / DEFINING CHARACTERISTICS	NURSING INTERVENTIONS / *RATIONALES*	EXPECTED OUTCOMES

Decreased cardiac output secondary to cardiac arrythmias (PVCs)
Related to:
Irritation of ventricular endocardium by catheter during insertion/ repositioning
Lodging of catheter tip in tricuspid valve
 	
DEFINING CHARACTERISTICS
Palpitation
Dizziness and fainting
Shortness of breath
Arrhythmia seen in ECG
Irregular apical pulse
	ONGOING ASSESSMENT
	• Document baseline precatheterization vital signs.
	• Observe patient for arrhythmias after catheter insertion.
	• Obtain catheter position on chest x-ray and whenever arrhythmias occur or inform physician of need for x-ray examination.
	• If arrhythmias occur:
	  Assess patient for complaints of dizziness, palpitations, lightheadedness, shortness of breath.
	  Observe contributing factors that may have potentiated arrhythmias (e.g., patient/catheter position; other medical problems) *to correct/intervene as early as possible.*
	
	THERAPEUTIC INTERVENTIONS
	• Inform physician of need for intervention.
	• Treat arrhythmias as indicated.
		Occurrence of ventricular arrhythmias will be reduced.

Potential for injury: pneumothorax *Related to:* Use of subclavian insertion site Patient movement during insertion **DEFINING CHARACTERISTICS** Shortness of breath Decreased breath sounds on affected side Unequal thoracic wall movement Shift of trachea toward unaffected side	**ONGOING ASSESSMENT** • Assess breath sounds, respiratory pattern, and chest movement before and immediately after insertion. • When checking for catheter placement on x-ray, note lung expansion. **THERAPEUTIC INTERVENTIONS** • Keep patient still during procedure. Provide sedative, local anesthesia, and reassurances as needed. • Provide optimal positioning at time of insertion (towel roll in back/ shoulder/subclavian region) *to minimize risk for accidental puncture of pleura.* • If pneumothorax symptoms noted, refer to physician and anticipate chest tube insertion.	Occurrence of pneumothorax will be reduced.

Pain
Related to:
Difficult/traumatic insertion
Tunnel phlebitis
Deep vein thrombosis
 	
DEFINING CHARACTERISTICS
Report of discomfort
Edema of neck and extremity
Limited movement of extremity
	ONGOING ASSESSMENT
	• Check insertion site q4h or prn for signs of inflammation or discomfort.
	• Check site for swelling. Compare with unaffected side.
	
	THERAPEUTIC INTERVENTIONS
	• Assist during insertion *so catheter positioned smoothly and rapidly.*
	• Maintain optimal position of extremity. Elevate distal portion of extremity.
	• Avoid tight bandaging of affected extremity. Use occlusive but nonconstricting dressing *to allow adequate circulation.*
	• *Promote circulation to affected extremity* by performing active/passive ROM, noting limitation of catheter.
	• If pain, phlebitis, or inflammation occurs:
	  Facilitate removal of catheter.
	  Apply warm compresses.
	  Elevate extremity.
	  Give pain medication prn.
		Pain in affected extremity is reduced/ relieved.

NURSING DIAGNOSES / DEFINING CHARACTERISTICS	NURSING INTERVENTIONS / *RATIONALES*	EXPECTED OUTCOMES
Potential for infection *Related to:* Indwelling catheter Manipulation of catheter connecting tubing Prolonged use of catheter **DEFINING CHARACTERISTICS** Redness at site Swelling Change in local temperature Drainage from catheter exit site Fever	**ONGOING ASSESSMENT** • Check insertion site for signs of infection. • Assess vital signs q4h as needed. **THERAPEUTIC INTERVENTIONS** • Change IV tubing per policy *to minimize possibility of contamination.* • Change Hickman catheter site dressing by sterile technique. • If infection occurs, notify physician for culturing, treatment, and possible catheter removal *to halt spread of infection.*	Occurrence of infection will be reduced.

Potential for injury: impaired catheter function
Related to
Mechanical impairment (e.g., clotting of catheter)
 	
DEFINING CHARACTERISTICS
Resistant or sluggish infusion of parenteral solutions and blood products.
Leakage of fluids from catheter or exit site
Inability to obtain blood return
	ONGOING ASSESSMENT
	• Check continuity of catheter.
	• Check for patency.
	• Flush line; note for leakage or resistance.
	• Observe gravitational flow (e.g., in transfusion of blood products).
	
	THERAPEUTIC INTERVENTIONS
	• Flush catheter per established policy/procedure *to prevent catheter clotting:*
	    At the end of every blood drawing procedure
	    At completion of each IV solution and blood product
	    Before capping catheter
	• Use mechanical IV pumps *to prevent "dry" IVs and backing up of blood into catheter.*
	• Repair external damage per manufacturing company recommendations or established procedures.
	• Notify physician for suspected internal catheter damage.
		Risk for injury is reduced.

Originated by: Neil Rey B. Bonje, RN, BSN

Sexually Transmitted Disease Care Plans

Acquired immune deficiency syndrome (AIDS)

Chlamydia

Gonorrhea

Herpes simplex virus: type II

Human papilloma virus

Syphilis

Acquired immune deficiency syndrome (AIDS)

(HUMAN IMMMUNODEFICIENCY VIRUS [HIV];
AIDS-RELATED COMPLEX [ARC];
OPPORTUNISTIC INFECTIONS)

Human immunodeficiency virus (HIV), either alone or in combination with other viral or idiopathic cofactors, causes acquired immune deficiency syndrome (AIDS). In 1988, HIV infected between 1.0 and 1.5 million Americans. The virus is spread in three ways: across the placenta, during sexual activity (heterosexual and homosexual), and by sharing of intravenous drug equipment. Early in the epidemic, blood products spread the virus, but measures to screen donors greatly improved the safety of blood products. Most of the early victims of the syndrome were gay men; however, in many cities today, infected IV drug users and their children outnumber infected gay men. Between 4 and 24 weeks after infection, an antibody to HIV appears in the adult patient's blood. Between 1 and 30 years later (8 years on average), the adult patient's immune system weakens enough to allow an opportunistic infection to develop. Some patients develop AIDS-related complex (ARC), a syndrome of weight loss, lymphadenopathy, night sweats, and fatigue, before the onset of an opportunistic infection, but other patients do not go through an ARC stage. Antiviral, vaccine, and immunity-enhancing therapies change rapidly and cannot be detailed in this care plan, nor does it outline local laws regarding conents for HIV testing, HIV reporting, and protection against discrimination, although these are significant concerns. It should also be noted that patients present at various stages of the disease.

NURSING DIAGNOSES / DEFINING CHARACTERISTICS	NURSING INTERVENTIONS / *RATIONALES*	EXPECTED OUTCOMES
Knowledge deficit: disease and transmission *Related to:* New condition **DEFINING CHARACTERISTICS** Multiple questions Lack of questions Confusion about disease, complications	**ONGOING ASSESSMENT** • Assess patient's knowledge of disease process, routes of transmission, complications, treatment, and modalities. **THERAPEUTIC INTERVENTIONS** • Instruct patient in dose, schedule, and side effects of antiviral, fungalstatic, and prophylactic medication. • Instruct patient regarding schedule of outpatient appointments and treatments. • Instruct patient in signs/symptoms of disease, opportunistic infections, and neoplasms and person to whom information should be reported. • Instruct patient in routes of HIV transmission. • Instruct patient in methods of preventing HIV transmission: Safe sex: Kissing Touching Mutual masturbation Probably safe: Vaginal or anal intercourse with latex condom and spermicidal lubricant *Nonoxyl-9 spermicide inactivates HIV in vitro; efficacy and side effects in vivo untested. Properly used, latex condom reduces HIV transmission risk for both partners.* Unsafe: Vaginal or anal intercourse without condom Sexual activities that cause bleeding Uncertain: Oral intercourse between man and woman, two men, two women *Although early studies indicated less risk during oral intercourse than vaginal or anal without condom, risk difficult to measure and unknown.*	Patient will verbalize understanding of disease process, transmission, complications, and treatment modalities.

Continued.

557

NURSING DIAGNOSES / DEFINING CHARACTERISTICS	NURSING INTERVENTIONS / *RATIONALES*	EXPECTED OUTCOMES
	• Role play to practice new behaviors in situations that may lead to transmission (e.g., saying no, or negotiating condom use).	
	• Explore possible benefits/drawbacks of sexual or needle-sharing partner's being tested for HIV. *Benefits include initiation of antiviral therapy if helper T-cell counts low. Drawbacks include possible discrimination and emotional depression.*	
	• Instruct patient/partners to avoid pregnancy. Instruct in birth control methods, including condom use. *Approximately 50% of infants of HIV-infected mothers are infected.*	
	• Encourage use of clean IV equipment with recreational drugs. *HIV is quickly killed by 10% hypochlorite solution. Flush syringe and needles with household bleach diluted ninefold with water; rinse with tap water. Refer to drug rehabilitation program.*	
	• Refrain from donating blood, semen, or organs.	
	• Do not share razors, toothbrushes.	
	• Clean blood or excreta containing blood with 10% hypochlorite solution. *Not necessary to use bleach to wash patient's dishes, clothes, or personal items.*	

	• Instruct patient to avoid exposure to infectious diseases:
	    Avoid contact with people who have infectious diseases.
	    Avoid sexual practices that lead to sexually transmitted diseases (STDs). *Used properly, condoms can help prevent STD spread during vaginal or anal intercourse. Immunocompromised people are especially vulnerable to viral infections (e.g., herpes or genital warts). Syphilis is more difficult to diagnose and treat in HIV-infected persons and progresses more rapidly. Normally nonpathogenic intestinal flora may cause disease in HIV-infected persons; therefore, they should refrain from anal-oral sexual activities. Dildoes and vibrators may act as fomites; therefore, should not be shared.*
	    Avoid changing cat's litter box. *Toxoplasmosis may be transmitted from stool of infected cat.*
	    Avoid raw vegetables, fish, milk, and meat *(harbor bacteria and protozoa that may cause infection in immuncompromized person).*	

	• Instruct patient to observe for signs of lactose intolerance; if present, change diet.	
Altered patterns of sexuality *Related to:* Physical limitation (chronic or time-limited, acute illness, fatigue or exercise intolerance Fear of AIDS/other STDs Knowledge deficit: safe sexual practices Altered self-concept Impaired relationships: loss of significant other, social isolation, or incomplete socialization to sexual orientation **DEFINING CHARACTERISTICS** Verbalized concern(s) about sexual functions	**ONGOING ASSESSMENT** • Assess for presence of Defining Characteristics. • Determine patient/significant other's concerns about AIDS. • Determine sexual orientation; number, kinds of sexual partners; recent, usual sexual activities. • Elicit patient's feelings about changed sexual behavior. **THERAPEUTIC INTERVENTIONS** • Explore ways to express physical intimacy during treatment that exclude vaginal, rectal, and pharyngeal intercourse. • Explore ways to express physical intimacy that will not lead to infection. • Explore patient's sexual partner's perceptions about his/her risk of HIV infection. *Fear of AIDS may alter sexual patterns.* • See Sexuality patterns, altered, p. 47.	Optimal means of satisfying sexual needs will be achieved.

Aquired immune deficiency syndrome—cont'd

NURSING DIAGNOSES / DEFINING CHARACTERISTICS	NURSING INTERVENTIONS / *RATIONALES*	EXPECTED OUTCOMES
Questions about "normal" sexual function Noncompliance with medications/ treatments with known risk of impaired sexual function Expressed decrease in sexual satisfaction Reported change in relationship with partner(s) Actual/perceived limitation secondary to diagnosis or therapy Sexually inappropriate behavior within setting Frequent seeking of confirmation of sexual desirability		

Infection
Related to:
Presence of HIV
 	
DEFINING CHARACTERISTICS
Decreased number of T_4 helper cells, altered T_4 helper cell function, reversed T_4/T_8 ratio, altered cellular immune response, altered humoral immune response, decreased response to antigens in skin testing
	ONGOING ASSESSMENT
	• Assess for presence of Defining Characteristics.
	• Obtain STD history.
	• Obtain tuberculosis (TB) history.
	• Screen for other STDs.
	
	THERAPEUTIC INTERVENTIONS
	• Wash hands before entering, after leaving room.
	• Administer antiviral agents and immune modulating therapies as ordered. *Antiviral agents prevent HIV from replicating and infecting additional cells. Immune modulators improve T-cell numbers/effectiveness and decrease risk of opportunistic infections.*
	• Prevent contact with other diseases:
	  If possible, assign to private room; if not possible, do not allow exposure to anyone with known infection.
	  Advise staff, visitors to avoid contact with patient if they suspect cold or influenza.
	• Do not serve raw fruits, vegetables, milk, or meat.
		Risk of future opportunistic infections will be reduced.

Potential for infection
Related to:
Accidental contact with HIV
 	
DEFINING CHARACTERISTICS
History of exposure to HIV-positive blood, semen, vaginal excretion, breast milk, amniotic fluid, wound drainages, blood-tinged body fluids, or fluids derived from blood
	ONGOING ASSESSMENT
	• Monitor CDC guidelines for prevention of spread/protection.
	
	THERAPEUTIC INTERVENTIONS
	• Use universal precautions to prevent HIV spread:
	  Avoid unprotected contact with blood, semen, vaginal secretions, blood-tinged body fluids, wound drainage, breast milk, and fluids derived from blood (e.g., amniotic fluid, pericardial effusion. *These body fluids harbor HIV in quantities that may cause infection.*
	  Wear gloves when exposed to potentially infectious fluids. *Latex gloves provide effective barrier against HIV.*
	  Wear gloves when handling specimens.
	  Label specimens with blood/body fluids precautions label; place specimen in plastic bag.
	  Wear gown when soiling anticipated.
	  Wear mask and goggles when potentially infectious body fluids may spray.
		Health care worker will not become infected with HIV through patient exposure.

Continued.

NURSING DIAGNOSES / DEFINING CHARACTERISTICS	NURSING INTERVENTIONS / *RATIONALES*	EXPECTED OUTCOMES
	Keep disposable Ambu bag and mask at bedside. Immediately clean spills of potentially infectious fluids with sodium hypochlorite (bleach) solution. *Bleach, cleaning solutions labeled tuberculocidal will kill HIV.* Prevent injury with needles or other sharp instruments. *Although most needle-stick injuries do not result in infection, risk exists.* Do not recap needles, resheath instruments. *Recapping needles most common cause of needle-stick injuries.* Dispose of sharps in rigid plastic container. Keep needle disposal container in patient's room. Obtain assistance to restrain confused or uncooperative patient during venipuncture or other invasive procedure. Take care to avoid needle-stick injuries during arrests/other emergencies. If accidental needle-stick injury occurs, complete incident report; notify employee health service.	
Ineffective individual coping *Related to:* Fatigue Social isolation from stigma Grave prognosis **DEFINING CHARACTERISTICS** Depression Withdrawal from relationships with significant others Anger Hostility Social isolation Inability to meet role expectations Suicidal gesture	**ONGOING ASSESSMENT** · Determine patient's previous coping patterns. · Assess patient's perception of self. · Determine suicide potential. · Assess patient's support network. · Observe and document expressions of grief, anger, hostility, and powerlessness. **THERAPEUTIC INTERVENTIONS** · Maintain nonjudgmental attitude when giving care. · Encourage patient to participate in own care. · Provide patient opportunity to express feelings. · Support patient's effective coping strategies. · Support patient's social network. *Lovers/nontraditional extended family may offer more support than traditional family.* · Provide opportunities for patient/family/significant other interaction. *Without intervention, hospitalizations may isolate patient and decrease ability to cope.* · Refer to psychiatric liaison or social worker as needed. · After discharge, refer to an AIDS support group. · See Grieving, anticipatory, p. 22.	Coping strategies will be identified, supported, and maximized.
Spiritual distress *Related to:* Pain, divorce, loneliness, hospitalization, surgery, terminal illness, chronic or debilitating illness Separation from religious ties and loved ones, loss by illness of loved one, and birth of unwanted, ill, or defective infant **DEFINING CHARACTERISTICS** Voiced guilt, loss of hope, spiritual emptiness, feeling of being alone, or questioning of belief system	**ONGOING ASSESSMENT** · Assess for presence of Defining Characteristics. **THERAPEUTIC INTERVENTIONS** · Structure interventions from patient's belief system. *Patients have right to beliefs that conflict with nurse's.* · Acknowledge and support patient's hope. · Do not provide logical solutions for spiritual dilemmas. · See Spiritual distress, p. 51; Hopelessness, p. 29.	Spiritual distress is acknowledged.

NURSING DIAGNOSES / DEFINING CHARACTERISTICS	NURSING INTERVENTIONS / *RATIONALES*	EXPECTED OUTCOMES
Anxious, depressed, discouraged, fearful, or angry appearance		
Potential fluid volume deficit *Related to:* Diarrhea Altered nutritional status Altered temperature regulation **DEFINING CHARACTERISTICS** Output > intake Sudden weight loss Decreased urine output Increased urine specific gravity Decreased skin turgor Increased serum sodium Dry mucous membranes Change in vital signs: increased heart rate, hypotension	**ONGOING ASSESSMENT** · Assess hydration status (see Defining Characteristics). · Monitor I & O every shift. · Record daily weight. · Monitor electrolytes, serum and urine osmolarity, and specific gravity. · Monitor and document vital signs, report abnormalities. **THERAPEUTIC INTERVENTIONS** · Encourage oral fluid intake. · Administer parenteral fluids as ordered. *Tachypnea, pain, nausea, and esophageal candidiasis may prevent oral intake. Vomiting, diarrhea, and night sweats may increase output.* · Administer antidiarrheal medication as ordered. · Administer antiparasitic medication as ordered.	Adequate fluid volume and electrolyte balance will be maintained.
Potential impairment of skin integrity *Related to:* Prolonged unrelieved pressure Altered nutritional status Presence of diarrhea Herpes infection Perianal *Candida* Infection Immobility from fatigue **DEFINING CHARACTERISTICS** Reddened skin Pain Numbness Blisters	**ONGOING ASSESSMENT** · Check skin color, moisture, texture, and temperature. · Assess for signs of ischemia, redness, pain. · Assess nutritional status. **THERAPEUTIC INTERVENTIONS** · Turn patient according to established schedule. · Provide prophylactic pressure-relieving devices: Alternating pressure mattress Stryker boots Elbow pads · Maintain functional body alignment. · *Increase tissue perfusion* by massaging around affected pressure area. · Keep skin clean and dry. *Night sweats and diarrhea macerate and damage skin.* · Maintain adequate hydration and nutrition. · See Skin integrity, impaired, p. 48. · Administer antiviral/antimonilial medication as ordered.	Skin breakdown will be prevented.
Altered nutrition: less than body requirements *Related to:* Loss of appetite Fatigue Oral or esophageal candidiasis	**ONGOING ASSESSMENT** · Document patient's actual weight on admission. · Obtain nutritional history. · Inspect mouth for *Candida* infection. · Document dietary and fluid I & O. · Obtain weight at least once a week. · Monitor serum/urine electrolytes, albumin, CBC, glucose, and acetone as necessary.	Optimal nutritional support will be maintained.

Continued.

Aquired immune deficiency syndrome—cont'd

NURSING DIAGNOSES / DEFINING CHARACTERISTICS	NURSING INTERVENTIONS / *RATIONALES*	EXPECTED OUTCOMES
DEFINING CHARACTERISTICS Weight loss (may be up to 20% of normal body weight) Calorie intake inadequate to meet metabolic requirements	**THERAPEUTIC INTERVENTIONS** • Provide dietary planning to encourage intake of high-calorie, high-protein foods. • Encourage participation in menu planning. • Assist with meals as needed. *Fatigue/weakness may prevent patient from eating.* • Encourage exercise as tolerated. • Administer dietary supplements/total parenteral nutrition (TPN) as ordered. *Despite supplements, HIV may cause wasting syndrome.* • Administer antimonilial medication as ordered. *Oral and esophageal candidiasis can cause sore throat, may cause lack of appetite.*	
Altered thought process *Related to:* Organic mental disorders associated with other physical disorders CNS infections Intracranial lesions HIV infection Ingestion of/ withdrawal from alcohol or other mood-altering substances **DEFINING CHARACTERISTICS** Disorientation to one/ more of the following: time, person, place, situation Loss of short-term memory Decreased cognitive functioning Altered behavior patterns Altered or labile mood states Impaired ability to perform ADLs without supervision caused by short attention span or confusion Altered perceptions of surroundings Poor judgment Short attention span	**ONGOING ASSESSMENT** • Assess for presence of Defining Characteristics. **THERAPEUTIC INTERVENTIONS** • See Thought processes, altered, p. 52. • Administer antiviral agents as ordered. *Dementia may herald acute CNS infection or chronic HIV infection. Anti-HIV treatment improves dementia caused by chronic HIV infection.* • *To provide safety,* supervise patient; remove potentially dangerous items from environment. • If dementia caused by substance abuse or withdrawal, refer to drug rehabilitation or start detoxification protocol.	Ability to behave and interact with others appropriately will increase.
Pain *Related to:* Medical problems Musculoskeletal factors Diagnostic procedures or medical treatment	**ONGOING ASSESSMENT** • Assess for presence of Defining Characteristics. **THERAPEUTIC INTERVENTIONS** • Respond immediately to complaint of pain. *During painful experiences, patient's time perception may be distorted. Prompt response to pain may decrease anxiety and demonstrate concern for the patient's welfare that fosters comfort .*	Pain will be relieved or reduced.

NURSING DIAGNOSES / DEFINING CHARACTERISTICS	NURSING INTERVENTIONS / *RATIONALES*	EXPECTED OUTCOMES
CNS HIV infection **Defining Characteristics** Patient/significant other report pain Self-focusing, narrowed focus (altered time perception, withdrawal from social or physical contact), depression, loss of appetite Moaning, crying, pacing, seeking out of other people or activities; restlessness, irritability, altered sleep pattern Facial mask of pain Altered muscle tone (listless/flaccid; rigid/tense) Autonomic responses not seen in chronic stable pain (e.g., diaphoresis, BP change, pulse rate, pupillary movements) Decreased respiratory rate, pallor, nausea	• Whenever possible, eliminate additional stressors and sources of discomfort. • Use alternative therapies: imagery, massage, distraction, or relaxation. • See Pain, p. 39.	
Ineffective breathing pattern *Related to:* Inflammatory process Decreased lung expansion Tracheobronchial obstruction Anxiety Decreased energy; fatigue **Defining Characteristics** Dyspnea Shortness of breath Tachypnea Fremitus Cyanosis Cough Nasal flaring Respiratory depth changes Altered chest excursion	**Ongoing Assessment** • Assess for presence of Defining Characteristics. • Monitor ABGs; note changes. **Therapeutic Interventions** • Position with proper body alignment for optimal breathing pattern. *Sitting position improves lung excursion and chest expansion.* • Administer anti-infectives as ordered. • Continue anti-infectives as prophylaxis. • See Breathing pattern, ineffective, p. 8.	Optimal respiratory status within limits of the disease will be achieved.

Continued.

NURSING DIAGNOSES / DEFINING CHARACTERISTICS	NURSING INTERVENTIONS / *RATIONALES*	EXPECTED OUTCOMES
Use of accessory muscles Pursed-lip breathing/ prolonged expiratory phase Increased anteroposterior chest diameter		

Self-care deficit
Related to:
Cognitive impairment
Fatigue
Exercise intolerance
 	
DEFINING CHARACTERISTICS
Inability to feed self
Inability to dress self
Inability to bathe and groom self
Inability to perform toileting tasks
Inability to transfer from bed to wheelchair (w/c)
Inability to ambulate
Inability to perform miscellaneous common tasks
   Telephoning
   Writing
	ONGOING ASSESSMENT
	• Assess for presence of Defining Characteristics.
	
	THERAPEUTIC INTERVENTIONS
	• Set realistic short-range goals with patient *to decrease frustration.*
	• Pace self-care tasks to allow rest.
	• See Self-care deficit, p. 44.
		Optimal level of independent self-care will be achieved.

Originated by: Martha Dickerson, RN, MS, CCRN
             Jeff Zurlinden, RN, MS

Chlamydia

(NONSPECIFIC URETHRITIS;
NONGONOCOCCAL URETHRITIS [NGU])

Chlamydia are bacteria that infect 3 to 5 million people in the United States each year. Teenagers and people in their early twenties are most commonly infected. Chlamydia usually creates a localized infection of the urethra, endocervical canal, nasopharyanyx, or rectum. The patient may have one site of infection or multiple sites. Although chlamydial infections may also spread through nonsexual routes, this care plan describes only adults infected through sexual transmission. The infection is spread by sexual contact with the infected site. Although symptoms abate without treatment, untreated chlamydia may lead to pelvic inflammatory disease (PID), epididymitis, or Reiter's syndrome. Chlamydia infections are one kind of nonspecific or nongonococcal urethritis (NGU).

NURSING DIAGNOSES / DEFINING CHARACTERISTICS	NURSING INTERVENTIONS / *RATIONALES*	EXPECTED OUTCOMES

Actual infection
Related to:
Presence of infectious organisms
 	
DEFINING CHARACTERISTICS
Positive culture from urethra, rectum, nasopharynx, or endocervical canal
Gram's stain with polymorphonuclear leukocytes and no gram-negative diplococci
Positive chlamydial test result on endocervical, urethral, or nasopharyngeal specimens
History of sexual contact with infected person
Persistent symptoms despite treatment for gonorrhea (GC) and negative GC cultures
	ONGOING ASSESSMENT
	• Determine sexual orientation, date of last sexual contact, number and sex of sexual partners, and recent and usual sexual activities.
	• Obtain history of sexually transmitted diseases.
	• Assess:
	    Urethral discharge
	    Painful urination
	    Urinary frequency
	    Rectal discharge
	    Endocervical discharge
	    Spotting between menstrual periods or after intercourse
	    Change in bowel movements
	    Tenesmus (rectal spasms)
	    Rectal itching
	    Mucous or blood in stools
	    Chlamydial infections are frequently asymptomatic; however, symptoms may occur within first 3 weeks after infection. If discharge present, less profuse, more mucoid than GC discharge.
	• Obtain menstrual history, including date of last period.
	• Determine method and compliance with birth control.
	• Perform pregnancy test.
	• Screen for other STDs *(patient with one STD at higher risk than general population for concomitant STDs).*
	
	THERAPEUTIC INTERVENTIONS
	• Administer antibiotics as ordered. *Tetracycline, usual drug of choice, contraindicated for children and pregnant women. Use other antibiotics.*
		Infection will be treated.

Knowledge deficit *Related to:* New diagnosis **DEFINING CHARACTERISTICS** Multiple questions or lack of questions Verbalized misconceptions	**ONGOING ASSESSMENT** • Assess patient/significant other's present level of understanding. • Assess patient/significant other's emotional readiness for learning. **THERAPEUTIC INTERVENTIONS** • Instruct patient about medication antibiotic schedule and side effects. *Administer tetracycline on empty stomach, avoid concomitant use of dairy products, and avoid exposure to sun unless protected with sunblocker.* • Instruct patient on mode of transmission. • Instruct patient in condom use or other "safe sex" means. *Condoms effective against chlamydia infections.* • Instruct patient to return for test of cure. • Instruct patient to return for routine screening if high-risk sexual behavior continues. • Instruct patient to inform all recent sex partners (last 3 weeks) of possible exposure to chlamydia, need for treatment. *Untreated asymptomatic sexual partners are common reinfection source.*	Patient/significant others will verbalize understanding of important aspects of chlamydia and its treatment.

Continued.

NURSING DIAGNOSES / DEFINING CHARACTERISTICS	NURSING INTERVENTIONS / *RATIONALES*	EXPECTED OUTCOMES
	• Instruct patient to report symptom persistence/recurrence. • Instruct patient to refrain from vaginal, rectal, or pharyngeal intercourse until results reported from test of cure *(may be infectious all or part of this time)*. • Explore possible benefits/drawbacks of HIV testing. *Benefits include initiation of antiviral therapy if helper T-cell counts low. Drawbacks include possible discrimination and emotional depression.*	
Noncompliance *Related to:* Complexity of treatment regime Unwillingness to participate in treatment regime **DEFINING CHARACTERISTICS** Recurrent infection Failure of urethral discharge, endocervical discharge, or proctitis to resolve Verbalized inability to comply with treatment, prevention, or informing of sexual partners	**ONGOING ASSESSMENT** • Compare actual therapeutic effect with expected effect. • Plot patient's pattern of returning for tests of cure or follow-up. • Assess patient's beliefs about current illness and treatment plan. **THERAPEUTIC INTERVENTIONS** • Suggest 1 dose/day tetracycline rather than q6h dose. *Simplifying treatment regimen increases compliance.* • Role play to practice informing sexual partners of possible exposure to chlamydia. • Follow-up with phone calls to remind patient of need for test of cure culture *(improves compliance)*. • Role play to practice new behavior in situations that may lead to reinfection. • See Noncompliance, p. 36.	Compliance will be maximized.

Altered patterns of sexuality
Related to:
Fear
Imposed restrictions
Risk of contagion
 	
DEFINING CHARACTERISTICS
Patient/significant others express concern about effect of chlamydial infection on expressions of physical intimacy
	ONGOING ASSESSMENT
	• Determine patient's/significant other's concerns.
	• Determine patient's/significant other's concerns about AIDS.
	• Assess whether patient/significant others appear:
	  Depressed
	  Unusually quiet
	  Repeatedly questioning despite adequate explanation
	  Reluctance to end encounter with nurse
	• Assess for recurrent infection.
	• Determine whether patient fails to return for test of cure.
	• Determine patient's compliance with treatment.
	
	THERAPEUTIC INTERVENTIONS
	• Explore ways to express intimacy during treatment, excluding vaginal, rectal, and pharyngeal intercourse.
	• Explore ways to express physical intimacy that will not lead to reinfection *(e.g., use of condoms and other techniques that prevent exchange of semen, vaginal secretions, or blood)*.
	• Elicit patient's feelings about limitations on sexual behavior *(sexual practices affected by feelings)*.
	• Explore patient's perceptions of HIV (AIDS) risk. *STD diagnosis may provoke fear of AIDS that alters sexual patterns.*
	• See Sexuality patterns, altered, p. 47.
		Expressions of physical intimacy will be satisfying.

Anxiety/fear *Related to:* Social or moral stigma Physical harm Potential harm to partner or self	**ONGOING ASSESSMENT** • Evaluate level of anxiety/fear. • Assess usual method of coping. • Assess perception of meaning of chlamydial infection.	Anxiety/fear will be reduced.

Chlamydia—cont'd

NURSING DIAGNOSES / DEFINING CHARACTERISTICS	NURSING INTERVENTIONS / *RATIONALES*	EXPECTED OUTCOMES
DEFINING CHARACTERISTICS Expressed shame, guilt, or need for atonement Restless, distracted, confused, demanding, or preoccupied with trivial detail Trembles, perspires, or fails to make eye contact.	**THERAPEUTIC INTERVENTIONS** · Display calm, accepting manner. · Encourage expression of concerns and feelings. *STTD diagnosis may provoke feeling of guilt or punishment or other anxiety-provoking thoughts unique to patient.* · Place patient in quiet, distraction-free environment. · Repeat information until patient verbalizes understanding of material. · Provide privacy; demonstrate respect for confidentiality.	

Originated by: Jeff Zurlinden, RN, MS

Gonorrhea (GC)

Gonorrhea (GC) is a bacterial infection that affects over 1 million people in the United States each year. Teenagers and adults in their early twenties are most commonly infected. GC usually creates a localized infection of the urethra, endocervical canal, rectum, or pharynx. The patient may have one site of infection or multiple sites. The infection is spread through sexual contact with the infected site. Although symptoms abate without treatment, untreated GC may lead to septicemia, PID, prostatitis, epididymitis, urethral stricture, or arthritis-dermatitis syndrome. This care plan does not describe gonorrhea of newborns.

NURSING DIAGNOSES / DEFINING CHARACTERISTICS	NURSING INTERVENTIONS / *RATIONALES*	EXPECTED OUTCOMES

Infection
Related to:
Presence of infectious organisms
 	
DEFINING CHARACTERISTICS
Positive culture from urethra, cervix, throat, or rectum
Gram-negative intracellular diplococci on smear
History of sexual contact with infected person
	ONGOING ASSESSMENT
	· Determine sexual orientation, date of last sexual contact, number and sex of sexual partners, and recent and usual sexual activities.
	· Obtain history of STDs.
	· Assess:
	    Urethral discharge (men and women)
	    Pain on urination
	    Urinary frequency
	    Sore throat
	    Rectal discharge
	    Cervical discharge
	    Changes in bowel movements
	    Mucus or blood in stools (*Rectal, pharyngeal, and cervical GC frequently asymptomatic. Heterosexual and bisexual men may have asymptomatic urethral GC. Urethral GC usually symptomatic in homosexual men. Discharge appears 2-5 days after infection.*)
	· Observe for possible anaphylactic reaction to antibiotics.
	· Screen for other STDs. *Patients with one STD at higher risk than general population for concomitant STD. Up to 45% of GC patients have simultaneous chlamydia infection that requires treatment with additional antibiotic.*
		Discharge will resolve, and test of cure culture will be negative.

Continued.

NURSING DIAGNOSES / DEFINING CHARACTERISTICS	NURSING INTERVENTIONS / *RATIONALES*	EXPECTED OUTCOMES
	• Screen for GC in additional sites. *Patients with GC in one site at higher risk than general population for GC in additional sites. Women frequently self-inoculate rectums with GC from urethral or endocervical discharges. Increasing number of sites cultured increases yield of positive cultures.* • Obtain menstrual history, including date of last period. • Determine method and compliance with birth control. • Perform pregnancy test. **THERAPEUTIC INTERVENTIONS** Obtain cultures: Warm culture plate to room temperature before inoculation. *Cold culture medium is bactericidal.* • After Thayer Martin culture plates inoculated, store in CO_2-enriched environment. *Neisseria gonorrhoea dies in room air O_2 concentrations.* • Administer antibiotics as ordered. Choice governed by patient's sexual orientation, drug allergies, and infection site(s).	
Knowledge deficit *Related to:* New diagnosis **DEFINING CHARACTERISTICS** Multiple questions or lack of questions Verbalized misconceptions	**ONGOING ASSESSMENT** • Assess patient's/significant other's present level of understanding. • Assess patient's/significant other's emotional readiness for learning. **THERAPEUTIC INTERVENTIONS** • Instruct patient about medication schedule and side effects of antibiotics used to treat infection. • Instruct patient on mode of transmission. • Instruct patient in condom use/other "safe sex" methods. *Condoms effective barrier against GC infection.* • Instruct patient to return for test of cure. *Antibiotic-resistant strains cause treatment failures (detected by test of cure).* • Instruct patient to return for routine screening if high-risk sexual behavior continues. • Instruct patient to inform all recent sex partners of possible exposure to GC and need for treatment. *Untreated asymptomatic sexual partners common source of reinfections.* • Instruct patient to report symptom persistence or recurrence. • Instruct patient to refrain from vaginal, or pharyngeal sexual intercourse until results are reported from test of cure. • Explore with patient the possible benefits and drawbacks of HIV testing. *Benefits include initiation of antiviral therapy if helper T-cell counts are low. Drawbacks include possible discrimination and emotional depression.*	Patient/significant others will verbalize understanding of gonorrhea and its treatment.
Noncompliance *Related to:* Complexity of treatment regimen Unwillingness to participate in treament regimen **DEFINING CHARACTERISTICS** Recurrent infection (Rule out [r/o] treatment failure caused by antibiotic-resistant strains)	**ONGOING ASSESSMENT** • Compare actual, expected therapeutic effect. • Plot patient's pattern of returning for tests of cure or follow-up. • Assess patient's beliefs about current illness and treatment plan. **THERAPEUTIC INTERVENTIONS** • Role play to practice informing sexual partners of possible exposure to GC. • Suggest IM medication if oral medication compliance poor. *IM medication eliminates need for patient compliance.* • Follow up with phone calls to remind of need for test of cure culture (*this improves compliance*). • Role play to practice new behavior in situations leading to reinfection (e.g., saying no, negotiating condom use). • See Noncompliance, p. 36.	Course of treatment and return for test of cure will be completed.

Gonorrhea—cont'd

NURSING DIAGNOSES / DEFINING CHARACTERISTICS	NURSING INTERVENTIONS / *RATIONALES*	EXPECTED OUTCOMES
Verbalized inability to comply with treatment, prevention, or informing of sexual partners No test of cure visit Incorrect pill count on return visit Inadequate blood level of antibiotic		

Altered patterns of sexuality
Related to:
Fear
Imposed restrictions
Risk of contagion
 	
DEFINING CHARACTERISTICS
Patient/significant others express concern about effect GC treatment has on expressions of physical intimacy
	ONGOING ASSESSMENT
	· Determine patient's/significant other's concerns.
	· Determine patient's/significant other's concerns about AIDS.
	· Assess whether patient/significant others appear:
	  Depressed
	  Unusually quiet
	  Repeatedly questioning despite adequate explanation
	  Apparent reluctance to end encounter with nurse
	· Assess recurrent infections.
	· Determine whether patient returns for test of cure.
	· Determine patient's compliance with treatment.
	
	THERAPEUTIC INTERVENTIONS
	· Explore ways to express intimacy during treatment, excluding vaginal, rectal, and pharyngeal intercourse.
	· Explore ways to express physical intimacy that do not lead to reinfection (e.g., *use of condoms, other techniques preventing exchange of semen, vaginal secretions, or blood).*
	· Elicit patient's feelings about sexual behavior limitations. *Sexual activities are influenced by feelings.*
	· Explore patient's perceptions of HIV (AIDS) risk. *STD diagnosis may provoke fear of AIDS that may alter sexual patterns.*
	· See Sexuality patterns, altered, p. 47.
		Expression of physical intimacy will be satisfying.

Anxiety/fear *Related to:* Social or moral stigma Physical harm Potential harm to partner and self **DEFINING CHARACTERISTICS** Expressed shame, guilt, or need for atonement	**ONGOING ASSESSMENT** · Evaluate level of anxiety/fear. · Assess usual method of coping. · Assess perception of meaning of GC infection. **THERAPEUTIC INTERVENTIONS** · Display calm, accepting manner. · Encourage expression of concerns and feelings. *STD diagnosis may provoke feelings of guilt or punishment or other anxiety-provoking thoughts unique to patient.* · Place in quiet, environment distraction-free. · Repeat information until patient verbalizes understanding of material. · Provide privacy; demonstrate respect for confidentiality.	Anxiety/fear will be reduced.

Originated by: Jeff Zurlinden, RN, MS

Herpes simplex virus: type II

(HSV-II; GENITAL HERPES)

Type II herpes simplex virus (HSV-II) is a virus transmitted by human-to-human contact of mucous membranes through intercourse or by contact with traumatized skin. The virus lives in the infected host permanently.

NURSING DIAGNOSES / DEFINING CHARACTERISTICS	NURSING INTERVENTIONS / *RATIONALES*	EXPECTED OUTCOMES

Knowledge deficit
Related to:
Condition recently diagnosed
Lack of knowledge about HSV-II, transmission, and prevention
 	
DEFINING CHARACTERISTICS
Verbalized deficiency in knowledge
Expressed inaccurate perception of health status
Noncompliance with prescribed health behavior
	ONGOING ASSESSMENT
	• Assess patient's knowledge of HSV-II:
	  Viral condition
	  Modes of transmission
	  Prevention of recurrences
	• Assess individual's history of disease:
	  Onset
	  Symptoms
	  Effects on life-style
	• Ask whether patient has recently experienced emotional stress, systemic infection, cold, fever, immunodeficient state, menses, or pregnancy.
	
	THERAPEUTIC INTERVENTIONS
	• Explain modes of virus transmission:
	  Direct contact with open lesion
	  Ascension into vaginal tract
	  Transplacental transmission
	• Explain importance of thorough health history, including previous history of symptoms, duration of outbreaks, and symptoms of partners.
	• Explain that virus needs dark, warm, moist environment to survive.
	• Explain that virus is unstable outside body. *(Patient may be afraid of transmitting disease through casual contact.)*
	• Explain that patient can be asymptomatic and still shed the virus (infect others). *By increasing knowledge of HSV-II, patient will actively participate in health behaviors to decrease recurrences and disease transmission.*
	• Explain that HSV-II is a permanent disease with remissions and exacerbations.
	• Explain that HSV-II management is supportive rather than curative.
	• Encourage patient to eat high-lysine, low-arginine diet. *Argenine thought to enhance virus growth, lysine to decrease growth. High-lysine diets may prevent/cure HSV-II. Some high-lysine foods: beef, pork, milk, cheese.*
	• Instruct patient about factors that reactivate HSV-II lesions: emotional stress, anxiety, colds, systemic infections, fevers, menses, friction and chafing, pregnancy, menses. *Virus believed to lie dormant in nerve roots and can be reactivated by these factors.*
	• Instruct women with genital herpes to have annual Pap smears *(higher cervical cancer rate than those without HSV-II).*
	• Instruct that pregnant women prone to HSV-II exacerbations. *HSV-II lesions may be exacerbated by hormonal changes during pregnancy. Accurate prenatal history important to ensure maternal, fetal health.*
		Patient will be able to describe the disease process, its causes, contributing factors, and symptom control.

Potential for infection
Related to:
Vesicle formation
Inflammatory process
 	
DEFINING CHARACTERISTICS
Localized:
Vesicle formation in genital area
Lesions:
  Bilateral distribution
  Infectious until crusted over
	ONGOING ASSESSMENT
	• Assess patient for symptoms (localized or systemic).
	• Determine when patient began to experience symptoms to determine whether patient experiencing primary, initial, or recurrent infection.
	  Primary:
	    Prodromal period 3-7 days (systemic symptoms)
	    Incubation 2-20 days, virus shed 3-33 days
	    Infection duration 3-6 weeks
	  Initial:
	    Prodromal period 1-7 days (localized symptoms)
	    Incubation, virus shed 4-20 days
	    Disease duration 1-3 weeks
		Risk of transmitting disease will be reduced.

Herpes simplex virus: type II—cont'd

NURSING DIAGNOSES / DEFINING CHARACTERISTICS	NURSING INTERVENTIONS / *RATIONALES*	EXPECTED OUTCOMES

Pruritus
Mild paresthesia
Inguinal lymphaden-opathy
Vaginal discharge
Systemic:
Fever
Chills
Headache
Malaise
Fatigue
	Recurrent:
	  Prodromal period 1-3 days (localized symptoms)
	  No incubation, virus shed 4-5 days
	  Disease duration 7-10 days
	
	THERAPEUTIC INTERVENTIONS
	• Instruct patient to avoid sexual activity from first feeling of tingling, before lesions appear, until after lesions have crusted over *(patient contagious during this period).*
	• Even when lesions are not present, encourage patient to use condoms during sexual contact and wash with soap and water after intercourse. *Virus may be shed during sexual contact even if patient asymptomatic.*
	• Encourage patient to wash hands after touching lesions.
	• Instruct patient to wash toilet seat with soap and water if vesicles break open when patient on seat. *If someone with traumatized skin comes in contact with toilet seat, viral transmission possible. Soap disintegrates virus.*
	• Encourage patient to tell health care providers they have come in contact with HSV-II. *Virus may be shed when patient symptomatic. Health care providers should wear gloves and practice good handwashing with all patients.*	

Pain *Related to:* Vesicle formation in-flammatory process **DEFINING CHARACTERISTICS** Tingling before lesions forms Painful lesions Burning when urine enters lesions Possible abrasion of lesions by clothing	**ONGOING ASSESSMENT** • Assess onset, duration, and intensity of patient's discomfort. • Assess for presence of lesions. • Observe for signs/symptoms of Acyclovir toxicity (i.e., altered renal output, decreased lethargy, tremors, confusion, hallucinations). **THERAPEUTIC INTERVENTIONS** • Administer analgesic medication, as ordered. • Administer Acyclovir IV, PO, or topically (apply with gloves). *Acyclovir does not cure disease but decreases pain associated with HSV-II; also decreases shedding time and speeds healing time.* • Encourage warm sitz baths 3 times/day. • Encourage patient to keep genital area clean and dry; wear cotton underwear.	Pain will be reduced.

Potential sexual dysfunction
Related to:
Active lesions, potential for recurrences, potential for transmission
 	
DEFINING CHARACTERISTICS
Depression
Reported limitations on sexual performance imposed by disease
Fears of future limitations on sexual performance
Withdrawn behavior
Patient report of perceived loss in sexual function and interpersonal relationships
	ONGOING ASSESSMENT
	• Assess patient's sexual history in private, relaxed setting ensuring confidentiality.
	• Provide open, objective, and reassuring environment.
	
	THERAPEUTIC INTERVENTIONS
	• Discuss with patient/significant other implications of HSV relationship.
	  Relate interrelation of stress and lesion recurrence.
	  Refer to professional counseling when appropriate.
	  High social support is correlated with fewer symptoms, increased self-esteem, better adjustment, and fewer social problems.
	• Encourage patient to use condoms during sexual contact.
	• Identify alternative methods if dispersing sexual energy when lesions present and sexual intercourse with others inadvisable:
	  Masturbate (if acceptable to individual).
	  Encourage regular physical activity (walking, jogging, or exercising 3 times/week).
	  Explore alternative physical contact (kissing, hugging, touching, massaging, etc.).
		Adjustments to changes in sexual function will be described by the patient.

Continued.

Herpes simplex virus: type II—cont'd

NURSING DIAGNOSES / DEFINING CHARACTERISTICS	NURSING INTERVENTIONS / *RATIONALES*	EXPECTED OUTCOMES
Ineffective individual coping *Related to:* Disease chronicity Change in life-style Lack of social support system **DEFINING CHARACTERISTICS** Feeling of emotional disruption related to HSV infection Verbalization of fear of condition Feeling of perceived loss of control over life-style Anger Guilt Depression Hopelessness	**ONGOING ASSESSMENT** • Ask how HSV interferes with life-style. • Ask whether fear of HSV has interfered with relationships. • Assess support systems. • Assess possible causative factors delaying patient's ability to cope (i.e., progression through grief process, lack of social support, denial, anger, depression, guilt, fear). • Assess past and present coping mechanisms. **THERAPEUTIC INTERVENTIONS** • Explain that there is no cure for HSV. Medical care supportive to prevent recurrences, decrease pain during recurrences. *Fear and anxiety may be reduced if patient knows what to expect.* • Attempt to reduce/eliminate causative factors. • Promote trusting relationship *(to increase self-esteem).* • Promote couple's cohesiveness *(to increase social support and strengthen relationship).* • Instruct patient about constructive outlets for anger (e.g., vigorous physical exercise). *With increased anger, patient may develop negative feelings toward intercourse.* • Instruct about coping mechanisms (e.g., stress reduction, proper nutrition, exercise, and adequate sleep).	Coping behaviors will be evident.

Originated by: Andrea Merkler, RN, BSN
　　　　　　　Monalisa S. Bron, RN, BSN

Human papilloma virus (HPV)

(VENEREAL WARTS)

Human papilloma virus (HPV) infections affects from 400,000 to 600,000 people in the United States each year. HPV causes warts on the penis, urethra, rectum, perineum, cervix, vagina, or labia. The patient may have one site of infection or multiple sites. The infection is spread through sexual contact with the infected site. Latent infections may be reactivated during pregnancy or during periods of immunosuppression. Even after treatment, otherwise healthy people frequently have recurrent growths of warts. Regardless of their age, women with warts on their cervix are at increased risk for cervical cancers. This care plan does not describe laryngeal papillomas of neonates after infection from the mother at the time of vaginal delivery.

NURSING DIAGNOSES / DEFINING CHARACTERISTICS	NURSING INTERVENTIONS / *RATIONALES*	EXPECTED OUTCOMES
Infection *Related to:* Presence of infectious organisms **DEFINING CHARACTERISTICS** Warts on penis, urethra, cervix, vagina, labia, perineum, or rectum	**ONGOING ASSESSMENT** • Determine sexual orientation, date of last sexual contact, number and sex of partners, and recent and usual sexual activities. • Obtain STD history. • Inspect: 　Penis 　Perineum 　Rectum 　Vagina 　Cervix *Genital warts are painless; usually appear 1-2 months after infection.*	Venereal warts will be effectively treated.

NURSING DIAGNOSES / DEFINING CHARACTERISTICS	NURSING INTERVENTIONS / *RATIONALES*	EXPECTED OUTCOMES
Cytologic abnormalities on Pap test	• Obtain menstrual history, including date of last monthly period (LMP). • Determine method and compliance with birth control. • Perform pregnancy test. • Screen for other STDs *(patients with one STD at higher risk than general population for concomitant STDs)*. **THERAPEUTIC INTERVENTIONS** • Assist with wart removal: cryotherapy with liquid nitrogen, surgical excision, direct injection of interferon into lesion, hyphrecation (electric cautery), topical podophyllin, or other topical medications.	
Knowledge deficit *Related to:* New diagnosis **DEFINING CHARACTERISTICS** Multiple questions or lack of questions Verbalized misconceptions	**ONGOING ASSESSMENT** • Assess patient's/significant others' present understanding. • Assess patient's/significant others' emotional readiness for learning. **THERAPEUTIC INTERVENTIONS** • Instruct patient to wash off podophyllin approximately 6 hr after application. *If applied too long, podophyllin causes excessive tissue damage.* • For all methods of removing warts, instruct to keep wounds clean and dry until healed. • Instruct in mode of transmission. • Instruct in condom use/other "safe sex" methods. *Condoms are effective barriers against HPV.* • Instruct patient to inspect for regrowth of warts. *Regrowth is common, may not indicate reinfection. Recurrence most common several months after treatment.* • Instruct patient to inform all recent (last 3 months) sex partners of possible HPV exposure. *Females partners need gynecologic exam and Pap test.* • Instruct to avoid vaginal, rectal, or pharyngeal intercourse until wounds healed. • Instruct women with cervical warts to receive regular gynecologic exams that include Pap test. *Cervical, other genital tract cancers more common in women with genital warts.* • Explore possible benefits/drawbacks of HIV testing. *Benefits include initiation of antiviral therapy if T-cell counts low; drawbacks include discrimination and emotional depression.*	Patient/significant others will verbalize understanding of important aspects of venereal warts and their treatment.
Noncompliance *Related to:* Complexity of treatment regime Discomfort during treatment regime Unwillingness to participate in treatment regime **DEFINING CHARACTERISTICS** Regrowth of warts (treatment failure approximately 40%, so regrowth may not represent noncompliance) Verbalized inability to comply with treatment, prevention, or informing of sexual partners Failure to keep return appointments	**ONGOING ASSESSMENT** • Compare actual with expected therapeutic effect. • Plot patient's pattern of returning for follow-up visits. • Assess beliefs about current illness and treatment plan. **THERAPEUTIC INTERVENTIONS** • Role play to practice informing sexual partners of possible HPV exposure. • Follow-up with phone calls to remind patient of need for return appointment. *Reminder phone calls improve compliance with return visits.* • Conduct role playing to practice new behavior in situations which may lead to reinfection. • See Noncompliance, p. 36.	Course of treatment will be completed.

Continued.

Human papilloma virus—cont'd

NURSING DIAGNOSES / DEFINING CHARACTERISTICS	NURSING INTERVENTIONS / *RATIONALES*	EXPECTED OUTCOMES
Altered patterns of sexuality *Related to:* Fear Imposed restrictions Risk of contagion **DEFINING CHARACTERISTICS** Patient's/significant others' expressed concerns about effects of treatment on expressions of physical intimacy	**ONGOING ASSESSMENT** • Determine patient's/significant other's concerns. • Determine patient's significant other's concerns about AIDS. • Assess whether patient/significant others appear: Depressed Unusually quiet Questioning after adequate explanation Reluctant to end encounter with nurse • Assess for recurrent infection. • Determine compliance with treatment. **THERAPEUTIC INTERVENTIONS** • Explore ways to express intimacy during treatment, excluding vaginal, rectal, and pharyngeal intercourse. • Explore ways to express physical intimacy that will not lead to reinfection *(e.g., use of condoms and other techniques that prevent exchange of semen, vaginal secretions, or blood).* • Elicit patient's feelings about sexual behavior limitations *(sexual behaviors affected by feelings).* • Explore patient's perceptions of HIV (AIDS) infection risk. *STD diagnosis may provoke fear of AIDS, altering sexual patterns.* • See Sexuality patterns, altered, p. 47.	Expressions of physical intimacy will be satisfying.
Anxiety/fear *Related to:* Social or moral stigmas Physical harm Potential harm to partner **DEFINING CHARACTERISTICS** Expressed shame, guilt, or need for atonement Restless, distracted, confused, demanding, or preoccupied (with trivial details) Trembles, perspires, fails to make eye contact	**ONGOING ASSESSMENT** • Evaluate level of anxiety/fear. • Assess patient's usual method of coping. • Assess patient's perception of meaning of syphilis infection. **THERAPEUTIC INTERVENTIONS** • Display calm, accepting manner. • Encourage patient to express concerns and feelings. *STD diagnosis may provoke feelings of guilt or punishment or other anxiety-provoking thoughts unique to patient.* • Place in quiet, distraction-free environment. • Repeat information until patient verbalizes understanding of material. • Provide privacy; demonstrate respect for confidentiality.	Anxiety/fear is reduced.

Originated by: Jeff Zurlinden, RN, MS

Syphilis

(LUES; SYPHILITIC CHANCRE; CONDYLOMATA LATA)

Syphilis is a bacterial infection; approximately 28,000 new cases appear each year. After an untreated infection, syphilis progresses over the remainder of the patient's lifetime through four stages: primary, secondary, latent, and tertiary. The defining characteristics of each stage are outlined in the care plan. Screening blood tests are vital to detect syphilis. Syphilis serology tests detect all the stages of the disease. These tests can also detect disease in a patient who may appear asymptomatic; however, syphilis serology will be falsely negative during the first 4 to 6 weeks after infection. Patients who are concurrently infected with HIV may remain falsely negative for syphilis serologies. Syphilis may take a more aggressive course, rapidly advancing to neurosyphilis, and be more difficult to treat in patients who are infected with HIV. This care plan does not describe congenital syphilis.

NURSING DIAGNOSES / DEFINING CHARACTERISTICS	NURSING INTERVENTIONS / *RATIONALES*	EXPECTED OUTCOMES
Infection *Related to:* Presence of infectious organisms **DEFINING CHARACTERISTICS** Fourfold increase in syphilis serology titer in a previously infected patient or any titer in patient with no previous infection history. *Low-titer biologic false-positive result possible during pregnancy, autoimmune disease, or infection. Confirmatory test will exclude biologic false-positive result in patients with no previous syphilis history.* History of sexual contact with an infected person. *Because infected person has negative syphilis serology for first 4-6 wk after infection, contacts are treated.* *Primary syphilis:* Chancre: solitary painless papule that eventually ulcerates at inoculation site 21-90 days after exposure; heals spontaneously in 1-6 wk	**ONGOING ASSESSMENT** ▪ Determine sexual orientation, date of last sexual contact, number and sex of partners, and recent and usual sexual activities. ▪ Obtain STD history, especially for previous syphilis infections. ▪ Assess syphilis serology results. ▪ Inspect skin, mouth, penis, vagina, rectum, and perineum for chancre, condylomata lata, and rashes. ▪ Obtain menstrual history, including date of last menstrual period. ▪ Determine method of compliance with birth control. ▪ Perform pregnancy test. ▪ Screen for other STDs. *Patient with one STD at higher risk than general population for concomitant STDs.* **THERAPEUTIC INTERVENTIONS** ▪ Administer antibiotics as ordered. *Choice and route of administration determined by disease stage.*	Syphilis titer will fall.

Continued.

NURSING DIAGNOSES / DEFINING CHARACTERISTICS	NURSING INTERVENTIONS / *RATIONALES*	EXPECTED OUTCOMES
Secondary syphilis: Highly variable, non-pruritic skin rash with lymphadenopathy that begins in untreated infection 6 wk after chancre heals. Rash spontaneously resolves in 2-6 wk *Latent syphilis:* Asymptomatic period after untreated infection may last decades before progressing to last stage *Tertiary syphilis:* Degenerative changes in heart, CNS, and skeletal system includes paresis, dementia, aortic insufficiency, and tabes dorsalis		
Knowledge deficit *Related to:* New diagnosis **DEFINING CHARACTERISTICS** Multiple questions or lack of questions Verbalized misconceptions	**ONGOING ASSESSMENT** · Assess patient's/significant other's present level of understanding. · Assess patient's/significant other's emotional readiness for learning. **THERAPEUTIC INTERVENTIONS** · Instruct about medication schedule for and side effects of antibiotics. · Instruct on mode of transmission. *Syphilis transmitted from chancre site to portion of partner's body that touches chancre.* · Instruct in condom use/other "safe sex" means. *Condoms prevent infection from chancres on penis or within vagina.* · Instruct patient to return for routine screening if high-risk sexual behavior continues. · Instruct patient to inform all sex partners (since time of infection) of possible exposure to syphilis and need for treatment. · Instruct to avoid vaginal, rectal, or pharyngeal intercourse until antibiotic therapy completed. *Patients with primary and secondary syphilis contagious.* · Inform patient of signs/symptoms of Jarisch-Herxheimer reaction (fever, chills, malaise, myalgia, and sore throat beginning 6-8 hr after antibiotic therapy; subsiding after 12-24 hr). May need aspirin for symptomatic relief. *Occurs in 50% of patients with primary syphilis and 75% with secondary syphilis.* · Instruct patient to return for repeat serology tests (usually performed at 1, 6, 12, 24 months after therapy). · Explore possible benefits/drawbacks of HIV testing. *Benefits include initiation of antiviral therapy if helper T-cell counts low; drawbacks include possible discrimination and emotional depression.*	Patient/significant others will verbalize understanding of important aspects of syphilis and its treatment.
Noncompliance *Related to:* Complexity of treatment regimen Unwillingness to participate in treatment regimen	**ONGOING ASSESSMENT** · Compare actual, expected therapeutic effect. · Plot patient's pattern of returning for follow-up visits. · Assess patient's beliefs about current illness and treatment plan. · See Noncompliance, p. 36.	Compliance will be maximized.

Syphilis—cont'd

NURSING DIAGNOSES / DEFINING CHARACTERISTICS	NURSING INTERVENTIONS / *RATIONALES*	EXPECTED OUTCOMES

DEFINING CHARACTERISTICS

Titer of syphilis serology that does not decrease after treatment

Verbalized inability to comply with treatment, prevention, or informing of sexual partners

Incorrect pill count on return visit

Inadequate blood level of antibiotic

Missed return visit

THERAPEUTIC INTERVENTIONS
- Role play to practice informing sexual partners of possible syphilis exposure.
- Suggest IM medication if compliance with oral medication poor. *IM medication removes need for patient compliance.*
- Role play to practice new behavior in situations that may lead to reinfection.
- Follow-up with phone calls to remind patient of next office visit *(improves compliance).*

Altered patterns of sexuality
Related to:
Fear
Imposed restrictions
Risk of contagion

DEFINING CHARACTERISTICS

Patient's/significant others' expressed concerns about effects of treatment on expressions of physical intimacy

ONGOING ASSESSMENT
- Determine patient's/significant other's concerns.
- Determine patient's significant other's concerns about AIDS.
- Assess whether patient/significant others appear:
  Depressed
  Unusually quiet
  Questioning after adequate explanation
  Reluctant to end encounter with nurse
- Assess for recurrent infection.
- Determine compliance with treatment.

THERAPEUTIC INTERVENTIONS
- Explore ways to express intimacy during treatment, excluding vaginal, rectal, and pharyngeal intercourse.
- Explore ways to express physical intimacy that will not lead to reinfection *(e.g., use of condoms and other techniques that prevent exchange of semen, vaginal secretions, or blood).*
- Elicit patient's feelings about sexual behavior limitations *(sexual behaviors affected by feelings).*
- Explore patient's perceptions of HIV (AIDS) infection risk. *STD diagnosis may provoke fear of AIDS, altering sexual patterns.*
- See Sexuality patterns, altered, p. 47.

Expressions of physical intimacy will be satisfying.

Anxiety/fear
Related to:
Social or moral stigmas
Physical harm
Potential harm to partner

DEFINING CHARACTERISTICS

Expressed shame, guilt, or need for atonement

Restless, distracted, confused, demanding, or preoccupied (with trivial details)

Trembles, perspires, fails to make eye contact

ONGOING ASSESSMENT
- Evaluate level of anxiety/fear.
- Assess patient's usual method of coping.
- Assess patient's perception of meaning of syphilis infection.

THERAPEUTIC INTERVENTIONS
- Display calm, accepting manner.
- Encourage patient to express concerns and feelings. *STD diagnosis may provoke feelings of guilt or punishment or other anxiety-provoking thoughts unique to patient.*
- Place in quiet, distraction-free environment.
- Repeat information until patient verbalizes understanding of material.
- Provide privacy; demonstrate respect for confidentiality.

Anxiety/fear is reduced.

Originated by: Jeff Zurlinden, RN, MS

Gynecologic Care Plans

DISORDERS

Bartholinitis
Infertility as emotional crisis
Pelvic inflammatory disease (PID)
Premenstrual syndrome (PMS)

THERAPEUTIC INTERVENTIONS

Dilatation and curretage (D & C) and cone
  biopsy
Hysterectomy, total abdominal
Infertility, diagnostic surgical procedures

Laparoscopy, hysteroscopy, and
  endometrial biopsy: postoperative care
Mastectomy: segmented and modified
  radical
Vulvectomy

Bartholinitis

An infection of the vulvovaginal or bartholin glands.

NURSING DIAGNOSIS / DEFINING CHARACTERISTICS	NURSING INTERVENTIONS / *RATIONALES*	EXPECTED OUTCOMES

Pain
Related to:
Infectious process
 	
DEFINING CHARACTERISTICS
Report of acute, throbbing pain between labia, especially during walking/sitting
Report of burning pain on urination and defecation
Unilateral or bilateral swelling over site of infected gland
Palpable, tender inguinal nodes
Redness and stretching of overlying skin
Edema of labia and surrounding tissues
Purulent drainage (spontaneous or expressed) from duct
Nonverbal physiologic expressions of pain (i.e., crying, grimacing, moaning, tenseness, extreme restlessness, or absolute stillness with body in protective position)
	ONGOING ASSESSMENT
	• Assess pain experience reported/manifested by patient:
	  Location: identify point of origin.
	  Intensity: identify on 0-5 scale, 5 most severe (mild, discomforting, intense, excruciating).
	  Record temporal pattern; time of onset and associated events; trigger zones.
	  Elicit description of quality of pain.
	  Assess effects of pain.
	  Assess effectiveness of relief measures; include undesired effects.
	
	THERAPEUTIC INTERVENTIONS
	• Accept and understand pain as patient describes it.
	• Anticipate need for analgesia.
	• Encourage bed rest *to prevent further irritation.*
	• Apply moist hot compresses/provide sitz baths *for symptom relief.*
	• Administer antibiotic therapy as ordered.
	• Prepare for possible incision and drainage.
		Comfort will be maximized.

Knowledge deficit *Related to:* Unfamiliarity with diagnosis **DEFINING CHARACTERISTICS** Verbalized lack of understanding of diagnosis and treatment plan Many questions or no questions Noncompliance with prescribed treatment Distrust; anger	**ONGOING ASSESSMENT** • Assess patient's perception and knowledge of symptoms, disease process, and specific treatment plans. • Identify learning needs. **THERAPEUTIC INTERVENTIONS** • Take time to explain procedures, policies, and hospital routines. • Describe infectious process, treatment involved, and probable outcome. • Provide reliable information about gonorrhea (if appropriate). • Ask questions; encourage verbalization of concerns. • Provide instruction in daily health and hygiene practices. • Teach patient to distinguish normal/abnormal vaginal discharge. • If patient sexually active, teach her to recognize infection signs in partner. • Stress importance of seeking medical attention as soon as infection signs develop. *Knowlege and understanding of health problem influence patient's ability to accept/reject care plan.*	Patient will be able to describe disease process, reasons and methods of treatment, and ways to prevent reinfection.
Sexual dysfunction *Related to:* Hospitalization and physical condition precluding sexual activity	**ONGOING ASSESSMENT** • Assess patient's perception of sexual function.	Optimal means of satisfying sexual needs will be achieved.

Continued.

Bartholinitis— cont'd

NURSING DIAGNOSES / DEFINING CHARACTERISTICS	NURSING INTERVENTIONS / *RATIONALES*	EXPECTED OUTCOMES
DEFINING CHARACTERISTICS Expressed concerns about ability to remain sexually active Verbalized concerns about social/sexual habits Verbalized fear of having venereal disease Report of dyspareunia	**THERAPEUTIC INTERVENTIONS** • Initiate discussion and explore issues of potential concern to patient, such as whether sexual abstinence possible and alternative methods to use (e.g., use of condom) until infection symptoms disappear. • Use careful, tactful questions. • Provide accepting atmosphere and understanding for patient's personal feelings. *Sexual dysfunction may affect previously satisfactory sexual relationship.* • Communicate through verbal/nonverbal cues knowledge and comfort in discussing sexuality. • Assure confidentiality. • See Sexuality patterns, altered, p. 47.	

Originated by: Fe Corazon R. Mendoza, RN, BSN

Infertility as emotional crisis

Feelings of failure, alienation, anger, and grief caused by inability to conceive a child.

NURSING DIAGNOSES / DEFINING CHARACTERISTICS	NURSING INTERVENTIONS / *RATIONALES*	EXPECTED OUTCOMES

Ineffective individual/ couple coping
Related to:
Childlessness
 	
DEFINING CHARACTERISTICS
 	
Verbalized inability to cope/ask for help
Inability to meet normal role expectations
Inability to meet basic needs
Inability to solve problems
Withdrawal
Crying
	ONGOING ASSESSMENT
	• Note expressed feelings of hopelessness, helplessness, and powerlessness.
	• Observe for expression of anger/hostility/loss of control.
	• Note weeping, irritability, and expressed feelings of incompetence.
	• Assess noncompliant/other problematic behavior.
	• Assess ability to plan/make decisions.
	• Note statements about work, social, or family withdrawal/incompetent performance.
	• Observe for evidence of decreased self-esteem:
	    Poor hygiene
	    Poor job performance
	    Poor sexual performance
	    Feelings of guilt and unworthiness
	• Assess ability to comprehend or follow through.
	• Observe for expressed overdependency.
	• Assess level of social/family acceptance; note descriptions of family pressures to have children.
	• Observe for isolation or statements of need to withdraw from child-centered family/friends/environments which have children.
	• Note descriptions reflecting secrecy about infertility/inability to discuss problem.
	
	THERAPEUTIC INTERVENTIONS
	• Provide emotional support:
	    Create environment conductive to expression of feelings.
	    Provide frequent unhurried contact.
	    Avoid excessive focus on physical tasks.
	    Emphasize patient's value as individual.
	    Offer feedback to patient.
		Couple will begin to cope with stress of childlessness.

Infertility as emotional crisis— cont'd

NURSING DIAGNOSES / DEFINING CHARACTERISTICS	NURSING INTERVENTIONS / *RATIONALES*	EXPECTED OUTCOMES
	Provide interest, concern, and understanding. *Emotional support allows patient to work through, resolve conflicts; provides them with a resource/support person.* • Encourage use of past adaptive coping mechanisms. *Patient often knows what works best.* • *Provide attention to concerns of each individual (husband/wife). Infertility affects both; husband also needs attention.* • Attempt to clarify feelings/behavior *to promote optimal communcation.* • Provide supportive silence to permit person to continue response when difficult. *This allows patient to verbalize feelings without nurse's interpretations/assumptions.* • Confront gently to focus attention on feelings/behavior. *Patient may try to avoid/hide feelings. Gentle confrontation by nurse may lead to productive dialogue.* • Refer to infertility support group, if available. *Patient may find it easier to relate to/speak with someone with similar experience. Patient may be referred to social service when individual therapy indicated.* • Facilitate communication between partners by including both in all aspects of care. *Often partners assume that other knows how they feel or hesitate to verbalize feelings. This may further strain the relationship.* • See Coping, ineffective individual, p. 15.	
Self concept/body image disturbance *Related to:* Belief that pregnancy critical to personal/social fulfillment as woman Psychosocial pressures to conceive Biophysical imperativeness to conceive while pregnancy physically possible Cultural/religious mandates that make pregnancy imperative. **DEFINING CHARACTERISTICS** Responses to actual/perceived change in structure/function: *Verbalization of injury to sense of self:* Feelings of bodily damage/invasiveness Feelings of incompetence (hampered work/family performance) Feelings of loss of identity; not feeling totally "female" or "male"	**ONGOING ASSESSMENT** • Assess level of social intellectual, intrapersonal, physical, and emotional function. • Observe for changes in affect, behavior, cognition, perception, level of function: 　Note quality and quantity of verbal expressions about self (see Defining Characteristics). 　Observe for help-seeking behaviors (e.g., crying, attention seeking, touching persons/objects, seeking someone to talk to). 　Observe for nonverbal behaviors (see Defining Characteristics). • Assess level/presence of grieving: children, genetic continuity, fertility, pregnancy experience. • Note religious/cultural background and potential conflicts with values or treatments. • Observe for statements that project psychologic inability to be good parent. ("I cannot conceive because God knows I will be a poor parent.") • Observe for statements of sexual behavior changes: 　Intercourse with prostitutes 　Extramartial affairs 　Impotence 　Frigidity 　Inability to achieve erection/orgasm 　Vaginismus 　Premature ejaculation 　Ejaculatory incompetence 　Statements of denial/loss **THERAPEUTIC INTERVENTIONS** • Discuss with the couple "usual" emotional reactions to childlessness *to allow couple to see that feelings are not uncommon.* • Provide accurate information. • When indicated, provide information/assistance about adoption as possible alternative. *Patient must realize alternatives.* • Promote warm, communicating relationship through effective verbal/nonverbal (touching) exchanges *to make patient feel more comfortable.* • Refer to sexual counseling as needed. • Stress importance of spouse support. Expressing acceptance of one another can be helpful to both. *Patient/spouse will need other's support during difficult waiting and testing of fertility treatment and afterward when infertility diagnosed.*	Couple begins to express positive self/body image.

Continued.

Infertility as emotional crisis— cont'd

NURSING DIAGNOSES / DEFINING CHARACTERISTICS	NURSING INTERVENTIONS / *RATIONALES*	EXPECTED OUTCOMES
Distorted perceptions: "everyone is pregnant except me" Obsession/ preoccupation with infertility and body function Grieving over loss of potential life-giving ability *Conflicts involving values:* Verbalization of threatened religious, cultural, or legal beliefs about infertility procedures/ treatments *Nonverbal response to actual/perceived change in structure/function:* Poor eye contact Preoccupation Discontent Noncompliance Self-destructiveness Nonparticipation in therapy Lack of responsibility for self-care Signs of initiation of grief: weeping, sobbing, physical symptoms (e.g., loss of appetite, exhaustion, choking or tightness in throat) Denial of role; refusal to verify actual change in reproductive capacity Negative feelings about body; increased verbalization of self-destruction;self-derogatory statements Verbalized change in personal identity and role performance Expressed inability to perform job	• Reinforce positive emotional responses; redirect negative responses. • Advise to give others' negative responses minimal significance. *Patient must realize that some disagree with choices for family building/parenting; they are entitled to personal decision.* • Help patient maintain positive attitude. *Patient needs balance between hope and truth.* • Provide safety from self-destructive behaviors. • Provide alternative methods for obtaining semen (seminal pouch) to patients with threatened religious/cultural values *to decrease anxiety/hesitancy about semen collection.* • Assist couple through grief: recognizing, working through, overcoming intense/painful loss feelings.	

Infertility as emotional crisis— cont'd

NURSING DIAGNOSES / DEFINING CHARACTERISTICS	NURSING INTERVENTIONS / *RATIONALES*	EXPECTED OUTCOMES
Inappropriately blaming of personal inadequacies for infertility Description of sexual inadequacies/ dysfunctions		

Knowledge deficit
Related to:
New diagnosis
 	
DEFINING CHARACTERISTICS
Verbalization of problem
Poor compliance with instructions
Inappropriate/ exaggerated behaviors (e.g., hysterical, hostile, anxious, apathetic)
Repetitive questions
	ONGOING ASSESSMENT
	• Assess understanding of disease process, treatments.
	• Assess level of anxiety, emotional reactions.
	• Assess level of education.
	
	THERAPEUTIC INTERVENTIONS
	• Help couple understand reproductive process, anatomy, and physiology. *Fertility patient needs good understanding of reproduction to provide information to fertility team and follow procedures through.*
	• Explain diagnostic test/procedures. *Patient who understands care less anxious; feels more in control.*
	• Relate diagnostic testing to normal physiology *to allow better understanding of treatment.*
	• Teach techniques for taking basal body temperatures, reading thermometer; correct recording measures. Encourage couple's involvement in care. *Accuracy of basal body temperature vital to infertility patient.*
	• Teach home care techniques:
	  Medications, side effects, mode of action, and method of administration
	  Rest and good nutrition
	  Menstrual calendar.
	  (Patient must be aware of what to expect, what to look for, and what to report. Good discharge teaching maximizes patient's chances of pregnancy.)
	• Observe response to teaching. *Patient may need some reinforcement.*
		Couple will demonstrate knowledge of diagnosis and its relation to treatment.

Originated by: Anita C. Houtsma, RN
              Margaret Hixson, RN, BSN

Pelvic inflammatory disease (PID)

(ACUTE SALPINGITIS)

A sexually transmitted process involving the endocervix, endometrium, and endosalpinx, with subsequent spill of tubal exudate into the peritoneal cavity, causing pain, inflammation, and tissue destruction. If untreated or frequently recurrent, can become a chronic condition; tissue destruction can lead to infertility.

NURSING DIAGNOSES / DEFINING CHARACTERISTICS	NURSING INTERVENTIONS / *RATIONALES*	EXPECTED OUTCOMES

Pain
Related to:
Pelvic cavity inflammation
	ONGOING ASSESSMENT
	• Assess patient for low abdominal and back pain:
	  Type: sharp/dull
	  Quality: severe/mild
	  Duration
	• Measure abdominal girth every shift.
		Pain will be reduced.

Continued.

NURSING DIAGNOSES/ DEFINGING CHARACTERISTICS	NURSING INTERVENTIONS/*RATIONALES*	EXPECTED OUTCOMES

DEFINING CHARACTERISTICS
Low abdominal pain and tenderness on rebound
Abdominal distention
Back pain
	• Assess bowel sounds q4h.
	• Assess for medication effects/side effects.
	
	THERAPEUTIC INTERVENTIONS
	• Administer analgesics for pain as ordered. *Some patients experience extreme discomfort; may require narcotic analgesia.*
	• Provide external comfort measures:
	  Heating pad at low temperature
	  Positioning with extra pillows	

Potential fluid volume deficit *Related to:* Vomiting **DEFINING CHARACTERISTICS** Abnormal electolyte values Decreased urine output (<30 ml/hr) Poor skin turgor Dry mucous membranes Increased urine specific gravity (>1.020), pH Hypotension Dizziness Pallor	**ONGOING ASSESSMENT** • Monitor patient for vomiting, test emesis for blood. • Assess emesis for amount, color, consistency. • Monitor I & O. • Check urine for specific gravity. • Monitor CBC and electrolytes. **THERAPEUTIC INTERVENTIONS** • Administer antiemetics *to prevent dehydration and electrolyte shift.* • Maintain NPO or give clear liquids until nausea and vomiting decrease. • Give small amounts of ice chips, sips of water, or carbonated beverages (not colas) until nausea and vomiting subside. • See Fluid volume deficit, p. 20.	Normal fluid volume will be maintained.

Actual infection
Related to:
Bacterial invasion:
  Fallopian tubes (salpingitis)
  Ovaries (oophoritis)
  Uterus (endometritis)
Gram-positive cocci:
  Chlamydia trachomatis
  Neisseria gonorrhoeae
  Mycoplasma hominis
Gram-negative cocci:
  Escherichia coli
  Hemophilus influenzae
 	
DEFINING CHARACTERISTICS
Edematous vaginal mucosa
Greenish yellow vaginal discharge
Malodorous discharge
Increased body temperature
Positive cultures
	ONGOING ASSESSMENT
	• Check vital signs q4h. Note spiking temperatures.
	• Assess for malodorous vaginal discharge (may be present, copious).
	• Assess for vulvovaginitis.
	• Monitor cultures.
	• Assess obstetric history for last menstrual period, abnormal menses, and sexual contacts.
	• Assess for past PID hospitalization.
	• Assess history of recent sexual contacts.
	
	THERAPEUTIC INTERVENTIONS
	• Institute precautions:
	  Discard soiled perineal pads in isolation containers.
	  Maintain strict hand washing technique for all persons in contact with patient.
	  Cleanse all equipment (i.e., bedpan, tub, and toilet seat) with disinfectant.
	  Use utensil/gloves when handling soiled materials.
	• Administer perineal care after each pad change and after bedpan used *to prevent skin excoriation.*
	• Administer antibiotics as ordered. *Aggressive antibiotic therapy may prevent tubal damage that will predispose patient to ectopic pregnancy/infertility.*
	• Ensure that patient does not use tampons (*can be medium for further bacterial growth; inhibit drainage*).
	• Position patient in sitting position *as often as possible to promote drainage.*
		Spread of infection will be reduced.

NURSING DIAGNOSES / DEFINING CHARACTERISTICS	NURSING INTERVENTIONS / *RATIONALES*	EXPECTED OUTCOMES

Potential anxiety/fear
Related to:
Negative family/
partner reactions
Hospitalizations
New treatments
 	
DEFINING CHARACTERISTICS
Expressed anger
Crying when discussing medical treatment or hospitalization
Agitation
Embarrassment
No questions or verbalized fears.
Withdrawal
	ONGOING ASSESSMENT
	· Assess normal coping patterns by patient/family/significant other interviews.
	· Assess behavior changes (see Defining Characteristics).
	· Assess urinary, reproductive tract infection history.
	· Assess past hospitalizations.
	· Assess treatment for gonorrhea or syphilis.
	· Assess use of contraceptives.
	· Assess whether patient is a minor; assess parental knowledge of sexual activity as appropriate.
	
	THERAPEUTIC INTERVENTIONS
	· After diagnosis confirmed, address patient's/family's feelings and concerns.
	· Elicit feelings about PID effects:
	    Recurrences
	    Normal sexual functioning
	    Surgical intervention
	    Normal childbearing
	· Be supportive and nonjudgmental about patient's behavior.
	· Explain all tests and procedures to patient before performed *to alleviate apprehension and promote cooperation:*
	    Blood and urine test
	    Pregnancy test
	    Gynecologic examination
	    X-ray studies
	    IV fluids
	    Medications
	· Provide physical and emotional support as needed during examinations.
		Level of anxiety/fear will be reduced.

Knowledge deficit
Related to:
Unfamiliarity with cause of disease, medical management, prevention
 	
DEFINING CHARACTERISTICS
Questioning
Silence during questioning about illness
Frequent complaints
	ONGOING ASSESSMENT
	· Assess level of knowledge.
	· Assess ability to learn.
	· Assess effectiveness of teaching.
	
	THERAPEUTIC INTERVENTIONS
	· Explain PID acquisition, prevention.
	· Explain that sexual contact(s) may have to be notified to obtain treatment.
	· Instruct on importance of proper administration of medication *to prevent ineffective treatment and recurrence of symptoms:*
	    Type of medication
	    Dosage
	    Side effects
	· Instruct patient to notify physician of:
	    Symptom reappearance
	    Lack of menstruation
	    Nonmenstrual bleeding
	    Severe abdominal cramps
	· Inform patient of importance of refraining from sexual intercourse until after follow-up visit.
	· Discuss contraceptive use if patient plans to continue sexual activities.
	· Inform patient of available resource personnel:
	    Family planning
	    Adolescent groups
	    Social worker
	· Use varied methods of providing information:
	    Verbal
	    Reading material
	    Pictures/film
		Patient will understand PID process, complications, medical treatment, and prevention of recurrence.

Continued.

Pelvic inflammatory disease— cont'd

NURSING DIAGNOSES / DEFINING CHARACTERISTICS	NURSING INTERVENTIONS / *RATIONALES*	EXPECTED OUTCOMES
Self concept disturbance *Related to:* Contagious infection Isolation during hospital stay **DEFINING CHARACTERISTICS** Withdrawal Crying Self-consciousness Anger Depression	**ONGOING ASSESSMENT** • Assess patient's level of self-esteem. • Assess PID impact on social activity. • Assess relationships with significant others. • Assess personal reaction and knowledge of isolation requirement during hospital stay. **THERAPEUTIC INTERVENTIONS** • Encourage patient to verbalize feelings, concerns about condition and further relationships *(helps identify patient's needs).* • Educate patient about PID effects on present, future relationships. *Patient's social skills and relationships may change if she becomes withdrawn and self-conscious.* • Allow patient privacy. Create environment conducive to communication. *Patient may exhibit natural reluctance to share feelings, particularly if confidence breached. Let trusting relationship develop before expecting her to "open up."* • Educate patient on reason for isolation. Give as much personal attention as possible *(may aid coping with negative feelings about isolation).* • Abolish misconceptions about sexually transmitted disease (STD). *Some people believe only "bad people" have STDs.* • Abolish misconceptions. *Patients may be private/secretive about sexual feelings, experiences; may see STD as punishment for transgressions.* • Describe other common uses for isolation/procedures. *Patients may feel isolation precautions draw attention to illness (contracted through sexual activity).*	Positive self-concept will be maintained.

Originated by: Mary Muse, RN,C, BSN
Caramen E. Billheimer, RN, BSN
Denise Talley-Lacey, RN, BSN

Premenstrual syndrome (PMS)

Premenstrual syndrome (PMS) is a cyclic occurrence of symptoms in the luteal phase (between ovulation and menses) for at least 2 consecutive months. The symptoms may begin or be exacerbated with the luteal phase. The number and the intensity of symptoms can vary from woman to woman and from cycle to cycle in an individual. PMS is a topic that lends itself to much more research. Studies conflict as to the etiology and treatment of PMS. It is known that there are over 150 and possibly close to 200 physiologic and psychologic symptoms.

NURSING DIAGNOSES / DEFINING CHARACTERISTICS	NURSING INTERVENTIONS / *RATIONALES*	EXPECTED OUTCOMES
Potential knowledge deficit *Related to:* Unfamiliarity with the topic Misconceptions Misinformation received from family/friends/media	**ONGOING ASSESSMENT** • Assess knowledge of topic. • Assess symptoms, especially in relation to menstrual cycle. **THERAPEUTIC INTERVENTIONS** • Familiarize patient with PMS by defining and discussing symptoms. *Broadened knowledge base increases patient's acceptance and ability to cope; may also decrease fear.*	Patient will be able to verbalize correct information and display understanding of PMS and symptoms.

NURSING DIAGNOSES / DEFINING CHARACTERISTICS	NURSING INTERVENTIONS / *RATIONALES*	EXPECTED OUTCOMES
DEFINING CHARACTERISTICS Feelings of isolation Fear Anger Frustration Confusion Multiple questions Lack of questions Expressed need for more information	• Provide patient with reading material; provide time later for questions *to supplement/reinforce teaching; allow learning at individualized pace.* • Have patient chart menstrual cycle using basal body temperature (BBT); chart incidence of symptoms at least 2 months *(will help differentiate PMS from dysmenorrhea, stress reactions, other medical/psychologic problems).* • Perform all interventions when patient not suffering with PMS symptoms.	
Potential for activity intolerance *Related to:* Fatigue Discomfort Indifference Mood swings **DEFINING CHARACTERISTICS** Change in role performance Inability to perform ADLs Inability to perform in social role Inability to work/go to school	**ONGOING ASSESSMENT** • Assess normal daily activities. • Assess level of activity during symptoms **THERAPEUTIC INTERVENTIONS** • Suggest patient anticipate time of intolerance, postpone activities/decisions, or make provisions ahead of time *(may relieve stress from inability to perform).*	Ability to perform roles/functions will be maintained or acceptance of inability to perform/ function will be established.
Altered nutrition: more than body requirements, less than body requirements *Related to:* Increased sugar intake Increased salt intake Increased appetite Decreased appetite **DEFINING CHARACTERISTICS** Excessive craving for certain food groups Consumption of more calories than usual/ suggested for daily requirements Consumption of fewer calories than usual/ suggested for daily requirements	**ONGOING ASSESSMENT** • Assess dietary intake daily and during luteal phase through patient log. • Assess dietary needs according to sex, age, body type. **THERAPEUTIC INTERVENTIONS** • Inform of foods with high salt content; suggest substitutes (e.g., herbal seasoning). *High salt intake increases H_2O retention, which increases edema and its discomforts. Educated patients may make better dietary decisions.* • Instruct patient to decrease sugar intake; increase protein and complex carbohydrate consumption; eat small, frequent meals. *PMS sufferers may display reactive hypoglycemia (sweating, nervousness) when blood sugar drops after high-carbohydrate meal.* • Review caloric needs and high-/low-calorie snacks as needed. *Education allows for informed choices; helps ensure consumption appropriate to needs.*	Intake will be balanced and food types thought to intensify PMS symptoms will be avoided.

Continued.

Premenstrual syndrome— cont'd

NURSING DIAGNOSES / DEFINING CHARACTERISTICS	NURSING INTERVENTIONS / *RATIONALES*	EXPECTED OUTCOMES
Potential ineffective individual coping *Related to:* Hormonal changes Reaction to other symptoms	**ONGOING ASSESSMENT**	Coping skills will be enhanced.

Potential ineffective individual coping
Related to:
Hormonal changes
Reaction to other symptoms

DEFINING CHARACTERISTICS
Depression
Fear
Feelings of actual/ potential loss of control
Anxiety
Edginess
Vulnerability
Mood swings
Decreased concentration
Crying

ONGOING ASSESSMENT
- Assess current coping mechanisms.
- Assess social support systems.
- Examine ability to use coping mechanisms. Teach alternate mechanisms.
- Assess effectiveness of coping mechanisms when patient not experiencing symptoms.
- Assess affect changes during PMS episode.

THERAPEUTIC INTERVENTIONS
- Give patient written material; or direct to source to explore coping techniques (e.g., assertiveness training, biofeedback, imaging, progressive relaxation, or breathing techniques). *This may give patient other constructive options for coping she may not have considered.*
- Help patient find local PMS support group if available; give the patient the PMS Hotline number (1-800-222-4PMS). *Peer support can help patient cope by decreasing feelings of isolation. Group experience allows opportunity for self-understanding and self-acceptance through others' understanding and acceptance.*
- Involve significant other in counseling/treatment. *Significant others increase their understanding of PMS and decrease possible pressure/negative feedback to patient.*
- Suggest regular exercise regimen *(may decrease stress/provide outlet for turbulent feelings)*.
- Instruct patient to take progesterone or birth control pills as prescribed *to provide stable hormonal environment. Hormone therapy may also decrease effects of low estrogen and progesterone levels in late luteal phase; may relieve PMS symptoms. Effectiveness of supplemental hormone therapy for PMS controversial.*
- Instruct patient to take mefenamic acid *(prostaglandin inhibitor)* as prescribed. *Relationship has been postulated between increased endometrial prostaglandin in late luteal phase and PMS symtoms.*
- Instruct patient to take prolactin inhibitors as ordered:
  Vitamin B$_6$
  Bromocriptine
  Some studies report increased prolactin levels in PMS sufferers. Use of inhibitor reportedly helps ease irritability and depression.
- Instruct patient to take tryptophan as prescribed. *PMS sufferers complaining of depression and mood swings found to have decreased serotonin levels. Tryptophan raises serotonin levels; may alleviate/reduce mood swings and depression.*

Coping skills will be enhanced.

Body image disturbance
Related to:
Weight gain
Skin eruptions

DEFINING CHARACTERISTICS
Abdominal distention
Swelling of fingers and hands
Swelling of ankles
Acne

ONGOING ASSESSMENT
- Assess weight gain 1 wk before menses; rule out dietary factors for weight increase.
- Assess patient for luteal phase edema.
- Assess severity of luteal phase skin eruptions.

THERAPEUTIC INTERVENTIONS
- Instruct patient on non-/low-sodium containing seasonings and foods. *Low sodium intake decreases H$_2$O retention, which can cause weight gain.*
- Instruct patient to take diuretics as prescribed *to reduce edema and, therefore, water weight gain.*
- Instruct patient to take prolactin inhibitor Bromocriptine as prescribed. See Diagnosis, Potential for ineffective individual coping, see above. *Some studies report relief of bloating with use of Bromocriptine.*
- Stress cyclic, temporary nature of weight gain. *Woman may be better able to accept weight gain if she realizes/remembers it is temporary and reversible.*
- Suggest patient explore fashion camouflages for weight gain times. *Person who perceives she looks good will feel better about self.*

Water weight gain decreases and comfort with body image is maintained.

Premenstrual syndrome— cont'd

NURSING DIAGNOSES / DEFINING CHARACTERISTICS	NURSING INTERVENTIONS / *RATIONALES*	EXPECTED OUTCOMES
	• Instruct patient to drink fluids with natural diuretic properties (e.g., cranberry or grapefruit juice) *to decrease edema.* • Instruct patient on skin hygiene, prescriptions, and over-the-counter drugs for acne treatment *to help alleviate/decrease breakouts.*	
Diarrhea/ Constipation *Related to:* Hormonal changes **DEFINING CHARACTERISTICS** Loose/frequent stools Difficult/no stools	**ONGOING ASSESSMENT** • Assess normal bowel function. • Assess bowel habits 1 wk before menses. **THERAPEUTIC INTERVENTIONS** • See Diarrhea, p. 16; Constipation/impaction, p. 12.	Normal bowel function will be maintained.
Pain *Related to:* Cramping Weight gain Breast tenderness Back pain Headache *Note:* These are most common factors; many others may also alter comfort **DEFINING CHARACTERISTICS** Crying Moaning Decreased mobility Grimacing Verbal reports	**ONGOING ASSESSMENT** • Assess quality/duration of pain. • Assess body areas affected by pain. • Assess response to pain. • Assess external factors that may aggravate pain. • Assess demographic factors (culture, religion, age, etc.) that may affect pain. **THERAPEUTIC INTERVENTIONS** • Instruct patient to take mefenamic acid as prescribed. *Some studies report decreased complaints of pain in PMS sufferers taking this medication.* • Instruct patient to take Bromocriptine or vitamin B_6 as prescribed. *Some studies claim breast pain lessened by medication.* • Instruct patient to take vitamin E as prescribed. *Some studies have attempted to link decreased reports of breast pain with PMS to vitamin E administration.* • Instruct patient to take oil of primrose as prescribed. *European studies have found that γ-linolenic acid, a fatty acid derived from oil of evening primrose, relieves complaints of breast tenderness, lumpiness, and pain.* • Instruct patient to decrease caffeine intake; inform patient of foods with high caffeine content. *Caffeine is a methylxanthine. Methylxanthines inhibit degradation of CAMP and CGMP to 5-Amp and 5-GMP; cause increased CAMP and CGMP concentration in cells. Increase results in production of fibrous tissue and cyst fluid.* • See diagnosis in this care plan: Potential for ineffective individual coping, p. 588. • See Pain, p. 39.	Pain will be decreased.

Originated by: Mary Sandelski, RN, MSN

Dilation and curettage (D & C) and cone biopsy

Dilation and curettage (D & C): a surgical procedure that involves dilating the cervix and scraping the inner lining of the uterus. Cone biopsy: surgical removal of tissue from the cervix for examination or treatment of a cervical condition.

NURSING DIAGNOSES / DEFINING CHARACTERISTICS	NURSING INTERVENTIONS / *RATIONALES*	EXPECTED OUTCOMES

Knowledge deficit
Related to:
New surgical procedure
 	
Defining Characteristics
Verbalized lack of knowledge of D & C and cone biopsy
Numerous questions or none
Call light used frequently
	Ongoing Assessment
	• Assess patient's knowledge of D & C and cone biopsy, including postoperative expectations.
	
	Therapeutic Interventions
	• Provide careful explanations of procedures, amount of vaginal drainage expected, and restriction on activity. *Level of knowledge and understanding of health problem can influence ability to accept/reject care plan.*
	• Instruct patient to notify staff of excessive, bright-red vaginal bleeding.
	• Provide discharge instructions:
	  Do not use tampons, douche, or have sexual intercourse until advised by physician.
	  Notify physician of vaginal bleeding more than normal period or bright red bleeding.
	  Notify physician if temperature elevated >24 h.
	  Do no strenuous work, exercise, or heavy lifting for 1 wk to 10 days.
	  Notify physician of foul-smelling vaginal discharge.
	• Take prescribed prophylactic medications until finished.
		Patient verbalizes understanding of D & C and cone biopsy procedure and post operative expectations.

Potential fluid volume deficit *Related to:* Excessive vaginal bleeding **Defining Characteristics** Report of faintness, dizziness, apprehension, and thirst Quick saturation of perineal pads (blood loss of at least 60 ml required to saturate perineal pad) Weak, rapid pulse and rapid respirations that become progressively shallow; early slight rise in BP Decreased urinary output	**Ongoing Assessment** • Assess vaginal bleeding; note volume lost (spotting, mild, moderate, or profuse) and number of perineal pads used. • Observe for changes that may indicate active bleeding (see Defining Characteristics). **Therapeutic Interventions** • Notify physician of excessive vaginal bleeding, marked changes in vital signs, and abnormal Hb and Hct values. • See Fluid volume deficit, p. 20.	Risk of fluid volume deficit will be reduced.
Potential anxiety *Related to:* New diagnosis New procedure **Defining Characteristics** Restlessness Increased awareness Increased questioning Withdrawal	**Ongoing Assessment** • Assess patient's anxiety (mild, moderate, severe). • Identify factors causing/contributing to anxiety. **Therapeutic Interventions** • Provide therapeutic climate; encourage patient to express feelings, ask questions. • Recognize uniqueness of surgical experience to patient. Listen to patient. • Provide reasonable, reality-based explanations. Correct misconceptions and misinformation. • Provide only information patient wants, needs, and can interpret. • See Anxiety, p. 4.	Anxiety level will be reduced.

Dilatation and curretage and cone biopsy— cont'd

RELATED FACTORS / DEFINING CHARACTERISTICS	NURSING INTERVENTIONS / *RATIONALES*	EXPECTED OUTCOMES
Pain *Related to:* Uterine cramping	**ONGOING ASSESSMENT** • Assess pain characteristics: pelvic, low back pain; duration; quality. • Assess effectiveness of pain relief measures.	Pain/discomfort will be relieved.
DEFINING CHARACTERISTICS Verbalized pain/ discomfort Restlessness, irritability Moaning, crying, facial grimace	**THERAPEUTIC INTERVENTIONS** • Explain cause of discomfort and expected duration. *Pain from procedure should be adequately relieved with analgesics.* • Provide analgesia and alternative comfort measures. • See Pain, p. 39.	

Originated by: Fe Corazon R. Mendoza, RN, BSN

Hysterectomy, total abdominal (TAH)

A surgical procedure that involves the complete excision of the uterus and the cervix through the abdominal wall.

NURSING DIAGNOSES / DEFINING CHARACTERISTICS	NURSING INTERVENTIONS / *RATIONALES*	EXPECTED OUTCOMES
Potential fluid volume deficit *Related to:* Excessive blood loss during surgery Excessive body fluid loss through nasogastric (NG) suction Bleeding from incision	**ONGOING ASSESSMENT** • Assess vital signs for hypovolemia; report deviations. • Monitor I & O records; report imbalances to physician. • Assess for signs of mental confusion, restlessness. • Monitor Hb, Hct; report changes. • Check incision for bleeding; change/reinforce dressings as needed. • Monitor blood loss by counting/weighing saturated perineal pads.	Fluid volume deficit is reduced/prevented.
DEFINING CHARACTERISTICS Increased pulse rate and rapid respirations Decreased BP Apprehension and restlessness Thirst and skin pallor Saturation of incisional dressing Decreased Hb/Hct	**THERAPEUTIC INTERVENTIONS** • Provide oral fluids as tolerated *to ensure adequate circulating blood volume.* • Administer parenteral fluids, blood, and blood components as ordered. • Maintain bed rest.	
Potential for infection *Related to:* Incision Indwelling catheter and IV site Surgical procedure	**ONGOING ASSESSMENT** • Inspect incision for redness, tenderness, and drainage. • Monitor and record vital signs; • Monitor blood count, especially WBC; note changes from preoperative levels. • Observe vaginal discharge for color, amount, and odor.	Risk of infection will be reduced.

Continued.

NURSING DIAGNOSES / DEFINING CHARACTERISTICS	NURSING INTERVENTIONS / *RATIONALES*	EXPECTED OUTCOMES
DEFINING CHARACTERISTICS Incision red, tender, and swollen Drainage from incision Increased pain at incision site Increased stress on suture line Increased pulse rate Fever Elevated WBC Frequency/pain upon urination	**THERAPEUTIC INTERVENTIONS** • Maintain good handwashing techniques before and after dressing changes. *Proper handling of incisional dressings greatly reduces wound infections.* • Change abdominal dressing, using aseptic technique. • Change perineal pads as needed. • Provide Foley catheter care. • Administer antibiotics and antipyretics as ordered.	

Ineffective airway clearance
Related to:
Anesthesia, immobility, pain
 	
DEFINING CHARACTERISTICS
Increased respiratory rate
Presence of rales, rhonchi
Diminished breath sounds, ineffective coughing
Feeling of chest tightness
Restlessness
Cyanosis and abnormal ABGs
Frequent, congested cough
	ONGOING ASSESSMENT
	• Assess quality of respirations.
	• Assess for signs of respiratory distress.
	
	THERAPEUTIC INTERVENTIONS
	• Instruct patient in:
	  Use of pillow or hand splinting when coughing *to minimize stress on incision*
	  Use of incentive spirometer
	  Importance of early ambulation
	• Encourage patient to turn, cough, and deep breathe at least q2h *to promote lung expansion and airway clearance.*
	• See Airway clearance, ineffective, p. 3.
		Airway is free of secretions.

Potential constipation *Related to:* Paralytic ileus Immobility Abdominal pain **DEFINING CHARACTERISTICS** Absence of flatus Emesis Nausea Abdominal distention Straining at stool Frequent nonproductive desire to defecate	**ONGOING ASSESSMENT** • Assess for presence or absence of bowel sounds, belching, or passing flatus *to determine onset of peristalsis.* • Assess dietary fluid intake and tolerance as client progresses from NPO to regular diet. **THERAPEUTIC INTERVENTIONS** • Restrict food and fluids until peristalsis resumes. • Administer laxatives as ordered. • Encourage fruit juice, high-roughage foods when tolerated. • Encourage sitting up and progressive ambulation *to relieve abdominal distention.* • Use rectal tube *to relieve flatus.*	Normal bowel elimination will be achieved.

Hysterectomy, total abdominal— cont'd

NURSING DIAGNOSES / DEFINING CHARACTERISTICS	NURSING INTERVENTIONS / *RATIONALES*	EXPECTED OUTCOMES
Urinary retention *Related to:* Bladder spasm Bladder manipulation during surgery Fluid volume deficit **DEFINING CHARACTERISTICS** Inadequate urine output Bladder distention Pain and restlessness	**ONGOING ASSESSMENT** · Inspect and palpate lower abdomen for distention. · Assess amount, frequency, character of urine output. · Assess indwelling catheter for patency, kinking. · Monitor I & O. **THERAPEUTIC INTERVENTIONS** · Administer fluids as tolerated *to enhance voiding, especially after Foley catheter removed.* · Provide catheter care per policy. · Remove catheter as soon as feasible. · See Urinary retention, p. 61.	Normal urine elimination will be achieved.
Pain *Related to:* Incisional pain Reduced mobility Ineffective pain control Patient's low tolerance **DEFINING CHARACTERISTICS** Verbal complaints of pain Tachycardia Facial grimacing Guarding of abdomen Withdrawal	**ONGOING ASSESSMENT** · Assess patient's experience of pain: location, quality, intensity, precipitating factors. · Assess response to pain medication. · Assess effectiveness of other pain-relief measures: position change, backrub, heat application. **THERAPEUTIC INTERVENTIONS** · Administer pain medications as needed; document response to therapy. *Individual patients react to pain differently; therefore, selection of pain relief individual.* · Initiate measures to reduce likelihood of pain (e.g., abdominal binder); compare behavioral responses before and after. · Teach ways to prevent tension on suture line during leg exercises, position changes, and ambulation. · See Pain, p. 39.	Pain will be relieved or reduced.
Body image disturbance *Related to:* Perceived body image changes Loss of childbearing capability Fears of loss of sexuality and femininity **DEFINING CHARACTERISTICS** Self-deprecating remarks Poor eye contact Weeping Decreased attention to grooming Verbalized negative feelings about body	**ONGOING ASSESSMENT** · Assess patient's feelings about self and body. *Loss of reproductive capability may cause disappointment and coping difficulties.* · Assess usual coping mechanisms and their previous effectiveness. · Assess patient's/spouse's understanding of effect of hysterectomy on sexual activity. *Physical recovery from hysterectomy requires abstinence from sex during healing period; psychosocial impact of hysterectomy may affect subsequent sexual relations.* **THERAPEUTIC INTERVENTIONS** · Provide accurate information about physiology, treatment, and recovery process. *Clarifying misconceptions may help women resume normal life.* · Encourage patient/significant other to express feelings. · Discuss physiologic and emotional influences on sexual functioning. · Stress the importance of spouse/significant other support. *Expressed acceptance can help the body image and self-image of the woman.* · See also Body image disturbance, p. 6; Self-concept disturbance, p. 46; Sexuality patterns, altered, p. 47.	Feelings about altered self-concept/body image will be acknowledged.
Knowledge deficit *Related to:* Unfamiliarity with surgical treatment and recovery process Lack of experience	**ONGOING ASSESSMENT** · Assess patient's knowledge. · Evaluate readiness for learning. *Knowledge and understanding of surgical procedure influence ability to respond and cooperate with care plan.* · Assess coping strategies.	Client verbalizes knowledge of operative experience and discharge instructions.

Continued.

Hysterectomy, total abdominal— cont'd

NURSING DIAGNOSES / DEFINING CHARACTERISTICS	NURSING INTERVENTIONS / *RATIONALES*	EXPECTED OUTCOMES

DEFINING CHARACTERISTICS
Verbalized lack of knowledge of procedures
Increased frequency of questions
Inability to respond to questions correctly
	THERAPEUTIC INTERVENTIONS
	• Provide preoperative teaching, careful explanations of procedures, and restrictions on activity.
	• Encourage patient to verbalize feelings and concerns.
	• Provide discharge teaching:
	  No vaginal invasion until instructed by physician
	  Physician to be informed of redness, bleeding from incision site, temperature elevation
	  Need for annual or more frequent gynecologic evaluations	

Originated by: Rosaline L. Roxas, RN

Infertility, diagnostic surgical procedures

(LAPAROSCOPY; HYSTEROSCOPY; ENDOMETRIAL BIOPSY)

Laparoscopy, hysteroscopy, and endometrial biopsy are important diagnostic aids for visualizing the pelvic organs, inspecting the uterine cavity, and performing histologic examination of the tissue.

NURSING DIAGNOSES / DEFINING CHARACTERISTICS	NURSING INTERVENTIONS / *RATIONALES*	EXPECTED OUTCOMES
Fear/anxiety *Related to:* Uncertainty about surgical diagnostic results **DEFINING CHARACTERISTICS** Restlessness Crying Expressed concern Increased questioning Withdrawal or excessive talking	**ONGOING ASSESSMENT** • Assess level of anxiety. **THERAPEUTIC INTERVENTIONS** • Maintain calm, nonthreatening manner with patient. *Patient develops security in presence of calm staff person.* • Encourage patient to verbalize concerns, questions. • Be with patient when physician explains findings *to reinforce, explain, and provide emotional support.* • See Fear, p. 18 and Anxiety, p. 4. • See also Infertility as emotional crisis, p. 580.	Fear/anxiety will be reduced.
Pain *Related to:* Surgical procedure **DEFINING CHARACTERISTICS** Report of pain at incisional site Evidence of decreased mobility	**ONGOING ASSESSMENT** • Assess location, duration, and intensity of pain. • Assess effect of pain relievers. **THERAPEUTIC INTERVENTIONS** • Provide pain medication as prescribed. • Assist with comfort measures (e.g., backrub, heating pad). *Patient comfort is nursing priority.*	Pain is relieved/ reduced.
Potential for wound infection *Related to:* Incision	**ONGOING ASSESSMENT** • Evaluate temperature and incision site for infection.	Risk of infection is reduced.

NURSING DIAGNOSES / DEFINING CHARACTERISTICS	NURSING INTERVENTIONS / *RATIONALES*	EXPECTED OUTCOMES
DEFINING CHARACTERISTICS Redness Swelling Pain Elevated temperature	**THERAPEUTIC INTERVENTIONS** • Change dressing as needed. *Keeping incision site clean and dry helps prevent infection.*	

Knowledge deficit
Related to:
Surgical procedure and follow-up home care
 	
DEFINING CHARACTERISTICS
Verbalized lack of knowledge
Repetitive questions
	ONGOING ASSESSMENT
	• Assess knowledge of procedure and follow-up care.
	
	THERAPEUTIC INTERVENTIONS
	• Provide preoperative teaching:
	    Pamphlets
	    Videotapes
	• Provide discharge instruction.
	    Nutritional needs
	    Activity level
	    Incisional care
	    Follow-up appointment with physician.
	Patient will adjust better from hospital to home care with specific instructions.
	• Encourage and respond appropriately to questions.
		Patient will verbalize understanding of preoperative teaching.

Originated by: Lydia Serra, RN, BSN

Laparoscopy, hysteroscopy, and endometrial biopsy: postoperative care

Laparoscopy: *Examination of the abdominal cavity, ovaries, and fallopian tubes with a laparoscope through a small incision in the abdominal wall. The procedure is used for both gynecologic diagnosis and sterilization.*
Hysteroscopy: *Direct visual inspection of the cervical canal, and uterine cavity through a hysteroscope. It is performed to examine the endometrium, to secure a specimen for biopsy, or to remove an intrauterine device or polyps.*
Endometrial biopsy: *Removal of a small piece of endometrial tissue from the uterus for microscopic examination to confirm or establish a diagnosis, estimate prognosis, or follow a course for a disease process.*

NURSING DIAGNOSES / DEFINING CHARACTERISTICS	NURSING INTERVENTIONS / *RATIONALES*	EXPECTED OUTCOMES
Knowledge deficit: surgical procedure and follow-up home care *Related to:* Indifference to learning Unfamiliarity with information resources	**ONGOING ASSESSMENT** • Assess need for teaching in terms of patient's understanding of procedure. • Assess level of education. **THERAPEUTIC INTERVENTIONS** • Provide preoperative teaching; use teaching manual and surgical program on closed-circuit television. • Discuss preoperative expectations in terms suited to intellectual/cognitive level of patient.	Patient will verbalize basic understanding of surgical experience.

Continued.

NURSING DIAGNOSES / DEFINING CHARACTERISTICS	NURSING INTERVENTIONS / *RATIONALES*	EXPECTED OUTCOMES

No requests for information
Information misinterpretation
 	
DEFINING CHARACTERISTICS
Verbalized lack of knowledge
Expressed need for more information
Repetitive questions
Inaccurate follow-through of instruction
	• Respond appropriately to questions and concerns.
	• Provide going-home instructions when patient demonstrates readiness to learn. Include information:
	    Nutritional needs
	    Activity level
	    Incision care
	    Vaginal discharge
	    Resumption of intercourse
	    Avoidance of tampons and douching
	    Follow-up appointment with physician
	• Provide information about warning signs. *Information will reduce possibility of complications.*	

Potential fluid volume deficit *Related to:* NPO/altered intake Poor appetite Nausea and vomiting **DEFINING CHARACTERISTICS** Decreased urine output Decreased venous filling Decreased skin turgor Concentrated urine Increased body temperature Weakness Thirst	**ONGOING ASSESSMENT** • Assess hydration status, skin turgor, mucous membranes as indicated. • Assess tolerance to oral fluids when instituted. • Monitor I & O. *Balanced fluid I & O essential to normal body functioning.* **THERAPEUTIC INTERVENTIONS** • See Fluid volume deficit, p. 20.	Adequate fluid volume balance will be maintained.

Pain
Related to:
Surgical procedure and intubation
Cultural implications
Inadequate pain relief from prn analgesics
Fear of drug dependence
 	
DEFINING CHARACTERISTICS
Report of pain in incisional site/shoulders
Evidenced decreased mobility
Reported sore throat
Autonomic responses: diaphoresis, BP or pulse rate change, increased/decreased respiratory rate, pupillary dilation
Guarding behavior
Self-focusing
Facial mask of pain
	ONGOING ASSESSMENT
	• Assess location, duration, quality, and intensity of pain.
	• Assess pain reliever(s) effect.
	• Use flow sheet to monitor pain (quality, intensity, duration, effects of narcotics, and comfort measures).
	
	THERAPEUTIC INTERVENTIONS
	• Apply heating pad for shoulder discomfort.
	• Offer throat lozenges and warm normal saline solution gargle for sore throat.
	• Teach relaxation techniques:
	    Slow chest breathing
	    Imagery *(provides alternative to chemical management of pain)*
	• See Pain, p. 39.
		Pain reduction after relief measures.

NURSING DIAGNOSES / DEFINING CHARACTERISTICS	NURSING INTERVENTIONS / *RATIONALES*	EXPECTED OUTCOMES
Potential for infection *Related to:* Altered skin integrity Traumatized tissue Inadequate acquired immunity Invasive procedures **DEFINING CHARACTERISTICS** Redness Tenderness Swelling Pain Elevated temperature Foul-smelling drainage	**ONGOING ASSESSMENT** ▪ Monitor results of CBC; report abnormalities. ▪ Assess vital signs, body fluids, and skin for signs of infection. ▪ Obtain cultures per order; report abnormalities. **THERAPEUTIC INTERVENTIONS** ▪ Utilize aseptic technique when performing invasive procedures. Use gloves when necessary. ▪ Encourage adequate rest. ▪ Describe symptoms that should be reported. ▪ Advise against removing scabs. ▪ Teach how to clean and dress wound.	Risk of infection is reduced.
Anxiety *Related to:* Threat to self-concept Threat of death Threat to/change in health status Situational or maturational crisis Unmet needs Lack of knowledge about diagnosis **DEFINING CHARACTERISTICS** Increased tension Apprehension Uncertainty Fearfulness Fear of unspecified consequences Distress Poor eye contact. Extraneous movements: foot shuffling; hand, arm movements Expressed concern about changes in life Worry Anxiety Facial tension Voice quivering Focus on self Inappropriate behavior	**ONGOING ASSESSMENT** ▪ Monitor level of anxiety. ▪ Assess knowledge of diagnosis and procedures. ▪ Assess support systems. **THERAPEUTIC INTERVENTIONS** ▪ Explain care, procedures to patient/family member. ▪ Encourage patient to discuss anxiety, fears, concerns. ▪ See Anxiety, p. 4.	Anxiety will be reduced.

Continued.

NURSING DIAGNOSES / DEFINING CHARACTERISTICS	NURSING INTERVENTIONS / *RATIONALES*	EXPECTED OUTCOMES
Potential ineffective individual coping *Related to:* Difficult adaptation to infertility Inadequate support systems Unmet expectations Inadequate coping method Chronic worry	**ONGOING ASSESSMENT** • Note expressed feeling of hopelessness, helplessness, powerlessness. • Observe for inappropriate expression of anger, hostility, loss of control. • Note weeping, irritability, and expressed feelings of incompetence. • Observe for expressed overdependency. • Assess noncompliance with treatment plan/other problematic behavior. **THERAPEUTIC INTERVENTIONS** • See Coping, ineffective individual, p. 15.	Calm approach to diagnostic testing will be demonstrated.
DEFINING CHARACTERISTICS Verbalized inability to cope Inability to meet basic needs Noncompliance with treatment plan Emotional tension Use of inappropriate defense mechanisms		

Originated by: Lydia Serra, RN, BSN

Mastectomy: segmented and modified radical

A segmented mastectomy involves removal of a quadrant of the breast or of only a tumor. A modified radical mastectomy involves removal of the breast and axillary contents, leaving the pectoral muscles intact to facilitate reconstruction. These procedures are currently done in the presence of malignant breast tumors. There is considerable controversy about the type of surgery and combination of therapies (i.e., radiation, chemotherapy, and surgical intervention) that ensure no recurrence of malignant disease.

NURSING DIAGNOSES / DEFINING CHARACTERISTICS	NURSING INTERVENTIONS / *RATIONALES*	EXPECTED OUTCOMES
Pain *Related to:* Contraction of tissue resulting from surgery and healing process Intraoperative arm position Possible injury to brachial plexus Lymphedema	**ONGOING ASSESSMENT** • Note subjective reports of pain/discomfort. • Assess neurovascular status of affected arm immediately after surgery and at regular intervals. • Measure arm circumference immediately after surgery and every shift. • Report signs of infections/phlebitis in affected arm. **THERAPEUTIC INTERVENTIONS** • Prevent constriction of affected arm. • Keep arm elevated on two pillows while patient in bed *to decrease edema.* • Protect affected arm from injury. Post notice at head of bed: No BP reading No blood drawing No IV • Instruct, encourage patient in straight extension and abduction exercise (straight elbow raises and wall climbing) on first postoperative day *to increase ROM progressively:*	Pain/discomfort will be reduced.
DEFINING CHARACTERISTICS Inability to move arm through full ROM		

Mastectomy: segmented and modified radical— cont'd

NURSING DIAGNOSES / DEFINING CHARACTERISTICS	NURSING INTERVENTIONS / *RATIONALES*	EXPECTED OUTCOMES
Increased circumference of affected arm Pain report	Perform exercises 5-10 times/hr as tolerated Continue for 1 month after surgery • Obtain elastic sleeve for affected arm with severe lymphedema (per physician's order).	
Potential for injury: seroma *Related to:* Altered lymph drainage Drain malfunction **DEFINING CHARACTERISTICS** Fluid accumulation under flap Flap tenderness Diminished/absent output from drain immediately after surgery	**ONGOING ASSESSMENT** • Immediately after surgery and at regular intervals, check drain for: 　Vacuum 　Clots 　Air leaks • Assess for presence of fluid accumulation beneath flap. • Document amount of output from drain. **THERAPEUTIC INTERVENTIONS** • Milk/strip drain tubing q1h *to maintain patency.* • Notify physician of: 　Drain malfunctions 　Fluid accumulation beneath flap	Potential for injury will be reduced.
Self-concept disturbance/body image disturbance *Related to:* Excision of breast and adjacent tissue Beginning scar tissue Asymmetric breasts caused by implant or prosthesis fit **DEFINING CHARACTERISTICS** Focusing behavior on altered body part Verbalized concerns about loss of femininity Negative feelings about altered body image described	**ONGOING ASSESSMENT** • Assess impact of change in patient's self-perceptions after surgery. **THERAPEUTIC INTERVENTIONS** • Encourage patient to verbalize feelings about effects of surgery on ability to perform roles: 　Woman 　Sexual partner 　Worker • Help patient get information about reconstruction. *Disfigurement caused by amputation need not be permanent; reconstruction techniques effective.* • Contact Reach-to-Recovery volunteer; facilitate visit. *Contact with women who have successfully dealt with mastectomy can help patients before surgery and afterward when they are struggling to adjust to its impact on life.* • Assist patient in wearing temporary, nonweighted prosthetic insert at time of discharge. *Weighted prosthesis can be worn after healing.* • Encourage family (especially husband) to provide positive input. • See Body image disturbance, p. 6.	Feelings about breast loss will be articulated.
Anxiety/fear *Related to:* Breast loss Diagnosis of cancer Uncertain prognosis **DEFINING CHARACTERISTICS** Questioning Crying Withdrawal Restlessness Inability to focus Insomnia	**ONGOING ASSESSMENT** • Assess anxiety level. • Assess previous successful coping strategies. **THERAPEUTIC INTERVENTIONS** • Encourage patient to verbalize feelings. • Reassure patient that anxiety normal. • Assist in use of previously successful coping measures; *(may need to be modified for this crisis).* • Involve other departments (psychiatry, social services) as indicated. • Support realistic assessment; avoid false reassurance. • See Fear, p. 18; Anxiety, p. 4.	Anxiety/fear will be manageable.

Continued.

NURSING DIAGNOSES / DEFINING CHARACTERISTICS	NURSING INTERVENTIONS / *RATIONALES*	EXPECTED OUTCOMES

Knowledge deficit
Related to:
Lack of similar experience
 	
DEFINING CHARACTERISTICS
Verbalized knowledge deficit
Demonstrated inability to grasp information
Questioning
	ONGOING ASSESSMENT
	• Assess knowledge of home care and health maintenance.
	• Determine ability to learn.
	
	THERAPEUTIC INTERVENTIONS
	• Teach about:
	  Wound/arm care:
	    Arm will be stiff and sore; stiffness will cease but armpit numbness will not if nodes dissected
	    Continue exercises at least 1 month
	    Protect arm from injury. Use electric razor when shaving, gloves when gardening or doing dishes, and mitts when handling hot dishes. No blood draws, IVs/injections during subsequent hospitalizations/visits.
	    Use of deodorant is safe
	    Avoidance of tight-fitting sleeves, watches
	    Brassier worn from time of discharge
	• Instruct regarding follow-up care:
	    Importance of monthly breast examination 1 wk after period
	    Annual mammogram of remaining breast *(increased risk of cancer)*
	    Reconstructive surgery (if desired) usually done within 3 months of surgery
	    Importance of being fitted for weighted prosthesis as soon as wound heals
	• Inform regarding family needs:
	    May be familial breast cancer tendency
	    All women in family over 20 should examine breasts monthly
	    Women over 35 should have annual mammogram
	• Explain activity guidelines:
	    Return to all activities as tolerated
	    Resumption of sexual activity as tolerated
	    Swimming permitted after prosthesis obtained
	    Driving resumed as tolerated
		Patient will verbalize importance of follow-up care and proper wound/arm care.

Originated by: Carol Burkhart, RN, BSN, CCRN
             Virginia Cabongon, RN, BSN

Vulvectomy

Surgical excision of the external female genitalia performed as treatment for cancer of vulva.

NURSING DIAGNOSES / DEFINING CHARACTERISTICS	NURSING INTERVENTIONS / *RATIONALES*	EXPECTED OUTCOMES

Knowledge deficit
Related to:
Unfamiliarity with disease process, treatment, and recovery
 	
DEFINING CHARACTERISTICS
Expressed lack of understanding of diagnosis and surgical intervention plan
	ONGOING ASSESSMENT
	• Identify learning needs and ability to comprehend.
	• Assess readiness to learn. *Teaching priorities based on patient need and preference.*
	
	THERAPEUTIC INTERVENTIONS
	• Provide information at the appropriate time about:
	  Diagnosis and reason for surgery
	  Preoperative preparation
	  Intraoperative procedure
	  Postoperative therapy
	• Involve family members in teaching as much as possible.
		Patient verbalizes understanding of nature and extent of disease, surgical treatment plan, and additional therapy.

Vulvectomy— cont'd

NURSING DIAGNOSES / DEFINING CHARACTERISTICS	NURSING INTERVENTIONS / *RATIONALES*	EXPECTED OUTCOMES
Many questions/no questions Expressed negative feelings	• Provide all explanations and information in supportive environment. *Adequate knowledge of disease process, treatment, and recovery ensures patient's/significant others' participation.*	
Potential anxiety/fear *Related to:* Diagnosis Surgical experience Fear of unknown **DEFINING CHARACTERISTICS** Poor eye contact Insomnia Facial tension Restlessness Altered vital signs (BP, pulse) Expressed concern Constant demands Feelings of inadequacy and uncertainty Fear Crying	**ONGOING ASSESSMENT** • Assess patient and family for anxiety signs/symptoms. • Note level of anxiety/fear (mild, moderate, etc.) **THERAPEUTIC INTERVENTIONS** • Encourage patient to express feelings about disfiguring, defeminizing surgery. • Support family members; help them cope with emotional disturbance. • Display confident, calm, tolerant, understanding attitude. • Establish rapport with patient, significant others. • Use other supportive staff (clergy, social worker) as needed. • See Fear, p. 18; Anxiety, p. 4.	Anxiety/fear is reduced/relieved.
Body image disturbance *Related to:* Disfiguring, defeminizing surgery Threatened change in sexuality **DEFINING CHARACTERISTICS** Verbalized feelings of helplessness, hopelessness in relation to body. Feelings of guilt, shame, grief related to physical disfigurement, loss of body part associated with sexuality Negative feelings about body (dirty, unsightly) Poor eye contact Weeping Noncompliance	**ONGOING ASSESSMENT** • Assess perception of body structure, function change. • Assess perceived impact of change on body image, role performance, and sexuality. **THERAPEUTIC INTERVENTIONS** • Acknowledge appropriateness of emotional response to perceived/actual change in body structure/function. • Encourage patient to verbalize feelings *to clarify misconceptions and provide basis for directing emotional support.* • Promote warm communicating relationship through effective verbal/nonverbal (touching) exchanges. Stress importance of spouse's/significant others support. • Reinforce appropriate emotional response; redirect inappropriate negative response. • Encourage self-care activities; provide positive reinforcement accordingly. • Refer to social services as needed. • See Body image disturbance, p. 6; Sexuality patterns, altered, p. 47	Feelings about altered body image are acknowledged.
Pain *Related to:* Surgical incision **DEFINING CHARACTERISTICS** Report of pain	**ONGOING ASSESSMENT** • Assess pain characteristics (quality, severity, location, duration, precipitating factor). • Evaluate pain medication effectiveness. **THERAPEUTIC INTERVENTIONS** • Administer pain medications *to provide analgesia and comfort; prevent unnecessary restlessness and trauma to suture line.*	Pain is relieved or reduced.

Continued.

Vulvectomy— cont'd

NURSING DIAGNOSES / DEFINING CHARACTERISTICS	NURSING INTERVENTIONS / *RATIONALES*	EXPECTED OUTCOMES
Guarded movement Self-focusing Distraction behavior (i.e., moaning, crying, pacing, seeking out other people) Insomnia Irritability	• Be meticulous in providing perineal care: *area very sensitive and friable.* Avoid straining suture line, causing increased pain. • See Pain, p. 39.	
Potential fluid volume deficit *Related to:* Loss of body fluid through nasogastric suction, drains Diuresis Excessive loss of blood during surgery NPO **DEFINING CHARACTERISTICS** Decreased urine output Concentrated urine Hypotension Increased pulse rate Dry mucous membrane Weakness Electrolyte imbalance Restlessness Excessive drainage from N/G tube Low Hb, Hct.	**ONGOING ASSESSMENT** • Assess vital signs. • Assess hydration status: skin turgor, mucous membranes, drainage from drains and N/G tube. • Maintain Hb, Hct, and electrolytes. **THERAPEUTIC INTERVENTIONS** • See Fluid volume deficit, p. 20.	Adequate fluid and electrolyte balance is maintained.
Potential for infection *Related to:* Wound site Surgical procedure Invasive catheters Perineal organisms **DEFINING CHARACTERISTICS** *Systemic:* Increased WBC Increased RBC Elevated temperature Increased respiratory rate *Wound:* Swelling and tenderness Drainage from incision with unusual odor and color	**ONGOING ASSESSMENT** • Assess vital signs, especially temperature. • Assess for wound infection signs/symptoms. **THERAPEUTIC INTERVENTIONS** • Maintain good hand washing technique. • Irrigate vulva with prescribed antiseptic solution; keep area dry. • Keep perineum free of rectal contamination. • Administer heat to perineal area *to promote healing of stitches.* • Maintain patency of Foley catheter; provide aseptic catheter care. • Administer antipyretics and antibiotics as ordered.	Wound and bladder infections are prevented/reduced.

NURSING DIAGNOSES / DEFINING CHARACTERISTICS	NURSING INTERVENTIONS / *RATIONALES*	EXPECTED OUTCOMES
Bladder: Urinary urgency and frequency (after Foley catheter discontinued) Hematuria, pyuria, bacteriuria		
Constipation *Related to:* Reduced physical activity Pain on defecation **Defining Characteristics** Reported feeling of rectal fullness/ pressure Straining for stool Abdominal pain Headache Decreased appetite Uneasiness	**Ongoing Assessment** · Assess abdomen for presence of bowel sounds. · Elicit usual constipation relief measures. · Review medications for side effects of constipation. **Therapeutic Interventions** · Modify dietary intake to include high-fiber foods. · Increase fluid intake. · Administer pain relief before defecation. *Fear of pain may inhibit desire to defecate.* · Provide privacy. · Increase physical activity as tolerated.	Constipation is relieved.

Originated by: Rosita Sortijas, RN, BSN

15

Psychosocial Care Plans

DISORDERS

Anorexia nervosa
Bipolar disorder/mania

Bulimia
Depression
Grief over long-term illness/disability

Isolation
Substance abuse
Suicidal attempt/suicidal gesture

Anorexia nervosa

Syndrome characterized by an intense fear of fatness, severe weight loss, and disturbed body image occurring in otherwise normal, healthy individuals.

NURSING DIAGNOSES / DEFINING CHARACTERISTICS	NURSING INTERVENTIONS / *RATIONALES*	EXPECTED OUTCOMES

Altered nutrition: less than body requirements
Related to:
Inability to allow for adequate nutritional intake caused by "fear of fatness"
 	
DEFINING CHARACTERISTICS
Body weight 20% or more below ideal for height and frame
Self-restricted food intake despite hunger
Excessive, irrational fear of fatness
Distorted body image
No other illness that would explain weight loss/prevent weight gain
	ONGOING ASSESSMENT
	- Document patient's actual weight and height on admission.
	- Obtain accurate weight history, including reason for weight loss.
	- Perform in-depth nutritional assessment:
	  Diet history (reconstruction of typical 24-hr intake)
	  Development of patient's beliefs and fears about food
	  Level of nutritional knowledge
	  Behaviors used to reduce energy intake (dieting), to increase energy output (exercising), and generally to lose weight (vomiting, purging, and laxative abuse)
	- Monitor and record daily I & O.
	- Weigh daily at same time, in same clothes, on same scale; record.
	
	THERAPEUTIC INTERVENTIONS
	- Closely supervise high-protein, high-calorie refeeding of approximately 1800 calories/day *to correct acute starvation phase.* Gradually increase daily caloric intake *to ensure steady weight gain until goal achieved.*
	- Closely supervise bathroom use after meals if required *to decrease opportunity to vomit/dispose of food.*
	- Be consistent. Present and remove food without persuasion *to help separate emotional issues (e.g., approval) from eating behavior.*
	- Set limits on excessive physical activity but allow daily activity (*overrestriction may induce severe/overwhelming anxiety*).
	- Provide accurate nutritional information *to correct false ideas about food and weight gain.*
	- Give assurances patient will not become overweight.
	- Acknowledge patient's anger and feelings of loss of control caused by established eating program.
	- In emergency refer to Enteral tube feeding, p. 308; Total parenteral nutrition p. 324.
		Optimal nutritional levels and normal body weight are attained.

Body image disturbance *Related to:* Failure to achieve unreasonable expectations of self **DEFINING CHARACTERISTICS** Disturbed body image Low self-esteem Alexithymia (channeling uncomfortable feelings into behaviors such as self-starvation)	**ONGOING ASSESSMENT** - Assess patient's perception of body image. - Elicit patient's assessment of strengths and weaknesses. - Assess patient's ability to identify feeling states. **THERAPEUTIC INTERVENTIONS** - Offer objective information about body shape and process of weight gain. - Help patient develop realistic, acceptable perception of body image and relationship with food. - Encourage patient to re-examine negative self-perceptions. - Encourage identification, expression, and tolerance of unpleasant feeling states. - Examine and deal with negative feelings about patient *to prevent interference with patient's care.*	Degree of body image disturbance is lessened.
Ineffective individual coping *Related to:* Inadequate repertoire of skills to deal with maturational crisis	**ONGOING ASSESSMENT** - Assess degree of social isolation. - Assess problem-solving abilities. - Observe behaviors (e.g., avoiding interaction with others, demanding behaviors) **THERAPEUTIC INTERVENTIONS** - Assist patient to assume control in areas other than dieting and weight loss *to decrease sense of "pseudoindependence" and regressive behaviors.*	Social integration and decision-making ability are improved.

Continued.

NURSING DIAGNOSES / DEFINING CHARACTERISTICS	NURSING INTERVENTIONS / *RATIONALES*	EXPECTED OUTCOMES
DEFINING CHARACTERISTICS Verbalized inability to cope Felt inability to meet role expectations Use of ineffective coping mechanisms to manage anxiety (e.g., rituals involving food/activity and preoccupation with thinness)	• Encourage and assist patient to make own decisions *to promote feelings of control through independent decision making.* • Encourage patient to reassess unrealistic self-expectations *as means of modifying self-critical thinking.*	
Altered thought processes *Related to:* Starvation state **DEFINING CHARACTERISTICS** Changed mental status Decreased attention span Impaired abstract thinking abilities Impaired judgment and decision-making capacity	**ONGOING ASSESSMENT** • Determine patient's degree of insight. • Assess patient's ability to acknowledge/appreciate physiologic, psychologic sequelae of starvation. **THERAPEUTIC INTERVENTIONS** • Provide frequent contact *to allay anxiety and establish trust.* • Provide accepting atmosphere. • Provide for nutritional restabilization by helping patient adhere to intake regimen. • Explain effects of starvation; emphasize its reinforcement of underlying feelings of helplessness through cognitive distortion. • Promote reality orientation *to provide factual, objective information about amount of food/liquid actually consumed and needed, but without challenging patient's irrational thinking.*	Marked cognitive improvement will be realized.
Knowledge deficit: *Related to:* Cognitive impairment secondary to starvation **DEFINING CHARACTERISTICS** Verbalized misconceptions about process of dieting and weight loss Apparent lack of concern about emaciated condition	**ONGOING ASSESSMENT** • Assess patient's knowledge of illness course. • Assess patient's cognitive readiness to learn and understand. **THERAPEUTIC INTERVENTIONS** • Instruct patient about the physiologic and psychologic sequelae of anorexia nervosa. • Allow and encourage patient to ask questions *to assess and promote improvement in patient's knowledge base.* • Identify improvement in cognitive/physical functioning secondary to nutritional restabilization.	Concentration and attention span improve.

Altered family process
Related to:
Developmental crisis of separation and family restructuring
	ONGOING ASSESSMENT
	• Assess type of interactional patterns used by family:
	  Enmeshment, *lack of generational boundaries between family members;*
	  Overprotectiveness, *demonstrated by exaggerated concern for welfare of others in family*
	  Rigidity, *emphasis on maintaining status quo*
	  Lack of conflict resolution via triangulation coalition (*parents collude with child to prevent conflict expression/resolution e.g., child becomes symptomatic to deflect parental conflict*)
	  Involvement of the anorectic child in unresolved parental conflict
		Family members appropriately address autonomy and conflict issues.

Anorexia nervosa— cont'd

NURSING DIAGNOSES / DEFINING CHARACTERISTICS	NURSING INTERVENTIONS / *RATIONALES*	EXPECTED OUTCOMES
DEFINING CHARACTERISTICS Family members' inability to relate to each other for mutual growth and maturation as evidenced by patient's self-starvation and weight loss	**THERAPEUTIC INTERVENTIONS** • Explore family's reasons for recurring problems *to de-emphasize family's notion of patient being problem.* • Explore with family members effects of each individual's behavior on others. • Identify interaction patterns among family members *to demonstrate how patterns engender dependence on environment for cues about regulation rather than fostering self-regulation.* • Acknowledge and offer feedback to family's expressed feelings *to encourage direct expression and ownership of feelings.* • Encourage participation in therapeutic group interaction, especially family therapy.	

Originated by: Nancy Staples, RN, BSN

Bipolar disorder/mania
(MANIC DEPRESSIVE DISORDER)

An altered psychologic state that may be characterized by excessive excitement and psychomotor activity markedly elevated mood, delusions of grandeur, excessive ideation, and impaired judgment.

NURSING DIAGNOSES / DEFINING CHARACTERISTICS	NURSING INTERVENTIONS / *RATIONALES*	EXPECTED OUTCOMES
Impaired verbal communication *Related to:* Altered thought processes Anxiety Drug effects Biochemical imbalance Impaired judgment **DEFINING CHARACTERISTICS** Rapid, pressured speech Intrusive behavior Verbal abusiveness Incessant verbalization Monopolizing of conversations Inappropriate speech Inattention Loose associations Flight of ideas Confusion Poor comprehension	**ONGOING ASSESSMENT** • Identify areas of communication difficulty (see Defining Characteristics). • Observe for contradictory verbal and nonverbal messages. **THERAPEUTIC INTERVENTIONS** • Provide atmosphere of acceptance. • Listen attentively. • Provide feedback about patient's communication: 　Restate what was communicated; allow patient to confirm/clarify. 　Correct misunderstandings immediately. • Assist patient in attempts to communicate effectively: 　Limit amount of stimulation. 　Keep conversations brief and concise. • Clearly communicate behavioral expectations. *Ambiguity and lack of concrete structure/guidance taxes resources of patient already overwhelmed by stimuli and experiencing significant anxiety; often produces further deterioration in communication.* • Encourage expression of feelings. • Assist with social/interactional aspects of communication process. Set limits on inappropriate behavior: 　Avoid agreeing with patient's deprecating or grandiose statements about self/others. 　Respond to verbally abusive comments calmly. 　Avoid engaging in power struggles or arguments. 　Model appropriate behavior in interactions with client, others: 　　Maintain respectful posture. 　　Demonstrate congruence between verbal and nonverbal messages.	Effectiveness of patient's verbal communication increases.

Continued.

NURSING DIAGNOSES / DEFINING CHARACTERISTICS	NURSING INTERVENTIONS / *RATIONALES*	EXPECTED OUTCOMES
Self-care deficit: bathing/grooming/ hygiene/dressing *Related to:* Perceptual and cognitive impairments Acute disorganization Hyperactivity Altered self-concept **DEFINING CHARACTERISTICS** Inappropriate, bizarre, or flamboyant dress/ grooming Failure to attend to hygiene Difficulty in completing grooming tasks/ rituals	**ONGOING ASSESSMENT** • Assess patient's hygiene practices (bathing, hair care, skin and nail care, and oral hygiene). • Assess preferences for types of grooming/hygiene products. • Assess ability to care for clothing (washing, ironing, minor repair, and appropriate storage). • Identify preferred clothing styles and patterns of makeup, grooming aids. **THERAPEUTIC INTERVENTIONS** • Establish routine for bathing, oral care, and dressing. • Assist patient (as needed) in performing basic personal hygiene. • Provide supervision with grooming activities. • Assist in clothing, makeup selection. • Assist with application of makeup/other grooming aids. • Give positive feedback for appropriate hygiene, grooming, and independent self-care practices. *Inappropriate/inadequate practices elicit social disapproval, further damage patient's self-concept; positive reinforcement may increase likelihood of adequate self-care.*	Hygiene, dress, and grooming practices will conform to reasonably acceptable social norms.
Potential altered nutrition: less than body requirements *Related to:* Increased caloric requirements caused by hyperactivity Decreased caloric intake Poor reality testing Indifference to food (too busy to eat) Idiosyncratic beliefs about food Socially inappropriate eating behavior **DEFINING CHARACTERISTICS** Inadequate food intake >10-20% below ideal body weight Loss of weight with/ without adequate caloric intake	**ONGOING ASSESSMENT** • Document admission weight. • Obtain nutritional history. • Monitor paient's eating patterns and behavior. • Monitor activity level; limit unnecessary/modifiable caloric expenditures when possible. **THERAPEUTIC INTERVENTIONS** • Provide quiet/nonstimulating setting during meals. • Assist patient in choosing realistic amounts, types of foods, fluids. • Provide portable high-calorie, nutritious foods (prepackaged items, sandwiches, fruit, shakes etc.) if patient unable to sit and eat. • Discourage use of non-nutritional/stimulating substances (i.e., coffee, cola drinks, simple carbohydrates) • Provide nutrition instruction as appropriate. *Excessively stimulated patients may not be able to use complex forms of information/attend to lengthy instruction.* • Limit inappropriate eating behaviors (e.g., gorging, stealing, or hording food items). • See Nutrition, altered: less than body requirements, p. 37.	Adequate nutrition and hydration levels are maintained.
Sleep pattern disturbance *Related to:* Psychologic stress Biochemical alteration Hyperactivity Anxiety/fear **DEFINING CHARACTERISTICS** Insomnia Frequent awakening	**ONGOING ASSESSMENT** • Assess past sleep/rest patterns • Assess past, present levels of activity. • Observe, document current sleep pattern. **THERAPEUTIC INTERVENTIONS** • Provide gradual transition between day and night activity levels. • Decrease environmental stimuli *to facilitate rest/sleep.* • Re-establish bedtime ritual *to help patient manage anxiety.* • Consider use of relaxation aids (e.g., warm bath, deep breathing exercise). • Administer sedating medications as ordered.	An adequate sleep-rest pattern will be established and maintained.

Bipolar disorder/mania— cont'd

NURSING DIAGNOSES / DEFINING CHARACTERISTICS	NURSING INTERVENTIONS / *RATIONALES*	EXPECTED OUTCOMES
Irritability Described/experienced need for little/no sleep Dozing during daytime hours Agitation	• Limit interaction with patient at night. *Important to reassure patient of availability of others but minimize unnecessary contacts to prevent stimulating highly reactive CNS.*	

Potential for injury: secondary to lithium toxicity
Related to:
Excessive lithium intake
Altered renal function
Altered fluid and electrolyte balance
Medication interactions
Altered cardiovascular status
Infection
Altered GI function
 	
DEFINING CHARACTERISTICS
Early:
Increased thirst
Muscle weakness
Increased fine muscle tremor
Poor coordination
Drowsiness/excitement
Nausea/vomiting
Diarrhea
Tinnitus
Late:
Muscle twitching/ spasm
Polyuria
Slurred speech
Confusion
Stupor
Seizures
Blurred vision
Nystagmus
Coma
	ONGOING ASSESSMENT
	• Assess patient's past/present medication history (drugs used, compliance with regimens, preferred forms or routes, etc.).
	• Note pre-existing medical condition/current factors that may influence lithium tolerance.
	• Document observed baseline mood and behavior and subsequent changes.
	• Monitor blood lithium levels every ___ days/weeks
	  Desired
	    Acute treatment phase 1.2-1.6 mEq/L
	    Maintenance/prophylaxis phase 0.8-1.2 mEq/L
	• Observe for lithium toxicity signs/symptoms (see Defining Characteristics). Inform physician to withhold lithium if necessary.
	
	THERAPEUTIC INTERVENTIONS
	• Administer lithium/other psychoactive drugs as ordered.
	• Attempt to minimize potential side effects/discomforts:
	  Reverse rapid dosage increases if possible.
	  Administer drug after meals *to decrease GI distress.*
	   Minimizing unpleasant side effects may increase likelihood of compliance with prescribed regimen.
	• Encourage consumption of balanced diet with "normal" Na^+ and K^+ intake. *Adequate fluid and electrolyte balance vital in preventing lithium toxicity.*
	• Educate patient/significant others about lithium therapy:
	  Action of medication
	  Prescribed dosage, need for regular blood level monitoring
	  Toxicity signs/symptoms
	  Possible side effects (mild, fine tremor, mild GI distress, etc.)
	  Illnesses or events that may alter lithium excretion
	  Importance of long-term maintenance in symptom control (i.e., not to be taken only when behavior/mood has escalated)
	• Use clear, simple language; provide written materials/instructions *to reinforce teaching.*
	• Provide nonjudgmental feedback on observed behavior changes since beginning use of lithium *to minimize denial.*
		Patient/significant other verbalizes understanding of use of lithium therapy and potential associated risks.

Knowledge deficit: illness
Related to:
Lack of adequate past explanations
Unfamiliarity with relevant terminology
New diagnosis
Stigma of mental illness
	ONGOING ASSESSMENT
	• Evaluate patient's knowledge of diagnosis:
	  Past exposure to information via teaching or informed learning
	  Role of hereditary, biochemical, and psychosocial factors
	  Recommended treatment:
	    Acute
	    Long-term management
	• Assess ability to comprehend, retain information.
	• Identify factors that may influence learning:
	  Communication problems; language barriers
	  Anxiety level
	  Acceptance of diagnosis by patient/significant others
	  Preferred learning methods (written material, informal discussion, etc.)
		Patient/significant other(s) verbalize basic understanding of diagnosis and recommended treatment.

Continued.

NURSING DIAGNOSES / DEFINING CHARACTERISTICS	NURSING INTERVENTIONS / *RATIONALES*	EXPECTED OUTCOMES

DEFINING CHARACTERISTICS
Denial of need for information
Noncompliance with prescribed regimen
Verbalized inaccurate perception of health status
Expressed needs for additional information about illness
	THERAPEUTIC INTERVENTIONS
	· Approach patient with acceptance.
	· Initiate basic information early in contacts with client by offering simple explanations and rationale for interventions.
	· As thinking processes become clearer, patient may be asked to use more traditional instructional methods. *Anxiety, decreased attention span, and impaired concentration all interfere with effective learning. Symptoms often in evidence during acute illness phases.*
	· Review with client:
	  Usual illness manifestations
	  Role of multiple factors in illness development and onset:
	    Biochemical
	    Hereditary
	    Psychosocial
	  Recommended treatment approaches:
	    Medications
	    Psychotherapy
	    Interpersonal/social implications
	· Include significant other(s) in teaching process as appropriate.
	· Offer patient/significant other(s) hope illness can be managed.
	· Connect episodes of illness to stressors/noncompliance with treatment regimen as appropriate *(may minimize denial).*	

Impaired socialization secondary to self-esteem disturbance
Related to:
Anxiety
Poor self-concept
Rejection/avoidance by others
Absence of gratifying interactions with others
Impaired communication
Hyperactivity
Inability to attend to others
Distorted perceptions
Impaired judgment
 	
DEFINING CHARACTERISTICS
Intrusive behavior
Tendency to monopolize conversations
Verbal abuse of others
Grandiose self-statements
Difficulty in expressing feelings/thoughts in logical/socially appropriate manner
Sexually provocative behavior
Observed discomfort of patient/others in social situations
	ONGOING ASSESSMENT
	· Assess for changes in usual style of relating to others.
	· Observe behavior in varied situations/settings:
	  Note tolerance for stimuli.
	  Monitor others' responses to patient's social behavior.
	  Observe congruence between verbal and nonverbal behavior.
	  Note comfort level in individual/group/community interactions.
	· Identify behavior suggesting increasing discomfort in social settings:
	  Tendency to distance/alienate others
	  Aloofness
	  Hyperactivity/agitation
	  Ignoring of others' verbal/nonverbal cues
	  Verbalized anxiety
	  See other Defining Characteristics
	
	THERAPEUTIC INTERVENTIONS
	· Assist patient in efforts to appraise socialization skills realistically.
	· Provide feedback on observed social interactions.
	· Limit nature, degree of involvement in activities that may be overstimulating.
	· Explore effect of behavior on others.
	· Set limits on inappropriate behavior. *Grossly inappropriate behavior elicits social disapproval and rejection; likely to lead to sense of isolation and further decrease in self-esteem.*
	· Support patient efforts to be effective group member (rather than center of attention).
	· Involve patient in interactions/activities that provide opportunities for success and improved self-concept:
	  Begin with simple; progress to more complex situations.
	  Build on patient's demonstrated strengths/pre-existing capabilities.
	· Provide role model for appropriate social behavior.
		Patient's ability to socialize improves.

NURSING DIAGNOSES / DEFINING CHARACTERISTICS	NURSING INTERVENTIONS / *RATIONALES*	EXPECTED OUTCOMES

Altered thought processes *Related to:* Biochemical abnormality Impaired individual coping Isolation Recent loss or stress Anxiety **DEFINING CHARACTERISTICS** Disorientation Distractability Impaired memory Inaccurate interpretation of stimuli; hallucinations; delusions Flight of ideas Loose associations Poor judgment Euphoria/elevated mood	**ONGOING ASSESSMENT**
	 • Assess current mental status in areas of judgment, orientation, memory, cognition, and affect.
	 • Note evidence in history suggesting distorted thinking processes (i.e., suspiciousness, unrealistic beliefs about self and own abilities, involvement in risky/fantastic ventures, sudden marked shift in behavior patterns).
	
	 THERAPEUTIC INTERVENTIONS
	 • Decrease environmental stimuli.
	 • Involve patient in simple, structured activities *to help focus attention.*
	 • Minimize ambiguity in interpersonal and environmental context. *Uncertainty may only heighten patient's sense of ineffectiveness and increase anxiety; may lead to further idiosyncratic thinking and impair problem-solving abilities.*
	 • Provide clear, concise instruction and direction.
	 • Assist with reality testing:
	   State own simple observations and views.
	   Avoid attempting to persuade patient that thinking/sensory experiences not true or real.
	   Assure of safety and security, particularly when he/she reports threatening/frightening delusions/hallucinations.
	 • Use antianxiety agents/other measures as ordered to assure patient safety if anxiety overwhelming.
	 • Orient as needed.
	 • Minimize number/complexity of decisions patient faces when thinking processes clearly impaired. Offer limited choices to *allow some sense of autonomy.*
	 • Teach problem-solving approach when appropriate:
	   Accurately appraising situation
	   Identifying problem to be solved
	   Listing possible solutions
	   Defining advantages/disadvantages of each
	   Selecting solution(s)
	   Implementing solutions
	   Evaluating outcome
		Thinking will be more organized.

Originated by: Ann Filipski, RN, MSN, CS, Psy D Candidate

Bulimia

Bulimia is a syndrome characterized by ego-alien episodes of binge eating involving rapid consumption of large quantities of food within a discrete time period. Feelings of guilt and pain follow from the lost sense of control, which trigger purging/dieting attempts to restore sense of control and weight mastery. The term normal weight bulimia *(NWB) refers to those individuals whose weight has always been in the normal range or above; the term* bulimia nervosa *(BN) refers to the subgroup who have experienced a previous episode of, but who no longer meet the criteria for, anorexia nervosa.*

NURSING DIAGNOSES / DEFINING CHARACTERISTICS	NURSING INTERVENTIONS / *RATIONALES*	EXPECTED OUTCOMES
Altered nutrition: potential for excess *Related to:* Intake may exceed metabolic needs because of episodic binge-eating activity **DEFINING CHARACTERISTICS** Unsuccessful attempts at severely restrictive dieting followed by episodic, secretive consumption of large to enormous amounts of food (usually sweets or carbohydrates) within discrete period Method of purging behavior (vomiting, laxatives, diuretics) results in weight fluctuations, often greater than 10 lb	**ONGOING ASSESSMENT** - Obtain accurate history of weight fluctuations - Assess height and weight; determine ideal body weight. - Obtain accurate diet history, including daily intake, number and methods of dieting, type and frequency of binge-purge behavior, and associated feeling states - Weigh patient twice weekly in same manner at same time; record. *More frequent weighing reinforces patient's preoccupation with body size.* **THERAPEUTIC INTERVENTIONS** - Establish reasonable weight range with patient. - Devise diet plan that specifies number of calories (but not less than 1600/day) and includes all food groups. Plan should include three meals plus a light evening snack *as adequate intake alleviates effects of starvation (e.g., sleeplessness or waking during the night), preoccupation with thoughts of food, and tendency to binge behavior.* - Give accurate information about nutrition and metabolic functioning *to correct faulty ideas.* Assure patient that all metabolic deficiencies can be corrected through proper nutrition. - Provide contact during, after meals *to encourage normal eating habits while interfering with potential impulse to vomit.* - Encourage reasonable physical activity *to regulate weight and promote sense of well-being and control.* - Be aware of potential for purging behavior, particularly weight shifts; if suspected, address issue directly. Use observation and supervision as necessary *to help patient interrupt cycle of purging behavior.*	Adequate dietary habits are developed while maintaining normal body weight.
Potential fluid volume deficit *Related to:* Fluid shifts caused by excess reliance on: Vomiting Laxatives Diuretics Severely restrictive dieting **DEFINING CHARACTERISTICS** Dehydration Thirst Electrolyte imbalance, particularly hypokalemia Edema Decreased urinary output	**ONGOING ASSESSMENT** - Accurately monitor I & O; and record. - Review lab results, especially for electrolyte imbalance. - Note ECG results. - Monitor vital signs *(patient may be prone to hypotension and tachycardia).* - Observe for signs of unexplained diarrhea or persistent hypokalemia *(usually indicates continued vomiting/use of diuretics/laxatives.* **THERAPEUTIC INTERVENTIONS** - Provide adequate fluid *to remedy imbalances of fluid and electrolytes;* limit amounts of diet sodas consumed *(generally high in sodium).*	Fluid volume, normal hydration, and electrolyte status are maintained.

NURSING DIAGNOSES / DEFINING CHARACTERISTICS	NURSING INTERVENTIONS / *RATIONALES*	EXPECTED OUTCOMES

Ineffective individual coping *Related to:* Deficit in introspective awareness (i.e., difficulty identifying, articulating, and modulating internal states, e.g., hunger, satiety, and their effects)
 	
DEFINING CHARACTERISTICS Binge/purge behavior is generalized to alleviate uncomfortable mood states (dysphoria)
Multiple impulse disorders (e.g., alcohol/drug abuse, sexual promiscuity, stealing, and self-harm) may be present in response to psychosocial stressors (e.g., depression, stress, and anxiety)
	ONGOING ASSESSMENT
	• Assess ability to differentiate and label mood states.
	• Obtain detailed history about type, duration, and intensity of impulsive behaviors.
	
	THERAPEUTIC INTERVENTIONS
	• Instruct patient to keep a food journal; include before-, during-, and after-binge/purge activities. *Self-monitoring activities can begin association of mood states with binge-purge behavior.*
	• Help patient develop list of alternatives to impulsive behavior (e.g., talking to someone, going for a walk). *By introducing technique of delay, impulse will lessen in strength; use of alternative strategies facilitates sense of mastery.*
	• Encourage and accept patient's verbal expression of feelings. *Maintain nonjudgmental attitude so as not to reinforce excessive feelings of guilt, shame, and helplessness.*
	• Review examples of cognitive distortion exhibited:
	    Magical thinking
	    Dichotomous/all-or-nothing thinking
	    Control fallacy; viewing self as externally controlled
	    Magnification
	    Overgeneralization
		Health coping skills are developed and utilized.

Body image disturbance *Related to:* Feelings of inadequacy, worthlessness, criticalness Shame and guilt caused by discrepancy between actual/ideal self **DEFINING CHARACTERISTICS** Lack of interpersonal confidence Body size dissatisfaction	**ONGOING ASSESSMENT** • Assess degree of impairment of life adjustments (i.e., work, interpersonal relationships) as result of symptomatic behavior. • Assess perception of body image as compared to ideal. **THERAPEUTIC INTERVENTIONS** • Explore and encourage patient to introduce into life self-enhancing activities (e.g., exercising) *to disrupt isolation and withdrawal; increase self-esteem.* • Encourage patient to use family/friends as source of support *to decrease social isolation and reduce fear of rejection from others.* • Encourage patient to develop and use problem-solving skills *as means of confronting perfectionistic self-expectations.* • Focus on healthy aspects of personality. Give examples of how patient magnifies weight-related issues while minimizing or discrediting other personal assets. • Listen to patient's concerns about self without minimizing them. *Maintaining positive regard can allow patient to experience self and others more acceptingly.* • Encourage patient to join appropriate support group as adjunct to other treatment interventions, *to reinforce sense of community and provide additional structure.*	Positive expressions of body image verbalized.

Continued.

NURSING DIAGNOSES / DEFINING CHARACTERISTICS	NURSING INTERVENTIONS / *RATIONALES*	EXPECTED OUTCOMES
Knowledge deficit *Related to:* Lack of information about illness caused by secrecy, feelings of guilt and shame about bulimia behavior **DEFINING CHARACTERISTICS** Lack of information about dieting and weight loss Misconceptions about appropriate, normal body size and weight	**ONGOING ASSESSMENT** ▪ Assess patient's knowledge of illness course. ▪ Assess readiness to learn and understand. **THERAPEUTIC INTERVENTIONS** ▪ Instruct patient about physiologic and psychologic aspects of bulimia. ▪ Provide information about effects of binge/purge behavior. ▪ Provide resource readings on dieting, set-point theory, and role of deprivation in triggering binges *to help patient see how struggles with food are culturally and biologically influenced rather than purely personal failures in "will-power"*	Understanding of disease process is verbalized.

Originated by: Nancy Staples, RN, BSN

Depression

An effective disorder characterized by feelings of unworthiness, profound sadness, guilt, apathy, and hopelessness. A loss of interest and pleasure in usual activities is evident. Behavioral characteristics may include slowing of physical activity or agitation and alterations in sleeping, eating, and libido. Depression differs from sadness in that it is a disease rather than a feeling. Depressive features are seen in postpartum depression, premenstrual syndrome, alcohol and/or drug withdrawal, and involutional melancholia. Depression may also be reactive and situational, associated with grief and loss of health, job, and/or significant other. Depression features can be a component of affective/mood disorders, including bipolar (manic-depressive) illness. Suicidal ideation and/or gestures, as well as psychotic thought processes, may be present.

NURSING DIAGNOSES / DEFINING CHARACTERISTICS	NURSING INTERVENTIONS / *RATIONALES*	EXPECTED OUTCOMES

Self-care deficits:
bathing/hygiene/
dressing/grooming,
feeding/toileting
Related to:
Psychomotor retardation/agitation
Energy depletion
Fatigue
Weakness
Low self-esteem
Apathy
Poor appetite
	ONGOING ASSESSMENT
	▪ Assess patient's current and past sleeping patterns. Determine whether patient has trouble falling asleep, wakes during sleep, or experiences difficulty with both. *Degree of psychomotor agitation/retardation impacts on particular sleeping pattern impairment.*
	▪ Assess the current and past:
	    Eating patterns
	    Energy level
	    Activity level
	▪ Monitor food and fluid intake.
	▪ Monitor weight regularly. Determine whether recent weight loss/gain.
	▪ Assess bowel and bladder elimination patterns.
		Self-care skills improve.

NURSING DIAGNOSES / DEFINING CHARACTERISTICS	NURSING INTERVENTIONS / *RATIONALES*	EXPECTED OUTCOMES
DEFINING CHARACTERISTICS Excessive sleeping/ interrupted sleeping patterns/lack of sleep Excessive eating/ interrupted eating patterns/lack of appetite Poor hygiene/ grooming Constipation	**THERAPEUTIC INTERVENTIONS** ▪ Encourage adequate balance of rest, sleep, and activity: ▪ Discourage daytime sleeping. ▪ Set firm but gentle limits on time spent in bed. ▪ Use prn medication to promote sleep. ▪ See Self-care deficit, p. 44. ▪ Assist in performing ADLs. *Depressed patient unable to define and balance needs for sleep, rest, and activity.*	
Impaired physical mobility *Related to:* Psychomotor retardation/agitation Energy depletion Fatigue Weakness Apathy (low self-esteem) **DEFINING CHARACTERISTICS** Feeling of heaviness Feeling of numbness (generalized) Restlessness Pacing Hand wringing Aimless walking Decreased motor activity Decreased energy for purposeful activities	**ONGOING ASSESSMENT** ▪ Assess current and past energy levels. ▪ Assess current and past activity/exercise levels. ▪ Assess ability to respond to staff contact when agitated. **THERAPEUTIC INTERVENTIONS** ▪ Emphasize importance of exercise/activity, relationship to improved mental and emotional status. *Depressed patient often believes he/she doesn't feel well enough to exercise; needs to understand importance of exercise/ activity. Do not wait to exercise until feeling better; exercise to feel better.* ▪ Structure schedule of exercise/activities; provide time alone and with others. Involve patient in development of schedule (*reinforces importance of input and degree of control*). ▪ Continue to expect patient to attend unit activities despite refusal.	Mobility is enhanced.
Social isolation *Related to:* Withdrawn and regressive behavior Impaired communication Low self-esteem Disrupted personal relationships Sexual dysfunction Fear of rejection Fear of failure **DEFINING CHARACTERISTICS** Feelings of numbness, emptiness, and hopelessness Verbalizations limited in spontaneity and quantity Depressed, dull affect	**ONGOING ASSESSMENT** ▪ Assess affect. ▪ Assess eye contact. ▪ Assess spontaneity and verbal frequency. ▪ Assess involvement with others. **THERAPEUTIC INTERVENTIONS** ▪ Encourage relationship with patient by spending time with him/her, providing supportive contact. *Patient's self-worth enhanced by consistent, supportive staff presence.* ▪ Encourage participation in group activities as tolerated. Allow patient to leave group situations when contact with others too anxiety-provoking. *Patient needs to feel some degree of control over environment.* ▪ Provide positive reinforcement when patient participates in group activities and interacts with others (*supports patient's efforts; helps augment feelings of self-worth*). ▪ Acknowledge patient's involvement in daily activities *to validate staff's awareness of attempts at help self.*	Social isolation diminishes.

Continued.

Depression— cont'd

NURSING DIAGNOSES / DEFINING CHARACTERISTICS	NURSING INTERVENTIONS / *RATIONALES*	EXPECTED OUTCOMES
Rumination and pre-occupation with negative thoughts Feelings of unworthiness Loss of interest in sexual activity		

Potential for violence: self-directed *Related to:* Low self-esteem Depressed mood Hopelessness Repeated failures in life activities Reality distortion Feelings of worthlessness Feelings of abandonment Anger Guilt Actual/perceived loss **DEFINING CHARACTERISTICS** Verbalized desire/plan to harm/kill self Self-destructive behavior Aggressive suicidal acts History of self-destructive behavior History of suicidal ideation/gestures Expression of hopelessness and powerlessness to improve life Preparation for "impending death" (i.e., putting family/business matters in order, giving away significant possession, writing will)	**ONGOING ASSESSMENT** • Interview patient to evaluate potential for self-directed violence. Ask: Have you felt like hurting yourself? *Suicidal ideation is process of thinking about killing oneself.* Did you ever attempt suicide? *Suicidal gestures are attempts to harm onself that are not considered lethal. Suicidal attempts are potentially lethal actions.* Do you currently feel like killing yourself? Have you recently attempted suicide? Do you have a plan to hurt yourself? What is your plan? Do you have the means to carry out your plan? *Development of plan and ability to carry it out greatly increase risk of patient's harming self.* • Assess for the presence of risk factors that may increase potential for patient to attempt suicide: Formulated plan Means to make plan reality History of suicidal attempts Mood/activity level that changes suddenly Giving away of personal possessions Young adult/adolescent male Divorced, widowed, or separated individual Early stage of treatment with antidepressant medication during which patient's mood/energy elevates *Remember that every patient has potential for suicide.* **THERAPEUTIC INTERVENTIONS** • Provide safe environment. *Suicide precautions are interventions taken to create safe environment for the patient; protect patient from acting on self-destructive impulses. Includes removing all potentially harmful objects: electrical appliances, sharp instruments, belts/ties, medication, glass items. Maintaining patient safety is priority.* • Provide close patient supervision. • Develop verbal/written contract stating the he/she will not act on impulses to harm self. Review and develop new contracts as needed. *Patient needs to verbalize suicidal ideations with trusted staff. Written/verbal agreement also establishes permission to discuss subject.* • Encourage verbalization of feelings within appropriate limits. *Depressed patient needs opportunity to discuss thoughts/intentions to harm self. Verbalization of these feelings may lessen their intensity. Patient also needs to see that staff can tolerate discussion of suicidal ideations; be available to cope with struggle.* • Develop agreement that patient will contact staff when experiencing suicidal ideations. • In addition to providing safe environment, taking suicide precautions, spend time with patient *to provide sense of security, reinforce self-worth.* • Refer to Suicidal attempt/Suicidal gestures, p. 627.	Potential for self-directed violence is reduced.

NURSING DIAGNOSES / DEFINING CHARACTERISTICS	NURSING INTERVENTIONS / *RATIONALES*	EXPECTED OUTCOMES
Altered thought processes *Related to:* Depression Psychotic depression **DEFINING CHARACTERISTICS** Difficulty in concentrating Rumination, preoccupation with negative, suicidal thoughts Fatigue Weakness Feelings of hopelessness Feelings of helplessness, powerlessness Difficulty in management of personal financial/household obligations Slowing of thought processes Impaired judgment, insight, and reality testing Withdrawn, regressive behavior Disruption in personal relationships Disruption in work performance	**ONGOING ASSESSMENT** · Assess cognitive functioning. · Assess for presence of psychotic thought processes. · Assess affect. · Determine whether patient can make eye contact. **THERAPEUTIC INTERVENTIONS** · See Thought processes, altered, p. 52.	Altered thought processes are identified and treated.

Knowledge deficit
Related to:
Lack of information about depression and treatment
Reluctance to explore depression, indicated treatment
 	
DEFINING CHARACTERISTICS
Questions about depression causes, course, treatment
Questions about specific treatment interventions: antidepressant medication, electroconvulsive therapy (ECT), hospitalization for increased protection
	ONGOING ASSESSMENT
	· Assess patient's understanding of depression and treatment.
	
	THERAPEUTIC INTERVENTIONS
	· Instruct patient, family, and significant others about depression:
	    Causes, related factors (emotional/physical)
	    Treatment
	    Antidepressant medication
	    ECT
	    Light therapy
	    Structured activity/exercise
	    Suicide precautions
	    Psychotherapy
		Patient will understand depression and its treatment.

Originated by: Ursula Brozek, RN, MSN

Grief over long-term illness/disability

(ANTICIPATORY GRIEVING; DYSFUNCTIONAL GRIEVING)

Intense mental anguish or a sense of deep remorse may be experienced by patients and their families as they face long-term illness or disability. This care plan discusses measures the nurse can use to help patient and family members begin the process of grieving.

NURSING DIAGNOSES / DEFINING CHARACTERISTICS	NURSING INTERVENTIONS / *RATIONALES*	EXPECTED OUTCOMES

Grieving *Related to:* Altered body structure/function **DEFINING CHARACTERISTICS** Anger Depression Denial Crying Guilt Disgust Hostility Withdrawal Excessive fatigue Disturbed sleep patterns Weight gain/loss Increased dependency	**ONGOING ASSESSMENT**
	• Identify:
	  Behaviors that suggest grieving (see Defining Characteristics)
	  Past response to loss
	  Stage of grieving that patient is experiencing (see Interventions)
	  Potential pathologic grieving responses (see Grieving, dysfunctional, p. 23)
	
	THERAPEUTIC INTERVENTIONS
	• Spend specific time period daily with patient.
	• Ensure privacy.
	• Encourage patient to discuss feelings; do not try to force disclosures. *Patients disclose feelings at pace comfortable to them.*
	• Help patients identify feelings. Ask for clarification when unclear.
	• Avoid personalizing patient's behavior (i.e., becoming angry if patient vents anger).
	• Recognize stages of grief; apply nursing measures aimed at that specific stage.
	Stages of grieving:
	• *Shock and disbelief are initial responses to loss. Reality is overwhelming; denial, panic, and anxiety may be seen.*
	  Provide safe environment for expression of grief.
	  Minimize environmental stresses/stimuli.
	  Remain with patient throughout procedures.
	  Accept need to deny loss as part of normal grief process.
	• *Realization occurs weeks to months after loss. Reality continues to be overwhelming; sadness, anger, guilt, hostility may be seen.*
	  Anticipate increased affective behavior.
	  Recognize need to maintain hope for future
	  Provide realistic information about health status without false reassurances, taking away hope.
	• *Defensive retreat occurs weeks to months after loss. Patient attempts to maintain what has been lost; denial, wishful thinking, unwillingness to participate in self-care, indifference may be seen.*
	  Recognize that regression may be adaptive mechanism.
	  Support, positively reinforce efforts to perform self-care.
	  Offer encouragement: point out strengths and progress to date.
	  Discuss possible need for outside support systems (i.e., peer support, groups, clergy).
	• *Acknowledgment occurs months to year after loss. Patient slowly realizes impact of loss; depression, anxiety, bitterness may be seen.*
	  Help patient list importance of rehabilitation needs.
	  Encourage patient's/significant others' active involvement with rehabilitation team.
	  Continue to reinforce strengths, progress.
	• *Adaptation occurs during first year, or later, after the loss. Patient continues to reorganize resources, abilities, and self-image.*
	  Recognize patient's need to review (relive) illness experience.
	  Facilitate reorganization by reviewing progress.
	  Discuss possible involvement with peers/organizations (e.g., stroke club, arthritis foundation) that work with patient's medical condition.
	• Recognize that each patient is unique, will progress at own pace. *Time frames vary widely. Cultural, religious, ethnic, individual differences impact on manner of grieving.*
		The grieving process is facilitated.

Grief over long-term/disability— cont'd

NURSING DIAGNOSES / DEFINING CHARACTERISTICS	NURSING INTERVENTIONS / *RATIONALES*	EXPECTED OUTCOMES

Body image disturbance/self-concept disturbance
Related to:
Biophysical:
Cognitive/perceptual disturbance
Psychosocial:
Changed body image
Changed role performance
Changed personal identity
 	
DEFINING CHARACTERISTICS
Neglect of body part
Refusal to discuss limitations/altered body function
Staring at affected body part
Unwillingness to look at/touch affected body part
Disparaging remarks about personal appearance
Refusal to accept/ participate in rehabilitation
Withdrawal from social/personal role responsibilities
Exaggerated attempts to direct own treatment
Orientation to past rather than present, future
Detached discussion of body part
Described disturbance in self-esteem
	ONGOING ASSESSMENT
	• Assess for:
	  Neurologic/cognitive impairments leading to self-concept distortion
	  Perceptions about altered body structure/function
	  Behavioral patterns suggesting altered self-concept (see Defining Characteristics)
	
	THERAPEUTIC INTERVENTIONS
	• Explain to patient/significant others that physical condition may affect emotional status.
	• Provide information, clarify misconceptions about health status.
	• Arrange for patient to meet individual successfully living with same condition.
	• Initiate discussion aimed at exploring condition's perceived significance.
	• Allow patient to verbalize negative feelings about changed self-image. Describe perceptions; explore why perceptions differ *(may be particularly useful when patient's perception is distorted)*.
		Self-concept, self-esteem are enhanced.

Potential ineffective individual coping
Related to:
Situational crisis
Maturational crisis
Inadequate support system
Inadequate coping methods
 	
DEFINING CHARACTERISTICS
Verbalized inability to cope
	ONGOING ASSESSMENT
	• Identify:
	  Behavioral cues suggesting ineffective coping (see Defining Characteristics)
	  Past coping mechanisms
	  Patient's support systems
	
	THERAPEUTIC INTERVENTIONS
	• Provide individualized approach to patient's care:
	  Respect need to be alone.
	  Demonstrate sensitivity to tolerance for information *(prevent sensory overload)*.
	  Encourage patient to participate in planning care. *Patients have greater investment in following care plan that meets own special needs as they see them.*
		Effective coping is evident.

Continued.

Psychosocial Care Plans

NURSING DIAGNOSES / DEFINING CHARACTERISTICS	NURSING INTERVENTIONS / *RATIONALES*	EXPECTED OUTCOMES
Change in usual communication patterns Inability to make decisions Altered behavior toward self/others Inability to meet basic needs of self/family Impaired concentration Inability to ask for help Emotional lability	Recognize tolerance for hearing emotionally charged information. Plan routine activities to meet patient's needs. • Encourage family/significant others to participate actively in patient's care. • Use other professional resources: clergy, social workers, psychiatric liaison, vocational counselor. • Encourage patient to identify factors over which they have control *to decrease sense of powerlessness*. • Encourage patient to participate in grooming, hygiene activities. • Point out aspects of patient's life in which they continue to function well *(decreases feelings of helplessness)*. • Foster sense of achievement by slowly giving increasingly complex tasks. • Assist patient in problem solving (e.g., identification of problem, alternative). • Encourage use of previously helpful coping mechanisms. • Support constructive coping behaviors. Point out something particularly effective in yielding desired results. • Continue to expect patient to meet realistic obligations (family, interpersonal, therapeutic). *Patient may refuse/be unable to meet these expectations.*	
Potential ineffective family coping *Related to:* Temporary/permanent changes of family members Family crisis Prolonged disability that exhausts supportive capacity of family members Prolonged disability that affects financial reserves Family disorganization that triggers old conflicts **DEFINING CHARACTERISTICS** Limited/noninvolvement with patient Expressed hopelessness Refusal to participate in rehabilitation Distortion of reality (about patient's health) Prolonged denial of patient's health status Verbalized inability to cope Emotional lability of family members Physical, emotional abandonment of patient	**ONGOING ASSESSMENT** • Identify: Behavioral cues suggesting ineffective coping (see Defining Characteristics) Past coping mechanisms **THERAPEUTIC INTERVENTIONS** • Create supportive environment for family: Orient family to hospital (e.g., visiting hours, cafeteria, way to contact the nursing unit and physician) Allow private time with patient • Acknowledge/allow expression of family's positive and negative feelings. *Ambivalence is common reaction to highly charged emotional experience.* • Provide realistic information about patient's health status; do not give false reassurances. • Encourage use of previously helpful coping mechanisms. • Acknowledge family's strengths *(will provide ready foundation to build upon when helping family restructure lives)*. • Encourage family members to discuss feelings about patient's hospitalization. *Remember that family may experience same stages of grieving at same/different time than patient.* • Teach family about patient's physical status. • Involve family in patient's care when possible. • Consider referring family to other sources (i.e., family therapist, psychiatric liaison, social workers, self-help groups, clergy) when problems exceed nursing expertise.	Coping skills are identified and used.

Originated by: Margaret Williams, RN

Isolation

(DIVERSIONAL ACTIVITY DEFICIT)

The limitation of movement and social contact of a patient who is being protected from disease or who has a communicable disease.

NURSING DIAGNOSES / DEFINING CHARACTERISTICS	NURSING INTERVENTIONS / *RATIONALES*	EXPECTED OUTCOMES

Anxiety
Related to:
Isolation procedures
Infectious disease progress
Unfamiliar procedures
 	
DEFINING CHARACTERISTICS
Absent/excessive questioning
Excessive anxiousness/seeming indifference
Inability to discuss new procedures
Avoidance of learning isolation techniques
Insomnia
Hostility/tearfulness
Repetitive, unnecessary requests
	ONGOING ASSESSMENT
	• Assess anxiety level:
	   Mood
	   Behavior
	   Previous illness experience
	• Assess level of understanding of need for isolation and hospitalization.
	• Assess support systems.
	• Assess normal coping patterns.
	
	THERAPEUTIC INTERVENTIONS
	• Plan daily schedule that alternates rest, activity. *Schedule affords knowledge that someone will be in at certain times to attend to needs.*
	• Encourage family calls/visits.
	• Provide desired/appropriate activities.
	• Encourage questions/conversation/ventilation of feelings.
	• Inform family of importance of maintaining physical, emotional contact. *Lack of physical, emotional contact reinforces feelings of anxiety, worthlessness, dirtiness, and punishment.*
	• Assure that optimal care provided for patients in isolation.
		Anxiety is reduced.

Knowledge deficit
Related to:
Unfamiliarity of procedure, need for infection control
 	
DEFINING CHARACTERISTICS
Multiple questions
Lack of questions
Apprehension
	ONGOING ASSESSMENT
	• Assess knowledge base, readiness for learning.
	• Assess current level of understanding:
	   Need for isolation
	   Meaning of isolation
	   Current disease process
	• Assess coping mechanisms being employed.
	• Assess current supports within family.
	
	THERAPEUTIC INTERVENTIONS
	• Provide explanations in simple, accurate terms appropriate to level of understanding.
	• Provide adequate time for explanations and demonstrations.
	• Explain isolation and appropriate procedures:
	   Rationale for isolation
	   Proper use of materials (i.e., gloves, masks, gowns, hand washing techniques)
	• Use variety of instructional methods/aids:
	   Demonstration
	   Discussion
	   Handouts/pamphlets on isolation procedures
	• Explain "normal" disease course, treatment, and follow-up.
	• Arrange public health/social work follow-up as needed.
	• Instruct family about special precautions/treatments necessary to prevent disease spread in community:
	   Refer to appropriate policy and procedure.
	   Consult infection control clinician as necessary. *Good knowledge base influences infection control, patient/family fears.*
		Patient verbalizes understanding of need for isolation.

Continued.

NURSING DIAGNOSES / DEFINING CHARACTERISTICS	NURSING INTERVENTIONS / *RATIONALES*	EXPECTED OUTCOMES
Diversional activity deficit *Related to:* Removal from normal interpersonal, social contact **DEFINING CHARACTERISTICS** Complaints of boredom, loneliness Lack of expression Regression in development Irritability Constant demands	**ONGOING ASSESSMENT** · Assess current physical abilities. · Assess past diversional preferences for adaptation to hospital/isolation. · See Diversional activity deficit, p. 17. **THERAPEUTIC INTERVENTIONS** · Obtain/provide diversional materials as appropriate to desires/abilities. · Spend time with patient. *Allowing large blocks of time supports conversation, rapport development.* · Arrange for others (e.g., volunteer, social workers, religious) to spend time with patient.	Complaints of boredom and loneliness will be reduced.

Originated by: Patricia Hasbrouck-Aschliman, RN, CCRN

Substance abuse

(ALCOHOL AND DRUG ABUSE/DEPENDENCY AND WITHDRAWAL)

Abuse is the inappropriate use of a potentially additive substance. Prescription, over-the-counter, and street drugs and alcohol may be abused. When the abuser becomes physically or emotionally dependent on the sensations that the drug causes, he or she is addicted. Commonly abused addictive substances include alcohol, narcotics, depressants, stimulants, hallucinogens, and cannobinols.

NURSING DIAGNOSES / DEFINING CHARACTERISTICS	NURSING INTERVENTIONS / *RATIONALES*	EXPECTED OUTCOMES
Knowledge deficit *Related to:* Denial of problem No experience with substance abuse Youth **DEFINING CHARACTERISTICS** Many questions No questions Incorrect information/ misconceptions	**ONGOING ASSESSMENT** · Assess knowledge of: 　Alcohol dependency (physical and emotional) 　Alcohol abuse and its effect on: 　　Body 　　Ability to think/process information 　　Life-style (work, interpersonal relationships, self-concept, ability to maintain home) 　Physical and emotional dependency on prescription, nonprescription, and street drugs 　Drug abuse and its effects on: 　　Body 　　Ability to think/process information 　　Life-style (work, interpersonal relationships, self-concept, ability to maintain home) · Assess readiness to learn (*necessary for taking in information*). · Ascertain which significant others would benefit from attending information sessions. Provide information to friends/family when appropriate. **THERAPEUTIC INTERVENTIONS** · Provide information about substance abuse in nonthreatening, matter-of-fact way. *Misconceptions/myths about substance abuse abound.* · State information simply. *Aim is to present information. Refrain from trying to convince of facts, frighten into sobriety.*	Patient verbalizes understanding of substance abuse and treatment.

Substance abuse— cont'd

NURSING DIAGNOSES / DEFINING CHARACTERISTICS	NURSING INTERVENTIONS / *RATIONALES*	EXPECTED OUTCOMES
	· Expect patient to alternate between acceptance, rejection of information. *Patient least likely to be able to absorb information while experiencing withdrawal/emotional longing for abused substance.* · Communicate that with correct information patient can choose detoxification, make decisions that will let him/her enjoy healthier life.	
Individual ineffective coping *Related to:* Coping behaviors never/inadequately learned No supportive others available Social outlets all revolve around drugs/alcohol **DEFINING CHARACTERISTICS** Frequent suicide attempts Frequent overdoses Binge drinking Drug binging Frequent psychiatric/medical hospitalizations Negative/counterproductive behaviors: hostility; aggression; inadequate behavior; physically abusive, lying, antisocial/criminal behavior Patient observed to verbalize inability to cope, meet role expectations	**ONGOING ASSESSMENT** · Assess for Defining Characteristics. · Assess how long Defining Characteristics present. · Assess whether patient has effective coping mechanisms. · Assess character strengths, deficits *to establish framework for coping mechanisms.* · Determine to what degree lack of coping behaviors results from alcohol/drug abuse/dependency. · Ask patient to identify behaviors that have most negative effects. *Work to develop successful coping mechanisms for these behaviors first.* **THERAPEUTIC INTERVENTIONS** · Confront patient with unacceptable behaviors. Enlist friends/family members in providing feedback *(provides immediate information). Patient may pause, reflect on impact on people in environment; also sets limits on behaviors others will tolerate.* · Affirm insight whenever patient displays insight into own behavior. *Positive reinforcement may encourage patient to display more of same behavior.* · Gently confront patient with reality when he/she attributes problem to others/circumstances beyond control. *Allowing rationalizations to be unchallenged sanctions behavior.* · Involve patient in support groups for recovering alcoholics/abusers. · Do not overwhelm patient with global expectations. Expect short-term behavior changes. *Do not make task impossible; realistic to expect patient to refrain from alcohol/drugs one day at a time.* · Help patient develop substitute (positive) behaviors in lieu of negative ones. · Help patient learn to identify feelings, express thoughts. *Articulating thoughts, feelings sometimes helps to diffuse them.* · Reward positive behaviors. · Praise patient when he/she successfully copes with problems. · Spend time with patient. Remain nonjudgmental. Avoid behaviors that reinforce already low self-esteem.	Successful coping is evident, one day at a time, without drugs/alcohol.
Potential for self-directed/other-directed violence: *Related to:* Withdrawal Hopelessness Depression **DEFINING CHARACTERISTICS** Reports of wanting to hurt self/others History of injuring self/others Psychosis/hallucinations that direct patient to hurt self/others	**ONGOING ASSESSMENT** · Determine degree of suicidal/homicidal risk. · Assess whether patient has means, plan to carry out act. **THERAPEUTIC INTERVENTIONS** · Remove dangerous objects from environment. · Approach patient nonthreateningly; take time to introduce self, describe procedures. · Tell patient when you are going to touch him/her. *Paranoid/delusional patients may fear physical contact; may perceive it as personal threat.* · Use medications to modify out-of-control behavior; treat delusional thinking; stabilize/reassure depressive features. · See Thought processes, altered, p. 52.	Risk for violence is reduced.

Continued.

Psychosocial Care Plans

NURSING DIAGNOSES / DEFINING CHARACTERISTICS	NURSING INTERVENTIONS / *RATIONALES*	EXPECTED OUTCOMES
Profoundly depressed affect Hostility to others Paranoid behaviors See Depression, p. 614 See Suicidal attempt/ Suicidal gesture, p. 627		

Altered health maintenance
Related to:
Alcohol/drug abuse/ dependency
Economic/fiscal mismanagement
Poor diet
Long-term substance abuse effects on mental, physical health
Presence of adverse personal habits
  Smoking
  Poor diet
  Morbid obesity
  Poor hygiene
  Lack of exercise
Withdrawal from physiologic dependence
Evidence of impaired perception
Lack of knowledge
Unavailability of services
Poor housing conditions
Inability to communicate needs adequately
Denial of need to change current habits
	ONGOING ASSESSMENT
	· Assess history of substance abuse.
	· Assess history of other adverse personal habits:
	  Smoking
	  Obesity
	  Lack of exercise
	· Assess last drug use; determine substance taken, amount, routes of administration. Assess amount of last alcohol ingestion, length of alcohol abuse.
	· Assess whether economic problems present barrier to maintaining health.
	· Assess patient's hearing; orientation to time, place, and person to determine perceptual abilities.
	· Assess for specific acute/chronic disease Defining Characteristics.
	· Assess patient's knowledge of health maintenance behaviors.
	· Assess past health history.
	· Assess to what degree, environmental, social, interfamilial disruptions/ changes correlate with poor health behaviors.
	· Assess appointment schedule to determine whether changed/skipped appointments associated with other symptoms of altered ability to maintain health.
	· Determine patient's specific questions about health maintenance.
	· Determine patient's motives for failing to report symptoms reflecting health status changes.
	· Discuss noncompliance with instructions/programs *to determine rationale for failure.*
	· Assess relationship with family/supportive others. Obtain home assessment from visiting nurse to determine accessibility, quality of living conditions.
	· Assess experience with stress/disruptors as they relate to health habits.
	
	THERAPEUTIC INTERVENTIONS
	· Provide rationales for importance of specific behaviors:
	  Cessation of alcohol and drug abuse *(In addition to physical addiction, physical consequences of substance abuse mitigate against abuse.)*
	  Regular exercise/rest *to promote weight loss, increase agility and stamina*
	  Proper hygiene *to decrease infection risk, promote maintenance and integrity of skin, teeth*
	  Regular physical and dental checkups *to identify, treat problems early*
	  Reporting of unusual symptoms to health professional *to initiate early treatment*
	  Proper nutrition
	  Regular inoculations
	  Balanced low-cholesterol diet *to prevent vascular disease*
	  Smoking cessation: *smoking directly linked to cancer, heart disease*
	· Follow up clinic visits with telephone/home visits *to develop ongoing relationships with patient, vocalize support for patient.*
	· Provide means of contacting health care providers available for questions/ problem solution.
	· Compliment patient on positive accomplishments to reinforce. Involve family/friends in health planning conferences.
		Health maintenance improves.

NURSING DIAGNOSES / DEFINING CHARACTERISTICS	NURSING INTERVENTIONS / *RATIONALES*	EXPECTED OUTCOMES

DEFINING CHARACTERISTICS
Frequent illness
Development of acute/ chronic illnesses (e.g., gastritis/ulcers, cirrhosis, esophagitis, esophageal varices, alcoholic cardiomyopathies, hallucinations, delirium tremors, dementia, cholelithiasis, pancreatitis, anemia, emphysema, leg ulcers, hepatitis, AIDS, electrolyte imbalance)
Frequent psychiatric hospitalizations
Frequent hospitalizations for drug overdose treatment
Frequent hospitalizations for alcohol abuse sequelae
Marital problems
Financial insolvency
Failure to keep appointments
Expressed interest in improving behaviors
Failure to recognize/ respond to important symptoms reflective of changing health state
Inability to follow health maintenance instructions/programs
Physical characteristics may include:
  Body/mouth odor
  Unusual skin color, pallor
  Physical dirtiness
  Soiled clothing
  Obesity/anorexia
  Anemia
  Chronic fatigue
  Apathetic attitude
	• Ensure that other agencies (i.e., Department of Children and Family Services, social services, Visiting Nurses' Association, Meals on Wheels) follow through with plans.
	• See Health maintenance, altered, p. 26; Cirrhosis, p. 275.	

Home maintenance *Related to:* Disrupted interpersonal relationships Lack of financial resources caused by expense of drug habit Lack of consistent employment to provide fiscal resources	**ONGOING ASSESSMENT** • Assess history of substance abuse; determine impact on ability to maintain home. • Determine areas of home management that represent greatest problems for patient/family. • Assess patient for poor personal habits. • Assess whether lack of money is cause of unclean, unsafe home. • Refer to visiting nurse for home assessment. Evaluate home for accessibility, physical barriers. • Evaluate each family member to determine whether basic physical, emotion needs met.	Home is maintained.

Continued.

NURSING DIAGNOSES / DEFINING CHARACTERISTICS	NURSING INTERVENTIONS / *RATIONALES*	EXPECTED OUTCOMES
Lack of consistent living arrangements Poor physical health Poor emotional health Inadequate/absent support systems Cognitive/emotional disturbance Helplessness Powerlessness **DEFINING CHARACTERISTICS** Patient/family expresses difficulty in maintaining home environment Poor personal habits (e.g., soiled clothing, frequent illness, weight loss, body odor, substance abuse, depressed affect) Mental confusion Poor fiscal management Vulnerable individuals in home (i.e., infants, children, elderly, infirm) neglected Patient's/family members' report of frequent injuries in home Unsafe home environment/lack of basic hygiene measures revealed by home visit Lack of knowledge of particular aspect of home management described by patient Presence of vermin in home Accumulation of waste in home Inappropriate environmental temperature	• Assess patient's emotional/intellectual preparedness to maintain home. • Enlist social worker assessment of community resources that may help family/individual. • Assess whether patient has all assistive devices necessary for safe home maintenance. **THERAPEUTIC INTERVENTIONS** • Begin discharge planning immediately after admission *to assure that discharge organized to meet individual family needs.* • Coordinate home assessment by visiting nurse, social services. • Integrate family/patient into discharge planning *to ensure patient-centered objectives, promote compliance.* • Plan home visit *to test patient's preparedness for discharge.* • Provide telephone/home visit support. • Demonstrate link between patient's interpersonal, financial, or employment problems and drug abuse *to prevent patient from rationalizing alcohol/drug abuse as function of overwhelming life problems.* • See Home maintenance/management, impaired p. 27.	
Noncompliance *Related to:* Denial of substance abuse/dependency Ability to rationalize substance use Lack of knowledge Fear	**ONGOING ASSESSMENT** • Assess to what degree patient uses denial, rationalization to sustain habit. • Assess secondary gains and reinforcement of maintaining present life-style (identify with fast/glamorous crowd, etc.). • Assess patient's insight into problem. • Perform blood/urine screens regularly *to test compliance.* • Help patient identify most effective motivating factors. • See Noncompliance, p. 36.	Compliance behaviors are evident.

Substance abuse— cont'd

NURSING DIAGNOSES / DEFINING CHARACTERISTICS	NURSING INTERVENTIONS / *RATIONALES*	EXPECTED OUTCOMES
Lack of resources (financial, social, personal) Physical limitations Mental disability Lack of satisfaction with outcomes Inconvenience Failure to recognize severity of problem/ need for treatment **DEFINING CHARACTERISTICS** Verbalized belief "I can quit anytime," "I'm not hooked," "I can take it or leave it" Use of rationalization to explain why use of abused substance should be sanctioned Verbalized belief that treatment program does not meet personal needs Verbalized wish to continue present lifestyle Demonstrated persistent lack of insight into problem	**THERAPEUTIC INTERVENTIONS** • Confront with laboratory findings that reflect ongoing drug use. • Consider inpatient treatment during withdrawal. • Enlist friends'/family members' aid in achieving compliance. • Follow up visits with telephone calls *to provide ongoing support.* • Provide phone numbers of crisis intervention lines. • Involve patient in Alcoholics/Narcotics Anonymous groups *to provide support.* • Encourage patient to take medications prescribed *to help minimize withdrawal symptoms.* • Encourage patient seek out other friendships/diversions *to reduce occasions for returning to abusive/addictive behaviors.*	

Originated by: Deidra Gradishar, RNC, BS

Suicidal attempt/suicidal gesture

A suicide attempt is an act that is carried out with the intent to end one's own life. A suicidal gesture is an act that is potentially self-destructive but not immediately life-threatening A gesture may be a precursor to an actual attempt.

NURSING DIAGNOSES / DEFINING CHARACTERISTICS	NURSING INTERVENTIONS / *RATIONALES*	EXPECTED OUTCOMES
Actual self-inflicted injury *Related to:* Wound, trauma, or poisoning **DEFINING CHARACTERISTICS** Open wounds Blood loss	**ONGOING ASSESSMENT** • Identify/locate injury and its course. • Assess patient's physical status. **THERAPEUTIC INTERVENTIONS** • Maintain open airway, air exchange. • Maintain cardiac function. • Treat physical injuries *in order of seriousness to preserve life.* • Refer to appropriate care plans based on physical findings.	Effects of injury are reduced.

Continued.

NURSING DIAGNOSES / DEFINING CHARACTERISTICS	NURSING INTERVENTIONS / *RATIONALES*	EXPECTED OUTCOMES
Altered state of consciousness Burns Cardiac/respiratory/ neurologic dysfunction		

Ineffective individual coping
Related to:
Low self-esteem
Hopelessness
Anger, depression
Known psychological illness
 	
DEFINING CHARACTERISTICS
Withdrawal
Tearfulness
Anger/hostility
Fatigue
Resignation
Disorientation
Wide mood swings (i.e., profound depression versus elation)
Inappropriate behavior
	ONGOING ASSESSMENT
	· Interview patient (if possible) and family. Assess for:
	   Behavior pattern, familiar coping mechanisms
	   Recent behavior, relationship changes
	   Alcohol/drug abuse
	   Physical illness
	   Social, family history of suicidal behaviors/attempts
	   Prior suicide attempts
	   Events surrounding attempts (i.e., planned or impulsive acts)
	   Recent losses: job, deaths, precious objects
	· Determine risk level and precautions necessary *to maintain patient safety.*
	· Have patient evaluated by psychiatrist *to determine need for transfer to psychiatric facility when physically stable.*
	
	THERAPEUTIC INTERVENTIONS
	· Orient to environment.
	· Develop primary nurse relationship.
	· Encourage ventilation of feelings when possible.
	· Maintain quiet, structured, safe environment:
	   Explain precautions.
	   Remove potentially harmful objects.
	   Provide sitter if necessary.
	   Provide room near nurses' station.
	   Maintain irregular contact *so patient cannot identify times when left alone.*
	   Use physical restraints if needed.
	· Provide suitable environment for psychiatric interviews/evaluation. *Quiet, private area with no interruption most conducive. Privacy should be maintained if interview conducted with patient in bed.*
	· Report behavior/mood changes.
	· Consult psychiatric liaison/nurse specialist as needed.
		Healthy coping skills are developed and used.

Self-concept disturbance *Related to:* Low self-esteem Worthlessness Poor body image Guilt Psychiatric disorder **DEFINING CHARACTERISTICS** Lack of self-care behaviors Self-deprecating remarks Verbalized hopelessness, guilt, worthlessness Suicidal ideation	**ONGOING ASSESSMENT** · Assess current behaviors. · Assess expressed feelings, self-perceptions. · See Hopelessness, p. 29; Self-concept disturbance, p. 46; Coping, ineffective individual, p. 15. **THERAPEUTIC INTERVENTIONS** · Allow expression of feelings. Do not make judgments about feelings *(may further damage self-concept).* · Provide supportive physical care when necessary. · Encourage positive activities; provide positive feedback when warranted. *Only honest expressions of positive accomplishment promote trusting relationship on which patient can rely.*	Positive expressions of self-concept are verbalized.

NURSING DIAGNOSES / DEFINING CHARACTERISTICS	NURSING INTERVENTIONS / *RATIONALES*	EXPECTED OUTCOMES
Knowledge deficit (patient and/or family) *Related to:* Lack of experience with suicide Hospital environment Diagnosis **DEFINING CHARACTERISTICS** Expressed lack of awareness Helplessness Questioning Avoidance/withdrawal Embarrassment Fear Anxiety Denial	**ONGOING ASSESSMENT** • Assess history. • Assess current understanding of problem, treatment, and prognosis. • Assess current ability to listen, discuss needs. **THERAPEUTIC INTERVENTIONS** • Provide information at appropriate time, comprehension level. • Provide referrals as necessary: Social work Psychological Hot line Self-help groups Clergy • Provide information about early warning signs of inability to adapt to loss: Insomnia Weight changes Agitation Guilt Thoughts of death Giving away of belongings No future objective/goals • Discuss suicidal gestures: Frequent accidents Overdoses Inadequate/no food intake • Discuss increased risk with decreased social network: No supportive relationships Changes in number/type of friends Perceived inability to ask for help • Discuss necessity of follow-up care. Provide appointments/phone numbers.	Understanding of problem and treatment options are verbalized.

Originated by: Janet McCants, RN, BSN
             Susanne DeFabiis, RN, MSN

General Surgery Care Plans

Patient-controlled analgesia
Routine perioperative care
Same-day surgery

Patient-controlled analgesia (PCA)

(PAIN MANAGEMENT)

Patient-controlled analgesia (PCA) is the IV infusion of a narcotic (usually morphine or Demerol) via an infusion pump that is controlled by the patient. This allows the patient to manage pain relief within prescribed units.

NURSING DIAGNOSES / DEFINING CHARACTERISTICS	NURSING INTERVENTIONS / *RATIONALES*	EXPECTED OUTCOMES

Pain
Related to:
Medical/surgical procedure/disease necessitating pain management:
  Surgery
  Sickle cell crisis
  Terminal pain
  Trauma
 	
DEFINING CHARACTERISTICS
Verbalized pain
Facial grimacing
Guarding behavior
	ONGOING ASSESSMENT
	• Assess appropriateness of patient as PCA candidate:
	  No history of substance abuse
	  No allergy to narcotic analgesics
	  Clear sensorium
	  Cooperative and motivated about use
	  No history of renal, hepatic, or respiratory disease
	  Manual dexterity
	  No history of major psychiatric disorder
	• Assess pain:
	  Location
	  Severity
	  Nature
	  Pattern
	• Assess PCA effectiveness.
	• Assess for changes that may negate patient's candidacy for PCA *because of anesthesia, general change in condition.*
	• Determine IV site patency.
	
	THERAPEUTIC INTERVENTIONS
	• Maintain PCA in functional condition.
	• Use nonpharmacologic pain control methods (e.g., distraction, touch).
	• Notify physician of inadequate pain control.
	• See Pain, p. 39.
		Consistent pain relief is experienced; sedation is prevented.

Knowledge deficit
Related to:
Unfamiliarity with PCA
 	
DEFINING CHARACTERISTICS
Multiple questions
Lack of questions
Observed inability to use PCA effectively
Uncontrolled pain
	ONGOING ASSESSMENT
	• Assess readiness, ability to learn.
	• Assess previous PCA experience.
	• Assess pain relief adequacy.
	
	THERAPEUTIC INTERVENTIONS
	• Teach patient preoperatively *so that anesthesia effects do not obscure teaching.*
	• Teach patient:
	  Purpose
	  Benefits
	  Techniques of use
	  Safety mechanism
	  Need for IV line
	  Other alternatives for pain control
	  Need to notify nurse of:
	    Machine alarm
	    Occurrence of untoward effects.
	• Teach patient to recognize PCA complications:
	  Excessive sedation
	  Respiratory distress
	  Urinary retention
	  Nausea/vomiting
	  Constipation
	  IV site pain, redness, or swelling
	• Teach patient effective timing of dose in relation to potentially uncomfortable activities and prevention of peak pain periods.
		Patient/significant other verbalizes/demonstrates effective PCA use.

Continued.

Patient-controlled analgesia— cont'd

NURSING DIAGNOSES / DEFINING CHARACTERISTICS	NURSING INTERVENTIONS / *RATIONALES*	EXPECTED OUTCOMES
Potential for injury *Related to:* Accidental overdose Inadequate assessment for appropriateness of PCA use Mechanical malfunction **DEFINING CHARACTERISTICS** Respiratory depression Sedation Urinary retention Constipation Nausea, vomiting Dependency Inadequate pain control	**ONGOING ASSESSMENT** • Assess for Defining Characteristics. • Monitor infusion setting. **THERAPEUTIC INTERVENTIONS** • Dedicate use of IV line for PCA only; consult pharmacist before mixing drug with narcotic being infused; *IV incompatibilities possible.* • Post "No additional analgesia" sign over bed *to prevent inadvertent analgesic overdosage.* • Keep Narcan/other narcotic-reversing agent readily available. • Notify physician of inadequate pain relief/other side effects. • See Breathing pattern, ineffective, p. 8; Urinary retention, p. 61; Constipation/impaction, p. 12.	Risk of injury is reduced.

Originated by: Marilyn Magafas, RN,C, BSN, MBA
Lori Luke, RN

Routine perioperative care

Although each surgical procedure varies by nature, a standard set of concerns is present for all procedures to assure safe operation.

NURSING DIAGNOSES / DEFINING CHARACTERISTICS	NURSING INTERVENTIONS / *RATIONALES*	EXPECTED OUTCOMES

Anxiety/fear
Related to:
Impending surgery
Perceived threat of pain, disfigurement, death
No operative experience/memories of negative experience
Concern about operative error
 	
DEFINING CHARACTERISTICS
Forlorn/upset appearance
Weeping
Avoidance of staff
Irritability
Aggression
Questioning reasons for procedures, delays
	ONGOING ASSESSMENT
	• Observe expressions of feelings: inadequacy, frustration, fear, hostility.
	• Assess comprehension level.
	• Assess degree of insight about surgical procedure.
	• Identify erroneous perceptions, exaggerated fears.
	• Review chart *to ensure smooth initiation of procedures.*
	• Verify surgical site with orders, OR schedule.
	
	THERAPEUTIC INTERVENTIONS
	• Visit patient preoperatively *to initiate nurse/patient interaction;* if preoperative visit not made on unit, use holding area to initiate interactions:
	    Demonstrate calmness.
	    Express warmth, friendliness.
	    Provide accepting atmosphere.
	    Use touch therapeutically.
	• Encourage patient to verbalize feelings, concerns:
	    Listen attentively.
	    Offer feedback to expressed feelings.
	• Solicit questions. Refer appropriate questions to surgeon; avoid leaving questions unanswered.
	• If family members present, encourage participation.
	• Confer with unit nurse *to share findings, exchange relevant data.*
	• Explain sensory experiences related to surgery: what client will see, hear, feel.
	• Describe what to expect in environment: holding area, attire, sounds, temperature, bright lights, personnel roles.
		Anxiety/fear is managed.

NURSING DIAGNOSES / DEFINING CHARACTERISTICS	NURSING INTERVENTIONS / *RATIONALES*	EXPECTED OUTCOMES
	• Provide printed material *to reinforce instructions.* • Prepare OR suite before patient arrives.	
Potential for injury *Related to:* Prolonged surgical procedure Use of electrical equipment Improper body alignment Improper padding/use of positioning apparatus Retained needles, sponges, instruments **DEFINING CHARACTERISTICS** Postoperative pain unrelated to incision site Prolonged pain complaints Denuded, discolored area(s) on skin corresponding with size, shape, and site of grounding pad placement X-ray positive for retained needle, sponge, or instrument Discovery of foreign object on subsequent procedure Foot drop Wrist drop Evidence of pressure sore(s)	**ONGOING ASSESSMENT** • Assess ROM and skin integrity before procedure. • Determine that all pieces of electrical equipment in safe working order. • Determine type of count appropriate to procedure being performed. **THERAPEUTIC INTERVENTIONS** • Place patient on table in anatomically correct position. • Pad bony prominences; use padded positioning devices as needed *to prevent skin breakdown, maintain correct body alignment.* • Remove, replace equipment that malfunctions during procedure. • Count instruments, needles, and sponges before, after, and through procedure according to policy. • Use only radiopaque sponges in wound; never remove instruments, sponges from room. • Account for pieces of broken instruments, needles, cut sponges. • Initiate x-ray procedure for incorrect count. • Ensure that area beneath patient remains dry through procedure. • Remind operative team to avoid leaning on patient. • Reposition patient as necessary during procedure.	Risk of injury during operative procedure is reduced.

Potential infection
Related to:
Surgical incision
Multiple portals for pathogen entry
 	
DEFINING CHARACTERISTICS
Redness, swelling, pain at incision site
Fever
Elevated WBC
	ONGOING ASSESSMENT
	• Identify patient at risk for infection:
	    Obesity
	    Extreme age
	    Poor nutritional status
	• Assess all incisions and other invasive sites 24-48 hr postoperatively.
	• Monitor housekeeping procedures in OR environment.
	• Monitor team for breaks in aseptic technique during procedure.
	
	THERAPEUTIC INTERVENTIONS
	• Ensure that team adheres strictly to aseptic technique/principles. *Members involved in procedure may be unaware that technique broken.*
	• Control OR suite traffic.
	• Assist with/ensure adequate preoperative scrub/surgical preparation.
	• Promptly communicate need for postoperative antibiotic therapy to Recovery Room/unit personnel
		Risk of infection is reduced.

Originated by: Katie Wyatt, RN
      Louise Rzeszewski, RN, BSN

Same-day surgery

(ONE-DAY SURGERY; SHORT-STAY SURGERY)

Many operative procedures previously requiring hospital admission/overnight stay are now performed as one-day surgeries. This reduces the cost of surgery and minimizes the stress that the patient and significant others experience.

NURSING DIAGNOSES / DEFINING CHARACTERISTICS	NURSING INTERVENTIONS / *RATIONALES*	EXPECTED OUTCOMES

Knowledge deficit
Related to:
Unfamiliarity with surgical procedure
Unfamiliar environment
 	
DEFINING CHARACTERISTICS
Repetitive questions
Anxiety
Silence
Hostility
Not seeking information about procedure/ cause of problem
Denial of need for surgery
Noncompliance with eariler therapy
Refusal to sign consent
	ONGOING ASSESSMENT
	• Assess knowledge of surgical procedure, preoperative care.
	• Assess available support system, usual methods of coping with stress.
	
	THERAPEUTIC INTERVENTIONS
	Before surgery:
	• Use appropriate teaching material.
	• Encourage questions.
	• Discuss/reinforce requirements of preoperative preparation:
	    NPO after midnight
	    Bath/shower night before surgery
	    Early arrival morning of surgery
	    Need for signing consent
	• Describe events that will occur postoperatively (in recovery room, on discharge).
	After surgery:
	• Discuss requirements for discharge:
	    Must have urinated
	    Surgical site free of excessive bleeding
	    Awake and responsive
	• Reinforce physician's discharge instructions:
	    Follow-up surgery clinic within 4-7 days
	    Wound closure strips not removed from incision
	    Area may be covered with bandage
	    Physical activity limited as instructed
	    Diet advanced from liquids to soft diet to normal diet
		Patient verbalizes understanding of surgical procedure and necessary preparation.

Altered comfort; post-operative pain
Related to:
Surgical incision
 	
DEFINING CHARACTERISTICS
Verbalized pain
Facial mask of pain
Guarded movement
	ONGOING ASSESSMENT
	• Assess pain:
	    Location
	    Quality
	    Severity
	    Precipitating factors
	• Determine history of analgesic use.
	
	THERAPEUTIC INTERVENTIONS
	• Instruct patient/significant other in appropriate analgesic use.
	• Instruct patient to notify physician if pain unrelieved by prescribed medication, *so that safe changes in drug/dosage/schedule can be made.* Discourage use of over-the-counter medications unless prescribed.
		Pain is relieved.

Potential infection
Related to:
Surgical incision
Invasive lines during surgery
 	
DEFINING CHARACTERISTICS
Redness, warmth, swelling of incision/ puncture sites
Fever
	ONGOING ASSESSMENT
	• Assess incision, other sites for redness, warmth, swelling.
	• Monitor vital signs.
	
	THERAPEUTIC INTERVENTIONS
	• Instruct patient/significant other in dressing change technique. *Clean technique easier, more likely to be followed.*
	• Encourage avoidance of crowds/individuals with infections.
	• Instruct patient/significant other to report:
	    Redness, swelling of incision
	    Fever
	    Loss of appetite
	    Feeling of malaise
		Risk of infection is reduced.

Originated by: Judith Kenney, RN, MSN
             Ruth Novitt-Schumacher, RN,C, MSN

Emergency and Trauma Care Plans

DISORDERS
Chest trauma
Hypovolemic shock: acute care
Lead poisoning

Near drowning
Rape trauma syndrome
Toxic ingestion

THERAPEUTIC INTERVENTIONS
Trauma patient: perioperative care

Chest trauma

(PNEUMOTHORAX; TENSION
PNEUMOTHORAX; FLAIL CHEST)

A blunt or penetrating injury of the thoracic cavity that can result in a potentially life-threatening situation secondary to pneumothorax and/or cardiac tamponade.

NURSING DIAGNOSES / DEFINING CHARACTERISTICS	NURSING INTERVENTIONS /*RATIONALES*	EXPECTED OUTCOMES

Ineffective breathing pattern
Related to:
Simple pneumothorax
Tension pneumothorax
Pain
Flail chest
Simple hemothorax (<400 cc blood)
Massive hemothorax (>1500 cc blood)
 	
DEFINING CHARACTERISTICS
Shortness of breath
Dyspnea
Tachypnea
Chest pain
Decreased breath sounds on affected side
Hyper-resonance on affected side (pneumothorax)
Dullness on affected side (hemothorax)
Unequal chest expansion
Abnormal ABGs
Anxiety, restlessness
Hypotension
Tachycardia
Cyanosis
Jugular venous distension
Tracheal deviation toward unaffected side
Subcutaneous emphysema
Paradoxical chest movements (flail chest)
	ONGOING ASSESSMENT
	• Assess airway for patency. *Maintaining airway always first priority.*
	• Assess for respiratory distress signs/symptoms:
	  Breathing patterns
	  Breath sounds (presence/absence)
	  Use of accessory muscles
	  Changes in orientation, restlessness
	  Skin color
	  Change in ABGs
	• Assess chest movements. *Paradoxical movement sign of flail chest. Decreased chest expansion on affected side sign of pneumothorax/hemothorax.*
	• Assess for pain, increase with inspiration (*sign of rib fracture*), decrease with inspiration (*sign of flail chest*).
	• Assess trachea position. *Deviation from midline sign of tension pneumothorax.*
	• Assess, inspect chest wall for obvious injuries that allow air to enter pleural cavity.
	• Monitor chest x-rays *to confirm correct placement of chest tubes, signs of improvement of pneumothorax or hemothorax.*
	
	THERAPEUTIC INTERVENTIONS
	• Suction *to clear secretions, optimize gas exchange.*
	• Insert oral/nasal airway as condition warrants *to maintain airway.*
	• Place in sitting position, if not contraindicated, *to assist lung expansion.*
	• Provide oxygen therapy in carefully metered doses to meet specific need.
	• If flail chest present, tape flail segment or place manual pressure over the flail segment *to stabilize. Patients with increasing respiratory distress may require external pressure until more definitive treatment (intubation, surgical stabilization) initiated.*
	• If open pneumothorax:
	  Cover chest wall defect with sterile vaseline and 4 by 4 dressing.
	  Tape on three sides with waterproof tape. *Untaped side allows air escape from pleural cavity (flutter-valve effect) so tension does not continue to increase.*
	• If patient *not* in severe respiratory distress, prepare for chest x-ray to determine pneumothorax/hemothorax size and/or confirm suspected diagnosis. *Patients with small pneumothoraces, hemothoraces, and minimal symptoms may not require chest tube.*
	• If tension pneumothorax, anticipate/prepare for emergency thoracentesis *to relieve air tension in pleural space on affected side.*
	• If severe respiratory distress/respiratory status steadily deteriorating, prepare for chest tube placement. *Larger chest tubes inserted for hemothorax than pneumothorax to help alleviate chest tube clotting. Chest tube then connected to underwater seal; closed drainage suction device applied to reinflate lung, remove secretions from the pleural space.* See Thoracotomy, p. 221.
	• Prepare for intubation if patient's condition warrants. *Note: Patients with flail chest may be stable initially because of compensatory mechanisms (e.g., splinting of flail segment, and shallow respirations). As these compensatory mechanisms fail, patient develops increasing respiratory distress. Intubation and positive-pressure ventilation are means of stabilizing flail segment by preventing patient from breathing independently.*
		Effective breathing pattern and gas exchange are restored.

Chest trauma— cont'd

NURSING DIAGNOSES / DEFINING CHARACTERISTICS	NURSING INTERVENTIONS / *RATIONALES*	EXPECTED OUTCOMES
Fluid volume deficit *Related to:* Trauma Hemothorax Chest tube drainage **DEFINING CHARACTERISTICS** Tachycardia Hypotension Cool, clammy skin Pallor Restlessness Anxiety Mental status changes Decreased urine output Possible jugular venous distention caused by mediastinal shifting toward unaffected side; >2 sec capillary refill	**ONGOING ASSESSMENT** • Assess vital signs q10-15 min until stable. Note heart rate; tachycardia early indication of fluid volume deficit. *Blood pressure not good indicator of early shock.* • Assess anxiety level. *Mild to moderate anxiety may be first early warning sign before vital sign changes. Anxiety may also indicate pain, psychological traumas, etc.* • Monitor I & O; document. *Decreased urine output indicates progressive shock.* • Obtain specimens; evaluate lab tests for CBC, electrolytes, BUN, creatinine, type, crossmatch. • Assess, measure, document amount of blood in chest tube collection chamber. Estimate blood lost to sterile towels, etc. • Monitor chest tube drainage q10-15 min until blood loss slows to <25 cc/hr. • Establish baseline Hct/Hb; monitor. **THERAPEUTIC INTERVENTIONS** • Attempt to control bleeding source by using direct pressure with sterile 4 by 4 bandage. • Insert one to two large-bore peripheral IVs. Administer crystalloid/colloid fluids as ordered. *Rule for fluid replacement: Infuse 3 cc IV fluid per 1 cc blood volume lost.* • Prepare patient for transfusions, if ordered, with typed and crossmatched blood if available and time permits. *Type-specific blood may be used if unable to obtain type and crossmatch. O negative blood may be used as last resort.* • Prepare patient for autotransfusion; *may be used in cases of blunt/penetrating injuries of chest only.* • Prepare for transfer to OR as condition warrants. • See Hypovolemic shock, p. 639.	Optimal fluid volume is restored.
Decreased cardiac output *Related to:* Acute pericardial tamponade from blunt/penetrating injury to heart; injury may cause pericardial sac to fill with blood. Eventually sac may fill to point that it compresses myocardium; causes decreased ability of heart to pump blood out/accept blood in **DEFINING CHARACTERISTICS** Decreased BP Narrow pulse pressure Pulsus paradoxus (systolic pressure falls >15 mm Hg during inspiration) Tachycardia	**ONGOING ASSESSMENT** • Monitor hemodynamic parameters (BP, HR, CVP, PAP, PCWP). Note equalization of pressures. • Assess for pulsus paradoxus and electrical alternans. • Assess for jugular venous distention. • Monitor serial chest x-rays; evaluate for widened mediastinum/increased heart size. • Monitor chest tube drainage q1h (if present). • Assess heart tones. • Assess chest pain quantity, quality. • Assess mental status. • Monitor Hb and Hct. • Assess peripheral pulses and capillary refill. • Assess I & O. • Assess ABGs. **THERAPEUTIC INTERVENTIONS** • Initiate O_2 therapy *to maximize O_2 saturation.* • Establish large-bore IV access. • Administer parenteral fluids are ordered. *Optimal hydration state increases venous return.* • Type and crossmatch as ordered. Anticipate blood product replacement *to correct existing hematology or coagulation factor alterations.* • Place patient in optimal position *to increase venous return.* • Have emergency resuscitative equipment, medications readily available.	Adequate cardiac output is maintained.

Continued.

NURSING DIAGNOSES / DEFINING CHARACTERISTICS	NURSING INTERVENTIONS /*RATIONALES*	EXPECTED OUTCOMES
Electrical alterans (decreased QRS voltage during inspiration) Equalization of pressures (CVP, PAP, PCWP) Jugular venous distention Widened mediastinum/ enlarged heart on chest x-ray Chest tubes (if present) suddenly stop draining (suspect clot) Distant/muffled heart tones Chest, back, or shoulder pain Restlessness, confusion, anxiety Fall in Hb, Hct Cool, clammy skin Diminished peripheral pulses Sluggish capillary refill Decreased urine output Decreased arterial, venous O$_2$ saturation Acidosis	• Assemble open chest tray for bedside intervention/prepare patient for transport to surgery. *Tamponade must be relieved to improve cardiac output; requires emergency bedside surgery or preferably emergency OR surgery.* • Maintain aggressive fluid resuscitation *(may be required as tamponade evacuated).* • Administer vasopressor agents (dopamine, levophed) as ordered *to maximize systemic perfusion pressure to vital organs.* • Administer sodium bicarbonate as ordered *to correct acidosis.*	
Pain *Related to:* Rib fractures Chest tube incision **DEFINING CHARACTERISTICS** Anxiety Wincing, grimacing Shallow respiration to minimize pain Tachycardia Agitation Verbalization of pain	**ONGOING ASSESSMENT** • Assess pain level. • Assess pain characteristics. • Evaluate effectiveness of all pain medication. *Unlike all other body fractures, rib fractures cannot be casted to reduce pain. Rib cage in continuous motion; therefore, more difficult to manage.* **THERAPEUTIC INTERVENTIONS** • Assist patient in splinting chest with pillow *to minimize discomfort, allow effective cough and deep breathing.* • Administer analgesia as ordered. • Assist with intrapleural catheter insertion for administration of long-acting Xylocaine. • Assist with intercostal nerve block. • Position patient for comfort. • Provide reassurance and emotional support. • See Pain, p. 39.	Pain is reduced or relieved.

Chest trauma— cont'd

NURSING DIAGNOSES / DEFINING CHARACTERISTICS	NURSING INTERVENTIONS /*RATIONALES*	EXPECTED OUTCOMES
Anxiety/fear *Related to:* Unfamiliar environment Dyspnea Pain Emergency **DEFINING CHARACTERISTICS** Apprehension Uncertainty Restlessness Expressed concerns Look of fear	**ONGOING ASSESSMENT** • Assess anxiety level (mild, severe). Note signs/symptoms, especially non-verbal communication. **THERAPEUTIC INTERVENTIONS** • Provide care in calm manner. • Orient patient/significant others to environment as feasible. • Encourage patient to ventilate feelings. • Explain procedures to be performed. • Remain with patient as much as possible. • See Anxiety, p. 4. • See Fear, p. 18.	Anxiety/fear is reduced.
Knowledge deficit *Related to:* New, acute experience Lack of experience **DEFINING CHARACTERISTICS** Questions Lack of questions Confusion about therapy	**ONGOING ASSESSMENT** • Assess patient's/significant others' level of knowledge of chest trauma. • Assess patient/significant others' physical/emotional readiness to learn. *During acute stages, family/significant others may receive the most teaching to minimize feelings of helplessness, assist in providing support to patient.* **THERAPEUTIC INTERVENTIONS** • When appropriate, provide information about disease process, reasoning for prescribed therapy *to help allay anxiety.* • Design teaching to involve patient participation.	Patient/significant other can verbalize basic understanding of disease process and therapy.

Originated by: Christine Jutzi-Kosmos, RN, MS
           Debbie Brooks, RN, MS
           Carol Ruback, RN, MSN, CCRN

Hypovolemic shock: acute care

Hypovolemia caused by blunt or penetrating trauma. May result from disruption of a major vessel, significant lacerations of soft tissue, internal chest or abdominal bleeding, and long bone fractures.

NURSING DIAGNOSES / DEFINING CHARACTERISTICS	NURSING INTERVENTIONS /*RATIONALES*	EXPECTED OUTCOMES
Fluid volume deficit *Related to:* Estimated blood volume loss up to 30% **DEFINING CHARACTERISTICS** Tachycardia BP normal Capillary refill normal or >2 sec Tachypnea Urine output may be normal (>30 cc/hr) or as low as 20 cc/hr	**ONGOING ASSESSMENT** • Evaluate, document extent of patient's injuries; use Primary Survey (or another consistent survey method) or ABCs: airway with cervical spine control, breathing, circulation. *Primary Survey helps identify imminent/ potentially life-threatening injuries. This is a quick, initial assessment.* • Perform secondary survey after all life-threatening injuries ruled out/ treated. *Secondary survey uses methodical head to toe inspection.* • Assess for early warning signs of hypovolemia. *Mild to moderate anxiety may be first sign of impending hypovolemic shock; unfortunately may also be easily overlooked, attributed to pain, psychological trauma, and fear. (BP not good indicator of early hypovolemic shock).* • Anticipate potential causes of shock state from ongoing assessment. • If only visible injury is obvious head injury, look for other causes of hypovolemia (i.e., long bone fractures, internal bleeding, external bleeding).	Fluid volume is maintained.

Continued.

NURSING DIAGNOSES / DEFINING CHARACTERISTICS	NURSING INTERVENTIONS / *RATIONALES*	EXPECTED OUTCOMES

Cool, clammy skin
Thirst
Dry mouth
Lightheadedness/ dizziness
Mild to moderate anxiety
	Isolated head injury does not usually lead to shock; extensive scalp lacerations, which can lead to exsanguination, are an exception.
	• Assess CVP to distinguish hypotension caused by hypovolemia (low CVP reading of <6cm H_2O) versus hypotension caused by pericardial tamponade/tension pneumothorax (high CVP reading of >10cm H_2O).
	• Monitor, document continued blood loss, chest tube drainage from hemothorax.
	• Record and evaluate I & O.
	• Obtain spun Hct, re-evaluate q30min-4h, depending on stability. Hct decreases as fluids administered because of dilution. *Rule of thumb: Hct decreases 1%/1L lactated Ringer's or NS used. Any other Hct drop must be evaluated as indication of continued blood loss.*
	• Obtain all initial baseline data: CBC, biochemistries, SGOT, and amylase; type and crossmatch, UA, ABG, CXR, ECG as ordered: *data help establish baseline for comparing future data, assist patient evaluation.*
	• Obtain baseline vital signs, Glasgow Coma Scale, trauma score, CVP. Recheck q15min as needed. Document, alert physician of changes from baseline data noted.
	• Monitor for arrhythmias. *Mild tachycardia (<120 beats/min) can be expected as sign of anxiety/mild hypovolemia.*
	
	THERAPEUTIC INTERVENTIONS
	• Try to control source of bleeding. If external, direct pressure most effective. *May also use pressure dressing; sterile 4 by 4 with elastic bandage wrapped around injury, making sure not to wrap too tightly, cause nerve damage to areas distal to pressure dressing from tissue hypoxemia. Never use hemostats to control bleeding; may damage tissue and nerves.*
	• If bleeding source internal (e.g., pelvic fracture), military antishock trousers (MAST)/pneumatic antishock garment (PASG) may be used *to tamponade bleeding. Hypovolemia from long bone fractures (e.g., femur fractures) may be controlled by splinting with air splints, Hare traction splints, or MAST/PASG trousers, to reduce tissue and vessel damage from manipulation of unstable fractures.*
	• Initiate IV therapy. Start two large-bore, shorter-length peripheral IVs *(amount of volume that can be infused inversely affected by length of IV catheter; best to use shorter-length, large-bore catheter).*
	  Replacement therapy: infuse 3 cc IV fluid /1 cc estimated blood loss.
	  Initiate IV therapy with lactated Ringer's solution. Colloidal expanders may also be ordered.
	• If patient hypotensive, prepare to bolus with 1-2 L IV fluids as ordered (normal adult dosage). *Patient's response to treatment depends on extent of blood loss. If blood loss mild (<20%), expected response is rapid return to normal blood pressure. If IV fluids slowed, patient remains normotensive. If patient has lost 20-40% of circulating blood volume or has continued uncontrolled bleeding, fluid bolus may produce normotension, but if fluids slowed after bolus, BP will deteriorate.*
	• Prepare for CVP insertion if ordered *to help evaluate fluid volume status.*
	• See Cardiac output, decreased, p. 9.	

NURSING DIAGNOSES / DEFINING CHARACTERISTICS	NURSING INTERVENTIONS / *RATIONALES*	EXPECTED OUTCOMES
Potential for altered tissue perfusion *Related to:* Volume loss ≥30% Late uncompensated hypovolemic shock **DEFINING CHARACTERISTICS** Pulse rate >120 beats/min Hypotension Capillary refill >2 sec Tachypnea (30-40 respirations/min) Urine output 0-15 cc/hr Cool, clammy skin Anxious, confused, lethargic attitude Decreased pulse pressure	**ONGOING ASSESSMENT** • Continue Ongoing Assessment as described in fluid volume deficit (p. 639). *Assess patient according to primary survey only; secondary survey only used when all life-threatening/potentially life-threatening injuries ruled out.* • Assess for CVP changes indicating improvement or deterioration in patient's condition. • Reassess all data accumulated in baseline assessment (e.g., CVP, Hct, urine output, vital signs, and ABGs) *for signs of improvement/deterioration.* **THERAPEUTIC INTERVENTIONS** • See Therapeutic Interventions for fluid volume deficit described on p. 640. • Maintain lactated Ringer's IV infusion wide open until BP 90 mm Hg systolic. • In addition to two established peripheral lines, prepare for additional peripheral lines, cutdowns. • Transfuse patient with whole blood/packed RBCs. Preparing fully crossmatched blood may take up to 1 hr in some labs. Consider using uncrossmatched or type-specific blood until crossmatched available. *If type-specific blood unavailable, type O blood may be used for exsanguinating patients. If available, Rh(−) blood preferred, especially for females of childbearing age.* • Apply MAST/PASG trousers when systolic BP below 90 mm Hg. Deflate *slowly* when systolic BP >100 mm Hg/patient in OR. • If possible, use fluid warmer/rapid fluid infuser *to keep core temperature warm, facilitate rapid IV fluids, blood infusion. Infusion of cold blood associated with myocardial arrhythimas, paradoxical hypotension. Macropore filtering IV devices should also be used to remove small clots, debris.* • Position patient with lower extremities elevated 20-30% *to help raise BP by shunting blood back into upper extremities.* • Prepare patient for possible chest tube(s) insertion, pericardiocentesis, peritoneal lavage, emergency thoracotomy, tracheostomy (if unable to secure airway). • Advise patient/significant others of possible surgery. • Initiate CPR, other lifesaving measures according to advanced cardiac life support (ACLS) guidelines.	Life sustaining tissue perfusion is maintained.
Anxiety/fear *Related to:* Acute injury Threat of death Unfamiliar environment **DEFINING CHARACTERISTICS** Restlessness Crying Agitation Increased pulse Increased BP Increased respirations Irrational thought process Admitted anxiety Questioning of patient's condition by patient/significant others	**ONGOING ASSESSMENT** • Assess level of anxiety/fear. **THERAPEUTIC INTERVENTIONS** • Reduce patient's/significant others' anxiety by explaining all procedures/treatment. Keep explanations basic. • Maintain confident, assured manner. *Staff's anxiety may be easily perceived by patient.* • Reduce unnecessary external stimuli (e.g., clear unnecessary personnel from room; decrease volume of cardiac monitor). • Reassure patient/significant others as appropriate. • Provide quiet, private place for significant others to wait. • Refer to other support systems, (e.g., clergy, social workers, other family/friends) as appropriate.	Anxiety/fear are reduced as much as possible.

Continued.

Hypovolemic shock: acute care— cont'd

NURSING DIAGNOSES / DEFINING CHARACTERISTICS	NURSING INTERVENTIONS / *RATIONALES*	EXPECTED OUTCOMES
Potential for injury: airway obstruction *Related to:* Chest trauma Pneumothorax Hemothorax Malpositioning of head/neck **DEFINING CHARACTERISTICS** Restlessness Agitation Absent/decreased breath sounds Rales Cyanosis Abnormal ABGs Respirations Stridor Use of accessory muscles	**ONGOING ASSESSMENT** · Assess respiratory rate, rhythm, quality. · Auscultate breath sounds before, after intubation. · Assess for respiratory distress. · Monitor ABGs. **THERAPEUTIC INTERVENTIONS** · Maintain patent airway by appropriate positioning. · Initiate basic CPR as needed. · Institute airway suctioning as appropriate. · Assist in intubation as necessary. · Provide supplemental oxygen. · See also Chest trauma, p. 636.	Effective airway is maintained.

Originated by: Christine Jutzi-Kosmos, RN, MS

Lead poisoning

(PLUMBISM)

Symptoms of lead poisoning are a result of chronic ingestion or inhalation of lead-bearing products. Lead poisoning is most commonly seen in children exhibiting pica behaviors but also occurs in adults who have chronically inhaled fumes from motor fuels, batteries, and paints. Accidental ingestion can occur from serving acidic liquids from lead-glazed pottery or antique pewter. Lead salts are absorbed by the blood, interfere with hemoglobin production, and destroy kidney and brain tissue. Mental retardation is permanent in children with CNS involvement.

NURSING DIAGNOSES / DEFINING CHARACTERISTICS	NURSING INTERVENTIONS / *RATIONALES*	EXPECTED OUTCOMES
Altered hematologic status *Related to:* Ingestion of substances containing lead **DEFINING CHARACTERISTICS** Decreased Hct Decreased Hb Increased lead level (>15-50 mg/100 ml) History of pica	**ONGOING ASSESSMENT** · Check vital signs with BP q4h. · Monitor daily lab values (i.e., CBC, lead levels). · Observe skin for pallor/anemia. · Monitor for side effects/complications of agents (see Urinary retention p. 643). **THERAPEUTIC INTERVENTIONS** · Administer chelating agents (e.g., dimercaprol [BAL in oil], edetate calcium disodium [CaEDTA]), *which form highly soluble compound that causes free lead to be readily excreted in urine.*	Blood lead level decreases.

NURSING DIAGNOSES / DEFINING CHARACTERISTICS	NURSING INTERVENTIONS / *RATIONALES*	EXPECTED OUTCOMES

Knowledge deficit
Related to:
Unfamiliarity with diagnosis, source of exposure
 	
DEFINING CHARACTERISTICS
Verbalized lack of understanding of diagnosis, cause
Multiple questions/ comments
Repeated episodes of ingestion
	ONGOING ASSESSMENT
	• Assess knowledge of lead poisoning, source of ingestion.
	• Assess for pica behavior.
	• Elicit information for possible lead sources.
	• If patient is child:
	    Screen all siblings for increased lead levels.
	    Observe family interaction/relationships.
	
	THERAPEUTIC INTERVENTIONS
	• Explain etiology of lead poisoning (i.e., pica, improperly glazed pottery, toxic fumes [paint], lead pipes).
	• Explain environmental factors that contribute to lead poisoning.
	    Poorly maintained older swellings
	    Fumes from toxic waste
	    Job-related (e.g., paint fumes)
	• Review, emphasize hazards of lead, signs of lead intoxication, and long-term complications.
	• Inform of importance of proper home medication administration.
	• Initiate referrals with social worker, public health nurse, Board of Health, and other agencies that can assist in overall management.
	• Emphasize need for continuing follow-up, lead level monitoring.
	• Provide telephone number for local emergency room, poison control.
		Understanding of lead poisoning, environmental hazards, long-term complications, medications, and resource people for follow-up is gained.

Urinary retention *Related to:* Toxic BAL/CaEDTA levels **DEFINING CHARACTERISTICS** Decreased urine output Proteinuria Hematuria	**ONGOING ASSESSMENT** • Monitor vital signs q4h (especially for increased heart rate and changed BP). • Monitor I & O q8h. • Check specific gravity and dipstick for protein/blood every void. • Monitor lab results (urinalysis, electrolytes, BUN, and creatinine); *chelating agents toxic to kidneys.* **THERAPEUTIC INTERVENTIONS** • Review potential renal side effects of all drugs used before administration. • Do not administer CaEDTA to dehydrated patients. *Decreased kidney function severely limits chelation therapy effectiveness.* • Ensure adequate PO/IV intake. *Fluids assure lead excretion via urine.* • Report significant change in I & O/urine output <30 ml/hr. *Chelating agents are nephrotoxic.*	Adequate urinary elimination is maintained.
Pain *Related to:* Multiple injections **DEFINING CHARACTERISTICS** Irritability Crying Swelling, inflammation, and redness at injection sites	**ONGOING ASSESSMENT** • Observe injection areas for swelling, redness, inflammation, abscess formation. **THERAPEUTIC INTERVENTIONS** • Palpate muscle area before preparing site to locate/avoid fibrous tissue from previous injections. • Rotate all injection sites; use large muscle groups. • Obtain order for use of local anesthetic with injection (draw up last in syringe; do not mix); *helps lessen pain during administration.* • Administer BAL and CaEDTA by deep IM injection as ordered *for adequate absorption.* • Apply warm soaks to injection sites as necessary *to relieve discomfort.*	Discomfort and complications from injections are reduced.

Continued.

Lead poisoning— cont'd

NURSING DIAGNOSES / DEFINING CHARACTERISTICS	NURSING INTERVENTIONS / *RATIONALES*	EXPECTED OUTCOMES
Potential altered levels of consciousness *Related to:* Chronic lead ingestion **DEFINING CHARACTERISTICS** Falling, clumsiness, loss of coordination Irritability Seizures Drowsiness Coma Peripheral nerve palsy	**ONGOING ASSESSMENT** • Assess level of consciousness (LOC) q4h/more frequently if deterioration, increased toxicity, or encephalopathy noted. • Assess vital signs, especially respiratory status, q2-4h. • Compare present neurologic assessment to previous level from history. Document serial assessments. **THERAPEUTIC INTERVENTIONS** • Use seizure precautions and safety measures (i.e., side rails up and padded); *seizure activity, loss of coordination, drowsiness may occur.* • If actual LOC alteration noted: Obtain emergency equipment; place Ambu bag at bedside. Report to physician. Initiate treatment for Consciousness, altered level of, p. 234. Consult neurology clinical specialist.	Maximum neurologic functioning is maintained.

Originated by: Karen Kushibab, RN, BSN
            Catherine Provenzano, RN, BSN

Near-drowning

Survival at least 24 hours after submersion in a fluid medium. Aspiration of salt water causes plasma to be drawn into the lungs, resulting in hypoxemia and hypovolemia. Freshwater aspiration causes hypervolemia resulting from absorption of water through alveoli into the vascular system. These fluids are further absorbed into the interstitial space. Hypoxemia results from the decreased lung surfactant washed away by the absorbed water. Severe hypoxia also results from the asphyxia related to submersion without aspiration of fluid.

NURSING DIAGNOSES / DEFINING CHARACTERISTICS	NURSING INTERVENTIONS / *RATIONALES*	EXPECTED OUTCOMES
Impaired gas exchange *Related to:* Surfactant elimination Bronchospasm Aspiration Pulmonary edema **DEFINING CHARACTERISTICS** Cyanosis Retractions Tachypnea Stridor	**ONGOING ASSESSMENT** • Assess breath sounds q2h. • Assess for respiratory distress signs: Retractions Stridor Nasal flaring Use of accessory muscles • Assess for signs of hypoxemia: Altered LOC Tachycardia Deteriorating serial ABGs Tachypnea Cyanosis Increasing respiratory distress • Assess serial chest x-ray examination reports. • Monitor for evidence of increasing pulmonary edema (*may indicate need for mechanical ventilation*). **THERAPEUTIC INTERVENTIONS** • Place patient in high Fowler's position *to allow maximum chest expansion.* • Notify physician of respiratory status changes.	Adequate gas exchange is maintained.

NURSING DIAGNOSES / DEFINING CHARACTERISTICS	NURSING INTERVENTIONS / *RATIONALES*	EXPECTED OUTCOMES
	· Administer humidified O_2 as ordered. · Suction only as needed; *hypoxia and Valsalva maneuver with suctioning may increase ICP, metabolic acidosis.* · See Mechanical ventilation, p. 213.	
Altered cerebral perfusion *Related to:* Impaired gas exchange Increased intracranial pressure (ICP) caused by fluid shifts with freshwater aspiration/hypoxia **DEFINING CHARACTERISTICS** Deficit in cranial nerve responses Altered LOC Inappropriate behavior Altered pupillary response	**ONGOING ASSESSMENT** · Assess neurologic signs q1h until stable; then q4h. · Monitor for increasing ICP: ICP monitor readings Narrowed pulse pressure; decreased heart and respiratory rates Altered pupil response Altered LOC since admission · Assess for seizure activity. · Assess environment for degree of stimulation. **THERAPEUTIC INTERVENTIONS** · Elevate head of bed (HOB) 30 degrees; maintain midline head, body alignment. · Notify physician of signs of increasing ICP. · Administer anticonvulsants as ordered *to prevent seizure activity.* · Maintain seizure precautions *to prevent patient from injuring self in event of seizure.* · Minimize frequency of suctioning. *Hypoxia, Valsalva maneuver associated with suctioning; may elevate ICP.* · Sedate patient before beginning procedures (i.e., blood drawing, invasive procedures) *to prevent ICP elevation.* · Administer medication as ordered to maintain patient in barbiturate coma *(protects brain from athetoid movements, grunting, and straining, which may increase ICP).* · Maintain body temperature at *30° C to reduce total O_2 requirements.*	Cerebral perfusion is maximized.
Fluid volume excess/ deficit: *Related to:* *Excess:* Aspiration of fresh water Fluid shift from interstitial to intravascular space *Deficit:* Aspiration of salt water Fluid shift from intravascular to interstitial space **DEFINING CHARACTERISTICS** Abnormal vital signs Poor peripheral vascular tone leading to edema Arrhythmias	**ONGOING ASSESSMENT** · Assess heart rate/rhythm. · Assess serial electrolytes. · Assess pH results for acidosis/alkalosis. · Assess Hct *to determine level of hemodilution/concentration.* · Assess urine output q1h; maintain accurate I & O. · Assess specific gravity. · Assess urine electrolytes, BUN, and creatinine. · Assess weight on admission, then every day when neurologic signs stable. **THERAPEUTIC INTERVENTIONS** · Notify physician of lab results, changes in output/cardiac function. · Administer IV fluids as ordered *to correct fluid imbalance.* · Place on cardiopulmonary monitor. · Administer sodium bicarbonate as ordered *to correct metabolic acidosis.*	Fluid volume imbalance is reduced.

Continued.

Emergency and Trauma Care Plans

NURSING DIAGNOSES / DEFINING CHARACTERISTICS	NURSING INTERVENTIONS / *RATIONALES*	EXPECTED OUTCOMES
Potential impaired skin integrity *Related to:* Imposed hypothermia Immobility Prolonged exposures **DEFINING CHARACTERISTICS** Reddened skin areas Rashes Edema Blisters	**ONGOING ASSESSMENT** · Assess rectal temperature q2-4h. · Assess patient q2h for pressure areas, redness, blisters, edema, rashes. **THERAPEUTIC INTERVENTIONS** · Maintain patient's temperature within normal range. · Reposition patient q2h to reduce risk of skin breakdown from pressure areas. · Protect bony prominence with padding. · Apply lotion to pressure areas. · See Skin integrity, impaired, p. 48.	Skin remains intact.
Potential for infection *Related to:* Aspiration of contaminated water **DEFINING CHARACTERISTICS** Increased temperature Rales, rhonchi in lungs Positive cultures	**ONGOING ASSESSMENT** · Monitor temperature q2-4h. · Monitor results of cultures and serial white blood cell counts *(may indicate infection).* · Assess for increased respiratory distress. · Obtain chest x-ray; *aspiration of contaminated water during near-drowning puts patient at risk for developing pneumonia.* · Record sputum color, odor, and amount. **THERAPEUTIC INTERVENTIONS** · Notify physician of fever; positive culture, x-ray, or clinical findings. · Administer antibiotics as ordered. · Position *for ease in lung expansion.* · Reposition *to promote drainage (postural drainage);* perform chest physical therapy as needed. · Encourage use of incentive spirometer.	
Knowledge deficit: family *Related to:* Near-drowning Patient's critical status Admission to ICU **DEFINING CHARACTERISTICS** Continuous questions Excessive talking Constant demands Inability to enter unit Pacing Withdrawal Inability to leave patient's bedside	**ONGOING ASSESSMENT** · Assess degree of stress. · Assess available support systems. · Assess level of understanding of patient's illness, hospitalization. · Assess degree of involvement in patient's care. **THERAPEUTIC INTERVENTIONS** · Establish good rapport. · Encourage expression of feelings about illness, hospitalization. · Reassure, support family. · Allow for questions; answer as honestly as possible. · Include family in patient's care. · Include clergy/social worker in meetings with family *so they may better answer questions, remember details of care.* · Assist family in anticipating mourning if applicable. · Provide information for follow-up, home care as necessary.	Patient and family understand treatments, prognosis, and follow-up care.

Originated by: Patricia Hasbrouck-Aschliman, RN, CCRN
　　　　　　　Catherine Provenzano, RN, BSN

Rape trauma syndrome

(SEXUAL ASSAULT)

Rape trauma syndrome is a response to the extreme stress and profound fear of death that almost all survivors experience during the sexual assault. It refers to the acute or immediate phase of disorganization and the long-term process of reorganization that occur as a result of attempted or forcible sexual assault. Although every survivor of sexual assault has unique emotional needs and responses, all experience rape trauma syndrome. Current literature now refers to victims as sexual assault as "survivors"; this term is used throughout this care plan.

NURSING DIAGNOSES / DEFINING CHARACTERISTICS	NURSING INTERVENTIONS / *RATIONALES*	EXPECTED OUTCOMES

Ineffective coping (survivor)
Related to:
Sexual assault trauma
 	
DEFINING CHARACTERISTICS
Acute:
Increased anxiety
Hostility, aggression
Guilt
Withdrawal
No verbalization of occurrence of rape/denial
Abrupt changes in relationships with men
Emotional outbursts (excessive crying)
Sense of humiliation
Long-term:
Repetitive nightmares/reliving of assault
Phobias:
  Fear of being indoors
  Fear of being outdoors
  Fear of crowds
  Fear of being alone
  Fear of men
  Fear of spouse
  Fear of lovers
Reactivated life problems (i.e., physical/psychiatric illnesses)
Reliance on alcohol/drugs
Sleep pattern disturbances
Eating pattern disturbances
GI irritability
Sexual dysfunctioning
Depression/loss of self-esteem
	ONGOING ASSESSMENT
	· Assess for signs of ineffective coping (see Defining Characteristics). *Defining characteristics are actually normal coping mechanisms that occur after sexual assault. However, if they persist and interfere with recovery, they become ineffective.*
	· Assess need for referrals.
	· Identify previous coping mechanisms.
	
	THERAPEUTIC INTERVENTIONS
	· Provide calm, supportive environment. Reassure survivor that he/she is now safe.
	· Encourage survivor to express feelings about experience.
	· Validate survivor's feelings; assist in channeling them appropriately.
	· Allow survivor time to cope. Help survivor identify coping skills used successfully in past.
	· Help survivor contact family/significant others (best support system).
	· Help survivor regain sense of control over self/life. *At each stage of interaction, explain what you would like to do, why; ask permission. Asking for permission helps survivor feel in control.*
	· Explain procedures, examinations.
	· Explain to survivor that in future mood swings, feelings of anger, fear, or sadness may be experienced; these are normal reactions.
	· Facilitate survivor's decision-making process; use active listening techniques.
	· Assure that survivor does not go home alone when discharged. If no significant other available, call Department of Human Services to escort patient.
	· Provide community referrals for physical, emotional care.
		Coping strengths are maximized.

Continued.

NURSING DIAGNOSES / DEFINING CHARACTERISTICS	NURSING INTERVENTIONS / *RATIONALES*	EXPECTED OUTCOMES
Ineffective coping (family/significant other) *Related to:* Sexual assault trauma	**ONGOING ASSESSMENT** • Assess family/significant others for Defining Characteristics. • Assess current knowledge of situation. • Observe family's current actions, effect on survivor. • Assess need for referrals. • Identify previous coping mechanisms.	Ineffective family coping is reduced.
DEFINING CHARACTERISTICS Family/significant other blames survivor for incident Expressions of guilt Inability to talk about incident Withdrawal Aggression, hostility Anger Embarrassment Humiliation Increased anxiety	**THERAPEUTIC INTERVENTIONS** • Provide supportive, calm environment. • Explain procedures. • Encourage family to verbalize concerns, feelings. Identify importance of support, understanding to recovery. *Verbalized negative feelings (i.e., blaming survivor for assault) must be addressed. Survivor should not feel responsible for assault; nothing justifies sexual assault.* • Validate family's feelings; help them to channel appropriately. Acknowledge stress that they are experiencing. • Provide support, counseling referrals. • Discuss with family/significant others ways to support survivor: Encouraging survivor to verbalize feelings Helping survivor resume usual life activities Avoiding overprotectiveness Being nonjudgmental Holding, touching survivor so as not to reinforce feelings of being unclean Helping mobilize survivor's anger; directing it at assailant *Studies indicate that type of emotional support sexual assault survivor receives initially has direct bearing on recovery.*	
Potential for associated physical injury *Related to:* Caused by sexual assault trauma	**ONGOING ASSESSMENT** • Assess for injury (see Defining Characteristics). • Assess for need for medication (pain, nausea, vomiting, muscle tension). • Identify evidence collection needed. • Identify orifices of sexual assault: oral/rectal/vaginal.	Complications from injuries are reduced.
DEFINING CHARACTERISTICS Survivor states he/she was raped Bruises/swelling Lacerations/abrasions Itching, burning on urination Bloody/stained clothing Pain Nausea/vomiting Muscle tension/ general soreness Vaginal/oral/rectal irritation Scratches	**THERAPEUTIC INTERVENTIONS** • Obtain patient's written consent for examination and treatment. • Collect, prepare evidence required by law. Refer to Rape Procedure in hospital policy. • Medicate as ordered for pain, nausea/vomiting, muscle tension, prevention of VD, pregnancy. *Urine pregnancy test should be done on all female sexual assault survivors in childbearing years to identify pre-existing pregnancy (alters type of medication ordered).* • Perform wound care as needed. • Give tetanus toxoid as ordered. • Provide follow-up care *to prevent complications (i.e., gonorrhea culture, Chlamydia culture, VDRL, pregnancy test in 4-6 wk, and HIV testing).*	
Knowledge deficit *Related to:* New situation/crisis	**ONGOING ASSESSMENT** • Assess ability to verbalize questions. • Assess current understanding of treatment, follow-up, etc. • Assess knowledge base.	Patient and family verbalize understanding of procedures, treatment modalities, and follow-up care.

NURSING DIAGNOSES / DEFINING CHARACTERISTICS	NURSING INTERVENTIONS / *RATIONALES*	EXPECTED OUTCOMES
DEFINING CHARACTERISTICS Verbalized lack of adequate knowledge of: procedures, follow-up care Confusion Questions Inaccurate instruction follow-through Improper performance Inappropriate/ exaggerated behaviors (hysterical, apathetic)	**THERAPEUTIC INTERVENTIONS** · Instruct patient/family as needed: Hospital procedures Police procedures Collection of evidence procedures Medications and side effects Possibility of sexually transmitted diseases, pregnancy Follow-up care Support referrals Patient's/family's potential emotions and feelings in future days/weeks *Providing this information lets survivor make informed choices.* · Provide written follow-up instructions. *Sexual assault survivor receives large quantity of information in emergency room. Printed instruction/ information sheets/booklets very helpful for review at home.* · Provide information to special patients. *For very young, old, or mentally impaired survivor, adapting instructions, information to level of understanding necessary. In some cases (depending on patient's age and mental capability) all information relayed directly to parent/guardian.*	
Self-concept/body image disturbance *Related to:* Sexual assault trauma **DEFINING CHARACTERISTICS** Embarrassment, humiliation Fear Anger Powerlessness Guilt Loneliness Mood swings Withdrawal Difficulty in relating to males Negative feelings about body	**ONGOING ASSESSMENT** · Assess patient's current self-image. · Assess reactions, feelings about sexual assault. · Assess need for referrals. **THERAPEUTIC INTERVENTIONS** · Provide private, supportive environment. · Show interest, respect, warmth, and nonjudgmental attitude. Avoid accusing, negative questions. *Much shame about sexual assault arises from mistaken belief that rape primarily sexual; thus survivor must in some way have provoked/enticed rapist. Rape is crime of violence—not passion.* · Listen attentively to convey belief in what survivor is saying. · Acknowledge survivor's feelings. *Many survivors filled with guilt, self-reproach. Remind survivor she/he in no way responsible for assault. Encourage survivor to direct negative feelings toward assailant, away from self.* · Be aware of your own feelings and attitudes and effect on survivor. · Interview significant other whom survivor wants present. · Provide anticipatory guidance to survivor/family. · Determine, address survivor's special concerns/immediate needs (i.e., concerns about physical injury, pregnancy, VD, AIDS). · Encourage female staff member to stay with female survivor if possible, as advocate. · Explain that patient's emotional, physical responses normal; may continue weeks after sexual assault trauma. *Rape is ultimate invasion of privacy; much time (and usually counseling) needed before survivor feels safe, secure, in control.* · Refer to Self-concept disturbance, p. 46; Body image disturbance, p. 6. · See Sexuality patterns, altered, p. 47. · See Powerlessness, p. 42.	Positive expressions of self-worth are acknowledged.
Anxiety *Related to:* Sexual assault trauma **DEFINING CHARACTERISTICS** *Mild:* Restlessness Increased awareness	**ONGOING ASSESSMENT** · Assess for anxiety symptoms (see Defining Characteristics). **THERAPEUTIC INTERVENTIONS** · Have support person stay with patient: If available, contact sexual assault victim advocate. *Role of sexual assault victim advocate is to provide nonjudgmental support, immediate crisis intervention to sexual assault survivor.*	Anxiety is reduced.

Continued.

Rape trauma syndrome— cont'd

NURSING DIAGNOSES / DEFINING CHARACTERISTICS	NURSING INTERVENTIONS / *RATIONALES*	EXPECTED OUTCOMES
Increased questioning Exaggerated startle response *Moderate/severe:* Restlessness Insomnia Glancing about/ increased alertness Facial tension/wide-eyed look Focus on self Poor eye contact Increased perspiration Anorexia/GI problems Overexcited/jittery Expressed concern Trembling Constant demands	Offer to call significant other. Contact U.S. Department of Human Resources if no one else available. • Complete most of history, treatment before police questioning, if possible. • Contact Social Service if acute anxiety experienced. • Send copy of record to hospital Social Service for follow-up of all sexual assault victims. • Provide calm, supportive environment. *Predominant emotion experienced by survivor is overwhelming fear/terror of death. Help to ease fear by assuring survivor of safety.* • Help survivor to talk through feelings, concerns about assault. • See also Anxiety, p. 4.	

Originated by: Evelyn Lyons, RN, BSN
Anita D. Morris, RN

Toxic ingestion

(POISONING)

Ingestion of substances (usually orally, but also intravenously or by inhalation) that cause cellular destruction and can be life-threatening.

NURSING DIAGNOSES / DEFINING CHARACTERISTICS	NURSING INTERVENTIONS / *RATIONALES*	EXPECTED OUTCOMES
Potential for injury: to self *Related to:* Accidental/intentional ingestion of potentially life-threatening substance **DEFINING CHARACTERISTICS** Decreased LOC Cardiac disturbance Tachypnea Dyspnea Respiratory failure Abdominal pain Decreased urinary output Hypotension/ hypertension	**ONGOING ASSESSMENT** • Monitor vital signs. • Elicit ingestion circumstances from patient/family. • Elicit initial ingestion symptoms. • Assess time of onset, estimated time of ingestion. • Assess prior treatment attempts. • Assess type, amount of drug ingested: Send blood and urine for toxicology screening immediately. Ask for empty bottles left nearby; question drugs missing from home. Ask whether patient takes any prescription drugs, type. Evaluate possibility of street drug use. • Monitor I & O. • Obtain patient's age and weight. • Repeat urine/blood toxicology levels as needed.	Risk of further injury is reduced.

NURSING DIAGNOSES / DEFINING CHARACTERISTICS	NURSING INTERVENTIONS / *RATIONALES*	EXPECTED OUTCOMES

	THERAPEUTIC INTERVENTIONS
	• Induce emesis as ordered:
	    Do not attempt if patient is convulsing or neurologic status is significantly depressed.
	    Do not induce if ingested substance caustic.
	    Provide ipecac, as ordered, for emesis induction.
	    Provide abundant clear liquids if ipecac given.
	• Provide gastric lavage as ordered (effective in patients with significantly depressed LOC; method of choice if ingested substance caustic):
	    Attempt nasogastric insertion after checking gag reflex; if sluggish, patient should be intubated first.
	    Provide appropriate-size nasogastric tube; check for placement before beginning lavage.
	• Administer absorption-inhibiting medications, as ordered and as appropriate for type of ingestion, at dosage safe for patient's age, weight:
	    Administer activated charcoal within one hr of aspirin ingestion.
	    Administer N-acetylcystein (Mucomyst) q4h for 24 hr if patient has ingested acetaminophen.
	• Promote catharsis as ordered *to decrease substance absorbed in gut:*
	    Provide medications as ordered; drug of choice magnesium sulfate solution.
	    Tell patient to expect abdominal cramping, diarrhealike symptoms.
	    Provide privacy, bedpan, cleaning materials.
	    Assist as needed.
	• Promote diuresis as ordered *to enhance renal excretion of toxic substance:*
	    Push oral fluids if patient alert.
	    Maintain IV fluids if LOC depressed (usually 1-1½ times maintenance fluid required for weight).
	    Assist with bedpan/urinal.
	    Catheterize if necessary.
	• If substance ingested is nephrotoxic, other elimination method (e.g., peritoneal, hemodialysis) should be considered. *Hypertension, decreasing urine output may indicate kidney failure.*	

Potential altered tissue perfusion: cardiopulmonary
Related to:
Drug ingestion:
  Street drugs
  Over-the-counter medications
  Psychological medications
  Seizure medications
  Other poison
 	
DEFINING CHARACTERISTICS
Change in LOC
Hyperventilation/ hypoventilation
Tachycardia, hypertension
Bradycardia, hypotension
	ONGOING ASSESSMENT
	• Assess respiratory function: rate, pattern, airway, lung sounds.
	• Assess cardiac function: rate, rhythm, and BP. *Most drug overdoses causes cardiac, respiratory depression. Ingestion of corrosive material may cause acute obstruction, necessitate emergency tracheostomy, intubation.*
	• Place patient on cardiorespiratory monitor.
	• Place patient in semi-Fowler's position *to assist lung expansion, prevent aspiration if vomiting occurs.*
	• Administer O₂ as necessary. Keep Ambu bag at bedside.
	• Maintain quiet environment.
	• Notify physician of vital sign changes.
	• Place crash cart at bedside if condition warrants or *prepare for possible intubation.*
	• See Mechanical ventilation, p. 213.
		Cardiorespiratory function is maintained.

Continued.

NURSING DIAGNOSES / DEFINING CHARACTERISTICS	NURSING INTERVENTIONS / *RATIONALES*	EXPECTED OUTCOMES
Altered levels of consciousness *Related to:* Toxic ingested drug levels **DEFINING CHARACTERISTICS** Restlessness Delirium Convulsions Marked pupil constriction/dilatation Lethargy, confusion, disorientation Coma (likely with ingestion of salicylate sedatives, narcotics, narcoticlike drugs, anticholinergic and cholinergic agents)	**ONGOING ASSESSMENT** • Assess neurologic status q2h: LOC Pupil size, reactivity Visual acuity Muscle strength Behavioral changes, irritability Headache Response to stimuli Orientation Tinnitus **THERAPEUTIC INTERVENTIONS** • Avoid excessive stimulation: Dim lights. Limit visitors. Maintain quiet environment. • Provide seizure precautions. Keep side rails up at all times; pad if necessary. Keep bed in lowest position. Keep HOB slightly elevated. • Record responses to questions; *may be useful during psychological evaluation.* • Reorient to environment as needed. • Provide antidote/perform procedures (lavage, dialysis) *that decrease amount of drug available to circulation.*	Consciousness will be maintained.
Potential fluid volume deficit *Related to:* Side effects of ingested toxins/ treatment modalities Decreased fluid intake **DEFINING CHARACTERISTICS** Tachycardia Hypotension Decreased urine output Increased urine specific gravity Elevated serum Na Dry mucous membranes Weakness	**ONGOING ASSESSMENT** • Assess hydration level q2h: Urine specific gravity Urine pH Skin turgor Mucous membranes I & O • Assess vital signs at least q2h. • Monitor for nausea, vomiting. • Measure, record type of emesis. • Check laboratory values: CBC Electrolytes Toxicology levels **THERAPEUTIC INTERVENTIONS** • Maintain fluid intake, oral if possible, or IV fluids as ordered *to prevent circulatory collapse. Plasma/blood may be required if patient severely dehydrated/losing blood in emesis/stool.* • See Fluid volume deficit, p. 20.	Risk of fluid volume deficit is reduced.
Ineffective family coping *Related to:* Temporary family separation/ disorganization Situational crisis Attempted suicide of family member New awareness of family member drug use/addictions	**ONGOING ASSESSMENT** • Assess family's immediate understanding of patient's situation/physical status. • Assess available coping mechanisms, supports. **THERAPEUTIC INTERVENTIONS** • Provide family with support personnel, clergy, ombudsman, volunteer, psychiatric nurse liaison, physician. • Keep family informed of patient's status, care provided *to decrease fear and anxiety, increase understanding of situation.* • Allow visits as soon as possible.	Effective coping mechanisms will be maximized.

Toxic ingestion— cont'd

NURSING DIAGNOSES / DEFINING CHARACTERISTICS	NURSING INTERVENTIONS / *RATIONALES*	EXPECTED OUTCOMES
DEFINING CHARACTERISTICS Verbalized inadequate understanding of situation Display of inappropriate/overly protective behaviors Withdrawn appearance Appearance of preoccupation with personal guilt, fears, and grief.	• Provide privacy during discussion of further treatment, hospitalization. • Support family's use of adaptive coping mechanisms. • See Coping, ineffective family, p. 14.	
Ineffective individual coping *Related to:* Circumstances of intentional ingestion: Suicide attempt Suicide gesture **DEFINING CHARACTERISTICS** Suicide ideation Depression Behavior changes	**ONGOING ASSESSMENT** • Assess type, amount of chemical ingested *(may indicate intentional versus accidental ingestion)*. • Assess previous behaviors, relationships. • Assess current coping mechanisms if possible. **THERAPEUTIC INTERVENTIONS** • Provide safe, structured environment, especially after initial physical crisis resolved. • Provide sitter if suicide suspected; transfer to psychiatric unit if possible. • Allow expression of feelings and concerns. • Obtain psychological consultant. *Intentional ingestion suggests psychiatric illness; counseling should be initiated before discharge.* • See Suicidal attempt/suicidal gesture, p. 627; Depression, p. 614.	Ineffective coping will be reduced.
Knowledge deficit *Related to:* *Circumstances of accidental poisoning:* Medications unlabeled; misunderstanding of label/directions Inability to read instructions Harmful substance within reach of children *Lack of knowledge of:* Prevention Emergency treatment Follow-up treatment **DEFINING CHARACTERISTICS** Verbalized lack of knowledge/ability of patient/family Demonstrated threat to self	**ONGOING ASSESSMENT** • Assess current level of understanding. • Assess cognitive abilities. **THERAPEUTIC INTERVENTIONS** • Provide information at level, in manner that best promote comprehension. • Initiate home/discharge teaching after crisis resolved. • Provide information on prevention/safety. • Provide consultation, follow-up as appropriate. • See Suicidal attempt/suicidal gesture, p. 627.	Patient verbalizes understanding.

Originated by: Janet McCants, RN, BSN

Trauma patient: perioperative care

An individual who sustained an injury as the result of an accident. Approximately 10% of patients who present themselves in the emergency room require a precise, rapid, systematic approach to initial management that is crucial to their survival. In these patients assessment and resuscitation must occur simultaneously. The American College of Surgeons have developed a system for orderly assessment that consists of a primary survey, resuscitation, a secondary survey, and definitive management. The definitive care phase of initial assessment is that period of the patient's treatment that is carried out in the operating room.

NURSING DIAGNOSES / DEFINING CHARACTERISTICS	NURSING INTERVENTIONS / *RATIONALES*	EXPECTED OUTCOMES
Knowledge deficit *Related to:* Emergency surgery Multiple injuries Fear of sudden death Concern for family **DEFINING CHARACTERISTICS** Nervous appearance Multiple questions Lack of questions Crying Increased BP Increased heart rate	**ONGOING ASSESSMENT** ▪ Assess patient's understanding of impending surgery. ▪ Assess anxiety level. **THERAPEUTIC INTERVENTIONS** ▪ Introduce self, other staff. *This assures the patient that a specialist is available for their injury and increases confidence.* ▪ Explain procedures as they are performed. *Because of the emergent nature of the condition, no time to explain OR sequence of events in advance. Informed patient can cope with psychological, physiological stress more positively.* ▪ Allow verbalization of feelings/concerns (*helps nurse identify fears, give appropriate psychological support*). ▪ Minimize OR activity. *Quiet environment reduces patient's stress.* ▪ Maintain calm, reassuring manner (*helps emotionally distressed patient mobilize psychological resources*). ▪ Include family/significant others as appropriate.	Knowledge of OR procedure is enhanced.
Potential for injury *Related to:* Hurried arrival/ undiagnosed patient with multiple injuries Emergent nature of impending surgery **DEFINING CHARACTERISTICS** Bruises, ecchymosis, abrasions (may indicate underlying organ damage) Swelling, large expanding hematomas with penetrating injuries and broken bones Deformed extremities; ischemic, open fracture(s) Abnormal laboratory results	**ONGOING ASSESSMENT** ▪ Obtain history using "AMPLE!" A: allergies M: medications P: past illness L: last meal E: events before injury *For trauma management, overall guide to rapid, dependable history in acute trauma setting.* ▪ Receive report from ER nurse/physician: Type of accident Injuries, treatment given, medications given Time/approximated time of injury *Report, though brief, guides nurse in assessment of patient's needs, plan for nursing care.* ▪ Identify conditions that are immediate threat to patient's life expeditiously. **THERAPEUTIC INTERVENTIONS** ▪ Maintain body alignment when moving/positioning patient (*prevents further injury, e.g., compounding simple fracture, compression of cervical spine injury*). ▪ Splint, support injured body part. *Sudden, unsupported movement may dislodge blood clot sealing a bleeder.*	Risk of injury is reduced.
Potential fluid volume deficit *Related to:* Blood loss from obvious/concealed bleeding	**ONGOING ASSESSMENT** ▪ Determine amount, type of blood loss as closely as possible. Document ongoing blood loss on sheets, OR bed, floor, suction, sponges. *Blood, IV infusion rate depends on severity of blood loss, clinical evidence of hypovolemia.*	Fluid volume deficit is prevented or corrected.

NURSING DIAGNOSES / DEFINING CHARACTERISTICS	NURSING INTERVENTIONS / *RATIONALES*	EXPECTED OUTCOMES
DEFINING CHARACTERISTICS Falling BP Increased heart rate Low CVP Markedly decreased urine output Pale, cool, clammy skin Confusion, disorientation Blood on bed, sheets Hematomas	· Closely monitor vital signs *to guide surgical team's decision making. Clinical course of injured patient not static.* · Monitor I & O. · Note behavior changes. · Observe closely for circulatory shock sign/symptoms. · Monitor flow rate of existing peripheral, central IVs *to replace fluid loss adequately, prevent overhydration.* **THERAPEUTIC INTERVENTIONS** · Stop obvious bleeding by pressure, tourniquet. · Inform anesthesiologist of approximated blood loss *so fluid replacement can be accurately calculated.* · Help start additional IV line *to provide venous access for rapid fluid loss replacement, restoration of intravascular volume.* · Keep additional lactated Ringer's and normal saline solutions on hand. *Isotonic solution choice for IV fluid because it rapidly equilibrates with total extracellular space.* · Determine fluid replacement needs on basis of weight and blood loss. · Administer blood/components. Use universal donor blood for critical patient. *Red blood cells indicated to maintain optimum O_2-carrying capacity.* · Obtain typed and crossmatched blood from blood bank as soon as possible.	
Potential altered body temperature *Related to:* Anesthetic agent(s) Family history of hyperthermic episodes Fluid/blood therapy Length of incision Exposure Shivering Blood loss **DEFINING CHARACTERISTICS** *Hypothermia:* Decreased body temperature Cool/warm skin Goose bumps on skin, pale to mottled Cold extremities Shivering *Hyperthermia:* Increased body temperature Increased heart rate Full/weak pulse Hyperventilation Chills, convulsions	**ONGOING ASSESSMENT** · Monitor patient's temperature throughout procedure via esophageal/rectal probe. **THERAPEUTIC INTERVENTIONS** *Hypothermia:* · Place aquamatic pad on OR bed; prewarm before patient arrives in OR. Prewarm OR suite. *Trauma victims with multiple injuries are left uncovered during surgical preparation to assess continuously for additional bleeding, clinical symptoms.* · Consult anesthesiologist about humidifiers, blood warmers. *Massive blood replacement has cooling effect; can cause cardiac arrest.* · Cover patient with warm blanket; expose only body part(s) surgical team will work on. · Use warm irrigation solutions *(to warm circulating blood).* *Hyperthermia:* · Assist anesthesiologist to discontinue anesthetic agents, administer emergency drugs. · Remove/discontinue all warming agents/devices. · Institute cooling measures (e.g., cold gastric lavage, cold packs, cold IVs).	Body temperature is maintained near baseline.
Potential excess fluid volume *Related to:* Aggressive fluid therapy Trauma	**ONGOING ASSESSMENT** · Assess vital signs. · Monitor I & O. · Assess extremities for swelling. · Monitor, document evidence of fluid excess *(to guide anesthesiologist in planning fluid therapy).*	Fluid volume excess is reduced.

Continued.

Trauma patient: perioperative care— cont'd

NURSING DIAGNOSES / DEFINING CHARACTERISTICS	NURSING INTERVENTIONS / *RATIONALES*	EXPECTED OUTCOMES
DEFINING CHARACTERISTICS Increased CVP Distended neck veins Increased pulmonary wedge pressure Swollen eyelids Peripheral edema	**THERAPEUTIC INTERVENTIONS** · Administer diuretic therapy as ordered *to enhance body fluid excretion through kidneys to correct/prevent circulatory overload.* Monitor results. · Anticipate, prepare for fasciotomy *(to relieve pressure in circulation; prevent nerve, muscle damage).*	

Potential ineffective airway clearance/ impaired gas exchange
Related to:
Misplaced/dislodged endotracheal tube
Pneumothorax/ hemothorax secondary to injury
Aspiration before/ during intubation attempts
Chest injuries
 	
DEFINING CHARACTERISTICS
Restlessness, agitation
Absent/decreased breath sounds
Rales
Cyanosis
Abnormal ABGs
Asymmetric chest movement
Dark blood (deoxygenated) observed from operative field
	ONGOING ASSESSMENT
	· Assess rate, rhythm, quality of respirations.
	· Auscultate breath sounds before, after intubation.
	· Note obvious chest injuries.
	· Note behavior changes, blood alcohol level. *Neurologic changes may be caused by alcohol intoxication rather than pathophysiologic conditions.*
	· Monitor blood gases.
	
	THERAPEUTIC INTERVENTIONS
	· Prevent/anticipate aspiration:
	    Verify NPO status with patient, ER nurse/physician.
	    Insert NG tube to empty stomach contents. *Because patient not on NPO at least 4-6 hr before surgery, gastric contents may be aspirated during intubation.*
	· Assist with intubation:
	    Encourage awake patient's cooperation. *Awake intubation minimizes aspiration, lessens amount of anesthesia use.*
	    Help anesthesiologist change endotracheal connections *(minimizes time patient is without oxygen).*
	    Obtain oxygen tank, Ambu bag for intubated patient *(provide continuous O_2 administration during transport from OR to RR/ICU).*
	    Obtain sterile tracaheostomy tray *in anticipation of cricothyroidotomy.*
	· Set up chest tube tray if indicated to perform closed thoracotomy if necessary.
	· Initiate, assist with, and document resuscitative measures as indicated. *Documentation communicates treatment, management.*
		Effective airway and gas exchange are maintained.

Potential for injury
Related to:
Incompatible blood products
Massive transfusion
 	
DEFINING CHARACTERISTICS
Increased body temperature
Chills
Hives, rash
Hemodynamic instability
Hematuria
Decreased urine output
	ONGOING ASSESSMENT
	· Monitor vital signs.
	· Monitor temperature via esophageal probe.
	· Note chills, rash.
	· Monitor I & O.
	· Note urine color, amount.
	· Send blood sample to monitor platelet count and hematocrit; report to anesthesiologist, surgeon *(helps anesthesiologist determine amount, type of blood component replacement).*
	
	THERAPEUTIC INTERVENTIONS
	· Administer blood, blood components according to hospital policy:
	    Obtain blood as soon as available. *Blood transfusions restore lost platelets and coagulation factor, oxygen-carrying capacity.*
	    Check blood identification number with patient identification according to policy. *Meticulous attention to details essential to prevent giving wrong blood to patient.*
	    Record all blood components administered, patient's reaction. *Documentation essential for furture reference as additional management planned.*
	    Set up cell saver. *Machine collects blood from operative field by suction; processes blood for transfusion to patient.*
	    Administer drugs as ordered.
		Potential for injury is reduced.

NURSING DIAGNOSES / DEFINING CHARACTERISTICS	NURSING INTERVENTIONS / *RATIONALES*	EXPECTED OUTCOMES
Potential anxiety *Related to:* Prolonged wait resulting from OR suite/ instrument/staff preparation **DEFINING CHARACTERISTICS** Patient questioning of delay in beginning procedure Patient interpretation of hurried preparation as lack of concern	**ONGOING ASSESSMENT** • Assess patient's anxiety level, concern(s). • Assess readiness of OR suite in view of patient's needs, condition. **THERAPEUTIC INTERVENTIONS** • See Routine perioperative care, p. 632. • Explain procedures/room preparation to patient as condition allows. • Plan for instrumentation, supplies, positioning, equipment, draping, as report received from ER nurse/physician. • Keep specialty cart(s) in room/just outside OR suite. *Carts contain additional supplies, instruments, medication(s) not stored in room. Keeping it close allows nurse to stay in OR suite, attend to needs of patient, surgical team.*	Anxiety is reduced.
Potential wound infection *Related to:* Penetrating traumas (stabs, gunshot wound) Unprepared surgical area **DEFINING CHARACTERISTICS** Wound drainage 24-72 hr surgery Red wound edges Fever Increased WBC	**ONGOING ASSESSMENT** • Assess wound/injury type, location. • Monitor aseptic technique throughout procedure. **THERAPEUTIC INTERVENTIONS** • Provide skin preparation *to remove dirt, transient microorganisms from skin; reduce resident microbial count as much as possible.* • Clean debris from wound. *If not removed, foreign matter, devitalized tissue, and dirt impairs ability to heal, resist infection.* • Administer antibiotics as ordered.	Potential for wound infection is reduced.

Originated by: Jacqueline Monaco, RN
                Remedios R. Manuel, RN

Index